SUDDEN CORONARY DEATH

ANNALS OF THE NEW YORK ACADEMY OF SCIENCES

Volume 382

SUDDEN CORONARY DEATH

Edited by Henry M. Greenberg and Edward M. Dwyer, Jr.

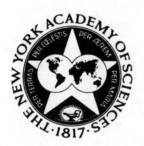

The New York Academy of Sciences
New York, New York
1982

Library of Congress Cataloging in Publication Data

Main entry under title:

Sudden coronary death.
    (Annals of the New York Academy of Sciences; v. 382)
    Proceedings of a conference sponsored by the New York Academy of Sciences, May 4–6, 1981.
    Bibliography: p.
    Includes index.
    1. Coronary heart disease—Congresses. 2. Sudden death—Congresses. I. Greenberg, Henry M. II. Dwyer, Edward M., 1936–   III. New York Academy of Sciences. IV. Series.

Q11.N5 vol. 382 [RC685.C6]   500s   82–3627
ISBN 0–89766–153–2   [616.1′2078]   AACR2
ISBN 0–89766–154–0 (pbk.)

PCP
Printed in the United States of America
ISBN 0–89766–153–2 (cloth)
ISBN 0–89766–154–0 (paper)

ANNALS OF THE NEW YORK ACADEMY OF SCIENCES

Volume 382

March 30, 1982

SUDDEN CORONARY DEATH *

Editors and Conference Chairmen
Henry M. Greenberg and Edward M. Dwyer, Jr.

———————◆———————

CONTENTS

Opening Remarks. *By* EDWARD M. DWYER, JR. AND HENRY M. GREENBERG ...   1

Part I. Epidemiology and Pathology of Sudden Coronary Death

Sudden Coronary Death: The Framingham Study. *By* WILLIAM B. KANNEL AND
    H. EMERSON THOMAS, JR.   3
Short-Term Risk Factors for Sudden Death. *By* LAWRENCE E. HINKLE, JR.   22
Pathology of Sudden Coronary Death. *By* WILLIAM P. NEWMAN III, RICHARD
    E. TRACY, JACK P. STRONG, WILLIAM D. JOHNSON, AND MARGARET C.
    OALMANN   39
Pathologic Changes in the Cardiac Conduction and Nervous System in Sudden
    Coronary Death. *By* LINO ROSSI   50
Collateral Anatomy and Blood Flow: Its Potential Role in Sudden Coronary
    Death. *By* WOLFGANG SCHAPER   69

Part II. Pathophysiology of Sudden Coronary Death—Electrical Instability

Introduction. *By* JOHN A. KASTOR   76
The Use of Animal Models in the Study of the Electrophysiology of Sudden
    Coronary Deaths. *By* JOSEPH F. SPEAR, ERIC L. MICHELSON, AND E. NEIL
    MOORE   78
Cellular Electrophysiology in Acute and Healed Experimental Myocardial In-
    farction. *By* ROBERT J. MYERBURG, KRISTINA EPSTEIN, MARION S. GAIDE,
    SAM S. WONG, AGUSTIN CASTELLANOS, HENRY GELBAND, JOHN S. CAMERON,
    AND ARTHUR L. BASSETT   90
Mechanisms in the Genesis of Recurrent Ventricular Tachyarrhythmias as Re-
    vealed by Clinical Electrophysiologic Studies. *By* LEONARD N. HOROWITZ,
    SCOTT R. SPIELMAN, ALLAN M. GREENSPAN, AND MARK E. JOSEPHSON 116
The Role of Intraventricular Conduction Disorders in Precipitating Sudden
    Death. *By* HEIN J. J. WELLENS, PEDRO BRUGADA, AND FRITS W. H. M.
    BÄR 136
Central Nervous System Risk Factors for Sudden Cardiac Death. *By* REGIS
    A. DESILVA 143
The Role of the Autonomic Nervous System in Sudden Coronary Death. *By*
    PETER J. SCHWARTZ AND H. LOWELL STONE 162
In Praise of Sudden Death. *By* HENRY GREENBERG 181

* This series of papers is the result of a conference entitled Sudden Coronary
Death, held by the New York Academy of Sciences on May 4–6, 1981.

Part III. Pathophysiology of Sudden Coronary Death—Ischemia and Altered Left Ventricular Function

Regulation of Calcium in Cardiac Muscle. By ARNOLD SCHWARTZ 183
The Role of Platelets in the Genesis of Ischemia. By ROBERT W. COLMAN 190
Role of Coronary Arterial Spasm in Sudden Coronary Ischemic Death. By ATTILIO MASERI, SILVA SEVERI, AND PAOLO MARZULLO 204
Sudden Cardiac Death: Role of Left Ventricular Dysfunction. By BERTRAM PITT 218
Effect of Infarct Size Limitation by Propranolol on Ventricular Arrhythmias after Myocardial Infarction. By JAMES R. STEWART, JOHN K. GIBSON, AND BENEDICT R. LUCCHESI 223

Part IV. Prevention of Sudden Coronary Death: Pharmacologic Studies

Drugs and Sudden Cardiac Death. By J. THOMAS BIGGER, JR. AND FRANCIS M. WELD 229
Pharmacokinetic Studies: Their Role in Determining Therapeutic Efficacy of Agents Designed to Prevent Sudden Death. By DAVID G. SHAND, EDWARD L. C. PRITCHETT, STEPHEN C. HAMMILL, W. WAYNE STARGEL, AND GALEN S. WAGNER 238
Clinical Efficacy of Antiarrhythmic Drugs in Prevention of Sudden Coronary Death. By ROGER A. WINKLE 247
Calcium Antagonists and Their Potential Role in the Prevention of Sudden Coronary Death. By DOUGLAS P. ZIPES AND ROBERT F. GILMOUR, JR. 258
Antiplatelet Agents: Their Role in the Prevention of Sudden Death. By J. HIRSH 289
Beta Blocking Agents: Current Status in the Prevention of Sudden Coronary Death. By Å. HJALMARSON 305

Part V. Prevention of Sudden Coronary Death: Nonpharmacologic Interventions

The Role of Organized Medicine in Providing Education About Cardio-pulmonary Resuscitation. By RICHARD CRAMPTON 324
Community-Based Cardiopulmonary Resuscitation: What Have We Learned? By LEONARD A. COBB AND ALFRED P. HALLSTROM 330
Exercise Conditioning Soon After Myocardial Infarction: Effects on Myocardial Perfusion and Ventricular Function. By ROBERT F. DEBUSK AND JOSEPH HUNG 343
Prevention of Ventricular Fibrillation by Use of Low-Intensity Electrical Stimuli. By RICHARD L. VERRIER AND BERNARD LOWN 355
Implantable Automatic Defibrillators: Their Potential in Prevention of Sudden Coronary Death. By M. MIROWSKI, MORTON M. MOWER, PHILIP R. REID, AND LEVI WATKINS, JR. 371
Surgery for Recurrent Sustained Ventricular Tachycardia Associated with Coronary Artery Disease: The Role of Subendocardial Resection. By MARK E. JOSEPHSON, LEONARD N. HOROWITZ, AND ALDEN H. HARKEN 381
Intraoperative Mapping and Surgery for the Prevention of Lethal Arrhythmias After Myocardial Infarction. By G. FONTAINE, G. GUIRAUDON, R. FRANK, R. COUTTE, C. CABROL, AND Y. GROSGOGEAT 396

Part VI. The Timing of Intervention: Its Role in the Control of Sudden Coronary Death

Large-Scale Clinical Trials: Are They Worth the Cost? By ROBERT I. LEVY AND EDWARD J. SONDIK 411
Primary Prevention of Sudden Coronary Death: A Community-Based Program in North Karelia, Finland. By JUKKA T. SALONEN 423

The Patient with Coronary Artery Disease without Infarction: Can a High-Risk Group Be Identified? *By* JAN ERIKSSEN AND REIDAR MUNDAL 438

Value of Early Thallium-201 Scintigraphy and Gated Blood Pool Imaging for Predicting Mortality in Patients with Acute Myocardial Infarction. *By* LEWIS C. BECKER, KENNETH J. SILVERMAN, BERNADINE H. BULKLEY, E. DAVID MELLITS, CLAYTON KALLMAN, AND MYRON L. WEISFELDT 450

The Chronology and Suddenness of Cardiac Death After Myocardial Infarction. *By* ARTHUR J. MOSS, JOHN DeCAMILLA, JONATHAN CHILTON, AND HENRY T. DAVIS 465

Sudden Coronary Death: A Look to the Future. *By* J. THOMAS BIGGER, JR. ... 474

Index of Contributors 483

Paper Presented at the Conference but not Submitted for Publication:

Part III.

Focal Border Zone of Ischemia and Infarction: Possible Role in Generation of Arrhythmias and Sudden Death. *By* EDWARD KIRK

Financial assistance was received from:

- ABBOTT LABORATORIES
- AMERICAN CRITICAL CARE
- BOEHRINGER INGELHEIM LTD.
- CIBA-GEIGY CORPORATION
- E.I. DUPONT DE NEMOURS & CO.
- ENDO LABORATORIES, INC.
- FOGARTY INTERNATIONAL CENTER, NIH
- HOECHST-ROUSSEL PHARMACEUTICALS, INC.
- HOFFMANN-LA ROCHE, INC.
- HONEYWELL, INC.
- IVES LABORATORIES, INC.
- LILLY RESEARCH LABORATORIES
- MC NEIL LABORATORIES
- THE MEDTRONIC FOUNDATION
- MERCK SHARP & DOHME
- NATIONAL INSTITUTE ON AGING
- NEW ENGLAND NUCLEAR CORPORATION
- NEW YORK HEART ASSOCIATION, INC.
- PFIZER, INC.
- G. D. SEARLE & CO.
- SURVIVAL TECHNOLOGY, INC.
- WARNER-LAMBERT COMPANY
- WYETH LABORATORIES

OPENING REMARKS

Edward M. Dwyer, Jr. and Henry M. Greenberg

Department of Medicine
St. Luke's-Roosevelt Hospital Center
New York, New York 10019

Department of Medicine
Columbia University
College of Physicians & Surgeons
New York, New York 10032

The major purpose of this conference on sudden coronary death is to bring together investigators, from diverse disciplines, who are contributing valuable data that provide important insights into the events surrounding sudden death. This forum will offer each of us an opportunity to gain a broad view of the ongoing research into this important medical problem. In addition, we hope to open the avenues of communication between those investigators who may not normally come together, but who are each actively working on various aspects of sudden death.

There is still a disturbing lack of agreement on the definition of sudden cardiac death, although some uniformity has begun to appear. The usual definition emphasizes the time from symptoms to death. Instantaneous death is clearly an acceptable category, but other definitions appear to be artificial and inappropriate. In some circumstances, a death is considered "sudden" when the patient dies within a very short time after symptoms have appeared, although he may have been admitted to a coronary care unit. On the other hand, others may die after a more extended period from the onset of symptoms without benefiting from medical attention; yet this is not considered "sudden death." The important feature of sudden coronary death is that death occurs unexpectedly in a situation which, for whatever reason, does not allow intervention by the existing health-care system.

This symposium rightly will stimulate more questions than it will answer. In this regard, it is important to recognize that considerable heterogeneity exists in those who suffer sudden death. In this conference we will concentrate on sudden coronary death; however, it is important to emphasize that although coronary artery disease may represent the most common cause of sudden death, it is not the only cardiac cause. Just as there are several cardiac disorders associated with sudden death, so too similar distinctions may also exist in the underlying mechanisms that characterize the pathophysiology of sudden coronary death.

Classification of all unexpected cardiac deaths under the single heading of "sudden death" has served to generate interest, enthusiasm, and community support, while furthering investigative goals which have immediate clinical benefit. However, as research efforts have yielded data suggesting multiple mechanisms, the time seems appropriate to expand our investigative efforts in each of these areas.

Sudden coronary death may occur within different settings and each of these settings may represent different pathophysiologic mechanisms of death.

1

0077-8923/82/0382-0001 $1.75/0 © 1982, NYAS

For example, some coronary patients die during acute ischemic events, while other patients with chronic coronary disease from prior infarctions die with or without an obvious ischemic event. Although our focus during this conference will be on the patient with coronary artery disease, sudden death is also prevalent in patients with primary myocardial disease, valvular disease, and primary malignant arrhythmias without structural heart disease.

In the recent literature on sudden death our attention has clearly been directed toward arrhythmias as the central mechanism leading to sudden death. But we must remember that ventricular tachyarrhythmias are not always the cause of sudden death: other mechanisms include acute ventricular failure, severe reflex hypotension, and malignant bradycardia, each of which may appear rapidly during acute ischemic events and lead directly to the patient's death. To a certain extent, the underlying mechanisms may dictate the temporal characteristics of sudden coronary death. Any contemporary definitions of sudden coronary death should take these mechanisms into consideration. We anticipate that the active exchange of ideas at this conference will help to clarify some of these definitional problems.

It is also important that we continue with our research efforts to reduce the population whom we consider to be at high risk of sudden death. Attempting to design interventions for the entire population with coronary artery disease is unwieldy, expensive, and frequently unrewarding. One portion of our program will address this aspect of the problem.

Until the pathophysiologic mechanisms are properly aligned with each of the high-risk subsets, we will not be able to offer the most effective and directed therapy. We hope that this conference will help us to develop a broader understanding of the mechanisms leading to sudden death and subsequently to improve our application of current and future therapies.

In conclusion, I would like to thank those people who have been instrumental in the development of this conference. First, thanks are due to The New York Academy of Sciences for its sponsorship, to Dr. Heinz Pagels, its President, and to Dr. Muriel Feigelson, the Chair of the Conference Committee. Drs. Kaden, Flanagan, and Kelly of the Academy have been especially helpful with their advice and aid in designing the program. We can't say enough for Ellen Marks and her staff, who have done the yeoman's work in handling all of the details and insuring the smooth conduct of this conference.

We owe a special debt of gratitude to the members and executive committee of our own post-infarction consortium, the Multicenter Postinfarction Project, who have been instrumental in gathering together the all-star team of conference participants.

SUDDEN CORONARY DEATH: THE FRAMINGHAM STUDY *

William B. Kannel and H. Emerson Thomas, Jr.

Division of Heart and Vascular Diseases
National Heart, Lung and Blood Institute
Bethesda, Maryland 20205

Evans Memorial Department of Clinical Research and
Department of Medicine
University Hospital
Boston University Medical Center
Boston, Massachusetts 02118

Sudden deaths abound in places with a high incidence of coronary heart disease. Epidemiologic studies agree that at least half of all coronary fatalities occur within 1 hour of onset of symptoms and that most occur outside the hospital. Most sudden deaths are unexpected and not preceded by symptoms of any duration or by overt coronary heart disease. The high rate of mortality from coronary heart disease can be substantially reduced only if sudden, unexpected coronary deaths can be prevented. Sudden death is now being studied seriously as an important feature of coronary heart disease. Epidemiologic studies have only recently shed some light on the natural history of this lethal manifestation of coronary heart disease.

THE ENTITY

Deaths occurring within 1 hour of onset of symptoms are usually associated with severe coronary atherosclerosis.[1, 2] When less rigorous temporal definitions for sudden death are accepted (for example, the definition recommended by the World Health Organization: death within 24 hours), the etiology is likely to be heterogeneous. The more restricted definition has been adopted in the Framingham Study. Data from this study form the basis for this presentation.

It is not clear how often sudden coronary deaths are an arrhythmic catastrophe of an evolving acute myocardial infarction or how often a mishap in a transient ischemic episode. Among persons resuscitated from sudden death only 10% go on to develop signs of myocardial infarction, suggesting that a substantial proportion of cases of sudden death are provoked by a transient ischemia.[3] However, this may only be true in cases of sudden deaths where resuscitation is possible. Sudden deaths in which resuscitation cannot be carried out may result from a more severe insult, and ventricular fibrillation may only represent an agonal event. Experience in coronary care units indicates that ventricular fibrillation is the usual mechanism causing death. MacWilliam first suggested that mechanism as early as 1889[4] and Halsey provided electrocardiographic documentation of this in 1915.[5] Animal experiments suggest that ventricular fibrillation is caused by reentry of the depolarization wave because

* This work was supported in part by contract numbers NIH–NO1–HV–92922 and NIH–NO1–HV–52971 from the National Institutes of Health, Bethesda, Maryland.

3

of altered conduction in the ischemic myocardium.[6] Although sudden death is almost invariably due to ventricular fibrillation, this may not always be a consequence of inadequate myocardial blood flow.

Severe coronary atherosclerosis is established as the most frequent anatomic substrate of sudden death. The frequency of antemortem thrombosis can be definitely incriminated in no more than 5 to 10 % of the incidences of sudden death.[7] No distinctive pattern of coronary artery involvement has been found among patients who have died suddenly, although left main coronary artery disease is alleged to predispose. There is little evidence that obstructive disease of the smaller intramyocardial branches of the arteries is an important feature.[8, 9] The denervated heart exhibits remarkable electrical stability, even during acute myocardial infarction, indicating the importance of neurohumoral influences.[10]

SIZE AND NATURE OF THE PROBLEM

Focus on the problem of sudden coronary death is amply justified. In persons between ages 35 and 64 years nearly one death in three is due to coronary heart disease.[11] There are more than 300,000 sudden coronary deaths each year, representing one-half of the annual toll of coronary mortality.[12] Death from a coronary attack is as likely as not to be sudden, unexpected, and unheralded by prior coronary heart disease or symptoms. The critical period in a coronary attack is the first few minutes. In patients in the age range of 45 to 74 years, more than half the deaths from initial coronary attacks at Framingham were sudden and unexpected (TABLE 1). Half of those with sudden death had no prior coronary heart disease and 17% of men and 13% of women with coronary attacks presented with sudden death as the first and last symptom.

Because of sudden death and unrecognized myocardial infarction, only 60% of patients with coronary attack are hospitalized and thus receive the benefits of coronary care units. Two-thirds of coronary fatalities occur outside the hospital, the majority suddenly. Even among persons with known coronary heart disease, nearly half of the deaths occurred outside the hospital, predominantly as sudden death (FIG. 1).

There is reason for optimism about the development of improved methods to safeguard the victim of a myocardial infarction by monitoring and early treatment of arrhythmias, measures to limit the size of the infarct, and the avoidance or better treatment of cardiogenic shock and heart failure. However, the natural history of coronary heart disease (CHD) indicates that most premature deaths from the disease cannot be avoided in this way. We are faced with a disease that is extremely common and highly lethal, one that frequently attacks without warning and in which the first symptom is too often sudden death. We must reduce the risk of sudden death.

WARNING SYMPTOMS

If premonitory symptoms of impending sudden death could be eliminated, some sudden deaths might be avoided by rapid transportation of the patient to a coronary care unit. Using a 24-hour definition of sudden death, Kuller found

TABLE 1

PROPORTION OF CORONARY DEATHS THAT WERE SUDDEN ASSOCIATED WITH PRIOR
EVIDENCE OF CORONARY HEART DISEASE: THE FRAMINGHAM STUDY
20-YEAR FOLLOW-UP OF MEN AGE 45–74 AT EXAMINATION PRIOR TO DEATH

Prior Coronary Heart Disease Status	No. of Sudden Deaths	No. of Coronary Heart Disease Deaths	Percentage of Coronary Heart Disease Deaths
Myocardial infarction	31	68	46%
Coronary insufficiency	1	4	25%
Angina pectoris	13	26	50%
Any form of coronary heart disease	45	98	46%
No coronary heart disease	57	101	56%

* Diseases are mutually exclusive categories: myocardial infarction means myocardial infarction with or without any other coronary heart disease; coronary insufficiency means coronary insufficiency, but not myocardial infarction; angina pectoris means angina pectoris only.

that 38 percent had recently sought medical attention for complaints of fatigue, breathlessness, cough, and chest pains.[13] An almost identical percentage of persons dying in Edinburgh (40%) had consulted a physician during the month prior to their demise.[14] The symptoms were, however, too vague to strongly infer coronary heart disease.

Meticulous inquiry in the Framingham and Albany studies, using the 1-hour definition of sudden death, failed to yield evidence that the sudden death victims had often reported either to their family or to a physician prodromata that could have been reasonably construed as symptoms of coronary heart disease.[15, 16] Thus, sudden deaths are usually unheralded by characteristic warning symptoms of any duration. Prevention is clearly the only way to cope with this problem.

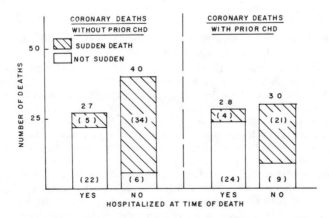

FIGURE 1. Hospitalization status of patients dying of coronary heart disease. The Framingham Study: 16-year follow-up of men aged 35–74 years at death.

THE CANDIDATE FOR SUDDEN DEATH

The incidence of sudden death increases with age in both men and women (TABLE 2). However, sudden coronary death occurs in women at only one-fourth the rate of men, and the occurrence in women lags that of men by 20 years. Although the incidence of sudden death tends to increase with age, the proportion of the coronary deaths that are sudden *decreases* with age (TABLE 2). However, at any age, in either sex, those who are especially vulnerable can be identified from their coronary risk profile. Although sudden death may result from several causes, coronary heart disease is by far the most common. In attempting to define the candidate for sudden death, emphasis is therefore placed on coronary disease and its precursors.

Prior Coronary Heart Disease

Angina pectoris has long been regarded as a harbinger of sudden death. The risk of sudden death among angina patients in the Framingham Study was four times that of the general population the same age (TABLE 3). However,

TABLE 2

INCIDENCE OF SUDDEN DEATH AND PROPORTION OF CORONARY DEATHS THAT WERE SUDDEN: THE FRAMINGHAM STUDY 20-YEAR FOLLOW-UP IN MEN AND WOMEN AGED 45–74

Age (yr.)	Men		Women	
	Incidence per 1000	Percent Sudden	Incidence per 1000	Percent Sudden
45–54	1.1	62%	0.3	63%
55–64	2.7	58%	0.4	33%
65–74	2.6	42%	1.2	33%
All ages	1.9	56%	0.5	42%

angina patients are no more likely than those without angina to die suddenly when a fatal attack occurs. The fraction of coronary deaths that are sudden is one-half, the same as in those who never had overt CHD (TABLE 1). It is alleged that the new onset of angina or an intensification of the frequency and duration of anginal attacks (unstable angina) may signify an impending myocardial infarction or a sudden death. However, all angina must begin sometime and angina is a variable condition. Studies of the natural history of unstable angina do not reveal that a myocardial infarction or sudden death is an alarmingly common sequela in patients with either recent onset or exacerbation of angina pectoris.[17-22]

Multiple myocardial infarctions, extensive damage to the heart, cardiomegaly, heart failure, and rhythm disturbances are all associated with a greater incidence of sudden death. However, it is not clear that death, when it comes, is more likely to be sudden in those with more myocardial damage (FIG. 2). We must seek more subtle evidences of preclinical CHD if we are to prevent sudden deaths.

TABLE 3

PROBABILITY OF SUDDEN DEATH IN UNCOMPLICATED ANGINA: THE FRAMINGHAM
STUDY 20-YEAR FOLLOW-UP IN MEN AGED 40–75

Years from Onset	Cumulative Percent Probability
1	—
2	2.6%
3	4.5%
4	4.5%
5	5.6%
6	6.8%
7	9.7%
Average annual rate	1.3 percent
Standardized mortality ratio	392 percent

Preclinical Coronary Heart Disease

In persons with a poor cardiovascular risk profile, the appearance of electro-cardiographic abnormalities at rest or after exercise, without other explanation, indicates a compromised coronary circulation, even in the absence of symptoms. Such persons are at greatly increased risk of both coronary attacks and sudden death (TABLE 4). And yet, except possibly for those with intraventricular block, there is no evidence of a disproportionate fraction of sudden deaths (TABLE 5). While electrocardiographic evidence of myocardial ischemia presages sudden death, such abnormalities preceded only 35 percent of the incidences of sudden death. However, the risk of sudden death associated with these electrocardiographic abnormalities is comparable to that in patients with a healed myocardial infarction or angina pectoris.

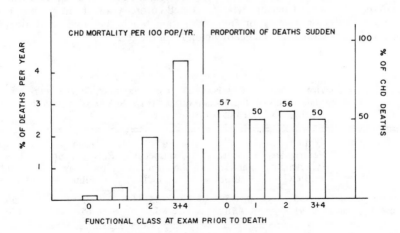

FIGURE 2. Coronary mortality according to functional class at examination prior to death (14-year follow-up). The Framingham Study: men and women aged 30–62 years at entry. (Adapted from Gordon and Kannel.[11])

TABLE 4

RISK OF SUDDEN CORONARY DEATH ACCORDING TO ELECTROCARDIOGRAPHIC
ABNORMALITY: THE FRAMINGHAM STUDY 20-YEAR FOLLOW-UP IN
MEN AND WOMEN AGED 45–74

	Age-Adjusted Average Annual Incidence per 10,000					
	Nonspecific S-T and T wave Abnormality		Intraventricular Conduction Defect		Left Ventricular Hypertrophy	
Electrocardiographic Abnormality	Men	Women	Men	Women	Men	Women
Negative	18.5	4.2	17.4	4.4	16.5	4.4
Positive	23.8	12.2	85.2	17.6	94.9	12.3
t-Value	0.49	1.67	3.61	1.34	4.24	1.10

Coronary Risk Profile

The risk profile of a candidate for a sudden death is virtually indistinguishable from that of persons who will manifest CHD in general (TABLE 6). There is a somewhat greater effect of obesity, the cigarette habit, abnormal heart rate, and intraventricular conduction disturbance in sudden death victims. Glucose levels and sedentary habits seem to have less effect. A comparison of the strength of the influence of these factors, using standardized regression coefficients to place them on equal footing as regards units of measurement, reveals the strongest impact for heart rate, cigarettes, and systolic blood pressure.

Risk profiles, constructed of some of these factors, allows an estimate of risk of sudden death over a 14-fold range and identifies a tenth of the population from which a third of the deaths will evolve (TABLE 7). When the risk factors of sudden death victims were compared by means of multivariate analysis with those of persons who developed coronary attacks in general, none of the risk factors, singly or in combination, could be used to distinguish accurately a potential sudden death victim from the rest.

TABLE 5

PROPORTION OF SUDDEN CORONARY DEATHS ACCORDING TO SPECIFIED
CARDIAC IMPAIRMENTS: THE FRAMINGHAM STUDY 20-YEAR FOLLOW-UP
IN MEN AND WOMEN AGED 45–75*

	Left Ventricular Hypertrophy on ECG †	Intra-ventricular Block	Nonspecific Abnormality on ECG	Cardiac Enlargement on X-ray Film	Low Vital Capacity ‡
Absent	55	52	55	52	56
Present	51	100	62	62	100

* Age-adjusted.
† Possible or definite.
‡ Low—less than 3.5 liters.

Kannel & Thomas: The Framingham Study 9

TABLE 6

REGRESSION OF CORONARY HEART DISEASE VERSUS SUDDEN DEATH INCIDENCE ON SPECIFIED RISK FACTORS: THE FRAMINGHAM STUDY IN MEN AGED 45–74*

	Standardized Coefficients	
	Coronary Heart Disease	Sudden Death
Systolic blood pressure	0.352	0.399
Blood glucose level	0.110	0.086 †
Relative weight	0.186	0.263
Cigarette-smoking	0.205	0.347
Left ventricular hypertrophy on ECG	0.205	0.432
Serum cholesterol level	0.255	0.303

* Source: Framingham Monograph #30.
† Not statistically significant.

CONTROLLABLE RISK FACTORS

In retrospective studies of sudden death, about half of the victims have known heart disease and are predominantly male, hypertensive, diabetic, and cigarette-smokers. Friedman found that most have a Type A (excessive sense of time-urgency) personality.[23] In this study a significant number had engaged in moderate or strenuous exercise shortly before collapsing. In contrast, other investigators have noted the physical indolence of the sudden death victims.[24] In Helsinki, life stress seemed to occur more often in sudden death victims than in survivors of a myocardial infarction, while at the same time occupational stress in aircraft pilots seems to play no role in sudden death.[25, 26] Firm

TABLE 7

INCIDENCE OF SUDDEN DEATH ACCORDING TO DECILE OF MULTIVARIATE RISK *: THE FRAMINGHAM AND ALBANY STUDIES COMBINED IN MEN AGED 45–64

Decile of Multivariate Risk	No. of Sudden Deaths	2-Year Incidence of Sudden Deaths per 1000
1	2	0.89
2	2	0.89
3	2	0.89
4	6	2.69
5	8	3.58
6	6	2.69
7	12	5.37
8	10	4.48
9	17	7.61
10	32	14.32
Total	97	4.34

* Risk variables: systolic blood pressure, left ventricular hypertrophy seen on electrocardiogram, relative weight, number of cigarettes per day, and serum cholesterol levels.

conclusions cannot be drawn from retrospective studies and the hypotheses derived from these must be tested prospectively. Prospective studies have confirmed some of the retrospective observations.[27-30]

Hypertension

Hypertension, a powerful contributor to coronary heart disease in general, is also a highly significant contributor to sudden death (FIG. 3), although for coronary heart disease in general, there is no indication that risk of sudden death is more closely linked to the diastolic component of the blood pressure.[28] Although the incidence of sudden death is distinctly related to blood pressure, the proportion of coronary deaths that are sudden is no different in hypertensive persons.

Cholesterol

The findings for cholesterol in prospective studies have been inconsistent. A combined Framingham-Albany report found no significant relationship,[28] whereas an earlier report from Framingham showed that such a relationship exists.[31] The latest data from Framingham, based on 20 years of follow-up study, show a significant relationship between cholesterol levels and coronary heart disease under age 55 (TABLE 8). The proportion of coronary deaths that were sudden was unrelated to cholesterol concentration.

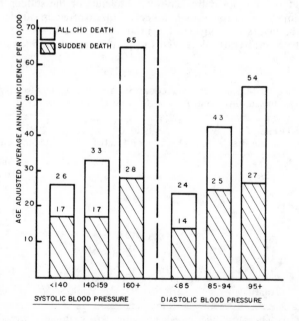

FIGURE 3. Risk of coronary mortality according to systolic and diastolic blood pressure. The Framingham Study 20-year follow-up in men aged 45–74.

TABLE 8

SUDDEN DEATH ACCORDING TO SERUM CHOLESTEROL LEVEL: THE FRAMINGHAM STUDY
20-YEAR FOLLOW-UP IN MEN AGED 45-74

Serum Cholesterol Level at Each Examination (mg/dL)	Proportion of Coronary Heart Disease Deaths That Were Sudden			Age-Adjusted Incidence Sudden Death (per 1000)
	No. of Sudden Deaths	No. of All Coronary Heart Disease Deaths	Percentage of Coronary Heart Disease Deaths That Were Sudden	
96–204	9	17	53%	26
205–234	19	35	54%	31
235–264	11	19	58%	36
265–294	7	10	70%	43
295–1124	6	14	43%	50
				t Value = 2.45

Diabetes

Diabetes is associated with atherosclerosis that is more severe. It has a greater relative impact for occlusive peripheral arterial disease and congestive heart failure than for coronary heart disease, although coronary disease is still on an absolute scale the chief vascular sequela.[32] Women tolerate diabetes poorly, so that it virtually eliminates their "immunity" to cardiovascular disease compared with that of men. In men, no significant relationship between sudden death and diabetes or impaired carbohydrate tolerance could be demonstrated.[28, 29]

Living Habits

There is a growing conviction that coronary disease results from a faulty lifestyle including a too-rich diet and too little exercise (leading to obesity) and the smoking of cigarettes.[33-36]

Obesity

Hippocrates pointed out some 2400 years ago that sudden death is more common in those who are naturally fat than in lean persons. In the Framingham cohort the risks of coronary mortality in general and sudden death in particular were significantly related to relative weight (TABLE 9). There was also a positive trend in the proportion of coronary deaths occurring suddenly in relation to relative weight. The mechanism by which obesity predisposes to sudden coronary death is uncertain.

TABLE 9

CORONARY MORTALITY ACCORDING TO RELATIVE WEIGHT: THE FRAMINGHAM STUDY
20-YEAR FOLLOW-UP IN MEN AGED 55–64

Weight (lbs.)	Relative Average Annual Incidence per 10,000 (smoothed)		
	Sudden Death	Death of CHD	Percentage of Sudden Deaths
65–104	12	31	39%
105–114	17	38	45%
115–124	23	43	53%
125–134	31	51	60%
135–272	43	61	70%
t value	2.93	1.91	

Physical Activity

Overweight can reflect not only gluttony, but also sloth: Those who are physically inactive are believed to have a higher coronary mortality. An examination of the risk of coronary heart disease in relation to physical activity at Framingham revealed a significant inverse relationship. A 20-year follow-up study in men showed a trivial and nonsignificant relationship for sudden death in particular, but examination of the relationship of physical activity to the *suddenness* of coronary fatality indicated a significant trend of a *higher* proportion of coronary fatalities that are sudden at higher levels of physical activity. Physical activity may protect against coronary attacks and even coronary deaths, but the death, when it comes, may be more likely to be a sudden death in those who are active.

A striking relationship of heart rate at rest to incidence of sudden death was noted in the Framingham cohort (TABLE 10). This was also true for coronary mortality in general and may reflect, among other things, physical fitness. However, no consistent trend in the fraction of deaths was noted in relation to heart rate.

TABLE 10

RISK OF CORONARY MORTALITY ACCORDING TO RESTING HEART RATE: THE
FRAMINGHAM STUDY 20-YEAR FOLLOW-UP IN MEN AGED 45–74

Heart Rate (beats/min)	Average Annual Incidence per 10,000		
	Death of CHD	Sudden Death	Percentage of Sudden Deaths
37–71	22	11	49%
72–83	32	18	56%
84–95	47	33	70%
96–170	83	38	45%

Cigarette-Smoking

It is now widely acknowledged that cigarette-smoking predisposes to coronary heart disease. Data from the Framingham Study continue to show that cigarette-smokers are at significantly higher risk of CHD and of sudden death in particular (FIG. 4). Risk of sudden death is increased almost three-fold in cigarette-smokers compared with nonsmokers. There is also a positive trend in the proportion of CHD deaths that are sudden that increases with the amount of cigarette-smoking.

Coffee

Coffee-drinking has been questioned as a risk factor for CHD by some retrospective studies.[37] However, its riskiness has not been confirmed by a

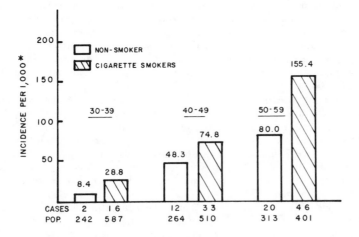

FIGURE 4. Risk of sudden death according to cigarette habit. The Framingham Study 24-year follow-up of men aged 30–59 at entry.

number of prospective studies.[38] In the Framingham Study, coffee intake could not be clearly associated with any manifestation of CHD: there was no trend in coronary fatalities among coffee drinkers.[38] The total number of CHD deaths and sudden deaths among non-coffee-drinkers was too few for a sound estimate.

VENTRICULAR PREMATURE BEATS

Ventricular premature contractions, particularly when they are frequent, multifocal, and have a short coupling interval,[39] are an established harbinger of sudden death because they lead to ventricular fibrillation, which in the setting of acute myocardial infarction is often fatal. A relationship between ventricular ectopy and subsequent death after recovery from a myocardial infarction has also been demonstrated. However, it remains unclear whether ventricular premature contractions are *specifically* related to sudden unexpected death.[40]

The prevalence of ventricular premature beats is greater in men and increases with age, with the prevalence of other electrocardiographically demonstrated ischemic abnormalities, and with the severity of the coronary risk profile.[41, 42] Angiographic study in coronary patients indicates that a higher prevalence and a more severe grade of ventricular premature contractions exist in patients with multivessel coronary artery disease than in those with only one vessel involved.[43] Thus, ventricular premature contractions, particularly when frequent or complex, often serve as an indicator of severe cardiac disease and left ventricular dysfunction. However, there is reason to question whether ventricular extrasystoles are invariably a marker of lethal electrical instability of the heart heralding ventricular fibrillation or are in themselves causal factors inducing instability. Data from Framingham indicate a three-fold increased risk of sudden death in subjects in the general population with ventricular premature contractions compared with those not exhibiting them on a standard electrocardiogram at rest. However, the electrocardiographic tracings on the examination prior to death showed that virtually all patients with ventricular premature contractions who died suddenly also had other abnormalities such as left ventricular hypertrophy, ventricular conduction disturbances, or myocardial infarction.

To determine whether ventricular premature contractions are specifically related to the *suddenness* of coronary fatalities, the fraction of CHD deaths that were sudden was examined in relation to the presence of ventricular premature contractions. In 22 years of follow-up study in the Framingham cohort, there were 216 coronary deaths, among which 105 were sudden. Of those who died of CHD, 29 had ventricular premature contractions on the standard resting ECG on the exam prior to death. This was distributed equally among those who died suddenly (14 out of 105) and those who died a more protracted death (15 out of 111). Thus, the proportion who died suddenly among those with ventricular premature contractions (14 out of 29) and those without (91 of 187) was virtually identical. Since the gender ratio and average age of the two groups were similar, there is no reason to believe that this negative finding derives from incomparable groups.

Even in the Coronary Drug Project, where ventricular premature complexes were shown to carry a doubled risk of sudden death, independent of other risk factors, including other electrocardiographic abnormalities, the proportion of deaths that were sudden was no greater in persons with ventricular premature contractions (FIG. 5).

PROSPECTS FOR PREVENTION

Risk factors for coronary attacks are inevitably related to the incidence of sudden death because most coronary fatalities occur suddenly. However, factors associated with an increased incidence of sudden death do not necessarily determine the suddenness of coronary fatalities. Hence, the potential sudden death victim cannot be confidently discriminated from the person destined for a less precipitous coronary death. Factors that determine the suddenness of coronary fatalities are still poorly understood. The data presented here suggest that overweight, cigarette-smoking, and physical activity may play a role, but this requires confirmation elsewhere.

In coronary patients, as in the general population, the key to prevention of sudden death appears to be measures to reduce coronary attacks. Limiting the size of a myocardial infarction offers some possibility of decreasing later sudden death, but this can do little to reduce the early sudden deaths that occur before such steps can be taken.[44] Coronary bypass surgery may play a role in stabilizing the myocardium of survivors of ventricular fibrillation without myocardial infarction, but this has yet to be determined. Although bypass surgery might be indicated for some candidates for sudden death with left main and three-vessel coronary artery disease, it is clearly not a practical solution for all of the 300,000 persons in whom sudden coronary death will occur each year.

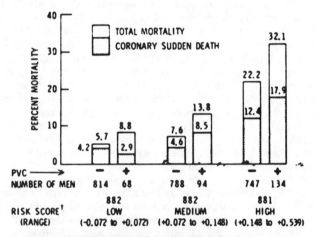

FIGURE 5. Three-year mortality rate for men with and without premature ventricular contractions according to the multivariate baseline risk score. Data from the Coronary Drug Project Research Group.

Encouraging subjects to seek medical attention promptly on the first indication that a coronary attack may be occurring might avoid some sudden deaths. However, there is much delay in seeking medical attention despite educational programs and many of those who do seek attention often have only ill-defined symptoms.[45, 46]

If ventricular premature contractions were in themselves factors inducing electrical instability of the myocardium, rather than a sign of an irritable, diseased myocardium, it would be logical to seek out and correct this condition. However, it has not been conclusively shown that suppression of ectopic ventricular activity *per se* will prevent sudden death in the chronic phase of coronary heart disease; furthermore, most suppressive drugs are too toxic for large-scale use over long periods. Among those with numerous, complex, severe grades of ventricular premature beats, the best candidates for drug therapy would appear to be those resuscitated from sudden death without myocardial infarction, those with coronary insufficiency without signs of myocardial infarction, and coronary patients with premature ventricular contractions at rest in the standard electrocardiogram. Beta adrenergic blocking agents have shown some promise in prolonging short-term survival after myocardial infarction in this circumstance.[47, 48]

Persons at high risk of sudden death can definitely be identified long in advance of the fatal coronary attack. The factors that predict coronary attacks, and presumably predispose to them, are even more predictive of sudden death. However, the sudden death victim cannot be confidently distinguished from those who experience a more protracted death. Thus, prophylaxis against sudden death must focus on preventing coronary deaths in general. Thus far, it has not been conclusively demonstrated that sudden death can be avoided by controlling risk factors. However, it seems logical to expect that by preventing coronary attacks they may do so. Some trials have suggested that overall mortality from CHD may be reduced by diet and clofibrate.[49-53] One study has suggested that sudden death in particular may be specifically reduced by dietary blood lipid control.[53] Trials of several lipid-lowering drugs to attempt to reduce mortality in the Coronary Drug Project suggest that short-term therapy of this sort in advanced disease will not reduce coronary mortality.[54] Short-term control of hypertension has not been consistently shown to reduce coronary mortality, but recent inclusion of beta adrenergic blocking agents seems to have been more efficacious.[55] This will require confirmation by other large-scale controlled studies.

Cessation of smoking seems to hold the most promise. Smoking may be specifically related to sudden death and studies have shown that quitting is associated with a decline in mortality, both in the general population and after myocardial infarction.[56] Ultimately, prevention of sudden death requires measures designed to delay the atherosclerotic process, which begins early in life, progresses insidiously, and finally becomes clinically manifest with distressing frequency from the fourth decade on. This process is multifactorial and requires public health measures to alter the national diet, encourage daily physical activity, and discourage cigarette-smoking. Hygienic measures along these lines taken by the public in their own behalf are also indicated. Physicians interested in prevention of sudden death would do well to counsel high-risk coronary candidates to reduce weight if necessary, quit smoking, restrict fats and cholesterol in their diet, and to remain under effective treatment for hypertension. While these precursors will not *specifically* reduce the risk of sudden death, it is hoped that they will reduce the occurrence of coronary attacks and hence the likelihood of a sudden death.

PROGNOSIS OF RISK

Because sudden death is such a prominent factor of coronary mortality there is considerable interest in factors that predispose specifically to its occurrence. Persons highly vulnerable to death from coronary heart disease, including sudden death, can be identified well in advance of the often unexpected precipitous demise. Prospective study reveals that risk of sudden death is related to antecedent hypertension, serum cholesterol levels, obesity, cigarette-smoking, the presence of electrocardiographic abnormalities, and resting heart rate.

The risk mounts with the number of these factors. From a coronary profile made up of these risk factors, the likelihood of sudden death can be estimated over a 14-fold range. One-third of the sudden deaths occur in men in the topmost decile of risk.

The same precursors are found in persons whose coronary attacks are fatal as in those that are not. A number of coronary risk factors are related to the *fraction* of coronary deaths that are suddenly fatal. These include physical activity, obesity, and cigarette-smoking. The other major coronary risk factors are not specifically related to the suddenness of coronary fatality. Persons with premature ventricular contractions have about a three-fold increased risk of sudden death. Virtually all of the persons with premature contractions who die suddenly have evidence of an ischemic myocardium, usually with other electrocardiographic abnormalities. The proportion of coronary deaths that are sudden is no greater among those with premature ventricular contractions than among those without them.

Persons with overt coronary heart disease are at a four-fold increased risk of sudden death, but only because of a greater incidence of coronary attacks. Fatalities are no more likely to be sudden than in the general population. Both in the patients with angina and in the general population, the proportion of coronary fatalities that are sudden is similar and decreases with age.

Factors related to the incidence of coronary attacks are inevitably related to the incidence of sudden death because most coronary fatalities occur suddenly. The potential sudden death victim cannot be confidently distinguished from the person destined for a less precipitous coronary death. Sudden coronary death would appear to be more of a consequence of the nature of the ischemic disease of the heart than of the factors that predispose to coronary atherosclerosis. The inescapable conclusion seems to be that prevention of sudden coronary death requires the prevention of coronary attacks by avoidance or correction of coronary risk factors.

SUMMARY

The occurrence of sudden death (within 1 hour of onset of symptoms) over a 26-year follow-up period in the Framingham Study has been studied. Of the 5209 subjects, 131 men and 49 women died suddenly and unexpectedly, 60% without prior indications of overt coronary heart disease (CHD). The incidence of these sudden deaths increased with age, averaging 35 per 1000. This incidence was related to blood pressure, serum cholesterol, glucose intolerance, left ventricular hypertrophy, heart rate, cigarette-smoking, and relative weight. Combining these risk factors quantitatively into a composite multivariate risk function, it is possible to estimate risk over more than a 14-fold range. In this way a tenth of the asymptomatic population can be identified from which 33% of the sudden deaths will arise.

Subjects with prior overt CHD are high-risk candidates for sudden death, with an incidence four times that of the general population. However, the proportion of coronary deaths that are sudden is 50%, no greater than that for the general population. Although the incidence of sudden death increases with age, the fraction of CHD deaths that are sudden decreases with age. Women lag men in incidence by 20 years.

The fraction of coronary deaths that are sudden was greater in subjects who were obese, cigarette-smokers, had rapid heart rates, and were physically active. When sudden death victims were compared by multivariate analysis with those who developed coronary attacks in general, none of the risk factors examined could be used to distinguish a potential sudden death victim from the rest. In men cigarette-smoking and relative weight were specific determinants of sudden death. The CHD risk profile for sudden death is very similar to that for CHD in general. They key to prevention of sudden death remains the reduction of risk of coronary attacks.

REFERENCES

1. SPAIN, D. M., V. A. BRADESS & C. MOHR. 1960. Coronary atherosclerosis as a cause of unexpected and unexplained death. An autopsy study from 1949–1959. J. Am. Med. Assoc. JAMA 174:384–388.
2. LAKE, J. L. & M. HELPERN. 1968. Sudden unexpected death from natural causes in young adults. A review of 275 consecutive autopsied cases. Arch. Pathol. 85:10–17.
3. BAUM, R. S., H. ALVAREZ, 3RD & L. A. COBB. 1974. Survival after resuscitation from out-of-hospital ventricular fibrillation. Circulation 50:1231–1235.
4. MACWILLIAM, J. A. 1889. Cardiac failure and sudden death. Br. Med. J. 1: 6–8.
5. HALSEY, R. H. 1915. A case of ventricular fibrillation. Heart 6:67–76.
6. HAN, J. 1969. Mechanisms of ventricular arrhythmias associated with myocardial infarction. 1969. Am. J. Cardiol. 24:800–813.
7. REICHENBACH, D. D., N. S. MOSS & E. MYER. 1977. Pathology of the heart in sudden cardiac death. Am. J. Cardiol. 39:865–872.
8. SCHWARTZ, C. J. & W. J. WALSH. 1971. The pathologic basis of sudden death. Prog. Cardiovasc. Dis. 13:465–481.
9. JAMES, T. N. 1967. Pathology of small coronary arteries. Am. J. Cardiol. 20:679–691.
10. HARRISON, D. C. 1975. Discussion: Electrophysiology of lethal arrhythmias. In: Sudden coronary death outside hospital. Circulation Suppl. III: 143.
11. GORDON, T. & W. B. KANNEL. 1971. Premature mortality from coronary heart disease: The Framingham Study. J. Am. Med. Assoc. 215:1617–1625.
12. GOLDSTEIN, S. 1974. Sudden Death and Coronary Heart Disease. Futura Publishing Co. Mount Kisco, NY.
13. KULLER, L., M. COOPER & J. PERPER. 1972. Epidemiology of sudden death. Arch. Intern. Med. 129:714–719.
14. FULTON, M., B. DUNCAN, W. LUTZ, et al. 1972. Natural history of unstable angina. Lancet 1:860–865.
15. DOYLE, J. T., W. B. KANNEL, P. M. MCNAMARA, et al. 1976. Factors related to suddenness of coronary death: Combined Albany-Framingham studies. Am. J. Cardiol. 37:1073–1078.
16. DOYLE, J. T. 1975. Profile of risk of sudden death in apparently healthy people. Circulation 52 Suppl. III: 176–179.
17. FULTON, M., B. DUNCAN, & W. LUTZ, et al. 1972. Natural history of unstable angina. Lancet 1:860–865.
18. KANNEL, W. B., P. M. MCNAMARA, M. FEINLEIB & T. R. DAWBER. 1970. The unrecognized myocardial infarction: Fourteen-year follow-up experience in the Framingham study. Geriatrics 25:75–87.
19. KRAUSS, K. R., A. M. HUTTER JR. & R. W. DESANCTIS. 1972. Acute coronary insufficiency. Course and follow-up. Circulation 45(Suppl. 1):66–71.
20. GAZES, P. C., E. M. MOBLEY, JR., & H. M. FARIS, JR., et al. 1973. Preinfarc-

tional (unstable) angina: A prospective study—ten-year follow-up. Prognostic significance of electrocardiographic changes. Circulation **48**:331–337.

21. HENG, M-K., R. M. NORRIS, B. N. SINGH & J. B. PARTRIDGE. 1976. Prognosis in unstable angina. Br. Heart J. **38**:921–925.

22. DUNCAN, B., M. FULTON, & S. L. MORRISON, *et al.* 1976. Prognosis of new and worsening angina pectoris. Br. Med. J. **1**:981–5.

23. FRIEDMAN, M., J. H. MANWARING & R. H. ROSENMAN, *et al.* 1973. Instantaneous and sudden deaths. Clinical and pathological differentiation in coronary artery disease. J. Amer. Med. Assoc. **225**:1319–1328.

24. BAINTON, C. R. & D. R. PETERSON. 1963. Deaths from coronary heart disease in persons fifty years of age and younger. A community-wide study. N. Engl. J. Med. **268**:569–575.

25. RAHE, R. H., M. ROMO & L. BENNETT, *et al.* 1974. Recent life changes, myocardial infarction and abrupt coronary death. Studies in Helsinki. Arch. Intern. Med. **133**:221–228.

26. JOKL, E. & J. T. MCCLELLAN. 1968. Sudden cardiac death of pilots in flight. Cardiologia **52**:235–238.

27. VEDIN, J. A., C. WILHELMSSON & D. ELMFELDT, *et al.* 1973. Sudden death: Identification of high risk groups. Am. Heart. J. **86**:124–132.

28. KANNEL, W. B., J. T. DOYLE & P. M. MCNAMARA, *et al.* 1975. Precursors of sudden coronary death: Factors related to the incidence of sudden death. Circulation **51**:606–613.

29. DOYLE, J. T., W. B. KANNEL, & P. M. MCNAMARA, *et al.* 1976. Factors related to suddenness of coronary death: Combined Albany-Framingham studies. Am. J. Cardiol. **37**:1073–1078.

30. CHIANG, B. N., L. V. PERLMAN & M. FULTON, *et al.* 1970. Predisposing factors in sudden cardiac death in Tecumseh, Michigan. A prospective study. Circulation **41**:31–37.

31. KANNEL, W. B., A. KAGAN & T. R. DAWBER, *et al.* 1962. Epidemiology of coronary heart disease: Implications for the practicing physician. Geriatrics **17**:675–690.

32. KANNEL, W. B. 1976. Diabetic and cardiovascular disease: The Framingham study: 18-year follow-up. Cardiology Digest **11**:11–16.

33. 1970. Report of Inter-Society Commission for Heart Disease Resources: Primary prevention of the atherosclerotic diseases. Circulation **42**:A55–A95.

34. 1976. Coronary Heart Disease. A progress report. National Heart Foundation of New Zealand.

35. 1976. Joint Working Party Report of the Royal College of Physicians and British Cardiac Society. J. Roy. Coll. Physicians London **10**:1–63.

36. KEYS, A. 1975. Coronary heart disease—the global picture. Atherosclerosis **22**:149–192.

37. JICK, H. & D. SLONE. 1972. Coffee drinking and acute myocardial infarction: Report from the Boston Collaborative Drug Surveillance Program. Lancet **2**: 1278–1281.

38. KANNEL, W. B. 1977. Coffee, cocktails and coronary candidates (editorial). N. Engl. J. Med. **297**:443–444.

39. KILLIP, P., III & J. T. KIMBALL. 1967. Treatment of myocardial infarction in a coronary care unit. A two-year experience with 250 patients. Am. J. Cardiol. **20**:457–464.

40. LAWRIE, D. M. 1969. Ventricular fibrillation in acute myocardial infarction. Am. Heart J. **78**:424–426.

41. HINKLE, L. E., JR., S. T. CARVER & M. STEVENS. 1969. The frequency of asymptomatic disturbances of cardiac rhythm and conduction in middle-aged men. Am. J. Cardiol. **24**:629.

42. VEDIN, J. A., C. E. WILHELMSSON & L. WILHELMSEN, *et al.* 1972. Relation of

resting and exercise-induced ectopic beats to other ischemic manifestations and to coronary risk factors. Am. J. Cardiol. **30**:25–31.
43. CALVERT, A., B. LOWN & R. GORLIN. 1977. Ventricular premature beats and anatomically defined coronary heart disease. Am. J. Cardiol. **39**:627–634.
44. MAROKO, P. R. & E. BRAUNWALD. 1973. Modification of myocardial infarction size after coronary occlusion. Am. Intern. Med. **79**:720–733.
45. SIMON, A. B., M. FEINLEIB & H. K. THOMPSON, JR. 1972. Components of delay in the pre-hospital phase of acute myocardial infarction. Am. J. Cardiol. **30**:476–482.
46. FULTON, M., W. LUTZ & K. W. DONALD, et al. 1972. Natural history of unstable angina. Lancet **1**:860–865.
47. WILHELMSSON, C., J. A. VEDIN & L. WILHELMSEN, et al. 1974. Reduction of sudden deaths after myocardial infarction by treatment with alprenolol. Lancet **2**:1157–1160.
48. 1975. A Multicentre International Study: Improvement in prognosis of myocardial infarction by long-term beta-adrenoreceptor blockade using practolol. Br. Med. J. **3**:735–740.
49. RINZLER, S. H. 1968. Primary prevention of coronary heart disease by diet. Bull. NY Acad. Med. **44**:936–949.
50. MIETTINEN, M., O. TURPEINEN & M. J. KARVONEN, et al. 1972. Effect of cholesterol-lowering diet on mortality from coronary heart disease and other causes. A twelve-year clinical trial in men and women. Lancet **2**:835–838.
51. LEREN, P. 1966. The effect of plasma cholesterol lowering diet in male survivors of myocardial infarction. A controlled clinical trial. Acta. Med. Scand. Suppl. **466**:1–92.
52. KRASNO, L. R. & G. J. KIDERA. 1972. Clofibrate in coronary heart disease. Effect on morbidity and mortality. J. Amer. Med. Assoc. **219**:845–851.
53. DEWAR, H. A. & M. F. OLIVER. 1971. Secondary prevention trials using clofibrate: A joint commentary on the Newcastle and Scottish trials. Br. Med. J. **4**:784–788.
54. 1975. The Coronary Drug Project Research Group: Clofibrate and niacin in coronary heart disease. J. Amer. Med. Assoc. **231**:360–381.
55. JULIAN, D. G. 1976. Toward preventing coronary death from ventricular fibrillation. Circulation **54**:360–364.
56. WILHELMSSON, C., J. A. VEDIN & D. ELMFELDT, et al. 1975. Smoking and myocardial infarction. Lancet **1**:415–420.

DISCUSSION

DR. RIBEIRO (*Browns Mills, New Jersey*): I'd like to know whether obesity by itself is a risk factor or whether obesity is a risk factor when it is associated with another risk factor.

DR. KANNEL: The data from Framingham have shown that many, but not all, of the associated risks for obesity are mediated through factors such as blood pressure, serum lipid elevation, or impaired glucose tolerance. In our data in multivariate analysis we see some residual effect for sudden death.

DR. RIBEIRO: Does coffee intake increase the risk of sudden death in patients with coronary artery disease?

DR. KANNEL: We could not find such a relationship in the general population, and we have not examined the relationship of coffee intake in persons with already established coronary disease. It is conceivable that coffee might enhance the irritability of a myocardium when it is ischemic. But such data still have to be gathered.

DR. ENGELBERG (*Beverly Hills, California*): In your data is there any level of obesity at which the incidence of sudden death sharply increases? Or is it a gradual change above the ideal weight?

DR. KANNEL: Our data show that it is gradual. We cannot define a critical value. Other sets of data I've seen suggest that it is the grossly obese who are at particular risk. Our own data suggest a graded, continuous variable effect.

UNIDENTIFIED SPEAKER: Was the increase in sudden death related to systolic or to diastolic blood pressure?

DR. KANNEL: The common clinical notion that all of the evil consequences of hypertension derive from the diastolic component cannot be supported by prospective epidemiologic data. The risk is as closely linked to the systolic pressure as to the diastolic.

DR. IRVING HERLING (*Philadelphia, Pennsylvania*): Does a family history of sudden death "separate out" as an independent risk factor for sudden death?

DR. KANNEL: We have only looked at this for coronary attacks in general. In the Framingham Study cohort, persons who have a family history of coronary disease (in siblings) are at a two- to three-fold increased risk. This increased risk persists even if one takes shared risk factors into account. There is something unique about having a strong family history of coronary disease. For sudden death, the data were inadequate to support analysis.

DR. BAHR (*Baltimore, Maryland*): What percentage of sudden deaths occur at night?

DR. KANNEL: Our study required that the death be within an hour, and that meant it had to be an observed death. If somebody were found dead in bed without any clear indication that the death had been a precipitous one, it was automatically excluded as a sudden death.

DR. A. HJALMARSON (*University of Göteborg, Göteborg, Sweden*): You said that one should try to eliminate the risk factors, Dr. Kannel. Is there any proof that it is worthwhile to stop smoking, to reduce the blood pressure, and to reduce weight?

DR. KANNEL: The evidence for that is not available. The evidence for lipid control, as you know, is equivocal. The evidence for physical activity is nonexistent. Aside from blood pressure and cigarette-smoking the evidence is rather thin. But remember, if you had to demand proof of efficacy in the practice of medicine, for most things you would be reduced to therapeutic nihilism.

The problem that we're facing is rather formidable. The chance of a person having a coronary attack in this country before the age of 60 is 1 in 5. We're not talking about a trivial matter and we cannot afford indefinite temporizing. After all, what we're recommending is worthwhile for other reasons, so we should not feel guilty about recommending a prudent diet, more exercise, and moderate weight. I can hardly see where that's going to be dangerous.

SHORT-TERM RISK FACTORS FOR SUDDEN DEATH

Lawrence E. Hinkle, Jr.

Department of Medicine
Division of Human Ecology
Cornell University Medical College
New York Hospital
New York, New York 10021

The investigations described in this report have been directed at ascertaining the factors that determine the risk of sudden death within 5 years among middle-aged American men, the conditions under which sudden deaths occur, and the factors that precipitate these deaths. Such information is of great importance for the secondary prevention of sudden death and for the clinical management of patients who have heart disease.

METHODS

The investigations have been based on a 5-year prospective survey of 1839 deaths attributed to coronary heart disease among 269,755 men aged 20 to 65 years employed in the telephone industry throughout the continental United States [1] and on 1023 5-year intensive prospective observations of men aged 40 to 65. These intensive observations included repeated (one to seven times) comprehensive medical histories and examinations; reviews of activities, medications, smoking, drinking, and time budgets; determinations of blood lipids, glucose tolerance, and serum uric acid; biochemical and hematologic profiles; chest X-ray films; 12-lead electrocardiograms and 24-hour recordings of electrocardiograms; and investigations of all deaths (total 142) that occurred. [2] The subjects, from 21 white- and blue-collar industries and two labor unions in New York, New Jersey and Connecticut, included 333 selected from medical records because of features thought to indicate "high risk," and 687 designated in random samples from age cohorts of employed men in which the sudden death rates and the incidence of coronary heart disease were determined to be similar to those of comparable men nationwide. The prevalence of coronary heart disease (CHD) and hypertension, the body-build, the rate of smoking and drinking, the serum cholesterol and serum uric acid levels, and the results on glucose tolerance tests in the random samples were also comparable to those of contemporary men nationwide. [2]

FINDINGS

"Sudden Deaths," "Arrhythmic Deaths," and "Deaths in Circulatory Failure"

Three-fifths (60.4%) of 1476 deaths attributed to coronary heart disease in the nationwide survey terminated final illnesses that lasted less than 2 hours. Forty-two and five-tenths percent of these "sudden deaths" (25.7% of all deaths

22

0077–8923/82/0382–0022 $1.75/0 © 1982, NYAS

attributed to coronary heart disease) occurred in men who had not previously been known to have coronary heart disease.[1]

On the basis of information from witnesses, rescue squads, physicians, hospitals, autopsy reports (31%), electrocardiograms and electrocardiographic recordings at or shortly after the time of collapse (20.4%), and our own previous examinations, 141 of the 142 deaths among men who were intensively observed could be classified into two major categories[3]: In 82 cases (58%) the pulse ceased abruptly without prior collapse of the circulation and did not return spontaneously. The adequacy of the circulation for perfusing the brain immediately before death was indicated by the fact that the subjects were conscious (often active) or asleep and readily aroused. Electrocardiograms obtained at or shortly after the time of collapse showed ventricular fibrillation or asystole. These deaths were classified as "arrhythmic." In 59 cases (42%) the peripheral circulation collapsed gradually, although sometimes rapidly, the subject lost consciousness and was not arousable, and the blood pressure could no longer be obtained, before the pulse finally ceased. These were classified as "deaths in circulatory failure." [3]

The primary cause of "sudden death" in these men was the sudden development of a cardiac arrhythmia. All "instantaneous deaths" that occurred in less than 5 minutes were "arrhythmic." Ninety-one and three-tenths percent of deaths in less than 1 hour were "arrhythmic," 84.8% of deaths in less than 24 hours were "arrhythmic," and 23.8% of deaths in which the final illness lasted more than 24 hours were "arrhythmic."

Noncardiac "Risk Factors" for Arrhythmic Death Within 5 Years

In the random samples the presence of vascular hypertension at the initial examination was associated with a slightly enhanced risk of arrhythmic death in 5 years, the risk increasing with the severity of the hypertension; present cigarette smoking was associated with enhanced risk of both arrhythmic death and death in circulatory failure, the risk increasing with the number of cigarettes being smoked; but the presence of a serum cholesterol concentration ≥ 250 mg/dL was associated only with an enhanced risk of death in circulatory failure (caused by deaths attributed to stroke and peripheral vascular disease) (TABLE 1).

Other noncardiac factors affecting a smaller proportion of the men were associated with a relatively larger proportion of deaths. Clinical diabetes mellitus was associated with deaths of both kinds. An enhanced risk of arrhythmic death was associated with a serum uric acid concentration ≥ 8 mg/dL; clinical evidence of arteriosclerosis of vessels other than the coronary arteries (calcification or aneurysm of aorta, intermittent claudication, stroke, or transient ischemic attacks); the consumption of five or more alcoholic drinks per day; and the presence of chronic obstructive pulmonary disease with severe airway disease ($FEV_1/VC < 60\%$).

Eighty-eight and eight-tenths percent of the men in the random sample had one or more of these noncardiac "risk factors" at the initial examination; the arrhythmic death rate of the men who had none of these was lower than that of the other men in the sample.

TABLE 1

RANDOM SAMPLES:
NONCARDIAC RISK FACTORS PRESENT AT INITIAL EXAMINATION

| | Men at Risk * | | Deaths in 5 Years | | | |
| | | | Arrhythmic † (n=38) | | Circulatory Failure ‡ (n=32) | |
	No.	%	No.	Rate per 100	No.	Rate per 100
All men in random samples	687	100	100	5.5	100	4.7
Hypertension						
Definite ($\geq$ 160/95)§	201	30.0	45.9	8.4 ‖	22.5	3.5
Borderline ($\geq$140/90, but < 160/95)§	156	23.3	21.6	5.1	25.8	5.1
None	312	46.6	32.4	3.8	51.6	5.1
Now smoking cigarettes						
More than 40/day	49	7.3	19.4	14.3 #	12.9	8.2 ¶
10–39/day	140	21.0	25.0	6.4	38.7	8.6
None	479	71.7	55.5	4.2	51.6	3.3
Serum cholesterol $\geq$250 mg/dL	265	41.3	37.5	4.5	62.1	6.8 ¶
Clinical diabetes mellitus	33	5.1	14.7	15.2 ¶	16.7	15.2 ¶
Serum uric acid $\geq$8.0 mg/dL	53	8.4	25.3	15.1 #	6.2	3.8
Arteriosclerosis of aorta or peripheral or cerebral arteries	131	15.4	37.8	10.6 ¶	16.7	3.8
Now drinking >5 drinks/day	31	4.5	12.8	16.1 ¶	3.1	3.1
Chronic obstructive pulmonary disease with FEV_1/VC <60%	12	1.8	16.7	33.3 #	0.0	0.0
Men with none of the above	77	11.2	2.9	1.3	10.0	3.9

NOTE: Estimates of probability are based on Chi square analyses, with Yates correction when indicated. Estimates relate to the probability that the indicated rate of arrhythmic deaths or of deaths in circulatory failure is different from the rate among other men at risk with data on this variable.

* This column represents all of the men at risk for whom complete data were available for the variable under consideration. A small and variable number of the men in the samples (range 0 to 88) did not have complete data on each variable. The % of men at risk is the percent of men with complete data on the variable under consideration who were at risk.

† This column represents arrhythmic deaths within 5 calendar years among the men at risk. A small and variable number of men (range 0 to 6) who suffered arrhythmic deaths did not have complete data on each variable. The % of arrhythmic deaths in this column is the percent of all the arrhythmic deaths that occurred among men who had complete data on the variable under consideration. Rate per 100 is the rate of arrhythmic deaths within five years among men who had complete data on the variable under consideration.

‡ The same considerations apply for deaths in circulatory failure as for arrhythmic deaths as stated in the preceding footnote.

§ References 2 and 4.

‖ $p < 0.1$.

# $p < 0.01$.

¶ $p < 0.05$.

Myocardial Disease Risk Factors for Arrhythmic Death in 5 Years

Clinical evidences of myocardial disease were, as single variables, the most potent risk factors for sudden death in 5 years. The 15.0% of men in the random samples who had definite clinical evidence of ischemic heart disease ("definite" or "probable" previous myocardial infarction, electrocardiographic evidence of old myocardial infarction, or definite clinical evidence of coronary insufficiency or angina pectoris) [2, 4] had a 5-year arrhythmic death rate of 16.5 per 100. Men with definite ischemic heart disease accounted for 44.7% of the arrhythmic deaths within 5 years. The risk of men with "probable" and "possible" ischemic heart disease was not significantly higher than that of other men with no clinical evidence of coronary heart disease, but it was three times as high as that of men with no evidence of any form of myocardial disease (p < 0.05) (TABLE 2).

Men with "definite" and "probable" electrocardiographic patterns of left ventricular hypertrophy (LVH),[2, 5] men with a transverse cardiac diameter on X-ray films ≥2 SD above the expected mean for height and weight,[2, 6] and men with definite clinical evidence of past or present congestive heart failure,[2] representing 2.4–4.6% of the men in the sample, had significantly enhanced risks of arrhythmic death (22.2–44.4 per 100) and accounted for 12.1–21.1% of the arrhythmic deaths in 5 years. Men with "possible" LVH patterns on the electrocardiogram (voltage abnormalities only) had an arrhythmic death rate not greater than that of all other men without LVH patterns, but three times as high as that of men with no evidence of myocardial disease.

One-half (49.4%) of the men in the random samples who had no clinical evidence of definite, probable, or possible myocardial disease at the initial examination experienced only 13.5% of the arrhythmic deaths in 5 years; the arrhythmic death rate among these men (1.6 per 100) was significantly lower than that of the other men in the sample (p < 0.001).

In all of the samples there was a significant enhancement of risk when two or more major indicators of myocardial disease were present. When "definite" or "probable" ischemic heart disease was associated with "definite" or "probable" LVH patterns on the electrocardiogram, the risk was 31.0 per 100 in 5 years; combined with cardiac dilatation ≥2 SD, the risk was 41.4 per 100; and combined with present or past evidence of congestive heart failure the risk was 31.0 per 100 (53.3 per 100 in the random samples).

Chronic Disorders of Heart Rate, Rhythm, Conduction, and
Repolarization as Risk Factors for Arrhythmic Death in 5 Years

Disorders of heart rate, rhythm, conduction, and repolarization were widely prevalent in the random samples. As single variables, major disorders in each of these categories, including sustained tachycardia, sustained bradycardia, disorders of the pacemaker, prolonged QRS conduction, prolonged repolarization, and very frequent supraventricular premature complexes, were associated with a significantly enhanced risk of arrhythmic death (TABLE 3).

One or more ventricular premature complexes (VPCs) were found in the tape recordings at the initial examinations of 71.6% of the men in the random samples. The arrhythmic death rate among these men (6.0 per 100 in 5 years) was higher than that of men without any VPCs (2.5 per 100), but the difference was of borderline significance (p < 0.1). After classification of the men by

TABLE 2

RANDOM SAMPLES:
CLINICAL EVIDENCE OF MYOCARDIAL DISEASE AT INITIAL EXAMINATION

	Men at Risk *		Deaths in 5 Years			
			Arrhythmic * (n=38)		Circulatory Failure * (n=32)	
	No.	%	%	Rate per 100	%	Rate per 100
All men in random samples	687	100	100	5.5	100	4.7
Clinical evidence of ischemic heart disease	139	20.8	51.3	13.7	15.6	3.6
"Definite" ischemic heart disease † ‡	103	15.0	44.7	16.5 §	12.5	3.9
"Probable" ischemic heart disease #	36	5.2	5.3	5.6	3.1	2.7
"Possible" ischemic heart disease ¶	81	12.8	14.7	6.1	10.3	3.7
LVH patterns on electrocardiogram	116	17.4	31.4	9.5	16.1	4.3
"Definite" and "probable" **	27	4.1	17.1	22.2 ‡	6.5	7.4
"Possible" ††	89	13.4	14.3	5.6	9.7	3.4
X-Ray evidence of dilatation ‡‡	62	9.9	24.2	12.9	7.1	3.2
≥2 SD above expected value	15	2.4	12.1	26.7 ‡	0.0	0.0
≥1 SD but <2 SD above expected value	47	7.5	12.1	8.5	7.1	4.2
Definite clinical evidence of congestive heart failure §§	18	2.6	21.1	44.4 ‡	3.1	5.6
Men with none of the above	313	49.4	13.5	1.6	41.1	3.8

* See the first three footnotes in TABLE 1.
† References 2 and 4.
‡ Definite or probable myocardial infarction, electrocardiographic evidence of myocardial infarction, definite coronary insufficiency, or definite angina pectoris.[2, 4]
§ p < 0.005 (see NOTE in TABLE 1).
# Probable angina pectoris or coronary insufficiency, ischemic S-T segments or T waves on standard electrocardiogram.[2, 4]
¶ Electrocardiographic evidence of possible myocardial infarction; transient "ischemic" S-T segments on tape recordings.[2, 4]
** Voltage and S-T segment and T wave abnormalities.[2, 5]
†† Voltage only.[2, 5]
‡‡ From insurance tables, based on height and weight.[2, 6]
§§ Reference 2.

TABLE 3

RANDOM SAMPLES

CHRONIC DISORDERS OF HEART RATE, RHYTHM, CONDUCTION, AND REPOLARIZATION AT INITIAL EXAMINATION

	Men at Risk *		Deaths in 5 Years			
			Arrhythmic * (n=38)		Circulatory Failure * (n=32)	
	No.	%	%	Rate per 100	%	Rate per 100
All men in random samples	687	100	100	5.5	100	4.7
Disorders of heart rate	16	2.7	12.5	25.0 †	0.0	0.0
Sustained tachycardia	14	2.3	9.4	21.4	0.0	0.0
Sustained bradycardia	2	0.3	3.1	50.0	0.0	0.0
Disorders of pacemaker	82	4.8	20.6	21.9 †	3.4	5.5
Atrial fibrillation	2	0.3	2.9	50.0	0.0	0.0
Ectopic or shifting atrial rhythms	19	2.8	11.8	21.1	0.0	0.0
A-V junctional rhythms	11	1.6	5.9	18.2	3.4	9.1
Supraventricular dysrhythmias SPCs ≥10/1000 complexes	40	6.5	15.6	12.5 ‡	14.3	10.0
Disorders of conduction QRS >0.11 sec	27	4.1	14.3	18.5 §	6.5	7.4
LBBB	5	0.8	5.7	40.0	3.2	20.0
RBBB	18	2.7	8.6	16.7	3.2	5.6
Ventricular dysrhythmias						
Any VPCs	435	71.6	86.7	6.0 ‡	64.3	4.1
VPCs ≥10/1000 complexes	61	10.0	26.7	13.1 §	3.6	1.7
Q form VPCs	146	24.0	53.3	11.0 †	28.5	5.5
Early-cycle VPCs R-R'/Q-T$_e$ <1	43	7.1	26.7	18.6 †	10.7	7.0
VPC pairs	81	13.3	13.3	4.9	0.0	0.0
Paroxysmal ventricular rhythms	29	4.8	10.0	10.3	3.6	3.4

Q-T$_c$ (Bazett) $\geq$440 msec ‖	46	6.9	14.2	15.2 §	10.0	6.5
Men with none of the above	194	32.4	9.4	1.5	14.8	2.1

NOTE: A-V=atrioventricular; LBBB=left bundle branch block; RBBB=right bundle branch block; SPCs=supraventricular premature complexes; VPCs=ventricular premature complexes.
* See first three footnotes in TABLE 1.
† p <0.005.
‡ p <0.1 (see NOTE in TABLE 1).
§ p <0.01.
‖ Reference 23.

the mean frequency of VPCs per 1000 complexes in the 24-hour recordings at the initial examinations, it was found that in all samples the risk of arrhythmic death increased stepwise as VPC frequency increased on a logarithmic scale, from <0.01 VPC/1000 complexes (arrhythmic death rate 2.3/100 men in 5 years in random samples) to >10 VPCs/1000 complexes (arrhythmic death rate 13.1/100 men in 5 years in random samples).[7] Men whose tape recordings contained VPCs at a frequency >1/1000 complexes had a subsequent risk of arrhythmic death that was significantly higher than that of all other men in the sample.

The frequency of bigeminal and trigeminal ventricular rhythms, paired VPCs, brief runs (1–15 complexes) of paroxysmal ventricular rhythms, and multiformal VPCs (two or more forms) increased with the frequency of all VPCs. When the effect of VPC frequency on risk of arrhythmic death was taken into account, no risk was added when complex VPCs were present.[7]

After classification of all VPCs by form, based on the configuration in the bipolar chest lead that was used for the recording (which had the positive electrode over the fifth rib in the nipple line), it was found that VPCs with a QS configuration in this lead were associated with a significantly enhanced risk of arrhythmic death (p < 0.01). Many of these VPCs probably originated in the left ventricle. They were present in 38.8% of all recordings. The risk associated with "Q form" VPCs was independent of VPC frequency. When multiformal VPCs were present in a recording, there was no added risk of arrhythmic death when the effects of VPC frequency and the presence of Q form VPCs were taken into account.

The presence of "early-cycle" VPCs in which the QRS complex of the VPC encroached upon the T wave of the preceding complex (R-R'/Q-T < 1) was associated with a significantly enhanced risk of arrhythmic death (p < 0.001). This risk was independent of VPC frequency and of VPC form.

A multiple logistic regression, including only the ventricular dysrhythmia variables mentioned earlier, indicated that among these variables only VPC frequency, Q form, and early-cycle VPCs contributed to risk of arrhythmic death independently of any risk associated with other dysrhythmia variables.[7]

The prognostic significance of ventricular dysrhythmias was significantly enhanced by the presence of definite or probable clinical evidence of ischemic heart disease (TABLE 4). In the absence of clinical evidence of ischemic heart disease, the risk of arrhythmic death associated with frequent VPCs, or with paroxysmal ventricular rhythms, was no greater than that of men with no VPCs at all. The risk of arrhythmic death associated with Q form VPCs and with early-cycle VPCs was higher in the presence of ischemic heart disease; but, even in the absence of ischemic heart disease, men with Q form VPCs and early-cycle VPCs had an arrhythmic death rate significantly higher than that of other men with VPCs.

Conditions Under Which Arrhythmic Deaths and Deaths in Circulatory Failure Occurred

Chronic Myocardial Disease Present Prior to Death

The men in these samples were examined one to seven times in the interval between their initial examination and their deaths, and information about them was obtained from physicians' records and from hospital records.

At the last examination prior to arrhythmic death, 92.5% of men in the random samples had clinically detectable chronic myocardial disease. Seventy-two and six-tenths percent had symptomatic or clinically evident chronic ischemic heart disease, 40% had LVH patterns on the electrocardiogram, 22.5% had cardiac dilatation on chest X-ray film, and 45% had evidence of chronic congestive heart failure. At autopsy, myocardial hypertrophy (80.0%) was as frequent as occlusive coronary arteriosclerosis (70.0%).[8]

In the random samples 51.6% of men who subsequently died in circulatory failure also had clinically detectable myocardial disease, but the number of men with manifestations in each category was smaller, fewer men had multiple manifestations, and a significantly larger proportion (48.4%) had no manifestations of myocardial disease.

TABLE 4

VENTRICULAR DYSRHYTHMIAS: EFFECT OF PRESENCE OF ISCHEMIC
HEART DISEASE ON RISK OF ARRHYTHMIC DEATH

	"Definite" or "Probable" Ischemic Heart Disease			
	Present		Absent	
	Men at Risk (No.)	Arrhythmic Deaths (Rate per 100)	Men at Risk (No.)	Arrhythmic Deaths (Rate per 100)
VPCs ≥ 10/1000 complexes	38	28.9 *	54	5.6
Q form VPCs	121	19.8 *	146	6.8 †
Early-cycle VPCs, R-R'/Q-T <1	22	40.9 †	40	15.0 *
Paroxysmal ventricular rhythms	29	31.0 †	26	3.8

NOTE: Probabilities of higher rates among men with ischemic heart disease (IHD) are based on comparison with the rates of similar men without IHD; probabilities of higher rates of men without IHD are based on comparison with rates of similar men without VPCs.
† p <0.05.
* p <0.005.

Acute Myocardial Disease at the Time of Death

In the random samples, 62.5% of men who had arrhythmic deaths, and 100% of men who died in circulatory failure had developed clinical evidence of acute abnormal conditions affecting the myocardium over a period of hours, days, or weeks immediately prior to death. The manifestations that preceded the two kinds of deaths were quite different.[8]

Sixty percent of men who experienced arrhythmic deaths had acute ischemic heart disease at the time of death. This was symptomatic in 35.3% of the cases and was "silent" (not reported by the subject and not suspected by his associates) in 22.5% of cases. In the "silent" cases it was represented by a recent acute myocardial infarction or coronary thrombosis discovered at autopsy. Only 3.2% of men who died in circulatory failure had symptomatic acute ischemic heart disease and no "silent" acute lesions were found at autopsy.

Ten percent of men who had arrhythmic deaths experienced prior exacerbations of chronic congestive heart failure. This was subacute in all cases and clinically "severe" (disabling) in only 2.5% of cases. Evidence of peripheral circulatory failure (shock) was present at the time of death in only 10% of men with arrhythmic deaths and was not severe in any case. On the other hand, 68% of deaths in circulatory failure were preceded by exacerbations of congestive heart failure, of which 8% were acute and 26% severe; and 100% of these deaths occurred in the setting of severe shock.

Evidence of acute anoxemia affecting the myocardium and arising from causes other than ischemic heart disease was present at the time of 25% of arrhythmic deaths. In 22.5% of the cases this was anoxic and was caused primarily by acute exacerbations of severe chronic obstructive pulmonary disease. Anoxic anoxemia, caused by central respiratory failure from stroke or brain tumor, or by obstructive respiratory failure from carcinoma of the lung, pneumonia, congestive heart failure, or acute airway disease was present at the time of death in 48% of men dying in circulatory failure. All of the hearts of men who died in circulatory failure were considered to have been anoxemic as a result of the profound circulatory collapse that was present at the time that the ventricular contractions ceased.

A larger proportion of the men who died arrhythmic deaths (57.5% as contrasted with 25.8%, $p < 0.01$) were receiving medications that had cardiac effects (such as digitalis glycosides, quinidine, other antiarrhythmic medications, vasodilators, antihypertensive agents, or diuretics) before the onset of the terminal illnesses. The only single category of medication which was associated with a greater than expected number of arrhythmic deaths was digitalis glycosides (30.0% versus 9.7%, $p < 0.05$).

Uremia (blood urea nitrogen level up to 41 mg/dL) was present prior to 5% of the arrhythmic deaths. Severe metabolic derangements were a feature of many of the terminal illnesses that preceded death in circulatory failure.[8]

Chronic Disorders of Rate, Rhythm, Conduction, and Repolarization Prior to Death

In the random samples, 92.5% of men who experienced arrhythmic death had chronic disorders of heart rate, rhythm, conduction or repolarization, and 51.6% of men who died in circulatory failure had similar abnormalities at the last examination prior to death. In every category except supraventricular dysrhythmias and prolonged repolarization, the abnormalities were significantly more frequent among men who died arrhythmic deaths. The single abnormalities that most significantly distinguished between the two kinds of subsequent death were early cycle VPCs ($p < 0.01$), sustained tachycardia ($p < 0.05$), episodes of sinus delay ($p < 0.05$), and Q form VPCs ($p < 0.1$) in that order.[8]

In the high-risk sample, for which the men were selected partly on the basis of preexisting disorders of rhythm and conduction, the only one of these variables that distinguished between arrhythmic death and death in circulatory failure at the last examination prior to death was sinus delay ($p < 0.01$). There was no overall difference with respect to the prevalence of any other variable. Although a greater proportion of the men with arrhythmic death had preceding supraventricular dysrhythmias, there was no significant difference between them and the men who died in circulatory failure with regard to any single kind of supraventricular dysrhythmia. A relatively larger proportion of the men who died in circulatory failure had evidence of prolonged repolarization shortly before death (p < 0.1).

Central Nervous System Arousal, Position and Activity of the Subjects Immediately Prior to Death

With the exception of those who were under anesthesia at the time of death, all of the men in these samples who experienced arrhythmic death were awake, or asleep and arousable, immediately before they collapsed and ventricular contractions ceased, whereas all of the men who died in circulatory failure were comatose and not arousable. Sixty-five and nine-tenths percent of men who experienced arrhythmic death were actively mobile, standing or sitting, at the time that they collapsed. All of the men who died in circulatory failure were lying immobile before the ventricular contractions ended.[8]

Precipitating Events

In all of the samples, 17.1% of the men with arrhythmic death collapsed while engaged in activities that are known to be associated with vagal effects upon the heart and have been reported to be associated with the onset of dysrhythmias.[9-14] Thirty-four and one-tenth percent of the arrhythmic deaths occurred during or immediately (<5 min) after the subject had been engaged in activities known to be associated with the occurrence of myocardial ischemia or with sympathetic effects upon the heart, such as tachycardia, or with an increase in ventricular dysrhythmias. All of these activities have also been reported to be associated with the occurrence of fatal arrhythmias.[14-18] Fourteen and six-tenths percent of arrhythmic deaths occurred within a period of a few minutes to not more than 4 hours after the onset of pain and other symptoms of acute myocardial ischemia.

In all of the samples, 86.5% of the deaths in circulatory failure were precipitated by conditions that led steadily and promptly (within minutes, hours, or a few days) to collapse of the peripheral circulation, and 13.5% of these deaths were precipitated by conditions that led promptly to myocardial failure.[8]

Mechanism of the Fatal Arrhythmia

We have observed four mechanisms by which sudden fatal (or potentially fatal) ventricular arrhythmias have occurred in men without prior collapse of the circulation: (1) An early-cycle VPC falling in the vulnerable period of repolarization and initiating ventricular fibrillation. This occurred immediately after physical activity that produced a sinus tachycardia of 165/minute.[17] (2) A marked widening of the Q-T interval during a symptomatic episode of myocardial ischemia, with an early cycle R-on-T VPC initiating ventricular fibrillation. (3) The apparently spontaneous appearance of a ventricular escape rhythm after a long R-R interval during a period of bradycardia, with rapid degeneration of the rhythm to ventricular fibrillation. This occurred in a man with a recent acute myocardial infarction. (4) A very rapid supraventricular tachycardia occurring during sleep, leading directly to the initiation of a rapid ventricular rhythm terminating in ventricular fibrillation.

SUMMARY AND CONCLUSIONS

In these random samples of middle-aged American men, 91% of the deaths within 1 hour and 85% of the deaths within 24 hours were precipitated by the sudden occurrence of a cardiac arrhythmia at a time when the peripheral circulation had not collapsed and was still adequate to support the function of the brain.

The multivariate analyses of the large number of highly interrelated variables from the first examination that represent potential risk factors for arrhythmic death in 5 years are still under way. The initial results reported here, based largely on single variable analyses, indicate that the most significant risk factors fall into four categories:

1. The major noncardiac risk factors for ischemic heart disease—hypertension, cigarette-smoking, and elevated serum cholesterol. These risk factors are widely prevalent in these samples. Hypertension and cigarette-smoking show a gradient of risk which increases with the severity of hypertension and with the number of cigarettes now being smoked, but only very frequent cigarette-smoking carried with it a relatively high degree of risk. An elevated serum cholesterol level was related to risk of death in circulatory failure caused by stroke or peripheral vascular disease but not to arrhythmic deaths.

2. Other noncardiac risk factors for arrhythmic death. These are not major risk factors for ischemic heart disease in younger people and are not highly prevalent in the sample. Among these, diabetes mellitus was related to deaths in circulatory failure as well as to arrhythmic death, and may be related to mortality in general. Evidence of arteriosclerosis of other vessels was probably an indicator of underlying and asymptomatic arteriosclerosis of the coronary arteries, which is frequently found at autopsy in arrhythmic deaths. Elevated serum uric acid levels may be related to chronically high levels of central nervous system arousal.[19] A heavy intake of alcoholic drinks was strongly associated with heavy cigarette-smoking and with chronic obstructive pulmonary disease, but alcohol also is toxic to the myocardium and it is sometimes arrhythmogenic.[20] Chronic obstructive pulmonary disease with severe airway disease was a risk factor by virtue of its frequent association with the subsequent development of acute respiratory obstruction and anoxic anoxemia.

3. Evidences of chronic myocardial disease. These were the most potent risk factors for arrhythmic death in these samples. Ischemic heart disease, LVH patterns on the electrocardiogram, evidences of cardiac dilatation, and congestive heart failure all carried with them a high risk of arrhythmic death. For each of the conditions, the risk became higher as the condition was more overt and advanced and as the evidence for it was more "definite." "Probable" or "possible" ischemic disease, "probable" LVH patterns, and cardiac dilatation >1 SD above the expected (but <2 SD), carried with them a risk of arrhythmic death that was only slightly higher than the average risk of all men in the samples, although it was significantly higher than the risk of men with no myocardial disease. Combinations of ischemic heart disease with LVH patterns, cardiac dilatation, or congestive heart failure increased risk significantly; but LVH patterns, cardiac dilatation, and congestive heart failure also appeared to be associated with increased risk independently of the presence of ischemic heart disease.

4. Disorders of heart rate, rhythm, conduction, and repolarization. Several kinds of these disorders were, as single variables, associated with a high risk of arrhythmic death. These variables were highly correlated and the extent to which they made independent contributions to risk is still to be ascertained. Among the ventricular dysrhythmia variables, which have been studied intensively,[7] only VPC frequency, Q form VPCs, and early-cycle VPCs made contributions to risk that were independent of those associated with the other ventricular dysrhythmias. The risk associated with ventricular dysrhythmias was strongly influenced by the presence of ischemic heart disease. In the absence of ischemic heart disease, the risk associated with frequent VPCs or with episodes of paroxysmal ventricular rhythms was not significantly different from that of men in the samples who had no ventricular dysrhythmias; but the risk of men with Q form VPCs and early-cycle VPCs was significantly higher than that of men with no VPCs, even in the absence of clinical evidence of ischemic heart disease.

In the interval between the initial examination and death, many men developed new manifestations of heart disease. At the time of death the great majority of those who died arrhythmic deaths had preexisting myocardial disease, but this was often asymptomatic. As the data from the nationwide survey had indicated, only 72% of the men who died arrhythmic deaths had previous clinically evident coronary heart disease. However, 92.5% of these men had been found at examination to have detectable clinical evidence of chronic myocardial disease prior to death. This myocardial disease included LVH patterns, cardiac dilatation, and chronic congestive heart failure as well as evidence of ischemic heart disease. At autopsy, hearts that were hypertrophied were almost as prevalent among these men (80%) as occlusive lesions of one or more major coronary vessels (70%).

One-half of the men in the random samples who died in circulatory failure had no clinical evidence of prior myocardial disease, but the other half had chronic myocardial disease similar to that of the men who experienced arrhythmic deaths. Some men with severe and far-advanced chronic myocardial disease died in circulatory failure, but in general the myocardial disease among these men was not so far advanced as that which was found in the men with arrhythmic deaths. There was only one man who had an arrhythmic death who did not have preceding clinical myocardial disease. All of the other men who had no clinical evidence of chronic myocardial disease died in circulatory failure.

Both arrhythmic deaths and deaths in circulatory failure usually occurred in the setting of an acute myocardial disorder that had developed within minutes, hours, or days immediately prior to death. The acute disorders that preceded the two kinds of deaths were different.

The majority of arrhythmic deaths occurred in the setting of acute ischemic heart disease or of myocardial anoxemia from other causes. In the random samples 60% of the arrhythmic deaths occurred in the setting of an episode of acute ischemic heart disease which was asymptomatic in 22.5% of the cases and took the form of a "silent" acute myocardial infarction or coronary occlusion found at autopsy. The proportion of "silent" myocardial infarctions in this series is like that which has been reported from Seattle and Miami.[21, 22] In addition, at least 70% of the arrhythmic deaths occurred in a setting of acute myocardial anoxemia from causes other than ischemic heart disease—chiefly anoxic anoxemia caused by acute exacerbations of chronic obstructive pulmonary disease, but in a few cases anemic anoxemia caused by severe chronic anemia.

In the random samples only 3.2% of the deaths in circulatory failure occurred in the setting of acute ischemic heart disease. Such deaths occurred, rather, in the setting of profound circulatory collapse ("shock"), and 68% of them occurred also in the setting of acute or subacute and severe exacerbations of congestive heart failure. The acute myocardial anoxemia and other metabolic abnormalities that undoubtedly affected the myocardium at the time of death in circulatory failure appeared to be primarily the result of failure of the general circulation.

The simple presence, absence, or frequency of chronic disorders of heart rate, rhythm, conduction, or repolarization at the last examination prior to death was not the final determinant of whether or not an arrhythmic death would occur. In the random samples a larger proportion of the men who died arrhythmic death had significant chronic ventricular dysrhythmias, sustained bradycardia or tachycardia, abnormal supraventricular rhythms, or prolonged QRS conduction; but this was not the case in the high-risk sample. In the high-risk sample, immediately prior to death, the men who died in circulatory failure exhibited all of the kinds of chronic disorders of rhythm and conduction that were exhibited by the men who died arrhythmic death, and, in general, these were equally prevalent.

The functional state of the central nervous system immediately prior to death was of great importance in determining the kind of death that would occur. Most of the arrhythmic deaths occurred in men who were awake, and often active and aroused. These deaths were in many cases precipitated by activities or conditions known to be accompanied by autonomic nervous effects—vagal or sympathetic—on cardiac function. The acute fatal arrhythmias that were observed to occur in these cases were initiated by mechanisms that might readily have been set in motion by the kinds of neural stimulation or the acute myocardial ischemia that was present at the time of the arrhythmic deaths.

Deaths in circulatory failure occurred in men who were unconscious and unarousable. The chain of events that led to these deaths was set in motion when the subject was conscious by acute events that led to circulatory collapse and unconsciousness—a major hemorrhage, trauma, or stroke for example. When such an event occurred in a man who had very severe or even acute myocardial disease accompanied by major abnormalities of rhythm and conduction, and who might therefore have been expected to die an arrhythmic death, the end result was not an arrhythmic death but a death in circulatory failure. This was true in all cases, except in those in which the subject was under anesthesia and an acute arrhythmia was precipitated by tracheal intubation.

The importance of the precipitating event in determining the nature of the fatal outcome places serious limits upon the extent to which the occurrence of an arrhythmic death can be predicted in advance from information based only upon features of the subject or his activities 5 years prior to the event.

REFERENCES

1. HINKLE, L. E., JR., L. H. WHITNEY, E. W. LEHMAN, J. DUNN, B. BENJAMIN, R. KING, A. PLAKUN & B. FLEHINGER. 1968. Occupation, education and coronary heart disease. Science 160:238.
2. HINKLE, L. E., JR. 1979. The Antecedents of Sudden Death: Prospective

Studies. (Report on Contract #NHL 70–02069, prepared for the Cardiac Diseases Branch, Division of Heart and Vascular Diseases, National Heart, Lung and Blood Institute; Bethesda, MD 20014.) Part I: Methods and Criteria. Copies available from National Technical Information Service, 5285 Port Royal Road, Springfield, VA 22151.

3. HINKLE, L. E., JR. & H. T. THALER. The clinical classification of cardiac deaths. Circulation. In press.

4. POLLACK, H. & D. E. KRUEGER, Eds. 1960. Epidemiology of Cardiovascular Diseases, Hypertension and Arteriosclerosis. Report of Conference held in Princeton, NJ, April 24–26, 1959. AHA-National Heart Institute. Am. J. Public Health & Nation's Health 50(10):1–24.

5. BLACKBURN, H., E. SIMONSON, A. KEYS, P. RAUTAHAJU & S. PUSAR. 1960. The electrocardiogram in population studies: A classification system. Circulation 21:1160.

6. UNGERLEIDER, H. E. & C. P. CLARK. 1939. A study of the transverse diameter of the heart silhouette with prediction table based on the teleroentgenogram. Am. Heart J. 17:92.

7. HINKLE, L. E., JR. & H. T. THALER. The prognostic significance of ventricular dysrhythmias in ambulatory middle-aged men. Submitted for publication.

8. HINKLE, L. E., JR. The immediate antecedents of sudden death. Acta Med. Scand. In press.

9. LITTLER, W. A., A. J. HONOUR & P. SLEIGHT. 1974. Direct arterial pressure, pulse rate and electrocardiogram during micturition and defecation in unrestricted man. Am. Heart J. 88:205.

10. LYLE, C. B., JR., J. T. MONROE, JR., D. E. FLINN & L. E. LAMB. 1961. Micturition syncope: Report of 24 cases. N. Engl. J. Med. 265:982.

11. SCHOENBERG, B. S., J. F. KUGLITSCH & W. E. KARNES. 1974. Micturition syncope—not a single entity. J. Amer. Med. Assoc. 229:1631.

12. GORLIN, R., J. H. KNOWLES & C. F. STOREY. 1957. The Valsalva manuever as a test of cardiac function. Am. J. Med. 22:197.

13. WOLF, S., R. A. SCHNEIDER & M. E. GROOVER. 1965. Further studies on the circulatory and metabolic alterations of the oxygen-conserving (diving) reflex in man. Trans. Assoc. Am. Physicians 78:242.

14. FRIEDBERG, C. K. 1966. Diseases of the Heart. 519, 524, 531. W. B. Saunders. Philadelphia, PA.

15. SCHARTUM, S. 1968. Ventricular arrest caused by the Valsalva maneuver in a patient with Adams-Stokes attack accompanying defecation. Acta Med. Scand. 184:65.

16. DEBACKER, G., D. R. JACOBS, JR., R. J. PRINEAS, R. S. CROW, H. KENNEDY, J. VILANDRE & H. BLACKBURN. 1980. Ventricular premature beats. Screening and induction tests in normal men. Cardiology 65:23.

17. HINKLE, L. E., JR. 1977. Pathogenesis of an unexpected sudden death: Role of early cycle VPCs. Am. J. Cardiol. 39:873.

18. LAHIRI, A., V. BALASUBRAMANIAN & E. B. RAFTERY. 1979. Sudden death during ambulatory monitoring. Br. Med. J. (June 23): 1676.

19. KASL, S. V., G. W. BROOKS & S. COBB. 1966. Serum urate concentrations in male high school students: A predictor of college attendance. J. Amer. Med. Assoc. 198:713.

20. REGAN, T. J., P. O. ETTINGER, B. HAIDER, S. S. AHMED, H. A. OLDEWURTEL & M. M. LYONS. 1977. The role of ethanol in cardiac disease. Annu. Rev. Med. 28:393.

21. BAUM, R. S., H. ALVAREZ, III & L. A. COBB. 1974. Survival after resuscitation from out-of-hospital ventricular fibrillation. Circulation 50:1231.

22. LIBERTHESON, R. R., E. L. NAGEL, J. C. HIRSCHMAN, S. R. NUSSENFELD, B. D. BLACKBOURNE & J. H. DAVIS. 1974. Pathophysiologic observations in prehospital ventricular fibrillation and sudden cardiac death. Circulation 49:790.

23. BAZETT, H. C. 1920. An analysis of the time-relations of electrocardiograms. Heart 7:353.

DISCUSSION

DR. LOCKHART (*New York, New York*): Did you notice any difference in risk between the VPCs that were occurring during the day with activity versus VPCs constantly through the day?

DR. HINKLE: I haven't examined that in great detail. My impression is that there is no difference.

DR. D. P. ZIPES (*University of Indiana, Indianapolis, Indiana*): I was intrigued by the Q in the PVC that you presented. Do you think that this is a different electrophysiologic mechanism that may be associated with an increased risk of sudden death? Or do you think it represents or marks a different patient, such as one who might have had an anteroseptal versus an inferior myocardial infarction?

DR. HINKLE: You know how difficult it is to say anything about VPCs from a single lead of a tape recording. My general thinking is that the latter of the two probabilities is the correct one. I think that we find these Q forms associated more with severe lesions of the left ventricle.

DR. R. CRAMPTON (*University of Virginia, Charlottesville, Virginia*): I was interested, but a little confused, about the predictive powers that you assign to the corrected Q-T intervals in sudden death in your population. Several studies in patients with acute myocardial infarction have shown that the Q-T interval is a predictor of ventricular fibrillation or ventricular tachycardia in the first 24 hours. We have done a prospective study in a very small group of patients. If we see an individual within 3 hours of onset of pain, a lengthened Q-T interval will predict ventricular tachycardia. None of the patients in our study died, so we can't say anything about predicting mortality. So how should we weight the Q-T interval within your population as a predictor?

DR. HINKLE: In those of the 687 men who in random samples had a prolonged Q-T interval, it was not shown to be a very strong predictor of sudden death. It is really not a very important indicator, even if you see it in persons at the last examination before death.

PATHOLOGY OF SUDDEN CORONARY DEATH *

William P. Newman III,† Richard E. Tracy,† Jack P. Strong,†
William D. Johnson,‡ and Margaret C. Oalmann†

† Department of Pathology and
‡ Department of Biometry
Louisiana State University Medical Center
New Orleans, Louisiana 70112

Sudden and unexpected death from coronary heart disease has been a major health problem throughout the world, especially in industrialized countries. Although progress has been made in determining the pathogenetic sequence of events leading to coronary heart disease and sudden death, many aspects of the process are still unknown. In our experience, most of these sudden deaths occur outside of the hospital or very shortly after the person's arrival. Autopsy materials from typical hospital-based studies do not include much of the information needed for a more complete description of the natural history of the disease.

Our team of investigators has been studying atherosclerosis, coronary heart disease, and sudden death from a high percentage of all 25–44-year-old men dying in a well-delineated geographic location during a specified time period. This community-wide survey was designed to include men dying both inside and outside of hospitals. A large number of heart specimens, collected from young men dying of all causes, was examined by a team of pathologists according to a standardized protocol which required objective evaluation of findings and uniform application of definitions. This report focuses on the findings in sudden and not-sudden deaths from coronary heart disease in this 10-year study.

MATERIALS AND METHODS

This study includes all 25- to 44-year-old black and white men who were residents of and who died in Orleans Parish (county), Louisiana, during the interval from October 1, 1968 to December 31, 1978. Results reported here represent findings of this 10-year investigation from individuals dying of coronary heart disease. Selected data from the first 4-year 3-month interval have been reported.[1-5] Effort was made to obtain autopsy materials and data from all men who died and were autopsied during the study period. Specimens were obtained from 1292 men, representing 52% of the total deaths. More than 95% of the autopsies were performed at the office of the Coroner, Orleans Parish, Charity Hospital of Louisiana, a large biracial community hospital, or the Veterans Administration Hospital. The remaining autopsies were performed at private hospitals. Records of vital statistics were used to confirm eligibility and to serve as a cross-check on subjects eligible for study but missed by protocol procedures.

* This work was supported by Grant HL08974 from the National Heart, Lung and Blood Institute, National Institutes of Health, United States Public Health Service, Bethesda, Maryland.

Specimen Preparation

Methods used to obtain and evaluate the hearts and arteries have been described in detail.[6-8] Briefly, the unopened heart was obtained at autopsy, taken to the laboratory, assigned a 4-digit code number, inspected, and radiographed. Both main branches of the coronary arteries were cannulated and sequentially injected with green (left) and red (right) barium sulfate-gelatin mixtures at pressures of approximately 120 mm Hg. The heart was X-rayed after each injection. After the gelatin mixture had set, the arteries were dissected free of the myocardium, X-rayed, and then opened longitudinally, cleaned, and fixed in a flattened position in 10% formalin. They were then stained with Sudan IV and sealed in plastic bags, as outlined in the procedures of the International Atherosclerosis Project (IAP).[6] The heart was machine-sliced from apex to base at 1.0 cm intervals and the slices were fixed in 10% formalin. The base was opened according to blood flow, the valves and atria were examined, and the base stored in a plastic bag. Sections of tissue from 12 standardized areas were stained with hematoxylin and eosin and Gomori's trichrome with aldehyde fuchsin.

Arterial Lesions

The coronary arteries were graded visually for the extent of fatty streaks, fibrous plaques, complicated lesions, and calcified lesions by procedures developed in the IAP.[6] The presence of occlusion, stenosis, hemorrhage, and thrombosis detected on postmortem angiograms and/or the opened processed arteries was recorded for each major branch of the coronary arteries.

Myocardial Lesions

Heart slices were examined grossly for the presence of myocardial lesions, myocardial rupture, ventricular aneurysm, mural thrombosis, and endocardial thickening. Size in millimeters, age, and location of myocardial lesions were recorded on a standardized grading form.[1] Age of lesions was recorded as necrosis, healing, and/or scar. Recent infarcts included lesions with necrosis or necrosis and healing. Old infarcts included lesions that were predominantly or all scar. The myocardium was visually divided into thirds from endocardium to epicardium for purposes of locating the lesions zonally. Grading was based on the following scores: 2 for dominant involvement, 1 for lesser involvement, and 0 for no involvement. Combinations in our study classified as "transmural" included those coded as 222, 221, 211, 121, 112, and 012 from inner to outer thirds of the myocardium; "subendocardial" included codes 210 and 200.

Histologic sections were examined for necrosis, granulation tissue, fibrosis, changes in small intramyocardial vessels, and other microscopic abnormalities.

Classification into Broad Disease Categories

For purpose of analysis all men studied were classified in one of the following disease categories:

1. CHD Group. This group was comprised of men whose cause of death was coronary heart disease. This determination was made from objective information pertaining to hearts and arteries, as well as other autopsy and medical information, including the circumstances of death. Coronary heart disease could have been present and not the cause of death; for example, one man with a healed myocardial infarction died of stomach cancer and another with an occlusive coronary thrombus died of a gunshot wound. These men were classified in the *Related Diseases* group.

2. Related Group. This includes men having an atherosclerosis-related disease such as hypertension, cerebrovascular events (excluding berry aneurysms), diabetes, or chronic renal disease, or men who had coronary heart disease but died of other causes. Thus, this group was comprised of men having diseases usually associated with an increased amount of atherosclerosis.

3. Uncertain Group. This group was made up of men for whom autopsy revealed no other disease process that might reasonably have been expected to cause death, for whom circumstances were suggestive of coronary heart disease, but for whom insufficient evidence of arterial occlusion and/or myocardial necrosis or scarring was found at autopsy for confident classification of the cause of death as coronary heart disease.

4. Basal Group. This included men whose cause of death could not be appropriately assigned to any of the foregoing three categories. This group included deaths due to external violence (accident, suicide, or homicide) and deaths due to natural causes other than those described above.

Definition of Sudden Death

Sudden death has been defined in many ways, such as death occurring within seconds, minutes, 1 hour, 2 hours, 12 hours or 24 hours after onset of symptoms in the terminal episode.[9–12] For our broadest definition of sudden death in this investigation we included all deaths occurring within 24 hours of onset of symptoms. Thus, men whose deaths were unwitnessed but who were seen alive and well within 24 hours of death were classified in the sudden death group.

Estimating and Controlling Observer Errors

Five pathologists during the first 4 years of the study and four pathologists during the last 6 years independently evaluated the hearts, arterial segments, and histologic sections. The pathologists attempted to standardize their grading techniques. Consistency of the graders was monitored by repeated independent gradings of selected coded specimens randomly interspersed within new materials. A consensus grading was used for most analyses. Consensus for extent of coronary arterial lesion involvement was defined as the unweighted average grading after eliminating "outliers" by a standard statistical procedure.[13] Consensus for "present" or "absent" observations (infarct, thrombus, hemorrhage, stenosis, and occlusion) was defined as the majority decision after discussion of recorded observations.

RESULTS

Of the 1292 men in the study for which we had specimens, the team of pathologists determined the cause of death as coronary heart disease (*CHD* group) in 36 black men and 38 white men and *uncertain* (possibly *CHD*) in two black men and six white men. Seventy-seven black men and 19 white men were classified as dying of atherosclerosis-*related diseases* such as hypertension, cerebrovascular events, diabetes, chronic renal disease, or *CHD* present but not cause of death. The largest number of cases (779 black and 335 white men) was classified in the *basal* group. From analysis of data from the first 4 years of study, we determined that the morphologic correlates (thrombus, occlusion, stenosis, extent of atherosclerotic lesions, and myocardial lesions) were nearly identical in the two races in the *CHD* disease category.[5] For these reasons, the findings in the races are combined in reporting observations concerning the sudden and not-sudden coronary deaths.

As shown in TABLE 1, 65 men (88%) in the *CHD* group died within 24 hours of onset of symptoms. Nine did not die suddenly (they died more than 24 hours after onset of symptoms) and were hospitalized at the time of death. Thirty-four men died in less than 1 hour after onset of symptoms and 13 within 1 to 24 hours, and 18 deaths were unwitnessed (TABLE 2). All of the 8 men in the *uncertain* group died suddenly. The most likely cause of death for each of the men in the *uncertain* group is shown in TABLE 3. Three men in the *uncertain* group probably died of CHD, but scanty clinical information and lack of sufficient evidence of arterial narrowing, plaque complications, or myocardial lesions led to the classification in this uncertain category. Four of the men in the *uncertain* group probably died of cardiovascular events other than CHD; however, clinical information and arterial findings did not allow us to conclusively assign a definite cause of death.

Raised Atherosclerotic Lesions

The coronary arteries of the vast majority of the *CHD* group had extensive involvement with atherosclerotic lesions regardless of whether or not death occurred suddenly (TABLE 4). The mean percentage of involvement with raised atherosclerotic lesions (mean $\pm$ SEM = 52 $\pm$ 3) for men who died suddenly was less than the corresponding mean (62 $\pm$ 5) for those who did not die suddenly, but the difference was not statistically significant. Although not shown in the tables, all of the men dying suddenly as well as those not dying suddenly had raised atherosclerotic lesions of some degree on the coronary arteries. Calcified coronary lesions were found in 62 (95%) men dying suddenly and in all of the 9 men not dying suddenly.

Occlusion and Stenosis

Occlusion of one or more coronary arteries was found in 26 of the 65 men (40%) in the *CHD* group who died suddenly (TABLE 5). Stenosis was found in at least one vessel of another 34 men (52%). No stenosis of greater than 50% of the cross sectional area of the lumen was found in five men. These five men with no occlusion or severe stenosis had varying degrees of advanced

TABLE 1
TIME FROM ONSET OF SYMPTOMS UNTIL DEATH

Time Until Death	No. of Patients	Percent
≤24 hours *	65	88%
>24 hours	9	12%
Total	74	100%

* Including those persons whose deaths were unwitnessed, but who were seen alive within 24 hours prior to death.

TABLE 2
CORONARY HEART DISEASE GROUP CLASSIFIED BY RACE AND TIME UNTIL DEATH AFTER ONSET OF SYMPTOMS

Race	≤1 hr	1–2 hr	3–24 hr	Unwitnessed *	Total No. of Sudden Deaths	Total No. of Not-sudden Deaths	Total No. of Cases
Black	22	3	4	5	34	2	36
White	12	2	4	13	31	7	38
Total	34	5	8	18	65	9	74

* Seen alive and well within 24 hours preceding death.

TABLE 3
UNCERTAIN CAUSE OF DEATH

Most Likely Diagnosis	No. of Cases	Race
Hypoplastic right coronary artery	1	W
Hypertrophic cardiomyopathy	1	B
Hypertensive cardiomegaly	2	W, W
CHD with no thrombus and no coronary occlusion	3	W, W, B
Drug abuse	1	W
Total	8	6W, 2B

TABLE 4
MEAN PERCENT (±SEM) SURFACE INVOLVEMENT WITH ATHEROSCLEROTIC LESIONS

Type of Lesion	Sudden Death (n=65)	Not-sudden Death (n=9)
Raised lesions	52±3	62±5
Fibrous plaques	32±2	33±3
Complicated lesions	2±0	8±2
Calcification	17±2	21±3

TABLE 5

CORONARY HEART DISEASE GROUP CLASSIFIED BY CORONARY ARTERIAL OCCLUSION
AND STENOSIS AND TIME UNTIL DEATH

| | Time Until Death | | | |
| | ≤24 hrs | | >24 hrs | |
Finding	No.	Percent	No.	Percent
Occlusion	26	40%	8	89%
3-vessel stenosis	6	9%	1	11%
2-vessel stenosis	17	26%	0	0%
1-vessel stenosis *	11	17%	0	0%
No stenosis	5	8%	0	0%

* Including borderline stenosis.

atherosclerotic lesions, and three of them had an ulcerated or ruptured plaque. Occlusions were found in eight of the nine men not dying suddenly and three-vessel stenosis was present in the ninth.

Thrombus and Occlusion

Thrombi were found in the coronary arteries of 44 men (67.7%) who died suddenly in the *CHD* group. When information on occlusion and thrombus was combined (TABLE 6), occlusive thrombi were found in 21 (32.3%) men who died suddenly; a thrombus without complete occlusion was present in 23 (35.4%); occlusion with no fresh thrombus in 5 (7.7%); and varying degrees of stenosis with no occlusion or thrombus in 16 (24.6%).

TABLE 6

CORONARY HEART DISEASE GROUP CLASSIFIED BY CORONARY ARTERIAL THROMBUS
AND OCCLUSION AND TIME UNTIL DEATH

| | Time Until Death | | | |
| | ≤24 hr | | >24 hr | |
Finding	No.	Percent	No.	Percent
Thrombus	44	67.7%	9	100.0%
Occlusion	21	32.3%	8	88.9%
No occlusion	23	35.4%	1	11.1%
No thrombus	21	32.3%	0	0.0%
Occlusion	5	7.7%	0	0.0%
No occlusion	16	24.6%	0	0.0%
Total	65	100.0%	9	100.0%

Myocardial Lesions

Grossly visible large (that is, 1 cm or greater in largest diameter) myocardial lesions (either necrosis, scarring, or both) were found in 47 of the men (72.3%) who died suddenly and in all 9 men who did not die suddenly in the *CHD* group (TABLE 7). Large myocardial lesions with necrosis and no scarring were found in six men (9.2%) who died suddenly; one man who died suddenly of *CHD* had only a small (<1 cm) area of necrosis. Of men who died suddenly with myocardial scarring as evidence of previous episodes of myocardial damage, 41 (63.1%) had large myocardial scars and an additional 6 (9.2%) had small (<1 cm) myocardial scars. Microscopic necrosis in the absence of grossly visible lesions was found in two of the men dying suddenly of *CHD*. In addition, five men dying suddenly had other forms of microscopic lesions, including

TABLE 7

CORONARY HEART DISEASE GROUP CLASSIFIED BY TYPE OF MYOCARDIAL LESION AND TIME UNTIL DEATH

	Time Until Death			
	≤24 hr		>24 hr	
Type of Lesion	No.	Percent	No.	Percent
Large lesions	47	72.3%	9	100.0%
Necrosis only	6	9.2%	1	11.1%
Necrosis and scar	21	32.3%	7	77.8%
Scar only	20	30.8%	1	11.1%
Small lesions only	7	10.8%	0	0.0%
Necrosis only	1	1.5%	0	0.0%
Necrosis and scar	0	0.0%	0	0.0%
Scar only	6	9.2%	0	0.0%
Microscopic lesions only	7	10.8%	0	0.0%
Necrosis	2	3.1%	0	0.0%
Other*	5	7.7%	0	0.0%
No lesions	4	6.2%	0	0.0%
Total	65	100.0%	9	100.0%

* Myocytolysis (1); fibrosis and/or granulation tissue, right ventricle (3); fibrosis and granulation tissue, anterior papillary muscle (1).

myocytolysis, fibrosis, or granulation tissue in the right ventricle or anterior papillary ventricle. Only four men who died suddenly in the *CHD* group had no myocardial lesions detected by gross or microscopic examination. Of the nine men in the *CHD* group who did not die suddenly, one had a large lesion with necrosis and no scar, seven had lesions of necrosis and scar, and one had a large myocardial scar and no necrosis.

The location of myocardial lesions was classified from endocardium to epicardium as previously described. "Subendocardial" infarcts were found in eight men (12.3%), "transmural" infarcts in 39 men (60.0%), and no grossly visible large infarcts in 18 men (27.7%) who died suddenly in the *CHD* group (TABLE 8). All men in the *CHD* group who did not die suddenly had transmural infarcts according to our system of classification.

DISCUSSION

We investigated autopsy findings in young men dying from all causes, both coronary- and noncoronary-related, after collecting autopsy specimens and data according to rigid protocol. Numerous studies of sudden death due to coronary heart disease have been conducted; [9-12, 14-22] some were based on deaths of hospitalized patients and others were based on persons clinically diagnosed or suspected of dying from coronary heart disease prior to autopsy review. Other studies excluded persons with pathologic evidence of myocardial infarction or otherwise restricted the study population.

This report is focused upon cardiac and arterial findings in young men with coronary heart disease as a cause of death. Most men in our *CHD* group died suddenly and did not reach a hospital or receive medical care prior to death. The number in this group who did not die suddenly was small. A majority of the men who died suddenly of coronary heart disease had extensive advanced atherosclerotic lesions within the coronary arteries. This finding is consistent with that of Roberts and Jones [23] and Oalmann.[9] Occlusive thrombi were found in 32.3% of the men dying suddenly. This frequency is much lower than that

TABLE 8

CORONARY HEART DISEASE GROUP CLASSIFIED BY LOCATION OF MYOCARDIAL FINDINGS AND TIME UNTIL DEATH

	Time Until Death			
	≤24 hours		>24 hours	
	No.	Percent	No.	Percent
Subendocardial infarct	8	12.3%	0	0.0%
Transmural infarct	39	60.0%	9	100.0%
No gross infarct	18	27.7%	0	0.0%
Total	65	100.0%	9	100.0%

reported by Friedman *et al.*[10] and comparable to the relative frequency of occlusive thrombi found by others who have used minutes to 2 hours as definition of sudden death.[11, 12, 19, 21, 22]

Several patients had nonocclusive or mural coronary thrombi. Strong [3] discussed the connection between nonocclusive thrombi and functional occlusion and sudden death. He suggested that the development of an atherosclerotic plaque is the initial step, with subsequent expansion and degeneration leading to softening, rupture, and ulceration of the plaque. Platelet aggregation then occurs as a result of loss of endothelial integrity and exposure of the flowing blood to collagen and other subendothelial substances. With growth and expansion of the platelet aggregate and mural thrombus formation, thromboxane A_2 is elaborated by platelets and this then invokes sustained coronary arterial spasm. Even though the plaque and developing thrombus did not completely occlude the lumen and no important abnormality could be demonstrated by angiography, this series of events could cause myocardial ischemia and its consequences. This theory does not preclude the possibility that distal microemboli, also containing platelets, may contribute to the problem.

On the other hand, as suggested by Baroldi *et al.*,[24] sudden death may be caused by metabolic factors that lead to myocardial necrosis and thrombosis may occur later. Our findings agree with those of Baroldi *et al.* as to the importance of atherosclerotic lesions in the pathogenesis of coronary heart disease and of sudden coronary death; yet the role of the occlusive episode versus metabolic causes of myocardial damage remains an issue for further research. Coronary spasm may cause variant angina and even myocardial infarction. Moreover, nonocclusive mural thrombi may result from the spasm (see Maseri *et al.*[25]). We feel that it is more likely that this sequence is reversed and that nonocclusive mural thrombi lead to coronary spasm, functional occlusion, myocardial ischemia, and sudden coronary death.

Most of the young men who died suddenly of coronary heart disease had large myocardial lesions of necrosis and/or scar; a much smaller number had only small gross lesions or microscopic lesions, and only four men had no detectable myocardial lesions. Seventy-two percent of the men dying suddenly had evidence of a previous episode of myocardial damage (scars, large or small), even though they had no previous history of cardiac disease. Lie and Titus[26] reported findings in 868 patients in four independent autopsy studies of pre-hospital sudden death. Twelve to 47% of the deceased persons had an acute myocardial infarct and 22 to 53% had an old myocardial infarct.

Evidence of recent myocardial injury was present in 46% of the men who died suddenly in the *CHD* group and recent lesions were superimposed on evidence of old myocardial damage (scar) in 32% of the subjects. These findings are important because they stress the necessity of developing methods for early detection and primary prevention. Further research is needed to determine why the preexisting myocardial damage that was detected in this and other autopsy studies was subclinical. An underlying abnormality in all cases of sudden coronary death is the atherosclerotic plaque. The possibility that there may be morphologic differences in plaques of individuals dying suddenly of CHD when compared to other deaths from CHD or deaths from other causes should be investigated.

Acknowledgments

We gratefully acknowledge the assistance of Pat Mangiaracina and Mary Taylor in preparing this manuscript.

REFERENCES

1. NEWMAN, W. P., III, J. P. STRONG, W. D. JOHNSON, M. C. OALMANN, R. E. TRACY & W. A. ROCK, JR. 1979. Community pathology of atherosclerosis and coronary heart disease in New Orleans: Pathogenic factors and racial comparisons. *In* Proceedings of the Florence International Meeting on Myocardial Infarction. G. G. Neri Serneri, Ed. Vol. **II**:748–750. Excerpta Medica. Amsterdam.
2. JOHNSON, W. D., M. C. OALMANN, J. P. STRONG, W. P. NEWMAN III, R. E. TRACY & W. A. ROCK. 1979. Implications of pathologic findings for prevention of sudden death in premature coronary heart disease. *In* Proceedings of the Florence International Meeting on Myocardial Infarction[1]: 599–601.
3. STRONG, J. P. 1979. Myocardial infarction in patients with patent coronary

bed—a pathologist's viewpoint. *In* Proceedings of the Florence International Meeting on Myocardial Infarction [1]: 647–659.

4. JOHNSON, W. D., J. P. STRONG, M. C. OALMANN, W. P. NEWMAN III, R. E. TRACY & W. A. ROCK, JR. 1981. Sudden death from coronary heart disease in young men: Pathologic findings. Arch. Pathol. Lab. Med. **105:** 227–232.

5. NEWMAN, W. P., J. P. STRONG, W. D. JOHNSON, M. C. OALMANN, R. E. TRACY & W. A. ROCK, JR. 1981. Community pathology of atherosclerosis and coronary heart disease in New Orleans: Morphologic findings in young black and white men. Lab. Invest. **44:** 496–501.

6. GUZMAN, M. A., C. A. McMAHAN, H. C. McGILL, JR., J. P. STRONG, C. TEJADA, C. RESTREPO, D. A. EGGEN, W. B. ROBERTSON & L. A. SOLBERG. 1968. Selected methodologic aspects of the International Atherosclerosis Project. Lab. Invest. **18:**479.

7. ROCK, W. A., JR., M. C. OALMANN, H. C. STARY, R. E. TRACY, M. T. McMURRY, R. W. PALMER, R. A. WELSH & J. P. STRONG. 1972. A standardized method for evaluating myocardial and coronary artery lesions. *In* The Pathogenesis of Atherosclerosis (Appendix): 247. R. W. Wissler and J. C. Geer, Eds. Williams & Wilkins. Baltimore, MD.

8. OALMANN, M. C., J. P. STRONG, W. D. JOHNSON, W. P. NEWMAN III, W. A. ROCK, JR. & R. E. TRACY. 1979. Community pathology of atherosclerosis, coronary heart disease, and sudden death: Study methods. *In* Proceedings of the Florence International Meeting on Myocardial Infarction [1]: 596–598.

9. OALMANN, M. C., R. W. PALMER, M. A. GUZMAN & J. P. STRONG. 1980. Sudden death, coronary heart disease, atherosclerosis, and myocardial lesions in young men. Am. J. Epidemiol. **112**(5):639–649.

10. FRIEDMAN, M., J. H. MANWARING, R. H. ROSENMAN, G. DONLON, P. ORTEGA & S. M. GRUBE. 1973. Instantaneous and sudden deaths: Clinical and pathological differentiation in coronary artery disease. J. Amer. Med. Assoc. **225:** 1319.

11. HAEREM, J. W. 1974. Mural platelet microthrombi and major acute lesions of main epicardial arteries in sudden coronary death. Atherosclerosis **19:**529.

12. JORGENSEN, L., J. W. HAEREM, A. B. CHANDLER & C. F. BORCHGREVINK. 1968. The pathology of acute coronary death. Acta. Anaesthesiol. Scand. Suppl. **29:**193.

13. DIXON, W. J. & F. J. MASSEY, JR. 1969. Introduction to Statistical Analysis. McGraw-Hill. New York, NY.

14. KULLER, L. 1966. Sudden and unexpected non-traumatic deaths in adults: A review of epidemiological and clinical studies. J. Chronic Dis. **19:**1165.

15. KULLER, L., A. LILIENFELD & R. S. FISHER. 1966. Epidemiological study of sudden and unexpected deaths due to arteriosclerotic heart disease. Circulation **34:**1056.

16. KANNEL, W. B., T. R. DAWBER & P. M. McNAMARA. 1966. Detection of the coronary-prone adult: The Framingham Study. J. Iowa Med. Soc. **56:**26.

17. SCHWARTZ, C. J. & R. G. GERRITY. 1975. Anatomical pathology of sudden unexpected cardiac death. Circulation **51**, **52**(Suppl. III):18.

18. ANDERSON, T. W., W. H. LE RICHE & J. S. MACKAY. 1969. Sudden death and ischemic heart disease: Correlation with hardness of water supply. N. Engl. J. Med. **280:**805.

19. ADELSON, L. & W. HOFFMAN. 1961. Sudden death from coronary disease: Related to lethal mechanism arising independently of vascular occlusion or myocardial damage. J. Amer. Med. Assoc. **176:**129.

20. RABSON, S. M. & M. HELPERN. 1948. Sudden and unexpected natural death. II. Coronary artery sclerosis. Am. Heart J. **35:**635.

21. SPAIN, D. M. & V. A. BRADESS. 1960. The relationship of coronary thrombosis to coronary atherosclerosis and ischemic heart disease (a necropsy study covering a period of 25 years). Am. J. Med. Sci. **240:**701.

22. Scott, R. F. & T. S. Briggs. 1972. Pathologic findings in pre-hospital deaths due to coronary atherosclerosis. Am. J. Cardiol. **29:**782.
23. Roberts, W. C. & A. A. Jones. 1979. Quantitation of coronary arterial narrowing at necropsy in sudden coronary death. Am. J. Cardiol. **44:**39.
24. Baroldi, G., G. Falzi & F. Mariani. 1979. Sudden coronary death. A postmortem study in 208 selected cases compared to 97 "control" subjects. Am. Heart J. **98:**20.
25. Maseri, A., A. L'Abbate, G. Baroldi, S. Chierchia, M. Marzilli, A. M. Ballestra, S. Severi, O. Parodi, A. Biagini, A. Distante & A. Pesola. 1978. Coronary vasospasm as a possible cause of myocardial infarction. A conclusion derived from the study of "preinfarction" angina. N. Engl. J. Med. **299:**1271.
26. Lie, J. T. & J. L. Titus. 1975. Pathology of the myocardium and the conduction system in sudden coronary death. Circulation **51, 52**(Suppl. III):41.

Discussion

Dr. El-Moraghi (*Toronto, Ontario*): Did you study the composition of the thrombus in these cases of sudden death in young people? Do you have any better data about the involvement of the microcirculation with thromboemboli that you alluded to? In a parallel study we did in Canada, the most impressive finding was that young people who die suddenly appear to have a thrombus, usually an occlusive thrombus that is composed predominantly of platelets and that is associated with extensive thromboembolism of the microcirculation. Did you confirm or otherwise support these findings in your study?

Dr. Newman: We have not done a microscopic study of the composition of thrombi. We have been able to identify in a small percentage of cases the presence of microembolization. However, we have not done extensive microscopic study of these particular thrombi.

PATHOLOGIC CHANGES IN THE CARDIAC CONDUCTION AND NERVOUS SYSTEM IN SUDDEN CORONARY DEATH

Lino Rossi *

*University of Milan
Milan, Italy*

The problem of sudden cardiac death, whether or not designated as coronary, has lately been epitomized by such dramatic expressions as "the major challenge to contemporary cardiology" [1] and "a statistician's nightmare" [2]; at postmortem examination, it is a Gordian knot to open, not to cut. Undoubtedly, ischemic heart disease and malignant arrhythmias are, respectively, the primary cause and the ultimate mechanism of most sudden cardiac deaths [3-5]; however, too-rigid anatomoclinical arguments, whetted by the current understanding of the pathogenetic sequence of "coronary arterial obstruction—catecholamine action —ventricular fibrillation" [6, 7] sometimes risk to sever, rather than unravel, the intricacies of the problem at issue. Only a few studies on sudden coronary death thus far have examined adequately the conduction and nervous system of the heart,[8-11] whose abnormalities are notoriously relevant to any discussion of the pathology of arrhythmias. Thus, today's basic information on this aspect of the subject is still poor.

To contribute to a more balanced assessment of arrhythmogenic substrates of sudden coronary death, the present morphologic research, preceded by a short pathophysiologic appraisal,[11] will focus upon the differential involvement of specialized and ordinary myocardium in severe acute ischemia and on intrinsic and extrinsic cardiac neuropathology. It is hoped that such evidence and discussions will prove useful to both the pathologist and the clinician confronted with actual or potential victims of sudden coronary catastrophe, in the autopsy room to explain death or on the spot to save life.

ARRHYTHMOGENIC MECHANISM FOR SUDDEN CORONARY DEATH

1. Severe acute myocardial ischemia, whether established or temporary (coronary arterial spasm), is liable to provoke electrical inhomogeneity, instability and desynchronization with impending risk of malignant arrhythmias; within a few minutes, reentry circuits may become functional and produce life-threatening tachyarrhythmias (namely, ventricular fibrillation). [12, 13, 14] In turn, in a matter of hours (up to 24), enhanced ectopic automaticity, within and around the damaged area, has been seen to become the major culprit in similar malignant arrhythmias.[12] Moreover, if the ischemic injury involves the conduction system, the patient undergoes the further risk of impairments in impulse formation and conduction, ranging from sinus arrest to heart block and asystole.[4, 15]

---

* Address correspondence to: L. Rossi, M.D., Via Annunciata 23/4, 20121 Milano, Italy.

0077-8923/82/0382-0050 $1.75/0 © 1982, NYAS

Consequently, malignant arrhythmias can suddenly kill during those 8-odd hours of "twilight" morphology [16] of ischemic injury. Lethal impairments of cardiac rhythm seem to depend more upon critical location than absolute extension and severity of damage from infarction. Therefore, signs of myofibrillar degeneration with contraction bands [17] and perhaps pronounced waviness of myocardial bundles [16] should be carefully looked for, particularly in the vicinity of the subendocardial layer of the ventricular septum and papillary muscles.[15, 17, 18] Later on, clearer microscopic changes from anoxia will allow more reliable study of arrhythmogenic pathology, besides the gross outlining and quantitation of the infarction itself.

2. Intrinsic neural abnormalities, either caused by or concomitant with acute ischemia, contribute to disorder and unbalance the autonomic input in the heart,[10] eventually triggering lethal arrhythmias. Emphasis has been laid on exaggerated catecholamine action that increases oxygen consumption by the myocardium (chrono- and inotropic stimulation) and reduces at the same time oxygen supply to the muscle by spasm and platelet aggregation in the small coronary arteries.[17, 19] Areas of absolute and relative anoxia result in electrical instability of the heart and often induce ventricular fibrillation, whose threshold is also lowered by sympathetic stimulation.[19] In turn, exaggerated cholinergic action,[20] mainly exerted on specialized cardiac tissue and enhanced by ischemia,[21] severely inhibits automaticity and conduction, eventually resulting in bradyarrhythmias and asystole.

In the domain of extrinsic cardiac innervation it has been demonstrated that left stellate ganglion discharge has a bearing on Q-T interval prolongation and/or ventricular ectopy and fibrillation in myocardial infarction.[22] Moreover, psychological stress from an acute coronary attack can trigger or take part in such neural mechanisms for lethal arrhythmias.[23]

3. Accessory atrioventricular communications are known to underlie life-threatening paroxysmal reciprocating arrhythmias, with or without evidence of preexcitation.[24] A few cases of postinfarction Wolff-Parkinson-White (WPW) syndrome have been tentatively explained by the hypothesis that concealed accessory arteriovenous pathways might have become functional during myocardial ischemia, with consequent imbalanced neural activity,[25] exposing the patient to the threat of reciprocating tachyarrhythmias.

Along these lines the present anatomoclinical investigation will focus upon the arrhythmogenic substrates for sudden coronary death.

MATERIALS AND METHODS

From 60 autopsy cases of coronary heart disease, 13 hearts were selected belonging to subjects who had died suddenly and unexpectedly within 24 hours (except case III) from the initial symptoms of myocardial infarction.

The two stellate ganglia included in the present study (by courtesy of Dr. P. J. Schwartz) had been surgically removed from patients with myocardial infarction to prevent life-threatening, recurrent bursts of ventricular fibrillation (cases XIV and XV [males, 52- and 40-years-old, respectively]). The mean age of the 15 subjects was 52 years (range 28–81 years); 12 were male and 3 female.

From each heart (after my usual technique [24]) two main blocks were removed—one for the study of the sinoatrial node and its approaches and ganglionated plexus, and the other for the study of the atrioventricular system, together with the ventricular septum (anterior papillary muscles included) and the intrinsic nerve networks. Sample sections of the free ventricular walls, atrioventricular groove, and main coronary arteries were also examined. The material was formalin-fixed, paraffin-embedded, and cut in series every 100 to 150 μ; the two left stellate ganglia were cut subserially. Sections were stained at varying intervals with hematoxylin-eosin (HE) or trichromic Heidenhein (Azan) and, occasionally, by silver impregnation (modified Bielschowsky). Clinicopathologic comparisons were made with available electrocardiographic documentation. TABLE 1 summarizes the main data concerning postmortem and clinical diagnosis, obstruction of major coronary arteries and of their conduction system ramifications, lesions of conduction system and abnormalities of nerve plexuses (with indication of the site). The findings in the stellate ganglia are referred to in the text.

The approximate mean incidence of significant pathologic changes is reported in TABLE 2.

RESULTS

The clinical diagnosis of acute myocardial infarction (TABLE 2), the most frequent diagnosis in the present series (69%), was histologically confirmed in the autopsied hearts and established beyond doubt in the two patients undergoing ganglionectomy; the infarction (in autopsied hearts) was anterior in 38%; posterior in 31%, and with septal involvement in 53%; in one case (II) it extended to the right atrium. In case VII the diagnosis was corroborated by the finding of pronounced waviness of myocardial bundles in the septum.

The exact nature of lethal arrhythmias is always difficult to ascertain; available final electrocardiograms and/or pertinent pathophysiologic considerations suggested A-V block-asystole in about one-third of the present cases, reentrant ventricular fibrillation in one-fourth, and either bradycardic or tachycardic arrhythmias, or both, in the others (mainly ventricular fibrillation). Coronary artery disease was atherosclerotic in nature and diffuse in location in 69% of the cases. Obstruction of the left coronary arterial tree was preeminent in 31% (always with acute occlusive thrombosis), of the right coronary arterial tree in 23% of cases, and of both coronary arterial trees in 46%. Severe obstruction of both coronary arteries was present also in a patient (case IV) without myocardial infarction. In the patient (case I) with arteriolar fibromuscular dysplasia[26] (FIG. 1) and in the two (cases XI and XII) with panarteritis nodosa (FIG. 2), the coronary arterial narrowing was segmentary and mainly affected the sinoatrial nodal area. Moderate to severe obstruction of conduction system arteries prevailed in the sinoatrial node (31%) (FIGS. 3 and 4) and in the atrioventricular node (23%) (FIGS. 5 and 6) of autopsied cases (TABLE 2).

Conduction system changes of different type and degree were observed in all hearts but one (95%), with an apparent relationship between the location and degree of coronary arterial obstruction. When marked and severe damage was taken as clinicopathologically significant, the sinoatrial node and its approaches were affected in 16% of cases and the common bundle and/or bundle branches in 30% of cases, whereas the atrioventricular node generally escaped major injury (TABLE 2).

Whether acute or chronic, the conduction system abnormalities were eminently ischemic in nature, especially considering that myofibrillar degeneration with contraction bands and so-called idiopathic fibrosis of conducting tissue can be ascribed, at least in part, to impaired blood supply [17, 24] (FIG. 7A). Extensive infarction necrosis of specialized tissue of the sinoatrial node was seen in case II (FIG. 3), and widespread ischemic degeneration and fibrosis were observed in cases IX and X. Patchy degeneration and necrosis, pronounced edema, and leukocytic infiltration were seen in the atrioventricular node (slightly in case X), the common bundle (case III), and the bundle branches (cases III, V, VI, VIII, and XIII); in the other cases only mild fibrosis was noticed.

In general, the impression was substantiated that the conduction system can withstand acute infarction injury much better than the adjacent working cardiac muscle,[18, 28] because of the lesser oxygen dependence of specialized tissue metabolism in comparison with that of the ordinary myocardium (FIG. 7B). Moreover, the location of the Purkinje-like fibers of the left bundle branch, close to the circulating blood in the left ventricle, further protects them against anoxia (transendocardial oxygenation) whenever coronary arterial supply is impaired.[17] Also, transitional and ordinary myocardial fibers in the subendocardium of the right ventricle (termination of the right bundle branch at the anterior papillary muscle) seemed to be less vulnerable to acute ischemia than the subjacent intramural fibers (FIG. 8).

Neural abnormalities, mainly affecting the sinoatrial nodal ganglionated plexus, the ventricular nerve network, and the atrioventricular groove's plexus were detected in 92% of the autopsied hearts (in a significant degree in 54% [TABLE 2]); the two left stellate ganglia exhibited pronounced alterations.

Cardiac neuropathologic changes were acute and chronic in nature, ranging from vacuolar swelling of nerve sheaths, epiperineural edema, inflammation (FIG. 9), hemorrhage or congestion (typical of infarction), with disruption of axons and/or neuronal degeneration (FIG. 10), to neural interstitial fibrosis (case XI), and proliferation of ganglionic capsular (satellite) cells (case III) (FIGS. 12, 13), accompanying neuronal loss (Terplan or Nageotte nodules) [29]; silver impregnation also demonstrates abnormal growth and disorder of neuronal processes.[24] The nature of these chronic changes is little known.

It is noteworthy that because of the difference between cardiac nerves and muscle with respect to metabolic requirements and sources, the nerves withstand early ischemic injury much better. So, damage to nerves from infarction is delayed with respect to that of the myocardium, and only seems to emerge when pronounced vessel engorgement and leukocytic infiltration inside and around the infarcted area take place. Sometimes a true infarct neuroganglionitis occurs, with multiple disruptions of the axons and/or severe neuronal damage (cases II, V, and VIII).

In the two patients with surgically ablated stellate ganglia, focal inflammation (case XIV) and chronic neuronal changes (case XV) were detected (FIG. 13).

DISCUSSION

The comparison between conduction system damage and related blocks agrees with current concepts: acute, severe ischemic lesions of the sinoatrial node resulted in suppression of pacemaker activity (case II), while patchy

TABLE 1

SUMMARY OF 13 AUTOPSIED CASES

Case No.	Age (yr) & Sex	Clinical & Postmortem Diagnosis	Main Coronary Arterial Obstruction	Conduction System Arterial Obstruction	Conduction System Changes	Neural Changes
I	29, M	Unexpected sudden death; slight cardiac hypertrophy	L±, R+	SAN++	SAN±	—
II	33, M	Buerger's disease; R atrial & posteroseptal AMI; SA arrest & AV junctional tachycardia	L+, R+++	SAN+++	SAN+++	SA plexus +++
III	55, M	Anteroseptal AMI; AVB, R on T ectopy; torsade de pointes	L++, R++	AVN+	Widespread ++	SA plexus +++ V plexus ++
IV	72, F	Aortic insufficiency; AF, R on T ectopy	L++, R++	SAN+ AVN++	SAN+	SA plexus +
V	71, F	Diabetes; anteroseptal AMI; RBBB & LAH; bradycardia	L+++, R+	SAN±	BB++	SA plexus ++
VI	63, M	Anteroseptal AMI; RBBB & LPH	L+++, R++	SAN+ AVN++	BB+	V plexus +

VII	53, M	Variant angina; initial postero-septal AMI; VF	L+, R++	—	—	V plexus +
VIII	55, M	Posterior AMI; 1st degree AVB, RBBB & LAH	L++, R++	AVN±	BB++	V plexus ++
IX	64, M	Anteroseptal AMI; RBBB & LAH	L+++, R++	—	BB+	V plexus ±
X	51, M	Anteroseptal AMI; complete AVB	L+++, R+	AVN++	AVN & BB+	V plexus ++
XI	28, M	Panarteritis nodosa; prolonged Q-T interval	L+, R+	SAN+++	SAN++	SA plexus ++
XII	39, M	Panarteritis nodosa; atrial arrhythmias	L+, R+	SAN+++	SAN++	SA plexus ±
XIII	81, F	Posteroseptal AMI; preexcitation; LBBB	L+, R+	AVN++	LBB++ Anomalous AV communication?	SA plexus + AV groove's plexus ++

NOTE: ± = minimal; + = moderate; ++ = marked; +++ = severe or total (whenever applied to coronary arterial obstruction + suggests <70%, ++ >70%, +++ occlusive thrombosis). A = atrial; AF = atrial fibrillation; AMI = acute myocardial infarction; AVB = atrioventricular block; AVN = atrioventricular node; BB = bundle branches; BBB = bundle branch block; L = left; LAH = left anterior hemiblock; LPH = left posterior hemiblock; R = right; SA = sinoatrial; SAN = sinoatrial node; V = ventricular; VF = ventricular fibrillation.

necrosis, with leukocytic infiltration and edema of the atrioventricular junctional tissue and/or bundle branches, accounted for heart block (cases III and IX), often preceded by electrocardiographic features of bilateral or homologous bundle branch block (cases V, VI, VIII, IX, and XIII). But such impairments in impulse formation and conduction and related life-threatening bradycardic heart action were apparently not the major culprit in sudden coronary death, which was more frequently due to tachycardic arrhythmias (ventricular fibrillation being the most frequent).

TABLE 2

APPROXIMATE MEAN INCIDENCE OF SIGNIFICANT PATHOLOGIC CHANGES
IN 13 AUTOPSIED HEARTS

Disorder		Percentage
Myocardial infarction		69%
Anterior	38%	
Septal	53%	
Posterior	31%	
Prevailing left coronary arterial obstruction		31%
Occlusive thrombosis	31%	
Prevailing right coronary arterial obstruction		23%
Occlusive thrombosis	8%	
Equivalent left and right coronary arterial obstruction		46%
Marked or severe conduction system arterial obstruction		54%
Sinoatrial nodal artery	31%	
Atrioventricular nodal artery	23%	
Marked or severe conduction system damage		46%
Sinoatrial node	16%	
Atrioventricular node	—	
Diffuse or peripheral	30%	
Marked or severe neural intrinsic abnormalities		54%
Sinoatrial plexus	23%	
Atrioventricular groove's plexus	8%	
Ventricular plexus	23%	

Accordingly, in the present group of cases, the incidence of right coronary arterial obstruction with posterior infarction (the common cause of acute ischemic heart block and asystole) [15] was lower than that of left coronary arterial occlusion with anterior infarction; however, the involvement of the septum in either left or right ischemic damage showed the highest incidence in relation to sudden coronary death. This is consistent with the fact that in the earliest stage of myocardial infarction the peripheral septoparaseptal radiations of the conduction system survive anoxia, while adjacent muscle undergoes severe damage, creating the substrate for lethal reentrant ventricular fibrillation. [12, 18]

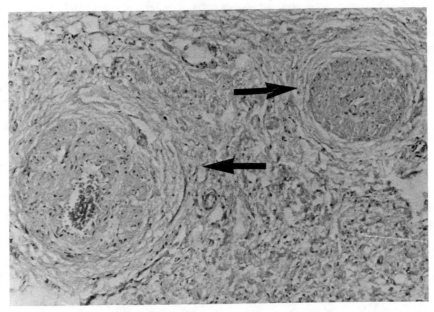

FIGURE 1. Case I. Fibromuscular dysplasia with subocclusion of the sinoatrial nodal arteriolae. (Hematoxylin and eosin stain; original magnification ×100.)

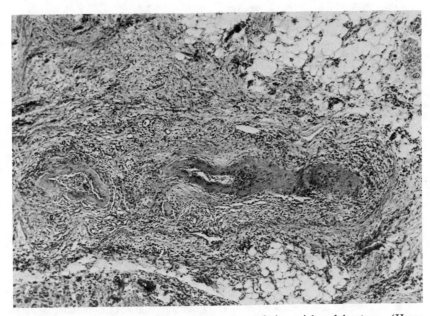

FIGURE 2. Case XI. Acute panarteritis nodosa of sinoatrial nodal artery. (Hematoxylin and eosin stain; original magnification ×60.)

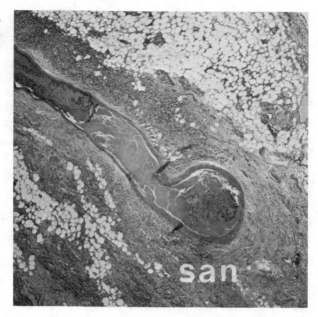

FIGURE 3. Case II. Occlusive thrombosis of sinoatrial nodal artery with acute infarction of sinoatrial node (san). (Hematoxylin and eosin stain; original magnification ×25.)

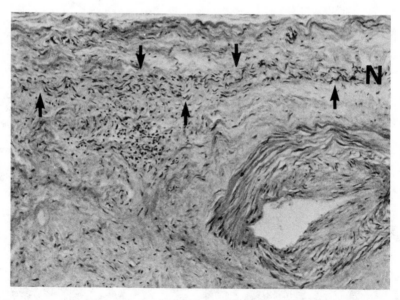

FIGURE 4. Case IV. Moderate stenosis of sinoatrial nodal artery and round cell infiltration close to a nerve (N) (arrows). (Hematoxylin and eosin stain; original magnification ×100.)

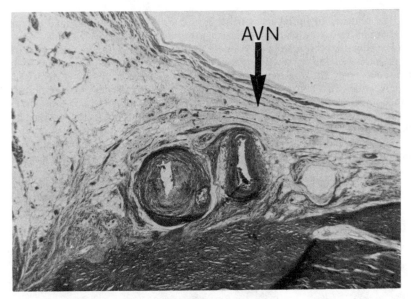

FIGURE 5. Case III. Marked and moderate stenosis of twin atrioventricular nodal arteriolae. (Azan stain; original magnification ×25.)

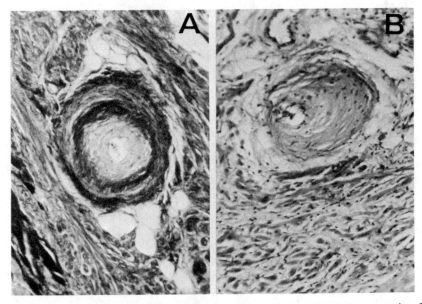

FIGURE 6. Case VI (A) and case XIII (B). Marked, subocclusive stenosis of atrioventricular nodal arteriolae. (Azan and hematoxylin and eosin stains; original magnification ×100; reduced by 15 percent.)

The features of initial myocardial infarction observed herein lend morphologic support to this pathophysiologic assumption: in cases IV, VI, and IX the Purkinje-like cells of the left bundle branch and the ultimate subendocardial ramifications of the conduction system were free of significant changes,[18] while the inner layer of working myocardium was already exhibiting myofibrillar degeneration with contraction bands (FIG. 8) as the earliest manifestation of severe anoxic injury. These two adjacent and interlaced fronts of, respectively, healthy, fast-conducting and damaged, slow-conducting myocytes together have the configuration of histopathologically ideal reentry circuits (FIG. 8).

The relevance of cardiac neuropathology to arrhythmogenic mechanisms for sudden coronary death derives from the pathophysiologic evidence presented

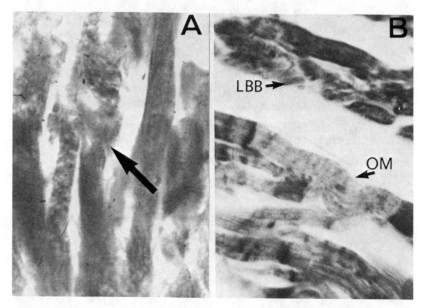

FIGURE 7. Case IX (A). Coagulative myocytolysis with contraction bands in some fibers of the right bundle branch. Case VI (B). Myofibrillar degeneration with contraction bands of septal ordinary myocardium (OM) side by side with the outer, well-preserved, filaments of the left bundle branch (LBB). (Azan stain; original magnification × 500; reduced by 15 percent.)

herein, but escapes any precise anatomoclinical assessment as yet. Correlative reasoning only permits suggestions as a premise and encourages further research.

In case II, sinoatrial nodal infarction severely damaged the local ganglionated plexus, which is mainly parasympathetic, thus provoking an imbalance of autonomic action on the heart in favor of orthosympathetic input: this, in turn, while preventing asystole from sinus arrest, by a prompt, even accelerated emergence of escape atrioventricular junctional beat,[30] could have facilitated simultaneously the triggering of lethal ventricular tachyarrhythmia.

The infarct involvement of the ventricular and/or the atrioventricular groove's plexus, somewhat retarded with respect to ischemic myocardial damage,

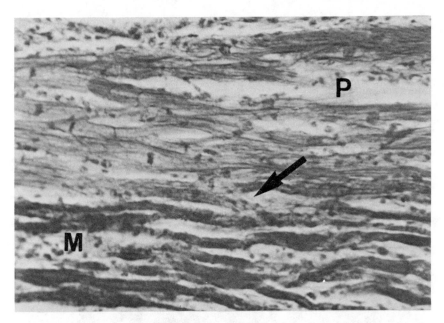

FIGURE 8. Case V. Anterior papillary muscle: the Purkinje-like (P) myocells beneath the endocardial surface (*top*) are well preserved and anastomose (*arrow*) with the deeper, infarcted myocardium. (Azan stain; original magnification ×250.)

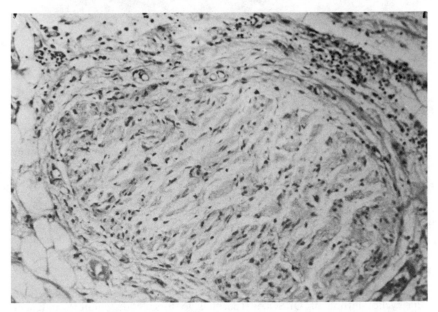

FIGURE 9. Case XIII. A nerve of the atriovascular groove's plexus exhibiting infarct epiperineuritis and edema. (Hematoxylin and eosin stain; original magnification ×250.)

perhaps has some bearing on the arrhythmias arising in a later phase that are ascribed to ectopic firing.[9] At this stage also, the previously preserved subendocardial fibers are likely to undergo anoxic damage, thereby suppressing the inhomogeneity in myocardial injury, which is initially responsible for reentry phenomena; it is during this phase that the intrinsic neural damage becomes more and more evident.

The chronic or subacute ganglionic changes, the cause of which is unclear, are yet likely to play a significant role in the autonomic neural imbalance that jeopardizes heart action as a consequence of myocardial infarction.

The high-risk prolongation of Q-T interval and/or the salvoes of ventricular ectopic beats could be attributed, at least in part, to those left stellate ganglion

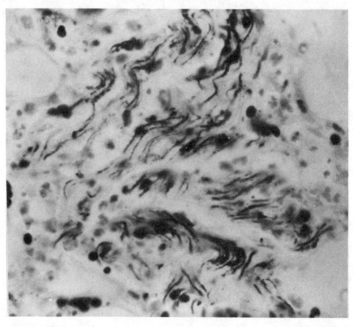

FIGURE 10. Case II. A nerve of the sinoatrial plexus undergoing severe infarct inflammation with multiple axonal disruptions. (Bielschowsky stain; original magnification ×500.)

abnormalities [22] that have been seen to accompany, if not to depend upon, acute myocardial ischemia. Anyway, it should be said that similar neurogenic rhythm disturbances can also be elicited apparently by lesions of lower autonomic cardiac ganglia (sinoatrial and atroventricular groove's plexuses) from either acute infarct or chronic origin, or both. This applies to case III, in which the patient was a victim of ventricular fibrillation, heralded by an ominous R on T phenomenon and torsade de pointes. The clinicopathologic correlation between the cyclic shifting of QRS axis (peculiar to torsade de pointes) and acute segmentary disruptions of the atrioventricular pathway (left bundle branch, particularly) [31] is now strengthened by the present evidence of severe neuropathologic changes in nerve plexuses, which confirms the importance of

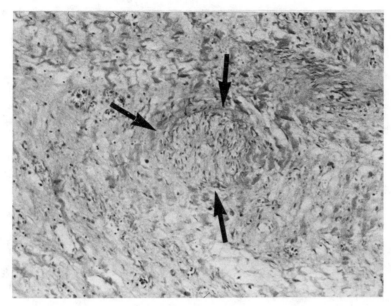

FIGURE 11. Case XI. Epiperineural fibrosis of a trunk, enmeshed in the sclerotic tissue replacing the sinoatrial node. (Hematoxylin and eosin stain; original magnification ×100.)

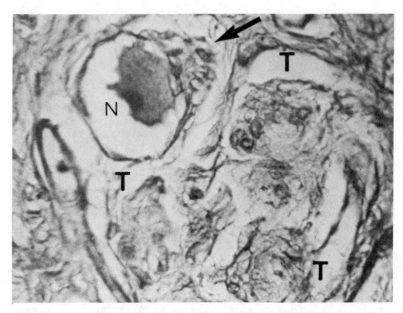

FIGURE 12. Case III. Sinoatrial plexus: eccentric proliferation of satellite cells (*arrow*) adhering to the neuronal body (N) or completely replacing three lost neurons (Terplan's nodules [T]). (Azan stain; original magnification ×500.)

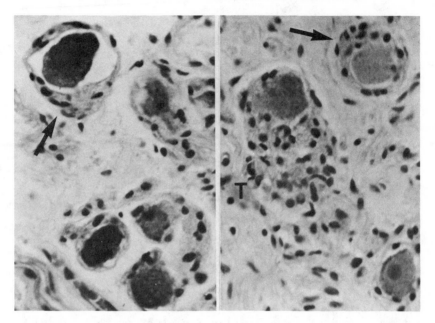

FIGURE 13. Case XV. Left stellate ganglion: proliferation of satellite cells (*arrows*) reducing the neuronal space and producing Terplan's nodules (T). (Hematoxylin and eosin stain; original magnification ×380; reduced by 15 percent.)

autonomic neural abnormalities in the etiology of this atypical ventricular tachycardia.[32]

The relevance of cardiac neuropathology to coronary arterial spasm is still debated; the finding (case VII) of juxtacoronary neuritis (FIG. 14), identical to that described by James *et al.* in eight hearts from patients with long Q-T syndrome who died from malignant tachyarrhythmias,[33] can thus be better correlated with the fatal ventricular fibrillation than regarded as a substrate for variant angina. But this unique association of coronary arterial spasm with intrinsic neural abnormalities seems, at least, to be worth attention.

It is also useful to take into consideration the possibility that stenotic nutritional arterioles of the conduction system with a well-preserved muscular layer and free from calcium deposition (cases I and IV), may suddenly undergo occlusive spasm, lethally impairing impulse formation or conduction, even without detectable lesions at postmortem examination of the specialized tissue. Autonomic neural imbalance may also be operative in sudden arrhythmic deaths of this kind, as suggested by case I, in which the patient died while having a meal. Swallowing is known to elicit intense vagal reflex activity (in the pharynx and esophagus) that can abnormally discharge on the heart [34] and suddenly impair pacemaking, particularly in such an ischemic sinoatrial node. Likewise, taking a prolonged Q-T interval as a hallmark of enhanced sympathetic action on the heart,[22, 33] one can reasonably surmise that this, combined with severe ischemic damage of the sinoatrial node (case XI) from panarteritis nodosa,[35] could have heralded a sudden-death-causing tachyarrhythmia.

A final remark pertains concerning the risk of sudden coronary death in relation to preexcitation and complicating tachyarrhythmias induced by myocardial infarction. In case XIII, the presence of multiple gaps in the atrioventricular anulus and of a defective central fibrous body can suggest the probable, if not proved, existence of accessory atrioventricular communications.[36] The neuropathologic involvement of the plexus of the atrioventricular sulcus in acute infarction may thus lend morphologic credibility to the hypothesized neural mechanism for activation by infarct of concealed atrioventricular anomalous pathways [25] with fatal arrhythmic outcome.

CONCLUDING REMARKS

The importance of histologic research on the conduction and nervous system of the heart for basic understanding of sudden coronary death is made clear by the data and arguments presented herein and should be given proper consideration.

Acute cardiac ischemia implies the risk of lethal bradycardic heart action from injury to the conduction system, but in turn the survival of the peripheral "radiations" of such injury may become critical to reentrant, killing tachycardic arrhythmias. This altogether endorses and extends the statement of Eliot and Edwards [5] that in myocardial infarction death often results from complications due to viable, rather than to necrotic muscle.

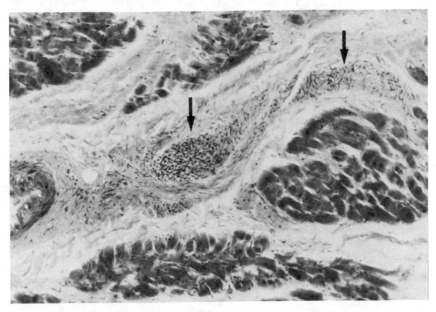

FIGURE 14. Case VII. Neuritis of trunk of ventricular septum (*arrows*) close to a perforating coronary artery (*left*). (Hematoxylin and eosin stain; original magnification ×100.)

Intrinsic and/or extrinsic cardiac neuropathologic changes, due either to ischemic heart disease or to poorly understood concomitant causes, significantly participate in the imbalance and asymmetry of autonomic control of the heart beat [8, 11, 24] and interact with the other and better known arrhythmogenic mechanisms for sudden coronary death.

SUMMARY

The arrhythmogenic substrates for sudden coronary death were studied in 13 autopsied hearts and in 2 left stellate ganglia (surgically excised). Diffuse or segmentary obstruction of nutritional arteries accounted for acute ischemic injury of the conduction system, which was the underlying cause of high-risk bradycardic arrhythmias in one-third of the cases. However, in one-quarter of the cases the survival of anoxia-resistant subendocardial specialized fibers was probably responsible for reentrant lethal tachycardic arrhythmias. In other cases, early infarct damage could have induced fatal arrhythmias of either type. Intrinsic and/or extrinsic neuropathologic changes, unbalancing the autonomic action on the heart, were often seen to participate in the arrhythmogenic features of sudden coronary death.

REFERENCES

1. LOWN, B. 1979. Sudden cardiac death: The major challenge confronting contemporary cardiology. Am. J. Cardiol. **43:** 313–328.
2. LOVEGRAVE, T. & P. THOMPSON. 1978. The role of acute myocardial infarction in sudden cardiac death—a statistician's nightmare. Am. Heart J. **96:** 711–713.
3. DAVIES, M. J. & A. POPPLE. 1979. Sudden unexpected cardiac death—a practical approach to the forensic problem. Histopathology **3:** 255–277.
4. MYEBURG, R. J., C. A. CONDE, R. J. SUNG, A. MAYORGA-CORTES, S. M. MALLON, D. S. SHEPS, R. A. APPEL & A. CASTELLANOS. 1980. Clinical, electrophysiologic and hemodynamic profile of patients resuscitated from prehospital cardiac arrest. Am. J. Med. **68:** 568–576.
5. ELIOT, R. S. & J. E. EDWARDS. 1978. Pathology of coronary atherosclerosis and its complications: Acute myocardial infarction. *In* The Heart. J. W. Hurst, Ed.: 1121–1134. McGraw-Hill. New York, NY.
6. BAROLDI, G. 1978. Coronary stenosis: Ischemic or non-ischemic factor? Am. Heart J. **96:** 139–143.
7. REICHENBACH, D. D. & N. S. MOSS. 1975. Myocardial cell necrosis and sudden death in humans. Circulation **52** (Suppl. III:III):60–62.
8. JAMES, T. N. 1973–1978. De Subitaneis mortibus (30 articles from Circulation [Vols. 48–57] privately bound by T. N. James, University of Alabama, Birmingham, Alabama).
9. LIE, J. T. & J. L. TITUS. 1975. Pathology of the myocardium and conduction system in sudden coronary death. Circulation (Suppl. III:III): 41–52.
10. JAMES, T. N. 1978. Neural pathology of the heart in sudden death. *In* Sudden Death. H. E. Kulbertus & H. J. J. Wellens, Eds.: 49–65. Martinus Nijhoff. The Hague.
11. ROSSI, L. 1980. Personal observations on the conduction system and nerves of the heart in patients dying with arrhythmias. Circulation **62** (Part II, Abstr. III): 4–5.
12. WIT, A. L. & J. T. BIGGER JR. 1975. Possible electrophysiological mechanisms for lethal arrhythmias accompanying myocardial ischemia and infarction. Circulation **52** (Suppl. III:III): 96–115.

13. DAVIS, J. H. & R. K. WRIGHT. 1980. The very sudden cardiac death syndrome. A conceptual model for pathologists. Hum. Pathol. **11**: 117–121.
14. VISMARA, L. A., V. ZAKUDDIN, J. M. FOERSTER, E. A. AMSTERDAM & D. T. MASON. 1977. Identification of sudden death risk factors in acute and chronic coronary artery disease. Am. J. Cardiol. **39**: 821–828.
15. TANS, A. C., K. I. LIE & D. DURRER. 1980. Clinical setting and prognostic significance of high degree atrioventricular block in acute inferior myocardial infarction: A study of 144 patients. Am. Heart J. **99**: 4–8.
16. BOUCHARDY, B. & G. MAJNO. 1974. Histopathology of early myocardial infarcts. Am. J. Pathol. **74**: 301–330.
17. ROSSI, L. 1980. Occurrence and significance of coagulative myocytolysis in the specialized conduction system: Clinicopathologic observations. Am. J. Cardiol. **45**: 757–761.
18. FENOGLIO, J. J., A. ALBALA, A. SILVA, P. L. FRIEDMAN & A. L. WIT. 1976. Structural basis of ventricular arrhythmias in human myocardial infarction: A hypothesis. Hum. Pathol. **7**: 547–563.
19. ABILDSKOV, J. A. 1975. The nervous system and cardiac arrhythmias. Circulation **52** (Suppl. III–III): 116–119.
20. ROTMAN, M., G. S. WAGNER & A. G. WALLACE. 1972. Bradyarrhythmias in acute myocardial infarction. Circulation **45**: 703–722.
21. BELLET, S. 1971. Clinical Disorders of the Heart Beat.: 583. Lea & Febiger. Philadelphia, PA.
22. SCHWARTZ, P. J. & L. STONE. 1980. Left stellectomy in the prevention of ventricular fibrillation caused by acute myocardial ischemia in conscious dogs with anterior myocardial infarction. Circulation **62**: 1256–1265.
23. LOWN, B., R. L. VERRIER & S. H. RABINOWITZ. 1977. Neural and psychologic mechanisms and the problem of sudden cardiac death. Am. J. Cardiol. **39**: 890–902.
24. ROSSI, L. 1979. Histopathology of Cardiac Arrhythmias. Lea & Febiger. Philadelphia, PA.
25. GOEL, B. & J. HAN. 1974. Manifestation of the Wolff-Parkinson-White syndrome after myocardial infarction. Am. Heart J. **87**: 633–636.
26. JAMES, T. N. & T. K. MARSHALL. 1976. De Subitaneis mortibus. XVII. Multifocal stenosis due to fibromuscular dysplasia of the sinus node artery. Circulation **53**: 736–742.
27. SCHERLAG, B. J., G. KOBELL, L. HARRISON, R. R. HOPE & R. LAZZARA. 1980. Mechanism of bradycardia-dependant arrhythmias in acute myocardial ischemia (abstr.). Am. J. Cardiol. **45**: 494.
28. ROSSI, L. 1963. Problems in histology and pathology of the intrinsic nerves of the heart. Am. Heart J. **66**: 838–839.
29. BENNINGTON, J. M. 1978. Pathology of Peripheral Nerve.: 246. W. B. Saunders. Philadelphia, PA.
30. KULBERTUS, H. E. & J. C. DEMOULIN. 1975. The conduction system: Anatomical and pathological aspects. *In* Cardiac Arrhythmias, the Modern Electrophysiological Approach. D. M. Krikler & J. F. Goodwin, Eds.: 16–38. Saunders. London.
31. ROSSI, L. & L. MATTURRI. 1976. Histopathological findings in two cases of torsade de pointes with conduction disturbances. Br. Heart J. **12**: 1312–1318.
32. COUMEL, P., J. FIDELLE, V. LUCET, P. ATTUEL & Y. BOUVRAIN. 1978. Catecholamine-induced severe arrhythmias with Adams-Stokes syndrome in children: Report of four cases. Br. Heart J. **40** (Suppl.): 28–37.
33. JAMES, T. N., P. FROGGAT, W. J. ATKINSONS, P. R. LURIA, D. G. MCNAMARA, W. W. MILLER, G. T. SCHLOSS, J. S. CARROLL & L. R. NORTH. 1978. De Subitaneis mortibus. XXX. Observations on the pathophysiology of the long Q-T syndrome with special reference to neuropathology of the heart. Circulation **57**: 1221–1232.
34. ARMOUR, J. A., R. D. WURSTER & W. C. RANDALL. 1977. Cardiac reflexes. *In*

Neural regulation of the heart. W. C. Randall, Ed.: 159–186. Oxford University Press. New York, NY.
35. THIENE, G., M. L. VALENTE & L. ROSSI. 1978. Involvement of the cardiac conducting system in panarteritis nodosa. Am. Heart J. **95:** 716–724.
36. VERDUYN LUNEL, A. A. 1972. Significance of annulus fibrosus of heart in relation to AV conduction and ventricular activation in cases of Wolff-Parkinson-White syndrome. Br. Heart J. **34:**1263–1271.

DISCUSSION

SIDNEY SCHERLIS (*Baltimore, Maryland*): Is it your thesis that the abnormal rhythm is a result of stimulation of nerves that have been affected by ischemia rather than the result of normal stimulation imposed upon an ischemic myocardium?

DR. ROSSI: This is a very complicated question to answer by pathology alone. I can only point out what the lesions are and where they are and just hypothesize, very feebly, what the function and dysfunction can be. It is up to the pathophysiologist to answer your question.

COLLATERAL ANATOMY AND BLOOD FLOW: ITS POTENTIAL ROLE IN SUDDEN CORONARY DEATH

Wolfgang Schaper

Max-Planck Institute for Heart Research
Bad Nauheim, Federal Republic of Germany

Exactly 100 years ago—in 1881—Cohnheim occluded the circumflex branch of the left coronary artery in anesthetized dogs. Because all animals died of ventricular fibrillation, the investigators concluded that the coronary arteries in mammals are true anatomic end-arteries. Although Cohnheim's conclusions were premature, a basis was laid for future research in the fields of sudden coronary death and collateral circulation. The interrelationship between fatal arrhythmias and collateral blood flow are to this day not particularly well known. It seems intuitively clear that collateral flow after sudden coronary occlusion must have some protective effect, but the opposite may also be true. If we assume that there is no collateral flow whatsoever, then we see that the afflicted myocardium would soon be rendered completely unexcitable and the danger of fatal arrhythmias would be minimal. Our own experiments in sheep, a species completely devoid of anastomoses, support this hypothesis.[1]

The pig is another interesting animal model of sudden coronary death, for it teaches us that the very little collateral blood flow that exists after coronary occlusion might in fact be dangerous because it facilitates the production of fatal arrhythmias. The area at risk is not immediately and completely electrically silent and it allows the dangerous conduction delays that lead to reentrant phenomena leading to ventricular fibrillation. But the most interesting species of experimental animal is the dog, because its collateral circulation, while sufficiently well developed to allow accurate measurement, is not too large to prevent infarction and arrhythmias. Furthermore, the conditions for the generation of arrhythmias and the production of infarcts can be manipulated to a surprisingly large extent by variation of the collateral blood flow and by variation of the myocardial oxygen demand.

We measured collateral blood flow with the tracer microsphere method [2, 3] after acute and chronic coronary occlusion. Great care was taken to ensure the presence of a sufficient amount of tracer microspheres in low-flow tissue samples. By dissecting rings of left ventricular myocardium into adjacent wedges in a continuous way, we were able to construct detailed maps of left ventricular blood flow distribution (FIGS 1 and 2).

EFFECTS OF ACUTE CORONARY ARTERIAL OCCLUSION

Acute and permanent coronary occlusion was produced in anesthetized large mongrel dogs in whom the left anterior descending coronary artery was occluded with a modified Judkins catheter that carried an occluding plug that could be released from the catheter after entrance into the coronary ostium. Proximal occlusion of the left anterior descending artery at a normal myocardial oxygen consumption of 7–8 ml O_2/min per 100 g produced the three well-known

69

0077–8923/82/0382–0069 $01.75/0 © 1982, NYAS

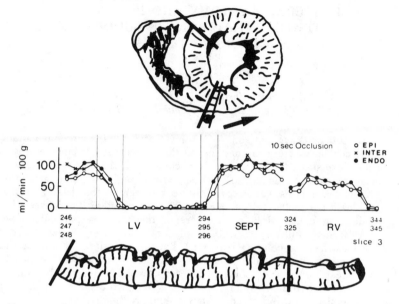

FIGURE 1. Construction of a blood flow map from the density distribution of tracer microspheres. A "bread loaf" heart slice is shown at *top*. "Unrolling" of the slice (*bottom*) and sectioning into adjacent wedges of myocardium is the basis for the abscissa-addresses (consecutive numbers). Density of microspheres in each tissue sample is plotted on the ordinate after translation into blood flow per unit tissue weight.

peaks of the frequency distribution of premature ventricular beats: the first between 3 and 6 minutes after occlusion, the second after about 30 minutes of occlusion, and the third starting 8 hours and reaching its maximum 16 hours after occlusion. The phases of arrhythmias, especially the first and third, were described by Harris in the 1950s. It is of note that the Harris type I arrhythmias, that is, the early ones, often lead to ventricular fibrillation. The late arrhythmias are almost never fatal, although they are also ventricular premature beats and much more numerous.

The just-described sequence of events is drastically altered when the occlusion is produced more distally, that is, when less myocardium is included in the risk region. The potentially dangerous Harris type I phase of arrhythmias almost disappears, the incidence of premature ventricular beats decreases, ventricular fibrillation becomes very rare, and only the Harris type II phase develops.

If we measure the collateral blood flow as a function of the area at risk, we find significant differences: the smaller the region of risk, the larger the collateral blood flow. By inference we arrive at the conclusion that the smaller-risk regions, which enjoy relatively better perfusion, develop fewer arrhythmias. The reasons for the relatively better perfusion of smaller-risk regions are probably purely geometric (FIG. 3).

On the other hand, even proximal occlusions involving large ischemic regions may not produce fatal arrhythmias when the myocardial oxygen consumption at the moment of coronary occlusion is very low. This is particularly true when a low myocardial oxygen consumption was produced by low heart rates. We create very low heart rates of around 40/min by giving high subcutaneous doses of synthetic morphine-like agents. Under these conditions blood flow to non-occluded myocardium is around 40 ml/min per 100 g and the blood flow deficit to subepicardial muscle is less than 50%. We believe that the magnitude

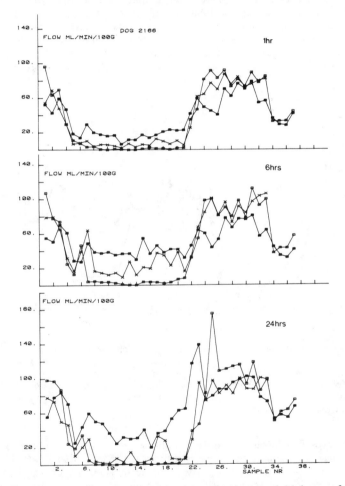

FIGURE 2. Blood flow map of the heart of a dog, 1, 6, and 24 hours after acute occlusion of the left anterior descending coronary artery. A significant blood flow deficit exists between tissue samples 5 to 21 that is particularly severe for the sub-endocardium (*open rectangles*) and less severe for the subepicardium (*closed rectangles*). At 6 hours after occlusion, subepicardial flow and that of the intermediate layer (*crosses*) has risen. At this stage most of the myocardium at risk could have been resuscitated by reperfusion. At 24 hours the entire subendocardium and the intermediate layer had become necrotic and intermediate layer blood flow had decreased again as a consequence of definite infarction. Only a subepicardial rim had survived, especially those samples where blood flow approached 60 ml/min per 100 g.

of the blood flow difference, that is, the deficit, between ischemic and well-perfused myocardium is the reason for the reduced incidence of dangerous arrhythmias as well as for the delayed transition from principally reversible ischemia to irreversible infarction. At first sight this does not appear very logical: the ischemic region receives an inadequate amount of blood flow and regardless of the situation in the normal myocardium this amount remains too low. If the rate of ischemic metabolism is influenced by the metabolic rate of the normal muscle, we must postulate an information transfer between normoxic and ischemic myocardium. The only way information can be passed is by way of the excitation process. Since ischemic tissue remains excitable for a while, the influence of heart rate on ischemic metabolism becomes understandable: at very low heart rates, ischemic tissue is relatively slow in breaking down

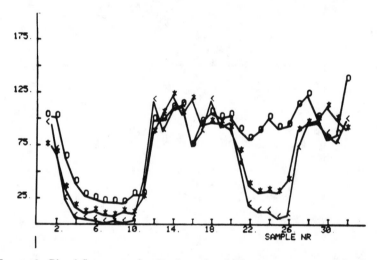

FIGURE 3. Blood flow map of a dog heart in which two coronary arteries (the left anterior descending and a smaller sidebranch) of the left circumflex were simultaneously occluded. Note that the larger risk region shows a greater blood flow deficit for all layers (subepicardial [*open circles*], intermediate [*crosses*], and subendocardial [*triangles*]) in comparison with the smaller region where there is no flow deficit for the subepicardium.

nucleotides and in accumulating metabolic waste; it survives longer and does not produce dangerous arrhythmias. In the extreme case, that is, at a heart rate of zero, the little available oxygen will suffice to keep the myocardium structurally alive. The best way to treat ischemic myocardium and to prevent dangerous arrhythmias would be to completely stop the information transfer, that is, to render ischemic myocardium unexcitable but still perfused at a lower than normal rate. Unfortunately, an agent for such purpose is, to my knowledge, not available.

Summarizing our experience with acute coronary occlusion, we can say that the early dangerous arrhythmias are produced by viable ischemic myocardial cells and when the ischemic myocardium is excitable. Excitation is a means to convey information from normal to ischemic myocardium. Total absence of collateral blood flow as in the sheep heart does not produce fatal arrhythmias, but maximal infarctions. The presence of collateral blood flow becomes dangerous with regard to fatal arrhythmias when the difference between ischemic and normal blood flow is great. This situation is normally present in the pig heart. The flow deficit is amenable to manipulation in the dog heart because collateral blood flow is somewhat higher, but usually almost always inadequate. By reduction of myocardial oxygen consumption, especially by reducing the heart rate, the flow deficit can be reduced, which has a salutary effect on ischemic metabolism and hence the generation of arrhythmias. If the speed of deterioration of ischemic metabolism can be retarded, fatal arrhythmias can be avoided, although the final infarct size remains unaltered.

CREATION OF A FLOW DEFICIT WITH PROGRESSIVE CORONARY ARTERIAL STENOSES

When a slowly swelling material like an ameroid constrictor is implanted around the left circumflex coronary artery, a progressive stenosis develops, which passes through different phases of constriction and goes on to total occlusion. The whole process from implantation to complete occlusion takes about 2½ weeks. Although the process of coronary occlusion occurs relatively slowly, about 30% of the animals die suddenly and unexpectedly of ventricular fibrillation around the fourteenth day after operation. The postmortem examination always reveals the same finding: a complete occlusion or a very tight stenosis and an insufficiently developed collateral circulation. In these cases the transition from a noncritical to a critical stenosis was too fast, a flow deficit developed, and ventricular fibrillation occurred.

We should explain here what we mean by development of a collateral circulation. Most mammals, including man, have preexistent interarterial connections between the coronary arteries that range between 10 and 500 μ in internal diameter.[1, 4] In the dog the statistical average[1] is around 40 μ and in normal human hearts it is between 100 and 200 μ. With the onset of episodes of ischemia, like those in angina pectoris or in experimental situations similar to angina pectoris, these vessels enlarge by virtue of active mitotic growth of all cellular constituents of the collateral vascular wall.[1, 5] The diameter of these collateral vessels in dogs increases up to a factor of 20 and the tissue mass by a factor of about 50 and sometimes more. It takes time for this growth process: about 24 hours are needed from the first transient episode of ischemia to the completion of the first cycle of cell divisions. It takes about 5 to 7 days for these vessels to reach final dimensions at a veinlike (that is, thin) vascular wall and it takes another 3 to 4 weeks until all typical morphologic dimensions and features of epicardial arteries have emerged from this growth transformation.

It is interesting that these greatly enlarged collateral vessels are able to completely prevent infarction in about 50% of all animals with chronic coronary occlusion.[6] In these animals the growth transformation stops when the myocardium at risk is adequately protected, that is, it receives enough blood to allow for the daily requirements of a normal sedentary dog. Heavy physical exercise, such as running on a treadmill at 8 miles per hour and at an inclination of 25%, produces again a flow deficit. The greatly enlarged collaterals act like a moderately severe stenosis and produce subendocardial ischemia.[7] Although the flow deficit can be quite large, depending on the severity of the exercise, it does not produce dangerous arrhythmias. Thus far we have exercised 50 dogs with chronic stable coronary occlusions at very severe loads and we have never seen ventricular fibrillation after the stable period of adaptation after chronic occlusion was reached. This high-flow ischemia is apparently much less dangerous than the low-flow ischemia of acute occlusion or when there are very tight stenoses. Exercise was started after closure of the coronary artery and continued for 4 months.

References

1. SCHAPER, W. 1971. The Collateral Circulation of the Heart. North-Holland Publishing Co. Amsterdam–New York.
2. SCHAPER, W., P. LEWI, W. FLAMENG & L. GYPEN. 1973. Myocardial steal produced by coronary vasodilation in chronic coronary artery occlusion. Basic Res. Cardiol. **68:** 3–20.
3. WINKLER, B. 1979. The tracer microsphere method. In: Schaper, W., Ed. The Pathophysiology of Myocardial Perfusion. Elsevier/North-Holland Biomedical Press. Amsterdam–New York–Oxford.
4. FULTON, W. F. M. 1965. The Coronary Arteries. Charles C Thomas. Springfield, IL.
5. SCHAPER, W., M. DEBRABANDER & P. LEWI. 1971. DNA-synthesis and mitoses in coronary collateral vessels of the dog. Circ. Res. **28:** 671–679.
6. FLAMENG, W., W. SCHAPER & P. LEWI. 1973. Multiple experimental coronary occlusion without infarction. Am. Heart J. **85:** 767–776.
7. SCHAPER, W., W. FLAMENG & B. WINKLER. 1976. Quantification of collateral resistance in acute and chronic experimental coronary occlusion in the dog. Circ. Res. **39:** 371–377.

Discussion

DR. RIBEIRO: First, I would like to congratulate Dr. Schaper for the nice data presented, and, second, ask this question: Since the arrythmias after coronary arterial occlusion are mainly due to reentry, is it possible that just decreasing the heart rate by itself decreases the chance of having reentry? Have you done the opposite? Did you increase the oxygen demand and increase the incidence of arrhythmias?

DR. SCHAPER: The last question is the easier to answer: Yes, we have increased oxygen demand, which greatly increased the incidence of fatal arrhythmias, especially when the increase in myocardial oxygen demand was stimulated by catecholamines.

It is very difficult to answer your first question because when the heart rate is reduced to a very low rate, say about 40 beats per minute, even a proximal occlusion of the left anterior descending artery will not produce a single premature ventricular beat, so it is difficult to speculate on reentry mechanisms.

DR. KIRK (*Albert Einstein Medical Center, Bronx, New York*): We collect similar data and I was pleased to see that you feel that the presence of collateral blood flow may be a double-edged sword. If it is not adequate, it could be worse than if it were altogether absent. That was certainly borne out in a recent experiment we performed. In an acute occlusion in the dog, we measured the ventricular fibrillation threshold and found that it actually increased as one bled "retrograde" the artery that had been occluded and drained the blood from the ischemic area, producing a much more severe ischemia.

The hearts of two animals were completely electrically unstable after simple occlusion and could only be maintained by retrograde bleeding. I think that there is a bi-modal distribution in which some collateral blood flow may be more dangerous than none whatsoever, while a lot of collateral flow is very good.

DR. SCHAPER: That completely confirms our view.

DR. ZIPES: I'd like to introduce a note of caution: The terms *reentry* and *automaticity* are being used with a great deal of finality; yet we don't really know that these early arrhythmias are reentrant, although much of the data supports that notion. It is quite clear that there is a triggered automaticity that can produce continuous diastolic activity that can simulate reentry. We cannot forget that these are presumptive diagnoses and that we do not have unequivocal electrophysiologic proof of reentry in these early or late arrhythmias.

DR. SCHAPER: I completely agree with you. It has become common to consider the early arrhythmias that end in ventricular fibrillation to be reentrant arrhythmias. In the models that I studied, early arrhythmias were dangerous, but the late arrhythmias—those occurring after about 8 to 16 hours—were not. Although the arrhythmias look quite similar, their mechanisms must be different.

DR. P. J. SCHWARTZ: Do you have any data or any thoughts on the influence of sympathetic activation on the function of these collateral vessels?

DR. SCHAPER: That is a very difficult question to answer. In acute occlusion these vessels, at least in my laboratory, do not respond to vasoactive substances; they do not constrict or dilate. These collateral vessels do not dilate, probably because they are already maximally dilated because of the stimulus of ischemia, and they may not be able to constrict because the dilatory stimulus of ischemia is just too intense.

The situation may be different in greatly enlarged collateral vessels. The enlarged collaterals can respond to vasoactive substances, notably to ergot by constriction and to nitrates by dilatation.

DR. MARCUS (*University of Arizona, Tucson, Arizona*): I would like to ask whether one can stimulate the collateral circulation, when one cannot see it, by the techniques that you mentioned. For example, can one stimulate collateral circulation in the sheep by gradual occlusion?

DR. SCHAPER: No, it is impossible; we have tried many times to do this, using various speeds of coronary occlusion ranging from 3 weeks to 3 months. The sheep heart that we investigated always developed large aneurysms that consisted only of fibrous tissue and no muscle. They are maximal infarctions.

DR. HERLING: Perhaps this question is better directed at Dr. Newman, but in the postmortem studies of collateral vessels, are the survivors of sudden death found to have normal amounts of collateral vessels or no collaterals or large collateral flow in the distribution of stenotic coronary arteries?

DR. SCHAPER: That is a really important, but very difficult question. In people dying suddenly, you can describe the anatomic system of vessels in the heart with great accuracy, but it does not mean that you know the blood flow going through these vessels. This is an inherent and principal difficulty that has not been solved.

INTRODUCTION

John A. Kastor

Cardiovascular Section
Department of Medicine
Hospital of the University of Pennsylvania
Philadelphia, Pennsylvania 19104

The word SUDDEN, which has roots in middle English via old French and Latin (*subitaneus*), means extreme quickness and unexpectedness. The dictionary, however, does not tell us *how* quickly the word *sudden* implies when it is used in that phrase so familiar to us at this conference—sudden death. Does it occur within seconds, minutes, or hours—and if hours, how many? The distinction is crucial if the phrase is to have a useful meaning. Despite the many definitions of the time course of sudden death, most of us think of an event that occurs dramatically and so rapidly that action must be taken at once to prevent nature taking its probable course. The treatment of sudden death is not a leisurely affair with time for deep reflection and evaluation of arcane laboratory data.

What produces such a rapid loss of useful human function? An occasional massive subarachnoid hemorrhage can kill in minutes, possibly seconds, but in nearly all other cases the culprit is the heart. If you will accept sudden death as an event measured in minutes rather than hours, then the *coup de grâce* is usually an electrical event, albeit one often occurring in a heart with severe myocardial disease. Except in the occasional patient with an isolated electrical malfunction (such as the long Q-T interval syndrome or preexcitation and atrial fibrillation with very rapid atrioventricular conduction), the electrical disorder which kills is part of a severe nonelectrical cardiac disease, usually coronary in this country.

In approaching the vital and most interesting topic of pathophysiology, we can look first of all at the natural history of the disease. Taking this approach and thinking back toward the beginning, we want to know what causes atherosclerosis or how the patient's myocardial infarction could have been prevented or limited. More proximal to the event, we might ask how the electrical event could have been prevented or rendered less ominous and more amenable to successful prevention. This last question brings us to the topic of this portion of the conference: what are the electrophysiologic causes of sudden death?

Fortunately, there are several animal models in which we can study this problem. Dr. Joseph F. Spear and his colleagues from the University of Pennsylvania School of Veterinary Medicine have been investigating this topic for many years. Their paper discusses the different arrhythmias that can develop during the three phases that occur in dogs who have had coronary occlusion. As we would expect, there are differences in addition to similarities between dog and man under these circumstances, and the authors will make these clear to us.

The second paper, by Doctor Robert J. Myerburg and his colleagues from

0077–8923/82/0382–0076 $01.75/0 © 1982, NYAS

the University of Miami, brings us further data about an important animal model of myocardial infarction—the cat. These studies show how micro-electrode techniques can be applied in the cat to study the electrophysiology of infarction and the effects of drugs on the damaged tissue.

Doctor Leonard N. Horowitz and his colleagues in the Clinical Electrophysiology Laboratory at the Hospital of the University of Pennsylvania will review their observations in 59 patients who were resuscitated from cardiac arrest occurring outside the hospital. In many cases, serious ventricular arrhythmias could be induced with ventricular stimulation, but that was not possible in one-third of the cases. The value of electrophysiologic studies will be described for us in such patients.

Although much importance is placed upon the role of ventricular tachycardia and fibrillation in the genesis of sudden death, bradyarrhythmias can also cause loss of adequate cardiac function. Intraventricular conduction disturbances warn the physician that atrioventricular block may follow. This topic is addressed in the paper by Doctors Wellens, Brugada, and Bär from the University of Limburg in Maastricht, the Netherlands.

"I'm scared to death." How often we have wondered whether that phrase has scientific accuracy in addition to its literary merit. Doctor DeSilva has some very provocative data, convincing to me at least, that the central nervous system plays a critical role in mediating ventricular arrhythmias in some patients who exhibit cardiac arrest. In a similar vein, Doctors Schwartz and Stone describe how autonomic neural activity can affect cardiac function as determined through elegant animal and human studies.

The papers in this section promote a better understanding of the electrical and neural factors that operate in patients who are at risk of sudden death. It is hoped that we can develop more successful methods of prevention and treatment of sudden cardiac arrest from just this type of information.

THE USE OF ANIMAL MODELS IN THE STUDY OF THE ELECTROPHYSIOLOGY OF SUDDEN CORONARY DEATHS *

Joseph F. Spear,* Eric L. Michelson,† and E. Neil Moore

*Department of Animal Biology
School of Veterinary Medicine
University of Pennsylvania
Philadelphia, Pennsylvania 19104*

*† Departments of Research and Medicine
Lankenau Hospital
Philadelphia, Pennsylvania 19151*

The natural history of ischemic heart disease in man is complex. This complexity poses a challenge in designing appropriate animal models to study mechanisms of human cardiac arrhythmias and to develop effective therapeutic approaches to prevent sudden cardiac death. Ideally an experimental animal model represents a less complex system while still exhibiting specific critical characteristics of the human situation. Then, by evaluating selected characteristics under controlled experimental conditions it is possible to gain insight into the functioning of the real system. The specific characteristics of an animal model are therefore determined by the experimental questions that are to be answered or the hypotheses to be tested. A valid model must be a reasonable analog of the human system, yet it must be sufficiently simple so that most variables can be controlled. The complexity of the problem of ischemic heart disease implies that no one animal model will provide all answers. This presentation will be restricted to a consideration of several recent *in vivo* canine electrophysiologic experiments that have clarified some of the mechanisms of arrhythmias associated with sudden coronary death in man.

Three major periods of ventricular arrhythmias in the dog occur after occlusion of a major coronary artery. In this discussion these periods will be referred to as acute, subacute, and chronic. They are distinguished both by the time of onset of the arrhythmias and by the specific characteristics of the arrhythmias.

ACUTE ARRHYTHMIAS

Within minutes after acute occlusion of a proximal artery, malignant ventricular arrhythmias occur. These persist for approximately 30 minutes and often lead to ventricular fibrillation.[1] There is evidence that the mechanism of the arrhythmias in this acute period is due to slow conduction and reentry within the ischemic epicardium.[2-8] Immediately after coronary occlusion there is a brief period of accelerated conduction within the ischemic zone.[8] This is

---

* Address for correspondence: Dr. Joseph F. Spear, Department of Animal Biology, School of Veterinary Medicine, University of Pennsylvania, 3800 Spruce Street, Philadelphia, Pennsylvania 19104.

followed by a dramatic slowing of conduction. Because of this slow conduction, activity may persist in the ischemic area sufficiently long to exit and reexcite the heart after the refractory period in the normal zone has subsided. During the arrhythmias the Purkinje system at the border of the ischemic zone is activated first, suggesting that the exit point for reexcitation of the heart may be by way of the subendocardial Purkinje system.[9] An additional mechanism for the acute arrhythmias has been suggested by studies in both dog and pig.[10] Ectopic impulses may be evoked at the border zone by electronically induced depolarization due to the current of injury that flows between the normal and ischemic myocardium. In addition, in the dog, the acute arrhythmias appear to be divided into "immediate" and "delayed" phases. The immediate phase occurs within 2 to 12 minutes and the delayed phase occurs from 14 to 30 minutes after ligation of the left anterior descending coronary artery. The delayed ventricular arrhythmias have as high an incidence of ventricular fibrillation as do the immediate ventricular arrhythmias, but are not accompanied by as severe an epicardial conduction delay.[6] The underlying reason for these two phases has not been clarified.

Release of an acute coronary arterial occlusion is also associated with malignant ventricular arrhythmias. The incidence of ventricular fibrillation is highest if release occurs after 20 to 30 minutes of occlusion, when ischemic alterations are apparently maximal and infarction still minimal.[11] The mechanisms for these arrhythmias are also complex; both reentry and altered automaticity have been implicated.[12, 13] No direct information is yet available in man with respect to either acute coronary occlusion or reperfusion phenomena to verify the applicability of these findings to the human situation.

SUBACUTE ARRHYTHMIAS

Approximately 15 to 24 hours after the arrhythmias of the acute period subside, a subacute period of spontaneous arrhythmias appears.[14] These arrhythmias, which last up to 72 hours, are rarely accompanied by fibrillation. Their mechanism is different from that of the ventricular arrhythmias of the acute period. Purkinje fibers removed from the infarcted region 24 hours after coronary occlusion exhibit enhanced automaticity.[15, 16] Studies using multiple recording and stimulation techniques in anesthetized dogs after occlusion of the left anterior descending coronary artery [4, 17] or the septal coronary artery [18] have verified that the arrhythmias have originated from the surviving subendocardial Purkinje system overlying the infarcted myocardium. The arrhythmias may be overdriven by electrical pacing and can be unmasked by slowing of the heart rate. While reentrant arrhythmias may be induced during this period, the dominant rhythm disturbance appears to be due to enhanced automaticity in the Purkinje system. In humans, arrhythmias that occur during this period after myocardial infarction appear to have a similar mechanism.[19]

FIGURE 1 is an example of the use of multiple recording and stimulation techniques to localize the origin of an arrhythmia occurring during this subacute period. This figure demonstrates the sequence of depolarization of the ventricular specialized conduction system in a dog 24 hours after two-stage occlusion of the left anterior descending coronary artery.[17] In FIGURE 1A, PF_i was recorded from the Purkinje system in the area of infarction during a spontaneous ventricular arrhythmia. During the ventricular tachycardia presented in the

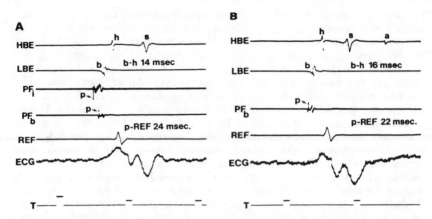

FIGURE 1. Depolarization of the ventricular specialized conduction system and electrocardiogram during spontaneous ventricular tachycardia (A) and ventricular pacing (B). One beat of each rhythm is shown. The records are bipolar recordings from the His bundle (HBE), the left bundle branch (LBE), border zone Purkinje fibers (PFᵦ), noninfarcted myocardium (REF), and lead II electrocardiogram (ECG). The time signal (T) denotes 100 msec intervals. In A, the interval between the activation of the left bundle branch and His bundle (b-h) was 14 msec. The interval between the border zone Purkinje fiber activation and normal myocardial activation (p-REF) was 24 msec. In B, during pacing from the infarct zone Purkinje fiber (PFᵢ) electrode site, these intervals were 16 and 22 msec, respectively. (From Horowitz et al.[17] Reproduced by permission.)

figure, this was the earliest site activated within the ventricles. Its activation preceded the activation of the proximal as well as the distal ventricular conducting system and ventricular muscle. Verification that this site was the origin of the arrhythmia is shown in FIGURE 1B. When the ventricle was paced through the electrode used to record PFᵢ, the sequence and timing of activation remained similar to those observed during the spontaneous arrhythmia. The surface electrocardiogram (ECG) also exhibited a similar configuration to that of the spontaneous arrhythmia. In 28 dogs in which ventricular arrhythmias were studied using these techniques 24 to 36 hours after occlusion, the site of origin of 26 spontaneous tachycardias was determined to be in the subendocardium. In these studies the earliest epicardial activation determined by epicardial mapping did not always correlate with the origin of the arrhythmia. The sites of epicardial breakthrough of the arrhythmias often were anatomically distant from the sites of origin on the endocardium and varied between 5 mm and 6 cm.[20] This finding points out that if a surgical approach to abolishing ventricular tachyarrhythmias is contemplated, epicardial mapping alone may not be sufficient to identify or predict their site of origin.

CHRONIC ARRHYTHMIAS

Approximately 3 days after coronary occlusion, spontaneous arrhythmias disappear. However, several investigators have recently described inducible sustained ventricular tachyarrhythmias in dogs that occur from 3 days to a number of weeks after experimental myocardial infarction.[21-25] In 38 animals studied in our laboratory[22] 3 to 30 days after undergoing two-stage coronary arterial occlusion followed 2 hours later by reperfusion, sustained ventricular tachyarrhythmias could be initiated in 35 by means of programmed stimulation methods similar to those routinely used in the human cardiac catheterization laboratory.[26-32] Fourteen dogs had inducible sustained ventricular tachycardia, nine had inducible flutter, and 12 had pacing-induced fibrillation. Ventricular tachycardia was defined as an accelerated ventricular rhythm with a basic cycle length of greater than or equal to 120 msec. At cycle lengths shorter than 120 msec, an organized regular arrhythmia was defined as ventricular flutter. Ventricular fibrillation was a chaotic incoordinate and irreversible ventricular arrhythmia confirmed electrocardiographically as well as visually. While different animals showed different patterns of ventricular tachyarrhythmias, in a given animal there was reproducibility in the rate and morphology of the arrhythmias that could be induced. FIGURE 2 presents records obtained from an animal 5 days after it had undergone coronary arterial occlusion followed by reperfusion. The left ventricle was paced at a basic cycle length of 300 msec, and after the introduction of two ventricular extrastimuli at 170 and 130 msec, respectively, a pleomorphic ventricular tachycardia was initiated that then stabilized as sustained ventricular tachycardia with a cycle length of 160 msec.

The ability to induce ventricular tachyarrhythmias in individual animals

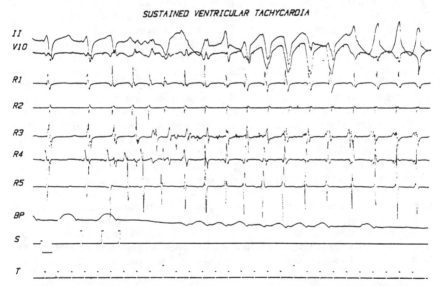

SUSTAINED VENTRICULAR TACHYCARDIA

FIGURE 2. Analog records demonstrating the initiation of sustained ventricular tachycardia in response to two ventricular extrastimuli. The lead II and V10 electrocardiograms are displayed along with multiple intramyocardial bipolar electrograms (R1–R5) recorded from the left ventricle. BP is the femoral arterial blood pressure. The left ventricle was paced at a basic cycle length of 300 msec. After the introduction of two ventricular extrastimuli at 170 and 130 msec, respectively, a pleomorphic ventricular tachyarrhythmia was initiated which then stabilized as sustained ventricular tachycardia with a cycle length of 160 msec. Sites R3 and R4 were located within the area of infarction. (From Michelson *et al.*[18] Reproduced by permission.)

depended on the site of stimulation.[33] When unipolar cathodal stimuli through intramyocardial wire electrodes were used, not all sites tested in a given animal permitted ventricular tachyarrhythmias to be induced. Also, some sites required a single ventricular extrastimulus for successful induction of the arrhythmia, while at other sites success could be achieved only when two or three ventricular extrastimuli were introduced. In 24 animals in which this was studied in detail, the most successful sites for the induction of tachyarrhythmias were those intramyocardial sites exhibiting normal excitability and refractoriness within 2 cm of the border of the area of infarction. Altogether, in 27 of 44 such sites tested ventricular tachyarrhythmias were successfully initiated. Normal left ventricular sites greater than 2 cm from the area of infarction, normal right ventricular sites, endocardial catheter sites, and left ventricular infarct sites were all less successful with respect to initiation of ventricular arrhythmias (which were induced in less than 25 percent of the sites attempted). The inability to induce arrhythmias in many of the sites located within the infarcted myocardium was found to be due in part to prolonged refractoriness in this area. FIGURE 3 presents four strength-interval curves obtained by unipolar cathodal stimulation from two normal sites and two infarct sites. The coupling intervals of the extrastimulus are plotted versus the maximal milliamperage failing to elicit a response at that coupling interval. At site 1, a stimulation intensity of twice diastolic threshold initiated ventricular tachycardia with two ventricular extrastimuli. Tachyarrhythmia could not be successfully initiated in the other sites. Notice that the sites located within the infarct (sites 3 and 4) had prolonged effective and relative refractory periods. An extrasystole at these sites could not be provoked at a sufficiently short coupling interval to induce ventricular tachycardia. That is, because of the prolonged duration of the refractoriness the prematurity of the evoked response was limited at these sites. Because site 2, which had a sufficiently short refractory period, was also not successful with respect to initiation of the tachycardia, additional factors such as the location of the electrode relative to the infarct must be involved in inducibility. Site 2, in which tachycardia could not be provoked, was located in normal myocardium at the base of the left ventricle, while site 1, in which the arrhythmia could be initiated, was 1 cm from the border of the infarct.

The evidence presently available indicates that the sustained ventricular tachyarrhythmias that can be induced and terminated in these animals by programmed stimulation are due to relatively localized reentry. Electrical recordings within the area of infarction often exhibit fractionated activity, which in some cases can be seen to bridge the diastolic period. In FIGURE 2 sites R3 and R4 are within the infarct, and fractionated activity can be seen in these recordings. The presence of this activity has been suggested to be due to slow conduction and reentry within ischemic tissue or surviving tissue in an infarcted area.[2-6, 25]

The phenomenon of concealed perpetuation described in human patients with inducible sustained ventricular tachycardia[31] can also be observed in these animals. During the tachycardia, electrical pacing of the ventricles may capture such a large part of the heart that electrograms recorded from widely separated regions of the ventricles become synchronized with the ventricular pacing. However, at the termination of ventricular pacing, the tachycardia resumes at its undisturbed rate. These findings indicate that the pathway involved in the reentry must be localized and relatively protected.

The effects of several antiarrhythmic agents have been studied in animals exhibiting sustained ventricular tachyarrhythmias. In 19 animals studied in our laboratory, 20 to 25 mg of procainamide (mean plasma level at the time of study 12.5 μg/ml) was administered intravenously after the basic pattern of ventricular tachyarrhythmia was determined.[34] In each case, the severity of the arrhythmia was reduced. FIGURE 4 summarizes our data. In four of nine animals in which ventricular fibrillation could be induced before procainamide was administered, no arrhythmias were inducible after procainamide. In the other five animals with ventricular fibrillation, only sustained ventricular tachycardia or nonsustained ventricular tachycardia could be initiated after

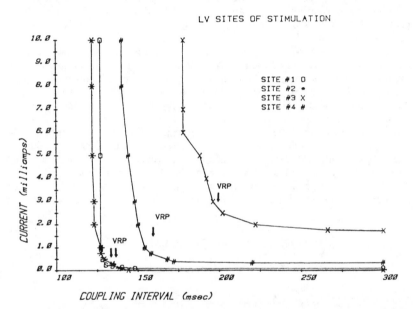

FIGURE 3. Strength-interval curves derived from measurements made at four left ventricular sites. Coupling intervals in msec are plotted versus the maximal milliamperage failing to elicit a response at that coupling interval. Site 1 was located in normal myocardium within 1 cm of the border of the left ventricular apical infarct; site 2 was located at the base of the left ventricle; and sites 3 and 4 were located within the area of infarction. VRP indicates the time of the ventricular refractory period, defined as the latest coupling interval at which a stimulus of twice diastolic threshold intensity was unable to evoke a premature beat. The cathodal current was 2 msec in duration and was delivered through an intramural electrode. (From Michelson *et al.*[38] Reproduced by permission.)

procainamide. This ability of procainamide to prevent the reinitiation, to convert sustained to nonsustained tachycardia, or to prolong the cycle length of the arrhythmia, was also true for the five animals that had ventricular flutter and the five animals with ventricular tachycardia.

In 10 other animals, a 2 to 3 mg/kg bolus of lidocaine was given intravenously followed by a 0.07 mg/kg per min infusion. After lidocaine administration, it was still possible to reinitiate the same ventricular tachyarrhythmias in each case. At higher doses (8 mg/kg bolus) the initiation of ventricular tachyarrhythmias was prevented in two of the ten animals. In individual animals, the cycle length of the tachyarrhythmia was either prolonged, shortened, or unchanged after lidocaine. These effects of procainamide and lidocaine in this model mimic closely effects reported in patients with recurrent sustained ventricular tachyarrhythmias studied in the catheterization laboratory.[26-32, 35]

Other laboratories using similar models have evaluated the effects of additional antiarrhythmic agents. TABLE 1 compares the efficacy of various drugs evaluated by programmed stimulation in chronic dog models [23, 34, 36-42] and man.[35, 43-45] Two investigational drugs that have not been used in man have been found to be effective in animals. Meobentine is a nonneuronal blocking bethanidine derivative and pranolium is a non-beta-blocking derivative of propranolol. A striking similarity is seen in drug efficacy between the dog with chronic infarction and man.

Thus, several chronic canine myocardial infarction models now exist that exhibit recurrent sustained tachyarrhythmias, and these are available for studying the mechanisms of arrhythmogenesis and for evaluating new antiarrhythmic agents. The advantages of these models are that the arrhythmias can be reproducibly and consistently induced, and often terminated, using routine programmed pacing. The arrhythmias are stable and reproducible over both the short- and long-term. The arrhythmia mechanisms appear comparable to those in patients with chronic coronary artery disease and the effects of antiarrhythmic drugs parallel those reported in man. However, these models are not yet ideal since they do not exhibit spontaneously occurring ventricular arrhythmias and do not undergo acute, spontaneously occurring sudden death. However, further development of this model may expand its capabilities in this direction.

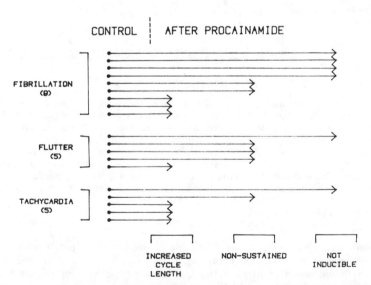

FIGURE 4. The antiarrhythmic effects of procainamide on inducible ventricular tachyarrhythmias. (*Left*) dots indicate the control ventricular arrhythmia induced in 19 animals. (*Right*) arrows indicate the change in the severity of the arrhythmia for each animal after intravenous administration of procainamide. See text for further discussion.

TABLE 1

COMPARISON OF ANTI-VT/VF DRUG EFFICACY EVALUATED BY PROGRAMMED PACING
IN CHRONIC DOG MODELS VERSUS MAN *

Drug	Efficacy in Chronic Dog Models	Efficacy in Man
Bretylium (chronic)	YES, ↓ VT rate	yes, ↓ VT rate
Diphenylhydantoin	yes	yes
Disopyramide	YES, ↓ VT rate	yes, ↓ VT rate
Lidocaine	+/−	+/−
Meobentine	YES, ↓ VT rate	?
Pranolium	YES	?
Procainamide	YES, ↓ VT rate	YES, ↓ VT rate
Propranolol	NO	NO
Verapamil	NO	NO

NOTE: YES=often: yes=occasional; +/−=infrequent; VT=ventricular tachycardia; ↓ = decrease; ? = unknown.
* From Michelson *et al.*[49] Reproduced by permission.

One experimental approach may be the superimposition of an acute, otherwise nonlethal ischemic event on the chronic infarction.[46, 47] In addition, the pathophysiology of the arrhythmia in animal models is different from that in man: notably the lesion is not due to atherogenic coronary artery disease.

In summary, animal models have advanced our knowledge of the mechanisms of cardiac arrhythmias associated with myocardial ischemia and infarction. While no one animal model ideally mimics the pathophysiology and natural history of coronary artery disease, the information generated by multiple models is beginning to produce meaningful insight into the mechanisms of life-threatening arrhythmias associated with coronary artery disease, and this has helped to develop new therapeutic modalities.

REFERENCES

1. HARRIS, A. S. & A. G. ROJAS. 1943. Initiation of ventricular fibrillation due to coronary occlusion. Exp. Med. Surg. 1:1–105–122.
2. WALDO, A. L. & G. A. KAISER. 1973. A study of ventricular arrhythmias associated with acute myocardial infarction in the canine heart. Circulation 47: 1222–1228.
3. BOINEAU, J. P. & J. L. COX. 1973. Slow ventricular activation in acute myocardial infarction: A source of reentrant premature ventricular contractions. Circulation 48:702–713.
4. SCHERLAG, B. J., N. EL-SHERIF, R. HOPE & R. LAZZARA. 1974. Characterization and localization of ventricular arrhythmias resulting from myocardial ischemia and infarction. Circ. Res. 35:372–383.
5. WIT, A. L. & J. T. BIGGER, JR. 1975. Possible electrophysiological mechanisms for lethal arrhythmias accompanying myocardial ischemia and infarction. Circulation 51, 52(Suppl III:III):96–115.

6. KAPLINSKY, E., S. OGAWA, C. W. BALKE, & L. S. DREIFUS. 1979. Two periods of early ventricular arrhythmia in the canine acute myocardial infarction model. Circulation **60:**397–403.
7. LEVITES, R., V. S. BANKA & R. H. HELFANT. 1975. Electrophysiologic effects of coronary occlusion and reperfusion: Observations on dispersion of refractoriness and ventricular automaticity. Circulation **52:**760–765.
8. ELHARRAR, V., P. R. FOSTER, T. L. JIRAK, W. E. GAUM & D. P. ZIPES. 1977. Alterations in canine myocardial excitability during ischemia. Circ. Res. **40:** 98–105.
9. KAPLINSKY, E., S. OGAWA, W. BALKE & L. S. DREIFUS. 1979. Role of endocardial activation in malignant ventricular arrhythmias associated with acute ischemia. J. Electrocardiol. **12:**299–306.
10. JANSE, M. J., J. L. VAN CAPELLE, H. MORSINK, et al. 1980. Flow of "injury" current and patterns of excitation during early ventricular arrhythmias in acute regional myocardial ischemia in isolated porcine and canine hearts. Evidence for two different arrhythmogenic mechanisms. Circ. Res. **47:**151–165.
11. BALKE, C. W., E. KAPLINSKY, E. L. MICHELSON, M. NAITO & L. S. DREIFUS. 1981. Reperfusion ventricular tachyarrhythmias: Correlation with antecedent coronary artery occlusion tachyarrhythmias and duration of myocardial ischemia. Am. Heart J. **101:**449–456.
12. PENKASKE, P. A., B. E. SOBEL & P. B. CORR. 1978. Disparate electrophysiological alterations accompanying dysrhythmia due to coronary occlusion and reperfusion in the cat. Circulation **58:**1023–1035.
13. KAPLINSKY, E., S. OGAWA, E. L. MICHELSON & L. S. DREIFUS. 1981. Instantaneous and delayed ventricular arrhythmias after reperfusion of acutely ischemic myocardium: Evidence for multiple mechanisms. Circulation **63:**333–340.
14. HARRIS, A. S. 1950. Delayed development of ventricular ectopic rhythms following experimental coronary occlusion. Circulation **1:**1318.
15. FRIEDMAN, P. L., J. R. STEWARD, J. J. FENOGLIO & A. L. WIT. 1973. Survival of subendocardial Purkinje fibers after extensive myocardial infarction in dogs. Circ. Res. **33:**597.
16. LAZZARA, R., N. EL-SHERIF & B. J. SCHERLAG. 1973. Electrophysiological properties of canine Purkinje cells in one-day-old myocardial infarction. Circ. Res. **33:**722.
17. HOROWITZ, L. N., J. F. SPEAR & E. N. MOORE. 1975. Subendocardial origin of ventricular arrhythmias in 24-hour-old experimental myocardial infarction. Circulation **53:**56–62.
18. SPEAR, J. F., E. L. MICHELSON, S. R. SPIELMAN & E. N. MOORE. The origin of ventricular arrhythmias 24 hours following experimental anterior septal coronary artery occlusion. Circulation **55:**844–852.
19. WELLENS, H. J. J., K. I. LIE & D. DURRER. 1974. Further observations on ventricular tachycardia. Circulation **49:**647.
20. SPIELMAN, S. R., E. L. MICHELSON, L. N. HOROWITZ, J. F. SPEAR & E. N. MOORE. 1978. The limitations of epicardial mapping as a guide to the surgical therapy of ventricular tachycardia. Circulation **57:**666.
21. KARAGUEUZIAN, H. S., J. J. FENOGLIO, M. B. WEISS & A. L. WIT. 1979. Protracted ventricular tachycardia induced by premature stimulation of the canine heart after coronary artery occlusion and reperfusion. Circ. Res. **44:**833–846.
22. MICHELSON, E. L., J. F. SPEAR & E. N. MOORE. 1980. Electrophysiologic and anatomic correlates of sustained ventricular tachyarrhythmias in a model of chronic myocardial infarction. Am. J. Cardiol. **45:**583–590.
23. GIBSON, J. K. & B. R. LUCCHESI. 1980. Electrophysiologic actions of UM-272 (pranolium) on reentrant ventricular arrhythmias in post-infarction canine myocardium. J. Pharmacol. Exp. Ther. **214:**347–353.
24. GARAN, H., J. T. FALLON & J. N. RUSKIN. 1980. Sustained ventricular tachycardia in recent canine myocardial infarction. Circulation **62:**980.

25. ElSherif, N., B. F. Scherlag, R. Lazzara & R. R. Hope. 1977. Reentrant arrhythmias in the late myocardial infarction period. II. Patterns of initiation and termination of reentry. Circulation **55**:702–719.
26. Denes, P., D. Wu, R. C. Dhingra, *et al.* 1976. Electrophysiologic studies in patients with chronic recurrent ventricular tachycardia. Circulation **54**:229–236.
27. Wellens, H. J. J., D. R. Duren & K. I. Lie. 1976. Observations on mechanisms of ventricular tachycardia in man. Circulation **54**:237–244.
28. Fisher, J. D., H. L. Cohen, R. Mehra, H. Altschuler, D. J. W. Escher & S. Furman. 1977. Cardiac pacing and pacemakers. II. Serial electrophysiologic-pharmacologic testing for control of recurrent tachyarrhythmias. Am. Heart J. **93**:658–668.
29. Josephson, M. E., L. N. Horowitz, A. Farshidi & J. A. Kastor. 1978. Recurrent sustained ventricular tachycardia. 1. Mechanisms. Circulation **57**: 431–440.
30. Wellens, H. J. J. 1978. Value and limitations of programmed electrical stimulation of the heart in the study and treatment of tachycardias. Circulation **57**: 845–853.
31. Josephson, M. E., L. N. Horowitz, A. Farshidi, S. R. Spielman, E. L. Michelson & A. M. Greenspan. 1978. Sustained ventricular tachycardia: Evidence for protected localized reentry. Am. J. Cardiol. **42**:416–423.
32. Mason, J. W. & R. A. Winkle. 1978. Electrode-catheter arrhythmia induction in the selection and assessment of antiarrhythmic drug therapy for recurrent ventricular tachycardia. Circulation **58**:971–985.
33. Michelson, E. L., J. F. Spear & E. N. Moore. 1981. Initiation of sustained ventricular tachyarrhythmias in a canine model of chronic myocardial infarction: Importance of the site of stimulation. Circulation **63**:776–784.
34. Michelson, E. L., J. F. Spear & E. N. Moore. 1981. Effects of procainamide on strength-interval relations in normal and chronically infarcted canine myocardium. Am. J. Cardiol. **47**: 1223–1232.
35. Greenspan, A. M., L. N. Horowitz, S. R. Spielman & M. E. Josephson. 1980. Large dose procainamide therapy for ventricular tachyarrhythmia. Am. J. Cardiol. **46**:453–462.
36. Glassman, R. D., J. C. Davis & A. L. Wit. 1978. Effects of antiarrhythmic drugs on sustained ventricular tachycardia induced by a premature stimulus in dogs after coronary artery occlusion and reperfusion (abstr.). Fed. Proc. **37**: 730.
37. Patterson, E., J. K. Gibson & B. R. Lucchesi. 1980. The electrophysiologic effects of disopyramide phosphate upon reentrant ventricular arrhythmias in conscious dogs after myocardial infarction. Am. J. Cardiol. **46**:792–799.
38. Patterson, E., J. K. Gibson & B. R. Lucchesi. 1981. Chronic canine ventricular tachyarrhythmias—prevention by bretylium tosylate administration. In press.
39. El-Sherif, N., B. J. Scherlag, R. Lazzara & R. R. Hope. 1977. Reentrant ventricular arrhythmias in the late myocardial infarction period. 4. Mechanism of action of lidocaine. Circulation **56**:395–402.
40. El-Sherif, N. & R. Lazzara. 1978. Reentrant ventricular arrhythmias in the myocardial infarction period. 5. Mechanism of action of diphenylhydantoin. Circulation **57**:465–472.
41. El-Sherif, N. 1979. Electrophysiologic basis of procainamide therapeutic and toxic effects on ischemia-related reentrant ventricular arrhythmias (abstr.). Am. J. Cardiol. **43**:429.
42. El-Sherif, N. & R. Lazzara. 1979. Reentrant ventricular arrhythmias in the late myocardial infarction period. 7. Effect of verapamil and D-600 and the role of the "slow channel." Circulation **60**:605–615.
43. Wellens, H. J. J., F. W. H. M. Bar, K. I. Lie, D. R. Duren & H. J. Dohmen. 1977. Effect of procainamide, propranolol and verapamil on mechanism of

tachycardia in patients with chronic recurrent ventricular tachycardia. Am. J. Cardiol. **40**:579–585.

44. HOROWITZ, L. N., M. E. JOSEPHSON, A. FARSHIDI, S. R. SPIELMAN, E. L. MICHELSON & A. M. GREENSPAN. 1978. Recurrent sustained ventricular tachycardia. 3. Role of the electrophysiologic study in selection of antiarrhythmic regimens. Circulation **58**:986–997.

45. ANDERSON, J. L., E. PATTERSON, J. G. WAGNER, T. A. JOHNSON, B. R. LUCCHESI & B. PITT. 1981. Clinical pharmacokinetics of intravenous and oral bretylium tosylate in survivors of ventricular tachycardia of fibrillation. In press.

46. SCHWARTZ, P. J. & H. L. STONE. 1980. Left stellectomy in the prevention of ventricular fibrillation caused by acute myocardial ischemia in conscious dogs with anterior myocardial infarction. Circulation **62**:1256.

47. LUCCHESI, B. R., K. HOLLAND & E. PATTERSON. 1981. Ventricular fibrillation resulting from ischemia at a distant site in a conscious canine model of sudden coronary death (abstr.). Fed. Proc. **40**:646.

48. MICHELSON, E. L., J. F. SPEAR & E. N. MOORE. 1981. Further electrophysiologic and anatomic correlates in a canine model of chronic myocardial infarction susceptible to the initiation of sustained ventricular tachyarrhythmias. Anat. Rec. **201**: 55–65.

49. MICHELSON, E. L., J. F. SPEAR & E. N. MOORE. 1981. Description of chronic canine myocardial infarction models suitable for electrophysiologic evaluation of new antiarrhythmic drugs. *In* The Evaluation of New Antiarrhythmic Drugs. Martinus Nijhoff. The Hague.

DISCUSSION

DR. LUCCHESI: Recently at the Federation ‡ meetings we presented a modification of the model that you described, Dr. Spear. The presence of stenosis in our experience is extremely important. The modification of the model that we have developed and reported on is the induction of a thromboembolic event in the circumflex artery, without occlusion of that circumflex vessel, in the ambulatory, conscious animal. In this model the animal has had occlusion and release of the left anterior descending artery with stenosis left in place. This model results in a 100% ventricular fibrillation.

Furthermore, we've noted that in our model the animal is extremely susceptible to stress, and the mortality is extremely high. In contrast to some of the other models without stenosis our model comes pretty close to what happens clinically.

DR. SPEAR: I'm not sure that the animals in our model are as susceptible to stress. We have been keeping some animals for a considerable time.

DR. KASTOR: How large a laboratory set-up is required? Can you give us a few practical points on setting up a laboratory to do this sort of work?

DR. SPEAR: The procedure is relatively simple. In a sterile operating space you make a small thorocotomy, occluding and dissecting free the coronary artery that you wish to occlude. Then apply the occlusion procedure, reinflate the lung and follow the animals for several days, using routine postoperative care.

DR. RICHARD CRAMPTON (*Charlottesville, Virginia*): Your model is elegant, but it is one in which the ventricle is stimulated. So we ought to bear

‡ Federation of Societies of Experimental Biology.

in mind that propranolol is ineffective in your assessment. Propranolol, in the Scandinavian and some other studies, has shortened the Q-T interval in the long-term patient, which is analogous to your model and has been shown to reduce late death in the human. This raises the question of neurogenic mechanisms in sudden death. We should keep this in mind with the chronic model because we are stimulating an end-organ and of course the programmed electrical stimulation may excite local nerves, giving afferent and efferent activity. We have to consider the role of the brain and the autonomic nervous system as well. Can we trigger arrhythmias from stimuli elsewhere in a chronic model to explain why a beta adrenergic blocking agent will work whereas another drug apparently won't or why the beta blocking drug won't work in another model.

DR. SPEAR: I agree. These dogs are easily studied in a chronic awake stage, which is important.

DR. CRAMPTON: It is interesting to note that these animals can drop dead when they are stressed.

DR. SPEAR: Our animals haven't died yet, but that's an excellent point.

DR. DWYER: Dr. Spear, would you comment on the lack of spontaneity of sudden death in animal models? Does this tell us something? Have there been any major efforts to further explore the development of spontaneity in these models?

DR. SPEAR: Yes, definitely. Dr. Lucchesi has pointed out experiments in which he is able to do this by superimposing an acute event in the chronic models, which produces a very high incidence of sudden ventricular fibrillation. In an acute model the intervention would not produce ventricular fibrillation.

Investigators are looking at this in terms of other kinds of stress, such as treadmill exercise. And I think that Dr. Schwartz will be talking about the role of the autonomic nervous system. He has several models in which he superimposes autonomic stimulation on chronic ischemia in which a large proportion of the animals show fibrillation.

DR. ZIPES: There is another point that you have referred to, Dr. Spear, that I think is important to stress: In these models, one can induce a sustained ventricular tachycardia that remains sustained in a certain percentage of the dogs. If the dog doesn't become hypotensive, it does quite well, which is quite different from the early sudden death seen in man as well as that in dogs after acute coronary arterial occlusion. You cannot produce a nice, stable, sustained ventricular tachycardia 5 minutes after tying a coronary artery. While patients with recurrent chronic sustained ventricular tachycardia have a great number of similarities to this chronic model, sudden death that occurs within minutes of the onset of symptoms may be quite different electrophysiologically.

DR. SPEAR: Yes, very possibly. I think that the patients whom you see are a lot sicker than the animals we're working with.

CELLULAR ELECTROPHYSIOLOGY IN ACUTE AND HEALED EXPERIMENTAL MYOCARDIAL INFARCTION *

Robert J. Myerburg,† Kristina Epstein, Marion S. Gaide,
Sam S. Wong, Agustin Castellanos, Henry Gelband,
John S. Cameron, and Arthur L. Bassett

*Departments of Medicine (Division of Cardiology),
Pharmacology, and Pediatrics (Division of
Pediatric Cardiology)
University of Miami School of Medicine
Miami, Florida 33101*

INTRODUCTION

Studies of the electrophysiology of experimental *acute* myocardial infarction, carried out during the past decade for the most part by the Harris ligation technique [1] in dogs, have yielded major new information about the electrophysiology of experimental arrhythmias occurring from the onset of ischemia through the first 48 to 72 hours.[2-17] Additional studies addressed the problem of the electrophysiologic changes that occur 5 to 10 days after experimental coronary ligation.[18-24] In these later experiments, there has been some controversy over the actual pathways and mechanisms of arrhythmias involved,[16, 19, 25] but most of the studies support a reentrant mechanism. The studies of early ischemia, and ischemia 5 to 10 days after ligation of a coronary artery, produced animal models that pathologically paralleled the *acute* and *early convalescent* phase of myocardial infarction in man. Initial attempts to identify persistent long-term electrophysiologic abnormalities or arrhythmias in these models were unsuccessful.

As an attempt to develop a model that paralleled the chronic, post-healing phase of myocardial infarction in man, we began to evaluate the long-term consequences of various ligation techniques in different species. We found that myocardial infarctions created in cats by ligation of distal tributaries of the left coronary system resulted in predictable infarction of 5 to 15% of the left ventricle, with persistence of spontaneous or inducible ventricular arrhythmias for up to 6 months after coronary ligation.[26-29] Spontaneous arrhythmias occurred in 25% of the animals and inducible arrhythmias in another 25%. In addition, histologic studies demonstrated survival of bands of subendocardial ventricular muscle cells overlying the myocardial infarction scars. The electrophysiologic characteristics of these surviving cells were abnormal,[27-29] and their histologic presence [27, 28] was different from that seen after the Harris

* This work was supported in part by Grants-in-Aid HL 21735–04 and HL 19044 from the National Heart, Lung and Blood Institute, by the American Heart Association, Greater Miami Affiliate, and the Miami Veterans Administration Hospital.

† Address for correspondence: Robert J. Myerburg, M.D., Professor of Medicine and Physiology, University of Miami School of Medicine, P.O. Box 016960, Miami, Florida 33101.

ligation technique in dogs.[3, 9, 11, 12]   Subsequently, other investigators, using coronary occlusion–reperfusion techniques, have also shown that late inducibility of arrhythmias persists, and that this capability is accompanied by survival of cells that have been exposed to acute ischemic injury.[24, 25, 30]

Since acute ischemia in hearts that have healed after previous ischemic injury is a common clinical event, we directed our subsequent studies to characterization of the electrophysiology of both acute and healed myocardial infarction preparations, to a comparison of their responses to membrane-active antiarrhythmic agents, and to the electrophysiologic consequences of superimposition of acute ischemia upon healed myocardial infarction in cats.

MATERIALS AND METHODS

Single-stage ligation of two or three distal tributaries of the left anterior descending and left circumflex arteries in domestic cats predictably infarcts 5 to 15% of the left ventricular muscle mass at the base of the anterior papillary muscle and adjacent areas of the apex, and the apical free wall and lower septum.[27]   The ligations are performed through a sterile left thoracotomy after the cats are anesthetized with sodium pentobarbital, 30 mg/kg intraperitoneally, and provided ventilatory support through endotracheal intubation and a Harvard respirator. A standard 6-lead electrocardiogram is recorded prior to and after the thoracotomy, and before and after ligation of the coronary arteries. Enough tributaries are ligated to produce a 50 to 100 mm^2 area of intense epicardial cyanosis. For acute myocardial injury studies in previously normal hearts (AMI preparations), the infarction was allowed to evolve for a period of 90 to 120 minutes before the heart was excised and mounted in tissue bath (see later). For preparations of healed myocardial infarction (HMI), the chest was closed and a postoperative electrocardiogram recorded. Surviving cats (approximately 85%) were maintained in a colony for 2 months or longer. On the day of terminal studies, the cats were anesthetized with sodium pentobarbital, a 6-lead electrocardiogram was recorded, and the rhythm monitored for 60 minutes prior to thoracotomy. Bilateral neck dissections were performed, the vagus nerves isolated and doubly ligated, and stainless steel wire probe electrodes attached with isolation from surrounding tissue by means of cotton jackets impregnated with mineral oil. Vagal stimulation, to allow identification of latent accelerated ventricular ectopic foci, was carried out during continuous electrocardiographic monitoring, as previously described.[27]

In cats in which acute myocardial ischemia was superimposed upon healed myocardial infarction (AMI/HMI), the left anterior descending or circumflex artery was ligated approximately 5 to 10 mm proximal to the site of the previous ligatures. Acute ischemia was identified by the development of an area of cyanosis adjacent to the old infarction scar. This was allowed to persist for up to 90 to 120 minutes, depending upon the stability of the preparation, before the heart was removed for tissue-bath studies. Continuous electrocardiographic monitoring was carried out, and the frequency and characteristics of ventricular arrhythmias were recorded. In those preparations in which ventricular fibrillation evolved, no attempt was made to defibrillate the heart; and it was removed at that point for tissue-bath studies. Studies were also carried out on a group of normal hearts in areas comparable to the AMI and/or HMI areas of the cats that had had experimental coronary ligation. Hearts from sham-operated cats were identical to normal cat hearts.

The atria and right ventricles of the isolated hearts were removed, and the left ventricle was opened by an incision through the free wall between the posterior papillary muscle and posterior paraseptal free wall.[27, 31] The mitral valve was excised and the aortic ring opened. The wet heart was weighed rapidly in a bottle of oxygenated Tyrode's solution, and the dimensions of the endocardial surface recorded. The left ventricle was mounted in a Lucite tissue bath and superfused in modified Tyrode's solution at 36 to 37° C.[31, 32] The preparations were driven through Teflon®-coated, fine silver-wire surface electrodes at cycle lengths ranging from 500 to 1000 msec. Stimuli were delivered to the left bundle branch at 1.2 times threshold current.[31] Surface electrograms were recorded through similar electrodes, and differential amplifiers were used to display these surface signals on an oscilloscope screen. The total surface area of the isolated endocardium was mapped initially with surface electrograms at 1- to 2-mm intervals to determine areas of infarction and the characteristics and pattern of ventricular activation. During other phases of the studies, premature stimuli were delivered to various sites on the endocardium overlying, bordering, and adjacent to the areas of myocardial infarction. Premature stimuli (S_2) were delivered at 2.0 times late diastolic threshold after every eighth drive stimulus (S_1). Local refractory periods were mapped over the entire endocardial surface at 1- to 2-mm intervals. The local refractory period was defined as the longest S_1–S_2 interval at a site of stimulation that did not result in a response to S_2. In some preparations (see RESULTS), attempts were made to initiate sustained ventricular activity by programmed stimulation techniques in the isolated preparations before mapping local refractory periods. In these preparations, premature stimuli were delivered to sites on 1- to 2-mm grids overlying healed and/or acute infarctions, and surrounding normal tissue, with varying S_1–S_2 intervals, and varying intensity of S_2 (from 2 to 10 times diastolic threshold). Prior to programmed pacing studies, maps of transmembrane action potential characteristics were made at 1-mm intervals over the endocardial surface using transmembrane action potential recording techniques as previously reported from our laboratory.[31–35]

Superfusion of isolated preparations with procainamide (PA) was performed by adding aqueous solutions of chemically pure procainamide hydrochloride (Sigma Chemical Co.) to Tyrode's solution in appropriate amounts to achieve desired concentrations. The smallest possible aqueous volumes were used, and never exceeded 10 ml/L of Tyrode's solution. In selected experiments, in which superfusion with tetrodotoxin (TTX) was performed, 1 mg of TTX (Sigma Chemical Co.) was dissolved in 5 ml of water and added to 500 ml of Tyrode's solution.

Statistical analyses of the relationships between experimental procedures and ventricular arrhythmias or inducible sustained activity in tissue bath were carried out by use of 2×2 tables with χ^2 analysis for each experimental contingency, as well as by a generalized χ^2 analysis for each category of data. Two-sample, two-tailed t-tests were used to test for differences between action potential durations or local refractory periods of acutely ischemic cells versus those of controls and of surviving cells from healed infarct preparations. Similar techniques were used to test for the differences in response to procainamide of AMI cells versus their controls, HMI cells versus their controls, AMI cells versus HMI cells, and the controls for both groups versus each other. To determine whether there was a significant differential between the responses of AMI and HMI cells to procainamide, analyses of variance and covariance, using repeated measures, were calculated throughout the time course of each of these studies.

RESULTS

The experimental coronary ligation technique produced predictable transmural myocardial infarction involving the base of the anterior papillary muscle and adjacent free wall or lower septum (FIG. 1). Histologically, the myocardial infarction scar was accompanied by bands of 2 to 10 cell layers of surviving ventricular muscle (VM) cells overlying the myocardial infarction scar (FIG. 2). Cellular electrophysiologic abnormalities, indicated by the characteristics of transmembrane action potential recordings, persisted in these surviving cell layers overlying the area of myocardial infarction (FIG. 2). The characteristics of the persistent abnormalities were a function of the period of time between coronary ligation and tissue-bath studies (see later).

In order to characterize and compare the electrophysiology of AMI versus HMI, studies were carried out in a total of 123 cats. Sixty-one cats were studied 2 to 4 months after *healing* of acute myocardial infarction (HMI), with no further interventions; and 38 cats were studied 90 to 120 minutes after creation of *acute* myocardial infarction (AMI). In 24 cats, the protocol called for studies carried out 90 to 120 minutes after *acute* myocardial ischemia was superimposed upon a 2- to 4-month *healed* infarction (AMI/HMI). In six cats, however, ventricular fibrillation (VF) occurred between 30 and 90 minutes after the second coronary ligation and the experiment was terminated at that point. The remaining three ventricular fibrillations occurred between 90 and 120 minutes. The incidence and type of *in situ* spontaneous ventricular arrhythmias, and of sustained ventricular activity inducible in tissue bath by premature stimuli, for each of the three groups (AMI, HMI, and AMI/HMI) is summarized in TABLE 1. Fifteen of the 24 AMI/HMI cats (62%) had spontaneous *in situ* ventricular arrhythmias prior to sacrifice, compared to 16 of 38 AMI cats (42%) and 19 of 61 HMI cats (31%). Moreover, TABLE 1 also indicates that the AMI/HMI cats had more advanced ventricular arrhythmias than did the other two groups. Thus, the hearts of the AMI/HMI cats were electrophysiologically more unstable than those of the AMI or HMI cats ($\chi^2 = 6.99$, $p < 0.05$). In tissue bath, the AMI/HMI hearts also had a greater incidence of inducibility of sustained ventricular activity by premature stimulation than did the hearts having AMI or HMI alone. Inducibility occurred in 16 of 24 AMI/HMI hearts (67%) compared with 13 of 38 (34%) and 20 of 61 (33%) in the AMI and HMI hearts, respectively ($\chi^2 = 8.85$, $p < 0.02$).

The correlation between spontaneous arrhythmias recorded *in situ* and inducibility of sustained ventricular activity in tissue bath for each of the three groups is shown in TABLE 2. The best correlation occurred in the HMI and the AMI/HMI preparations. In the AMI/HMI group, negative correlations were observed in 7 of the 24 preparations, and positive correlations in 14. In only 3 of the 24 preparations (13%) was there discordance between electrocardiographic arrhythmias and inducibility of sustained ventricular activity ($\chi^2 = 12.8$, $p < 0.001$). This compares with discordance rates of 25% in the AMI group ($\chi^2 = 6.0$, $p < 0.02$) and 21% in the HMI group ($\chi^2 = 15.9$, $p < 0.001$).

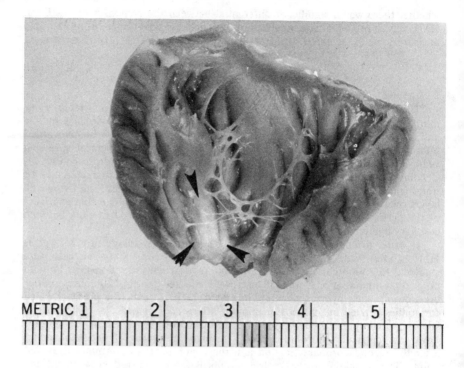

FIGURE 1. Endocardial surface of healed myocardial infarction in cat heart. The left ventricle has been opened by an incision through the free wall in a heart removed 3 months after coronary ligation by the technique described in the text. The three *arrows* identify a pale area of healed myocardial infarction at the base of the anterior papillary muscle and adjacent paraseptal free wall.

Transmembrane Action Potential Characteristics After Acute Myocardial Ischemia Compared with Surviving Cells in Healed Myocardial Infarction

The cellular electrophysiologic characteristics of AMI and HMI preparations were compared by recording maps of transmembrane action potentials from the endocardial surface of isolated left ventricles. Complete 1–2-mm grids of action potentials recorded at drive-cycle lengths of 630 msec were obtained during tissue-bath studies of 29 AMI, 41 HMI, and 13 AMI/HMI hearts. Representative points from a grid on the endocardial surface are seen in FIGURE 3 for one AMI heart and in FIGURE 4 for one HMI heart. In FIGURE 3, the middle two transmembrane action potentials in row C and the middle three transmembrane action potentials in row D were recorded from the acute ischemic zone. Action potential duration at 90% repolarization (APD_{90}) is noted under each transmembrane action potential. In FIGURE 4, HMI, the first action potential in row B and each of the first two action potentials in both rows C and D were recorded from cells overlying the HMI scar. APD_{90} of cells recorded from the ischemic zone was shorter than that of control cells in AMI hearts. In contrast, APD_{90} recorded from surviving cells over the infarct scar of HMI hearts was longer than that of the controls. In the 29 AMI hearts, the mean APD_{90} at a cycle length of 630 msec was 124 ± 18 msec (mean $\pm$ SD) in cells recorded from the region of the AMI, and 151 ± 12 msec in cells recorded from normal zones of the same hearts ($p < 0.01$). In contrast, the mean APD_{90} for surviving cells overlying 41 healed myocardial infarction scars was 178 ± 21 msec, while mean APD_{90} for the normal control cells of the same hearts was 145 ± 13 msec ($p < 0.01$). In 13 AMI/HMI hearts, APD_{90} varied considerably, ranging from 70 msec to >200 msec, with a mean of 143 ± 44 msec.

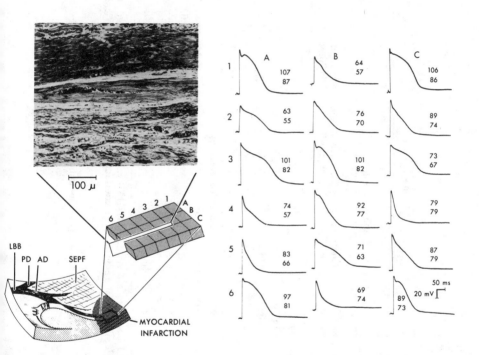

FIGURE 2. Cellular electrophysiology and histology 1 month after myocardial infarction (MI). The surface of the myocardial infarction is indicated by the shaded area. The grid is in the center of the infarction, and the cutaway view of the papillary muscle is for demonstration purposes only. The left ventricle was mounted as described in the text, and the recordings on the grid represent the first impalement from the surface of the preparation at each site. The dimensions of the grid were $0.6 \text{ mm} \times 1.2 \text{ mm}$. The schematic diagram, the grid, and the histologic section are not illustrated in scale to one another. The histologic section was cut through the center of the region of the grid and demonstrates a layer of surviving cells overlying the area of scar formation in the infarct zone. The measured upstroke amplitudes (top numbers) and resting potentials (bottom numbers) of the action potentials shown on the grid are printed adjacent to each action potential. Cycle length of stimulation= 630 msec. (From Myerburg *et al.*[27] Reproduced by permission.)

TABLE 1*

	Electrocardiographic Monitoring					Tissue Bath Studies	
	No VEA	Unifocal PVCs	Complex PVCs	Ventricular Tachycardia	Ventricular Fibrillation	No Inducible SVA	Inducible SVA
AMI (n = 38)	22 (58%)	16 (42%)	—	3† (8%)	—	25 (66%)	13 (34%)
HMI (n = 61)	42 (69%)	13 (21%)	6 (10%)	4† (7%)	—	41 (67%)	20 (33%)
AMI + HMI (n = 24)	9 (38%)	—	9 (38%)	6 (25%)	9† (38%)	8 (33%)	16 (67%)

Statistical Analysis

	Arrhythmias on ECG	Inducible Activity in Tissue Bath
Generalized χ^2	$\chi^2 = 6.99$, $p < 0.05$	$\chi^2 = 8.85$, $p < 0.02$
AMI versus AMI/HMI	$\chi^2 = 1.70$, $p = $ NS	$\chi^2 = 4.99$, $p < 0.05$
HMI versus AMI/HMI	$\chi^2 = 5.81$, $p < 0.02$	$\chi^2 = 6.77$, $p < 0.01$
Both versus AMI/HMI	$\chi^2 = 4.83$, $p < 0.05$	$\chi^2 = 7.62$, $p < 0.01$

NOTE: AMI = acute myocardial ischemia/infarction; AMI/HMI = acute ischemia superimposed on healed infarction; HMI = healed myocardial infarction; PVCs = premature ventricular contractions; SVA = sustained ventricular activity; VEA = ventricular ectopic activity.

* From Myerburg et al.[37] Reprinted with permission.

† These arrhythmias occurred in addition to other arrhythmias indicated.

TABLE 2 *

		Inducible Sustained Ventricular Activity in Tissue Bath					
		AMI (n = 38)		HMI (n = 61)		AMI/HMI (n = 24)	
		No	Yes	No	Yes	No	Yes
Ventricular Arrhythmias on ECG	No	18	4	35	7	7	2
	Yes	7	9	6	13	1	14
		$\chi^2 = 6.0$ $p < 0.02$		$\chi^2 = 15.9$ $p < 0.001$		$\chi^2 = 12.8$ $p < 0.001$	

NOTE: AMI = acute myocardial ischemia/infarction; AMI/HMI = acute ischemia superimposed on healed infarction; HMI = healed myocardial infarction.
* From Myerburg *et al.*[37] Reprinted with permission.

Local Refractory Periods

Local refractory periods were determined at basic driving cycle lengths of 630, 800, and 1,000 msec by delivering premature stimuli over 1–2-mm interelectrode grids on the endocardial surface of isolated left ventricles from 13 normal cats, 21 AMI cats, 33 HMI cats, and 18 AMI/HMI cats. A mean of 27 points per heart was recorded from the 85 endocardial surfaces studied. FIGURE 5 summarizes local refractory period data from the four groups of cats (normal, AMI, HMI, AMI/HMI) recorded during studies at a basic driving cycle length of 800 msec. Mean local refractory periods were shortest in the AMI group (150.3 ± 18.0 msec) and longest in the HMI group (196.6 ± 19.8 msec). The mean values were similar in the normal group (179.4 ± 15.0

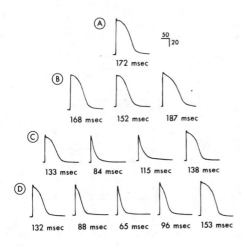

FIGURE 3. Examples of transmembrane action potentials recorded from sites on an endocardial grid from a 90-minute acute myocardial infarction (AMI). Transmembrane action potentials at 90% repolarization are indicated below each recording. The middle two recordings from row **C** and the middle three recordings from row **D** were recorded from cells overlying the AMI zone. Row **A** is toward the base of the heart and row **D** is toward the apex. The AMI cells have shorter APD_{90}s than do normal cells from the same preparation. (Modified from Myerburg *et al.*[37])

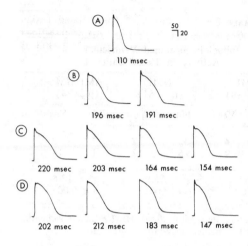

FIGURE 4. Transmembrane action potentials recorded from sites on the endocardial grid from a 2-month healed myocardial infarction (HMI). Transmembrane action potential durations at 90% repolarization are indicated below each recording. The first transmembrane potential in row **B** and the first two transmembrane action potentials in rows **C** and **D** were recorded from surviving cells overlying the HMI zone. Row **A** is toward the base of the heart and row **D** is toward the apex. The cells overlying the HMI zone have longer APD_{90}s than do normal cells from the same preparation. (Modified from Myerburg et al.[37])

msec) and the AMI/HMI group (172.9 ± 27.9 msec). However, the mean *range* of refractory periods, from shortest to longest, among the four groups was *greatest in the AMI/HMI group* (mean range = 107.9 msec). This indicates a greater dispersion of recovery of excitability in AMI/HMI hearts compared with the hearts under the other experimental conditions.

Sustained Ventricular Activity Initiated in Tissue Bath

Sustained ventricular activity could not be induced by premature stimulation in normal hearts, using the same stimulation procedures applied to the experimental preparations. In three of the normal hearts, repetitive responses to a single premature stimulus (1 to 5 repetitive depolarizations after a premature

FIGURE 5. Range of local refractory periods for each of the four experimental conditions. Rectangles indicate normal left ventricle acute myocardial infarction (AMI), healed myocardial infarction (HMI), and acute myocardial infarction superimposed on healed myocardial infarction (HMI/AMI). Within each rectangle the mean±standard deviation is indicated. The mean refractory periods were shortest in AMI preparations, longest in HMI preparations, and intermediate (and nearly equal) in the normal preparations and HMI/AMI preparations. However, the HMI/AMI preparations had the greatest dispersion of refractoriness, with an average range of 107.1 msec compared with 59.0, 62.7, and 64.6 for normal, AMI, and HMI preparations, respectively. (From Myerburg et al.[37] Reproduced by permission.)

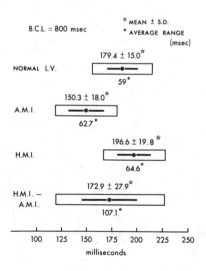

impulse) were observed during periods of stabilization of the isolated tissue. Automatic firing at cycle lengths ≤630 msec was recorded in four preparations from normal cats; and in two of the four, the activity ceased after a period of 30 to 40 minutes of stabilization.

Sustained ventricular activity was initiated by early premature stimuli in 20 of 61 (33%) HMI preparations (FIG. 6). In order to initiate sustained activity, however, the premature stimuli had to be delivered to the layer of endocardial cells overlying or bordering the HMI area. Premature stimulation

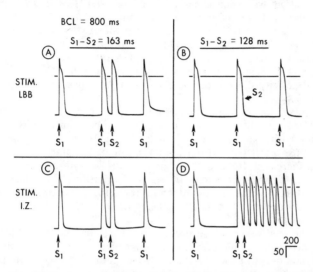

FIGURE 6.   Induced sustained ventricular activity in an isolated HMI preparation. The action potential was recorded from a ventricular muscle cell on the endocardial surface of the HMI zone. In panels **A** and **B** the recordings are made during stimulation of the left bundle branch at 1.2-times threshold. At an S_1-S_2 interval of 163 msec, the response to the premature stimulus (S_2) is propagated to the recording electrode and initiates a single response to the premature stimulus. At a coupling interval of 128 msec (panel **B**), S_2 is blocked, presumably in the specialized conducting tissue, and no response occurs at the site of the recording electrode overlying the healed myocardial infarction. In panels **C** and **D** the stimulus is delivered to the infarct zone; and at a coupling interval of 163 msec (panel **C**), a single response to the premature stimulus again occurs. In panel **D**, the premature stimulus delivered 128 msec after the drive stimulus initiates a run of sustained ventricular activity. Delivery of stimuli at other sites on the preparation (not overlying the HMI) did not initiate sustained ventricular activity, even if a response to S_2 occurred. *Calibrations:* vertical, 50 mV; horizontal, 200 msec. (From Myerburg *et al.*[37] Reproduced by permission.)

of normal areas, even in the range of coupling intervals sufficient to initiate sustained activity over the infarct area, did not initiate sustained activity. In addition, premature stimulation of the proximal specialized conducting system generally resulted in block because of physiologic refractoriness before a coupling interval was reached that was short enough to initiate sustained ventricular activity. As demonstrated in FIGURE 6, sustained ventricular activity was achievable only when an S_2 encroached upon phase 3 of transmembrane

action potentials overlying the surviving tissue in the HMI zone. In panels A
and B of FIGURE 6, coupling intervals of 163 msec and 128 msec were unable
to initiate sustained activity when delivered to the left bundle branch. In panels
C and D, however, when the stimuli were delivered to muscle over the HMI, a
short coupling interval (panel D, 128 msec) initiated sustained activity.

We were *unable* to terminate prematurity-induced sustained activity by
burst-pacing over the area of the myocardial infarct or normal tissue anywhere
on the endocardial surface once sustained activity was initiated. In every
instance, termination was spontaneous, occurring after 1.63 ± 0.71 minutes.
In contrast to the HMI preparations, the site of stimulation for initiation of
sustained ventricular activity was not critical in the AMI preparations. Sustained activity was initiated in 13 of 38 AMI preparations, and the site of
stimulation resulting in initiation of sustained activity was over the acute
myocardial infarct in 8 and over normal tissue in the remaining 5. Furthermore, sustained activity did not persist as long in AMI preparations (mean =
29.1 ± 14.3 sec).

The superimposition of acute myocardial ischemia on healed myocardial
infarct (AMI/HMI) resulted in a greater ability to initiate sustained ventricular
activity in tissue bath than in preparations having AMI or HMI alone (16 of
24 preparations [67%]). This greater ability to initiate sustained activity correlated with the increased frequency of spontaneous arrhythmias seen on the
electrocardiogram (TABLE 2) and with greater dispersion of local refractory
periods in AMI/HMI than recorded from the other experimental settings
(FIGURE 5). The duration of initiated sustained activity was similar to that with
HMI preparations (1.45 ± 0.59 minutes).

FIGURE 7 shows a series of recordings from a representative AMI/HMI
tissue-bath experiment in which sustained ventricular activity was initiated by
premature stimulation. In panel A, at a cycle length of 800 msec, simultaneous
transmembrane action potentials are recorded from a surviving cell in the
region of *acute* myocardial ischemia (V–1), from a surviving cell overlying
the *healed* myocardial infarction scar (V–2), and from a *normal* cell on the
adjacent left ventricular septum (V–3). The APD_{90} recorded from the AMI
cell is short compared with that of the normal cell, and the APD_{90} from the
tissue overlying the HMI is long compared with that of the normal cell. When
a premature stimulus is delivered to a site overlying the AMI region at an
$S_1–S_2$ coupling interval of 99 msec (panel B), a short period of irregular chaotic
activity is recorded from the three sites, with subsequent stabilization into a
run of sustained ventricular activity (panel C) at a cycle length of 110 msec.
After 1.3 minutes, the cycle length spontaneously lengthened for three cycles,
and the sustained ventricular activity ceased (not shown on illustration). The
effects of superfusion with procainamide (panels D and E) will be discussed
below.

Comparison of Effects of Procainamide on Action Potential
Duration and Local Refractory Periods in AMI and HMI Preparations

Representative illustrations of the effects of procainamide (PA) on transmembrane action potentials recorded from cells in an AMI ventricle and from
an HMI ventricle are shown in FIGURES 8 and 9, respectively. In both experiments, recordings from the normal and infarct zones were carried out simul-

taneously, and the impalements for these recordings were maintained throughout the experiments. In the AMI preparation (FIGURE 8), APD_{90} of the normal cell was 121 msec, compared with an APD_{90} of 100 msec in the AMI zone cell. After 45 minutes of exposure to procainamide (40 $\mu g/ml$), the APD_{90} of the cell in the normal zone increased 30 msec to 151 msec (+25%). At the same time, the APD_{90} of the cell in the AMI zone increased 62 msec to a duration of 162 msec (+62%). After a 90-minute period of wash with

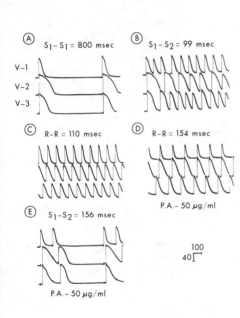

FIGURE 7. AMI superimposed on HMI. Panel **A** demonstrates three transmembrane action potentials recorded from ventricular muscle during stimulation of the preparation at a cycle length of 800 msec. V–1 is recorded from the site overlying acute myocardial infarction (AMI); V–2 is recorded from a surviving cell overlying a healed myocardial infarction (HMI); and V–3 is recorded from an endocardial cell in a normal zone. Drive stimuli and subsequent premature stimuli were delivered to a site overlying the AMI. In panel **B**, at an S_1–S_2 interval of 99 msec, S_2 initiates a response in the AMI zone that causes irregular activity through the preparation for a few seconds before stabilizing into a run of sustained ventricular activity (panel **C**) at a regular cycle length of 110 msec. In panel **D**, 15 minutes after introduction of procainamide (PA) to the system (approximately 10 minutes after procainamide reaches tissue bath), at a concentration of 50 $\mu g/ml$, the cycle length of inducible sustained ventricular activity has lengthened to 154 msec. Panel **E**, recorded after an additional 20 minutes of superfusion, demonstrates lengthening of the refractory period of the preparation to 156 msec. The inducibility of sustained ventricular activity has been lost at this point. *Calibration:* Vertical, 40 mV; horizontal, 100 msec. (Modified from Myerburg *et al.*[37])

Tyrode's solution, the APD_{90} of the normal cell shortened to 118 msec, 2% less than control value, while the APD_{90} of the cell from the AMI zone shortened to 135 msec, still longer than control, but 17 msec less than the duration at the time of maximal drug effect. Thirty minutes later the APD_{90} of the AMI cell had further shortened to 120 msec.

In contrast to those of the AMI preparation, the control recordings in the HMI preparation (FIGURE 9) demonstrated a longer APD_{90} recorded from

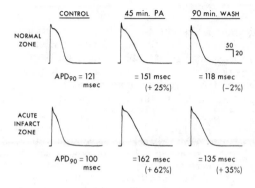

FIGURE 8. Effects of procainamide on transmembrane action potentials recorded from a 90-minute acute myocardial infarction (AMI) preparation. Simultaneous recordings of transmembrane action potentials from a normal zone cell and an AMI zone cell prior to superfusion with procainamide (PA) 45 minutes after beginning procainamide superfusion at 40 μg/ml, and after 90 minutes of washing with Tyrode's solution. The action potential durations printed under each transmembrane action potential were measured at 90% repolarization, and the percentages in parenthesis during and after procainamide superfusion represent percent change compared with control value for each recording. *Calibration:* horizontal, 50 msec; vertical 20 mV. (Modified from Myerburg *et al.*[38])

FIGURE 9. Effects of procainamide (PA) on transmembrane action potentials recorded from a 2-month-healed myocardial infarction (HMI) preparation. Simultaneous recordings of transmembrane action potentials from a normal cell and from a cell overlying an HMI area prior to superfusion with procainamide 45 minutes after beginning procainamide superfusion at 40 μg/ml, and after 90 minutes of washing with Tyrode's solution. Action potential durations under each transmembrane action potential were measured at 90% repolarization (APD$_{90}$) and the percentages in each parenthesis under the APD$_{90}$s indicate comparison during and after procainamide superfusion with control values for each recording. *Calibration:* horizontal, 50 msec; vertical, 20 mV. (Modified from Myerburg *et al.*[38])

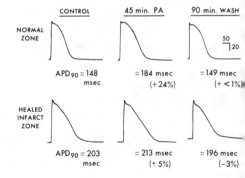

the cell within the HMI zone (203 msec) compared with that of the normal zone (148 msec). After 45 minutes of exposure to procainamide, the APD_{90} of the cell in the normal zone had increased by 36 msec to 184 msec (+24%). The percent increase is similar to that recorded from the normal cell in the AMI preparation. However, the cell in the HMI zone had an APD_{90} increase of only 10 msec, to 213 msec (+5%). After a 90-minute washing, both the control cell and the HMI cell had returned to nearly normal levels (+<1% and −3%, respectively). These two experiments demonstrate that in AMI and HMI preparations, relative and absolute changes in response to superfusion of procainamide differ in normal, AMI, and HMI tissues. APD_{90} of the AMI cell is shorter than normal prior to superfusion of procainamide, and the relative and absolute responses to procainamide are greater in the AMI cell than in the normal cell, decreasing the absolute differences in APD_{90} between ischemically injured and normal tissue. In contrast, in HMI preparations, the control APD_{90}s are longer in HMI cells than in normal cells, and the magnitude of the response to superfusion with procainamide is less in HMI cells than in normal cells, again decreasing the absolute differences between cells from the infarct zone and normal zone.

The cumulative data on absolute and relative change in APD_{90} at a drive-cycle length of 630 msec for the series of 14 AMI preparations and 17 HMI preparations are shown in FIGURE 10. Panel A shows a mean control APD_{90} of 136 ± 6 msec recorded from normal cells in the AMI cat hearts, and a mean control APD_{90} of 114 ± 4 msec recorded from cells in the infarct areas of the AMI hearts before superfusion with procainamide. The middle two pairs of bars demonstrate the response to superfusion with procainamide, 40 μg/ml, at 30 and 60 minutes, respectively. The data show that the APD_{90} of both the normal cells and acute infarct area cells is prolonged during superfusion with procainamide, but that the prolongation is greater in the AMI cells (mean = +40 msec or +35% at 60 min) than in the normal cells (mean = +30 msec or +22% at 60 min). In panel C, which is based on similar data recorded from HMI preparations, the control APD_{90}s recorded from cells in the HMI zone were longer than those recorded from normal zones, with the HMI cells having relatively less responsiveness than normal cells to procainamide at 30 and 60 minutes of superfusion. The percent change at 60 minutes of procainamide superfusion in *normal* cells was nearly identical in both AMI and HMI preparations (+22% versus +21%). However, the mean change for HMI cells (+19 msec or +13% at 60 min) was *less* than that of normal cells (+29 msec or +21%) (panel D) in contrast to the results in AMI preparations. The overall effect of these variations in responsiveness to procainamide is a tendency to make the absolute values of APD_{90} less disparate in the three types of tissue. In AMI preparations, mean APD_{90} *differences* between cells in the infarct zone and normal zone decreased from 22 msec before procainamide to 12 msec during procainamide administration (−45%). In HMI preparations, the mean differences decreased from 19 msec before to 11 msec during procainamide superfusion (−42%).

In the AMI preparations, the data were derived only from cells in which resting membrane potentials and upstroke velocities were maintained in the range of normal. The major effect of ischemia in these cells was shortening of the duration of repolarization. This selection process was carried out in order to have a population of AMI cells that had resting potential and upstroke velocity characteristics comparable to those of healed cells from HMI preparations.

Statistical analyses of APD_{90} changes were carried out using a two-tailed, two-sample t test. There was a small but significant difference in APD_{90} between normal cells in AMI preparations (mean $= 136 \pm 6$ msec) and normal cells in HMI preparations (mean $= 140 \pm 3$ msec) prior to procainamide superfusion (p $= 0.024$), but there were no significant differences between the two normal cell groups at 30 and 60 minutes of procainamide superfusion and at 30 and 60 minutes of wash in Tyrode's solution after

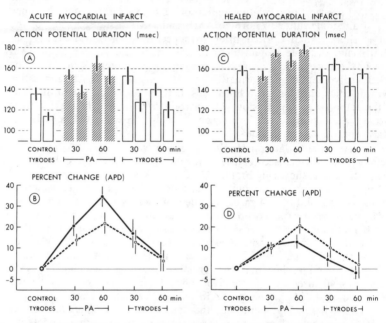

FIGURE 10. Cumulative data on the effects of procainamide on 14 AMI experiments and 17 HMI experiments. Panel **A** compares mean APD_{90} from AMI preparations, the left bar in each pair demonstrating data (mean±SD) from normal cells, and the right bar of each pair demonstrating data (mean±SD) from AMI cells. The *cross-hatched bars* depict the mean APDs for normal and AMI cells at 30 and 60 minutes of superfusion with procainamide (PA). Panel **B** demonstrates the percentage change in APD_{90} for AMI cells (*solid lines*) and normal cells (*dashed lines*). Panels **C** and **D** demonstrate the same information for HMI preparations. In panel **C** the left bar of each pair represents mean APD_{90} for normal cells and the right bar of each pair represents the data from surviving cells overlying HMI scars. Panel **D** shows percent change of APD_{90} with the *solid lines* representing HMI cells and the *dashed lines* normal cells. (Modified from Myerburg *et al.*[38])

superfusion. In contrast, the differences in APD_{90} between AMI cells and their controls, HMI cells and their controls, and AMI cells compared with HMI cells, were highly significant before procainamide superfusion, at 30 and 60 minutes of procainamide superfusion, and at 30 and 60 minutes of wash in Tyrode solution (p < 0.001). In all three comparisons, the t values were maximum before superfusion and minimum at 60 minutes of superfusion with procainamide, although the differences remained significant throughout the time courses of the experiments. By means of analysis of variance and co-variance, with repeated measures, it was determined that there was a significant differential between the response to procainamide of AMI cells compared with their controls, HMI cells compared with their controls, and AMI compared with HMI cells, throughout the overall time course of each group of studies. The results of these analyses suggest fundamental differences in both the quantitative and qualitative responses to procainamide of AMI cells, HMI cells, and normal cells.

It was possible to measure local refractory periods by premature stimulation in the region of the microelectrodes, recording action potentials from the AMI and HMI zones, and their respective controls, in 9 of the 14 AMI experiments and in 10 of the 17 HMI experiments. Local refractory periods paralleled APD_{90}s in both groups before superfusion of procainamide, while during superfusion there was a tendency for the relationship between APD_{90}s and local refractory periods of AMI cells to be more dissociated than in HMI cells. In the 9 AMI refractory period experiments, refractory periods of *normal* cells lengthened from a control value of 149 ± 17 msec to 178 ± 12 msec after 60 minutes of procainamide superfusion ($+19\%$). The ischemically injured cell's refractory periods lengthened from a mean of $126 + 11$ msec to 169 ± 21 msec after 60 minutes of superfusion ($+34\%$). In the 10 HMI refractory period experiments, the refractory period in normal cells lengthened from a mean control value of 151 ± 8 msec to 184 ± 13 msec after pro-cainamide superfusion ($+21\%$), while that of HMI cells lengthened from 165 ± 15 to 192 ± 20 msec ($+16\%$).

Delivery of Procainamide to HMI Cells During Superfusion

One possible explanation for the lesser responsiveness of HMI cells to superfusion with procainadide is failure of delivery of the test substance due to the interstitial fibrosis that occurs as a consequence of the ischemic injury.[27] We, therefore, compared the effects of procainamide and tetrodotoxin (TTX) on the same HMI cells in four experiments. Since the process of *de*polarization returns to normal after acute ischemic injury with healing, and the process of *re*polarization often shows persistent abnormalities manifested by prolongation of APD_{90}, we carried out these studies on the basis of the hypothesis that unimpaired superfusion of the superficial cells would result in similar effects of TTX on depolarization of both HMI and normal cells. FIGURE 11 demon-strates one of the four experiments carried out for this purpose. The left panel demonstrates the effect of procainamide on a cell from the normal zone and a cell from the HMI zone, the latter having a longer control APD_{90} (143 msec versus 177 msec). After superfusion with procainamide, 40 μg/ml for 30 minutes, the APD_{90} in the normal zone had increased by 31 msec or 22%, while that in the HMI cell had increased by 24 msec or 14%. Both values returned to within 1% of control after wash with drug-free Tyrode's solution. In both the cell from the normal zone and the cell from the HMI zone, there was little change in time from the stimulus to the response ($+3$ and -5 msec) during procainamide superfusion. The panel on the right shows the effects of TTX, 2 μg/ml, on the same cells after 90 minutes of superfusion with Tyrode's solution to wash out residual procainamide. Control action potential duration in the HMI cell again was longer than in the normal cell; and both cells showed

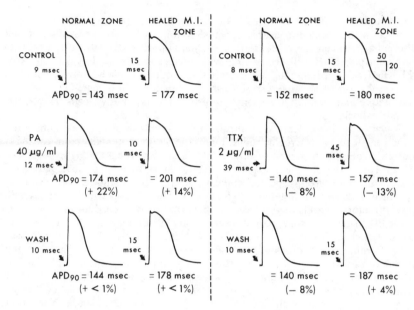

FIGURE 11. Comparison of effectiveness of procainamide (PA) and tetrodotoxin (TTX) on normal and HMI cells in 2-month-healed myocardial infarction. (*Left*) effects of procainamide, 40 μg/ml, on a cell from a normal zone and a cell from the HMI zone in an isolated preparation. The normal zone cell has a shorter control APD$_{90}$ and a greater percent response to procainamide. (*Right*) exposure of the same preparation to tetrodotoxin shows equivalent prolongation of conduction time from the stimulus site to the recording site in the cells in both the normal (+31 msec) and the HMI zone (+30 msec). These data suggest that delivery of test substances to the cell membranes is equivalent in a normal and an HMI zone, and that the differential response to procainamide is due to a membrane change rather than to impaired delivery. (From Myerburg *et al.*[38] Reproduced by permission.)

shortening of APD$_{90}$ after exposure to TTX for 20 minutes. In addition, both cells showed *equivalent prolongation of conduction time* from the site of stimulation to the recording microelectrode (+30 msec in the recording from the HMI cell, and +31 msec in the recording from the normal cell). Both values returned to control values after washing with Tyrode's solution for 60 minutes. Thus, equivalent effects of TTX were recorded on the normal zone cells and on the HMI zone cells in this and the other three experiments.

Effect of Procainamide on Inducibility of Sustained Ventricular Activity in HMI Ventricles

We had observed inducibility of sustained ventricular activity by premature stimulation of surviving subendocardial ventricular muscle cells overlying scars in isolated HMI ventricles,[36, 37] and we next evaluated the influence of superfusion with procainamide on inducibility.[38] In seven experiments, sustained ventricular activity in tissue bath was present before superfusion with procainamide and was not inducible during procainamide superfusion. In five of the seven experiments, inducibility returned after cession of superfusion. FIGURE 12 demonstrates a preparation in which superfusion with procainamide at a concentration of 25 μg/ml prevented the inducibility of sustained ventricular activity in an HMI ventricle. Prior to exposure to procainamide (top row of recordings), the cell from the HMI zone had a longer APD_{90} (123 msec) than the cell recorded from the normal zone (95 msec) at a driving cycle length of 630 msec. Sustained ventricular activity at a cycle length of 108 msec (middle panel, top row) was initiated by premature stimulation close to the refractory period of the HMI zone. The second row, recorded after exposure to procainamide at a concentration of 25 μg/ml for 30 minutes, shows only a 12 msec prolongation of the APD_{90} of the cell recorded from the HMI zone (from 123 to 135 msec), but an 80 msec prolongation of the APD_{90} of the cell recorded from the normal zone (from 95 to 175 msec). At this time, S_2 resulted in repetitive ventricular responses (RVR), but no sustained activity could be induced. The third row shows that 5 minutes after procainamide superfusion was stopped, no sustained activity was inducible, but an RVR again

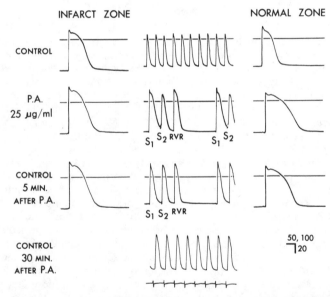

FIGURE 12. Effect of procainamide on transmembrane action potentials and response to premature stimulation in a healed myocardial infarction preparation. The *left* column demonstrates the response of cells in the HMI zone to procainamide (PA), 25 μg/ml; and the *right* column shows its effects on a cell in the normal zone. The *center* column demonstrates the response to premature stimulation close to the refractory period before, during, and after superfusion with procainamide. Prolongation of APD_{90} during exposure to procainamide is much greater in the cell from the normal zone than from the HMI zone; and in addition, the ability to induce sustained ventricular activity disappears during superfusion with procainamide and reappears after washing. Repetitive ventricular responses (RVR) still occur during superfusion with procainamide, however. See text for further details. (From Myerburg *et al.*[38] Reproduced by permission.)

occurred. The APD_{90} of the HMI cell had shortened to 130 msec and that of the normal cell to 151 msec. The bottom panel shows that 30 minutes after cessation of procainamide superfusion, sustained ventricular activity was again inducible. Thus, the greater relative and absolute effects of procainamide on APD_{90} of *normal* cells, compared with its effects on HMI cells, occurred in parallel with loss of inducibility of sustained ventricular activity.

Panels D and E of FIGURE 7 demonstrate the effects of superfusion of procainamide (50 μg/ml) on an AMI/HMI preparation. Sustained ventricular activity still was inducible after 10 minutes of superfusion, but the cycle length had increased to 154 msec (panel D). After 30 minutes of superfusion, the shortest S_1–S_2 interval achievable in the preparation was 156 msec (panel E), and sustained ventricular activity could not be reinduced. The *two effects* of procainamide on this preparation (*a direct slowing of conduction in the reentrant circuit, thereby increasing the cycle length from 110 to 154 msec; and prolongation and decreased dispersion of refractory periods so as to interfere with inducibility of sustained ventricular activity*) were representative of the effects in the nine other preparations in which these studies were carried out.

DISCUSSION

Considerable information has been accumulated on the electrophysiologic properties of experimental acute myocardial infarction in both anesthetized [2-16] and conscious [17, 30] animals, and on the actively healing myocardial infarction studied up to 5 to 10 days after coronary arterial ligation.[18-23] Less information has been available on the cardiac electrophysiologic characteristics of animals that have survived experimental myocardial infarction and the infarct allowed sufficient time to heal completely.[24, 25, 27, 30] Nor is there much information on the interaction of the acutely ischemic tissue and tissue healed after ischemic injury.[30, 36-38]

We have reported the development of an experimental myocardial infarction preparation which maintains electrophysiologic abnormalities for at least 6 months after healing,[26-29] and other investigators also have reported techniques that induce spontaneous or inducible arrhythmogenesis after complete healing of myocardial infarction.[24, 25, 30] We have recently reported our observations on the correlation of spontaneous arrhythmias *in situ* with findings in isolated tissue bath of AMI and HMI preparations, and we have compared these observations with those in preparations in which acute ischemia is superimposed upon healed infarction (AMI/HMI).[37] The early cellular electrophysiologic changes that we observed in the AMI preparations are similar to those reported by other investigators, and serve, along with findings in normal cats, as one form of control for the present studies. It is significant that the cells that overlie healed myocardial infarction scars on the endocardial surface, which we know from the AMI studies were exposed to ischemic injury during the period of time shortly after coronary ligation, have abnormal action potential characteristics. The persistent abnormalities occur predominantly during the period of repolarization. The AMI cells have APD_{90}s that are shorter than normal, while the HMI cells overlying an infarct scar have APD_{90}s that are longer than normal. The combination of acute injury and healed infarction produces populations of cells with a very wide dispersion of action potential durations and corresponding dispersions of local refractory periods. The latter theoretically should produce the most unstable form of preparation on the basis of previous observations by Han and coworkers.[39, 40] As shown in TABLES 1 and 2 and FIGURE 7, the AMI/HMI preparations had the most predictable tendency towards spontaneous arrhythmogenesis and ability for sustained ventricular activity to be initiated in tissue bath. *We consider this observation on the AMI/HMI preparation particularly intriguing because spontaneous potentially lethal arrhythmias in man, whether or not occurring in the presence of an acute myocardial infarction, tend to occur in individuals who have evidence of preexisting ischemic injury with healing, and presumption or evidence of transient or recent acute ischemia.* This model, and the electrophysiologic characteristics that we have observed, parallel the pathologic setting in which clinical potentially lethal arrhythmias occur in man.

The requirement for stimulation at selected sites in surviving tissue overlying HMI scars in order to initiate sustained ventricular activity in isolated hearts is consistent with recent data reported by Michelson *et al.*[41] These investigators demonstrated that the greatest success rate for initiating sustained ventricular tachycardia in *in situ* hearts studied 3 to 30 days after myocardial infarction occurred with stimulation of tissue within 2 cm of the myocardial infarct. Attempts at stimulation of more distant sites were less successful.

The mechanism underlying prolongation of action potential duration in cells overlying healed areas of myocardial infarction has not yet been elucidated. The possibilities include changes in ionic movements across membranes that are irreversibly injured as a consequence of the ischemic injury, uncoupling of the endocardial cells from underlying cells in these preparations, or permutations of the two factors. Data showing decreased responsiveness of the surviving cells overlying HMIs during exposure to membrane-active antiarrhythmic agents during superfusion in tissue bath [38] suggest the possibility of a membrane abnormality rather than uncoupling as the underlying mechanism. However, further studies are needed to validate this hypothesis.

Evaluation of the effects of antiarrhythmic agents on the cellular electrophysiology of this model has been a natural extension of the initial studies. Most prior studies of drug effects on experimental models have focused on acutely ischemic or early healing tissue.[42-55] The data presented herein demonstrate different effects of a membrane-active antiarrhythmic agent (procainamide) on acutely injured ventricular muscle cells compared with cells that have survived prior injury and overlie the scar of a healed myocardial infarction. The experiments demonstrating comparable delivery of another test substance (TTX) to the healed myocardial infarct and to the normal zone indicate that the differences are due to true abnormalities in the process of repolarization rather than to failure of delivery of test substances due to interstitial fibrosis between surviving cells in the HMI preparations.

Since it is common in clinical settings to have coexistence of tissue that has healed after ischemic injury and superimposed acute ischemia, the tendency for procainamide to show a greater prolonging effect on the short action potential durations of AMIs and a lesser prolonging effect on the longer action potential durations of HMIs, with resultant tendency towards more uniformity of action potential duration, is a theoretically desirable effect. This may explain, in part, its stabilizing influence on arrhythmias. Han and coworkers [39, 40] have demonstrated the importance of dispersion of action potential durations and refractory periods in arrhythmogenesis. The data in our current studies suggest that procainamide theoretically has the capability of decreasing dispersion in a setting in which there is bidirectional deviation of APD_{90} and local refractory periods during the coexistence of acute ischemia and healed myocardial infarction. Our observations on the effect of procainamide on inducible sustained ventricular activity in isolated AMI/HMI ventricles (FIG. 7) provide some support for this theoretical consideration. Exposure to procainamide did in fact decrease the dispersion of APD_{90}s and refractoriness between normal, AMI, and HMI cells in these preparations, and this was associated with the loss of the ability to induce sustained ventricular activity (FIG. 7, panels D and E). Procainamide appeared to slow conduction in the presumed reentrant circuit (prolonged cycle length of sustained ventricular activity) before prolonging refractory periods to the point where sustained ventricular activity could no longer be induced. *Several of our other experiments* (FIG. 12) *also suggested that the experimental antiarrhythmic effects of procainamide may be two-fold: (1) prolongation of refractory periods, resulting in loss of ability to induce sustained activity by premature stimulation; and (2) slowing of established sustained ventricular activity, presumably due to a change in refractory period and/or conduction properties in reentrant circuits. The two interdependent effects may explain some observations on dissociation of effects of membrane-active drugs on various forms of clinical arrhythmias.*[56, 57]

Finally, the observation that effects of procainamide on normal tissue are greater than on surviving tissue from infarct zones in HMI preparations may be of fundamental importance to concepts of experimental cardiac electropharmacology. In recent years less attention has been paid to the cellular electrophysiologic effects of membrane-active drugs on normal tissue because it has been hypothesized that significant drug effects must be on abnormal tissue and that these might differ qualitatively from effects on normal tissue. Our data support the latter point, but also suggest that effects of drugs on normal tissue might be an important influence against sustained ventricular activity.

REFERENCES

1. HARRIS, A. S. 1950. Delayed development of ventricular ectopic rhythms following experimental coronary occlusion. Circulation 1:1318–1328.
2. SCHERLAG, B. J., R. H. HELFANT, J. I. HAFT & A. M. DAMATO. 1970. Electrophysiology underlying ventricular arrhythmias due to coronary ligation. Am. J. Physiol. 219:1665–1671.
3. FRIEDMAN, P. L., J. R. STEWART, J. J. FENOGLIO & A. L. WIT. 1973. Survival of endocardial Purkinje fibers after extensive myocardial infarction in dogs. Circ. Res. 33:597–611.
4. FRIEDMAN, P. L., J. R. STEWART & A. L. WIT. 1973. Spontaneous and induced cardiac arrhythmias in subendocardial Purkinje fibers surviving extensive myocardial infarction in dogs. Circ. Res. 33:612–662.
5. LAZZARA, R., N. EL-SHERIF & B. J. SCHERLAG. 1973. Electrophysiological properties of canine Purkinje cells in one-day old myocardial infarction. Circ. Res. 33:722–734.
6. BOINEAU, J. P. & J. L. COX. 1973. Slow ventricular activation in acute myocardial infarction: A source of re-entrant premature ventricular contraction. Circulation 48:702–713.
7. WALDO, A. L. & G. A. KAISER. 1973. A study of ventricular arrhythmias associated with acute myocardial infarction in the canine heart. Circulation 47:1222–1228.

8. SCHERLAG, B. J., N. EL-SHERIF, R. R. HOPE & R. LAZZARA. 1974. Characterization and localization of ventricular arrhythmias resulting from myocardial ischemia and infarction. Circ. Res. **35**:373–383.

9. LAZZARA, R., N. EL-SHERIF & B. J. SCHERLAG. 1974. Early and late effects of coronary occlusion on canine Purkinje fibers. Circ. Res. **35**:391–399.

10. WILLIAMS, D. O., B. J. SCHERLAG, R. R. HOPE, N. EL-SHERIF & R. LAZZARA. 1974. The pathophysiology of malignant ventricular arrhythmias during acute myocardial ischemia. Circulation **50**:1163–1172.

11. FRIEDMAN, P. L., J. J. FENOGLIO & A. L. WIT. 1975. Time course of reversal of electrophysiological and ultrastructural abnormalities in subendocardial Purkinje fibers surviving extensive myocardial infarction in dogs. Circ. Res. **36**:127–144.

12. FENOGLIO, J. J., A. ALBALA, F. G. SILVA, P. L. FRIEDMAN & A. L. WIT. 1976. Structural basis of ventricular arrhythmias in human myocardial infarction: A hypothesis. Human Pathol. **7**:547–563.

13. HOROWITZ, L. N., J. R. SPEAR & E. N. MOORE. 1976. Subendocardial origin of ventricular arrhythmias in 24-hour old experimental myocardial infarction. Circulation **53**:56–63.

14. DOWNAR, E., M. J. JANSE & D. DURRER. 1977. The effect of acute coronary occlusion on subepicardial transmembrane potentials in the intact porcine heart. Circulation **56**:217–224.

15. KAPLINSKY, E., S. OGAWA, W. BALKE & L. S. DREIFUS. 1979. Two periods of early ventricular arrhythmia in the canine acute myocardial infarction model. Circulation **60**:397–403.

16. KAPLINSKY, E., S. OGAWA & L. S. DREIFUS. 1978. Central role of subendocardial activation in the genesis of malignant ventricular tachycardia and fibrillation. Am. J. Cardiol. **41**:427.

17. STEWART, J. R., J. K. GIBSON, B. PITT & B. R. LUCHESE. 1979. Post-infarction arrhythmias in the conscious dog: Electrophysiologic observations. Circulation **60**(Suppl. III):115.

18. EL-SHERIF, N., B. J. SCHERLAG, R. LAZZARA & R. R. HOPE. 1977. Re-entrant ventricular arrhythmias in the late myocardial infarction. 1. Conduction characteristics in the infarction zone. Circulation **55**:686–701.

19. EL-SHERIF, N., B. J. SCHERLAG, R. LAZZARA & R. R. HOPE. 1977. Re-entrant ventricular arrhythmias in the late myocardial infarction. 2. Patterns of initiation and termination of re-entry. Circulation **55**:702–719.

20. EL-SHERIF, N., R. LAZZARA, R. R. HOPE & B. J. SCHERLAG. 1977. Re-entrant ventricular arrhythmias in the late myocardial infarction period. 3. Manifest and concealed extrasystolic grouping. Circulation **56**:225–234.

21. EL-SHERIF, N. 1978. Re-entrant ventricular arrhythmias in the late myocardial infarction period. 6. Effect of the autonomic system. Circulation **58**:103–110.

22. EL-SHERIF, N. & R. LAZZARA. 1979. Re-entrant ventricular arrhythmias in the late myocardial infarction period. 7. Effect of verapamil and D–600 and the role of the "slow channel". Circulation **60**:605–615.

23. KARAGUEUZIAN, H. S., J. J. FENOGLIO, B. F. HOFFMAN & A. L. WIT. 1977. Sustained ventricular tachycardia induced by electrical stimulation after myocardial infarction. Circulation **56**(Suppl. III):79.

24. SPEAR, J. F., E. L. MICHELSON & E. N. MOORE. 1979. Excitability of cells within a mottled infarct of dogs susceptible to sustained ventricular tachyarrhythmias. Circulation **60**(Suppl. III):158.

25. KLEIN, G. J., R. E. IDELSER, W. M. SMITH, L. A. HARRISON, J. KASELL, A. G. WALLACE & J. J. GALLAGHER. 1979. Epicardial mapping of the onset of ventricular tachycardia initiated by programmed stimulation in the canine heart with chronic infarction. Circulation **60**:1375–1384.

26. MYERBURG, R. J., H. GELBAND, K. NILSSON, R. J. SUNG, R. J. THURER, A. R. MORALES & A. L. BASSETT. 1976. Long-term electrophysiologic abnormali-

ties resulting from experimental myocardial infarction. Circulation 54(Suppl. II):17.

27. MYERBURG, R. J., H. GELBAND, K. NILSSON, R. J. SUNG, R. J. THURER, A. R. MORALES & A. L. BASSETT. 1977. Long-term electrophysiologic abnormalities resulting from experimental myocardial infarction in cats. Circ. Res. 41: 73–84.

28. BASSETT, A. L., H. GELBAND, K. NILSSON, A. R. MORALES & R. J. MYERBURG. 1977. Electrophysiology following healed experimental myocardial infarction. In Proceedings of International Conference on Re-entrant Arrhythmias. :242–255. MTP Press. Lancaster.

29. BASSETT, A. L., R. J. MYERBURG, K. NILSSON & H. GELBAND. 1978. Characterization of persistent membrane abnormalities in ventricular cells surviving myocardial infarction. Proc. Int. Union Physiol. Sci. 13:58.

30. SCHWARTZ, P. J. & H. L. STONE. 1980. Left stellectomy in the prevention of ventricular fibrillation due to acute myocardial ischemia in conscious dogs with an anterior myocardial infarction. Circulation 62:1256–1265.

31. MYERBURG, R. J., K. NILSSON & H. GELBAND. 1972. The physiology of canine intraventricular conduction and endocardial excitation. Circ. Res. 30:217–243.

32. MYERBURG, R. J., J. W. STEWART & B. F. HOFFMAN. 1970. Electrophysiologic properties of the canine peripheral A-V conducting system. Circ. Res. 26: 361–378.

33. MYERBURG, R. J., J. W. STEWART, S. M. ROSS & B. F. HOFFMAN. 1970. On-line measurements of the duration of cardiac action potentials and refractory periods. J. Appl. Physiol. 28:92–93.

34. GELBAND, H., R. J. MYERBURG, S. M. ROSS & B. F. HOFFMAN. 1970. Digital monitoring of cardiac transmembrane potential characteristics. J. Appl. Physiol. 29:894.

35. MYERBURG, R. J., K. NILSSON, B. BEFELER, A. CASTELLANOS & H. GELBAND. 1973. Transverse spread and longitudinal dissociation in the distal A-V conducting system. J. Clin. Invest. 52:885–895.

36. MYERBURG, R. J., A. L. BASSETT, K. NILSSON, A. CASTELLANOS, R. J. SUNG & H. GELBAND. 1978. Electrophysiologic interactions between acute ischemia and healed experimental myocardial infarctions in cats. Am. J. Cardiol. 41: 365.

37. MYERBURG, R. J., K. EPSTEIN, M. S. GAIDE, S. S. WONG, A. CASTELLANOS H. GELBAND & A. L. BASSETT. Electrophysiologic consequences of experimental acute ischemia superimposed upon healed myocardial infarction in cats. Am. J. Cardiol. In press.

38. MYERBURG, R. J., A. L. BASSETT, K. EPSTEIN, M. S. GAIDE, P. KOZLOVSKIS, S. S. WONG, A. CASTELLANOS & H. GELBAND. Electrophysiologic effects of procainamide in acute and healed experimental ischemic injury of cat myocardium. Circ. Res. In press.

39. HAN, J. & G. K. MOE. 1964. Non-uniform recovery of excitability in ventricular muscle. Circ. Res. 14:44–60.

40. HAN, J. 1961. Ventricular vulnerability during acute coronary occlusion. Am. J. Cardiol. 24:857–864.

41. MICHELSON, E. L., J. F. SPEAR & E. N. MOORE. 1981. Initiation of sustained ventricular tachyarrhythmias in a canine model of chronic myocardial infarction: Importance of the site of stimulation. Circulation 63:776–784.

42. ALLEN, J. D., F. J. BRENNAN & A. L. WIT. 1978. Actions of lidocaine on transmembrane potentials of subendocardial Purkinje fibers surviving infarcted canine hearts. Circ. Res. 43:470–481.

43. BRENNAN, F. J. & A. L. WIT. 1973. Effects of lidocaine on electrophysiological properties of Purkinje fibers surviving acute myocardial infarction. Circulation 48:149.

44. BRENNAN, F. J., P. F. CRANEFIELD & A. L. WIT. Effects of lidocaine on slow

response and depressed fast response action potentials of canine cardiac Purkinje fibers. J Pharmacol. Exp. Ther. **294:**312–324.

45. CARDINAL, R. & B. I. SASYNIUK. 1978. Electrophysiological effects of bretylium tosylate on subendocardial Purkinje fibers from infarcted canine hearts. J. Pharmacol. Exp. Ther. **204:**159–174.

46. EL-SHERIF, N., B. J. SCHERLAG, R. LAZZARA & R. R. HOPE. 1977. Re-entrant ventricular arrhythmias in the late myocardial infarction period. 4. Mechanism of action of lidocaine. Circulation **56:**395–402.

47. EL-SHERIF, N. & R. LAZARRA. 1978. Re-entrant ventricular arrhythmias in the late myocardial infarction period. 5. Mechanism of action of diphenylhydantoin. Circulation **57:**465–472.

48. HONDEGHEM, L. M., A. O. GRANT & R. A. JENSEN. 1974. Antiarrhythmic drug action: Selective depression of hypoxic cells. Am. Heart J. **87:**602–605.

49. KUPERSMITH, J., E. M. ANTMAN & B. F. HOFFMAN. 1975. In vivo electrophysiological effects of lidocaine in canine acute myocardial infarction. Circ. Res. **36:**84–91.

50. KUS, T. & B. I. SASYNIUK. 1975. Modification by disopyramide phosphate (DP) of the electrophysiological characteristics of canine subendocardial Purkinje fibers surviving infarction. Proc. Can. Fed. Biol. Soc. **18:**74, 1975

51. LAZZARA, R., R. R. HOPE, N. EL-SHERIF & B. J. SCHERLAG. 1978. Effects of lidocaine on hypoxic and ischemic cardiac cells. Am. J. Cardiol. **41:**872–879.

52. SASYNIUK, B. I. & T. KUS. 1973. Alterations in electrophysiological properties of cells from infarcted ventricular tissue. Pharmacologist **15:**178.

53. GUSE, P. A., M. S. GAIDE, R. J. MYERBURG, K. EPSTEIN, H. GELBAND & A. L. BASSETT. 1980. Electrophysiological effects of alprenolol on depressed canine myocardium. Cardiovasc. Res. **14:**654–660.

54. SASYNIUK, B. I. & T. KUS. 1974. Comparison of the effect of lidocaine on electrophysiological properties of normal Purkinje fibers and those surviving acute myocardial infarction. Fed. Proc. **33:**476.

55. WANG, C. M., C. A. JAMES & R. A. MAXWELL. 1979. Effects of lidocaine on the electrophysiological properties of subendocardial Purkinje fibers surviving acute myocardial infarction. J. Mol. Cell. Cardiol. **11:**669–681.

56. MYERBURG, R. J., CONDE, C., SHEPS, D. S., APPEL, R. A., KIEM, I., SUNG, R. J. & A. CASTELLANOS. 1979. Antiarrhythmic drug therapy in survivors of pre-hospital cardiac arrest: Comparison of effects on chronic ventricular arrhythmias and recurrent cardiac arrest. Circulation **59:**855–863.

57. MYERBURG, R. J., K. M. KESSLER, I. KIEM, K. C. PEFKAROS, C. A. CONDE, D. COOPER & A. CASTELLANOS. 1981. The relationship between plasma levels of procainamide, suppression of premature ventricular contractions, and prevention of recurrent ventricular tachycardia. Circulation **64:** 280–290.

DISCUSSION

DR. KASTOR: In your excellent model you keep referring to repetitive ventricular activity. Are you avoiding using the term tachycardia for some reason?

DR. MYERBURG: I don't like to use the term ventricular tachycardia for isolated preparations in tissue bath; it just doesn't seem pure enough. I'm trying to find a term that will not be confusing; I don't think that we can make the jump from ventricular tachycardia with an intact ventricle to a piece of tissue sitting flat in tissue bath in which we're inducing sustained activity. I hope that the situation is analagous, but I don't know.

DR. P. J. SCHWARTZ: I would like to know something more about those nine cats in which you obtained spontaneous ventricular fibrillation by the superimposition of acute myocardial ischemia. Did the acute myocardial ischemia last for about 120 minutes?

DR. MYERBURG: That's what I said, but let me amplify that. The experimental design was to wait 90 to 120 minutes before terminating the experiments. However, six of the nine had fibrillation in less than 90 minutes and three of the nine had fibrillation between 90 and 120 minutes.

DR. SCHWARTZ: What kind of acute myocardial ischemia did you produce?

DR. MYERBURG: We ligated the left ventral artery, between 5 and 10 mm proximal to the original ligation. Where it wasn't feasible, we went to the circumflex artery.

DR. SCHWARTZ: What kind of anesthesia do you use?

DR. MYERBURG: For those preparations we used Pentothal; when we were monitoring for the arrhythmias we used chloralose.

DR. SCHWARTZ: This makes a difference because of a differential effect on vagal outflow, of course. What was the level of blood pressure just preceding onset of ventricular fibrillation?

DR. MYERBURG: Blood pressure remained stable throughout the experiment because the infarct was never large enough for it to cause low output. We were careful about that because we didn't want the left ventricular dynamics to become a confounding influence.

DR. LUCCHESI (*University of Michigan, Ann Arbor, Michigan*): Dr. Myerburg has brought up the very important matter of drug delivery to the site of abnormal activity. Recently, using programmed electrical stimulation in the conscious dog with previous myocardial injury, we have noted with most of the antiarrhythmic drugs, such as disopyramide or lidocaine, that an animal that was previously nonprogrammable can now be programmed for the first time. Other researchers have seen the same phenomenon in human subjects. In order to abolish programmed electrical stimulation, many times we have to use extremely high serum concentrations of the drug. In your studies, Dr. Myerburg, you used about 25 to 50 μg/ml of procainamide. Taking into consideration plasma protein binding, which does not occur in the organ bath in Dr. Myerburg's experiments, we're talking about even higher concentrations relative to man. So, Dr. Myerburg, would such concentrations be possible in man over the long term?

DR. MYERBURG: I don't think that you can make that transition. If you look for drug effects at a cellular level with quinidine rather than procainamide in tissue bath you can work in the same range or perhaps slightly higher than you do clinically. In contrast, with procainamide, in the range of 8 to 12 μg/ml, you are not going to see much in terms of equivalent electrophysiologic changes. I don't know the reason for this and I can't find anyone who does; I've been asking this question for a long time. In order to work with procainamide in tissue bath you have to increase the dosage to 40 to 70 μg/ml. In order to get unexcitability, you sometimes have to go to 150 μg/ml. I don't know the reason for this or what the difference is, but I don't consider this equivalent to a clinical setting in terms of drug concentrations, particularly with procainamide. I wish somebody could give me a clue as to why there is a very real difference and why it seems to be specific for procainamide.

DR. CRAMPTON: Dr. Myerburg, you've shown some very interesting heterogeneity in the behavior of the cells and also in their response to procainamide. Did you observe any heterogeneity in velocity of upstroke in resting potentials? In other words, were these all depressed fast responses or are we looking at some induced slow responses? If so, were they slow responses, depressed fast responses, or fast responses and slow responses? How would you characterize them?

DR. MYERBURG: Let me briefly summarize what we've done in regard to that problem. In the healed myocardial infarction preparation, those cells that survive and are in the center of the endocardial surface over the infarct scar have normal upstroke velocities and resting potentials. But around the border of the infarct there are some very interesting action potential changes that we are in the process of analyzing.

In terms of the acute experiments there is a different problem. You cannot compare a cell markedly depressed by drugs to the action potential changes that we see in chronic cells, which have good upstroke velocities in their resting potentials. Those cells that haven't died are like the border zone cells and have very strange action potentials and low resting potentials, that is, very slow upstroke velocities. They are not included in this analysis. If you do include them, then you don't have something that is comparable to the upstroke velocity and resting potential of the healed myocardial infarction. Most of the abnormal cells are probably depressed fast responses, but some slow responses are also present.

To answer the question you asked regarding the cells that we are talking about, there are no differences in upstroke velocity, but that is by selection.

MECHANISMS IN THE GENESIS OF RECURRENT VENTRICULAR TACHYARRHYTHMIAS AS REVEALED BY CLINICAL ELECTROPHYSIOLOGIC STUDIES

Leonard N. Horowitz,* Scott R. Spielman,† Allan M. Greenspan,†
and Mark E. Josephson ‡

Clinical Electrophysiology Laboratory
Hospital of the University of Pennsylvania, and
Cardiovascular Section
Department of Medicine
University of Pennsylvania School of Medicine
Philadelphia, Pennsylvania 19104

Sudden cardiac death has been presumed to be caused primarily by ventricular tachycardia and ventricular fibrillation.[1-4] Study of the mechanism of these tachyarrhythmias in man, however, has been limited. The development of intracardiac electrophysiologic techniques for evaluation of ventricular tachyarrhythmias in man and the availability of a large population of survivors of cardiac arrest have now made such studies possible. A more precise understanding of the mechanisms of these tachyarrhythmias may lead to more accurate techniques for predicting vulnerability in individual patients and more specific therapies. The data presented in this report were obtained during electrophysiologic studies performed to define therapeutic regimens in patients who survived out-of-hospital cardiac arrest and were at high risk for recurrence.

PATIENT POPULATION AND METHODS

Electrophysiologic studies were performed in 59 patients who had been resuscitated from out-of-hospital cardiac arrest. The entry criteria into this study included: (1) the absence of symptoms compatible with acute myocardial infarction or angina at the time of cardiac arrest; (2) absence of evidence of acute myocardial infarction in the immediate post-arrest period; (3) absence of severe hemodynamic impairment (hypotension, low output state, etc.) or immediately life-threatening arrhythmias requiring acute antiarrhythmic therapy during the interval between cardiac arrest and the electrophysiologic study (at least 48 hours); (4) the absence of an identifiable and correctable cause of the cardiac arrest (such as drug toxicity or electrolyte disturbance); (5) written, informed consent. Acute myocardial infarction was diagnosed by the presence

* Recipient of Young Investigator Award from the National Heart, Blood, and Lung Institute. Present address and address for correspondence: Likoff Cardiovascular Institute, Hahnemann Medical College & Hospital, Philadelphia, Pennsylvania 19102.

† Present address: Likoff Cardiovascular Institute.

‡ Recipient of Research Career Development Award from the National Heart, Lung, and Blood Institute.

0077-8923/82/0382-0116 $01.75/0 © 1982, NYAS

of at least two of the following criteria: (1) new diagnostic Q waves; (2) a rise in cardiac enzyme levels to 150 percent or greater than normal with classic enzyme patterns; and (3) typical symptoms of prolonged ischemic pain and persistent T wave inversions. All patients underwent 48 hours or more of continuous computer-assisted electrocardiographic monitoring prior to study.

The patient population included 44 men and 15 women whose ages ranged from 18 to 75 years. Fifty-four patients had structural heart disease. Forty-six of these patients had coronary artery disease and 37 had sustained a previous myocardial infarction.

Electrophysiologic studies were performed in the postabsorptive state. All antiarrhythmic medications had been discontinued for more than five half-lives prior to study and plasma concentrations of the drugs at the time of study were below routinely measurable levels by standard laboratory techniques. Clinical status was stable and electrolyte measurements were normal and stable. During the study no patient exhibited clinical or electrocardiographic evidence of acute myocardial ischemia.

Two to four electrode catheters were inserted percutaneously or by cutdown and positioned in the heart under fluoroscopic guidance. In each patient, a catheter was positioned in the right ventricular apex. In selected patients, catheters were positioned in the coronary sinus, right ventricular outflow tract, and left ventricle. Standard quadripolar catheters (10-mm interelectrode distance) were used when recording and stimulation at the same site were required. Stimulation was performed using a specially designed programmable stimulator and optically isolated constant current source. The stimuli were 1-msec rectangular pulses with current intensity of 0.5 to 2.5 mA, but in each patient did not exceed twice diastolic threshold. Leakage current was carefully monitored and never exceeded 6 μA.

The protocol of programmed stimulation included: (1) atrial pacing at decremental cycle lengths (600–250 msec); (2) premature atrial stimulation during normal sinus rhythm and/or atrial pacing at several drive-cycle lengths; (3) ventricular pacing at decremental cycle lengths (600–250 msec); (4) premature ventricular stimulation during normal sinus rhythm and/or ventricular pacing at several drive-cycle lengths; (5) atrial and/or ventricular pacing and programmed atrial and/or ventricular stimulation during induced ventricular tachyarrhythmias whenever feasible. Single and double premature extrastimuli were used in all patients, and in 10 patients triple extrastimuli were used. The protocol of the scanning with multiple extrastimuli has been previously described.[5] Stimulation was performed at the right ventricular apex in all patients. In each patient in whom no ventricular tachyarrhythmia was induced by right ventricular stimulation, the stimulation protocol was repeated in the left ventricle.

After base-line studies, either procainamide (1–2 g at a rate of 50 mg per minute) or quinidine (600–1200 mg at a rate of 20 mg per minute) was infused intravenously and programmed stimulation was repeated.

Whenever cardioversion was required, it was accomplished within 10 seconds of loss of consciousness and in no case were neurologic or cardiac sequelae observed.

Intracardiac recordings were filtered at 30–500 Hz and displayed simultaneously with two or three electrocardiographic leads and 10-msec time lines on an oscillographic recorder (Electronics for Medicine, VR-16). Analog data were displayed on a spray ink recorder (Mingograf) for real-time analysis.

All data were stored on magnetic analog tape and the data retrieved on photographic paper at speeds of 75–200 mm/sec for illustrative purposes.

RESULTS

Sustained Ventricular Tachycardia: Initiation and Termination

Sustained ventricular tachycardia (VT) was initiated by programmed stimulation in 23 patients. The electrocardiogram at the time of resuscitation in these patients showed VT in 8 patients and ventricular fibrillation (VF) in 15 patients. Induction of VT was accomplished by a single premature stimulus in 5 patients, double premature stimuli in 16 patients and triple premature stimuli in 2 patients (FIG. 1). Ventricular tachycardia was initiated by right ventricular stimulation in 21 patients, but required left ventricular stimulation in 2 additional patients. Initiation was reproducible in each patient.

In eleven patients, VT could be terminated by programmed stimulation during the control state. Termination was accomplished by premature extrastimuli in three patients and rapid ventricular pacing in eight patients. In 12 patients VT produced prompt hemodynamic collapse and required immediate termination by cardioversion. In 10 of these latter patients in whom cardioversion had initially been required, the VT could be terminated by programmed stimulation after administration of procainamide or quinidine. The procainamide or quinidine typically increased the ventricular tachycardia cycle length, thus ameliorating the symptoms, but did not change the QRS morphologic pattern of the tachycardia. Ventricular tachycardia was terminated by programmed stimulation during either the control study or after antiarrhythmic drug administration in a total of 21 of the 23 patients.

Observations During Ventricular Tachycardia

Fragmented systolic and diastolic electrical activity or continuous fragmented electrical activity were observed at the area of origin of VT during the arrhythmia in 11 patients. Initiation and maintenance of the tachycardia were shown to be dependent upon this fragmented activity in each of these cases (FIG. 1).

In four patients, ventricular tachycardia spontaneously degenerated into ventricular fibrillation. In three, VF had been recorded at the time of resuscitation from out-of-hospital cardiac arrest. In these four patients, the onset of VF was preceded by spontaneous acceleration of the VT. During this acceleration, ventricular electrograms recorded at individual sites revealed disorganization and independent fibrillatory activity. When most or all of the ventricular electrograms showed local fibrillatory activity, the surface electrocardiographic pattern was that of typical ventricular fibrillation (FIG. 2).

Torsade de Pointes: Initiation and Termination

Torsade de pointes (TdP) was initiated by programmed electrical stimulation in 10 patients. The electrocardiogram at the time of resuscitation showed ventricular fibrillation in all 10 patients. Induction of TdP required a single extrastimulus in one patient and two extrastimuli in the other nine. Torsade de pointes was initiated by right ventricular pacing in nine patients and required

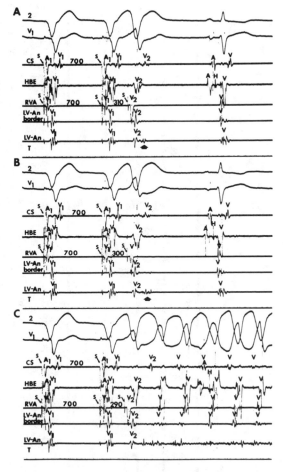

FIGURE 1. Initiation of ventricular tachycardia by programmed stimulation. In each panel, electrocardiographic leads II and V_1 are shown with electrograms recorded in the coronary sinus (CS), His bundle area (HBE), right venticular apex (RVA) at the border of a left ventricular aneurysm (LV-AN border), and within a left ventricular aneurysm (LV-An). Right ventricular pacing at a cycle length of 700 msec was performed as indicated by the stimulus artifact(s). In panel **A**, a premature extrastimulus was delivered at a cycle length of 310 msec. A single response occurred, and fragmentation noted during pacing and normal sinus rhythm in the LV-An electrogram increased (*broad solid arrow*). In panel **B**, the premature extrastimulus was delivered at a coupling interval of 300 msec and again a single response occurred. The fragmentation in the LV-An electrogram was increased still further. In panel **C**, the premature extrastimulus was delivered at a coupling interval of 290 msec, and fragmentation noted in the LV-An electrogram extended through diastole became continuous and ventricular tachycardia was initiated. Ventricular tachycardia was not initiated until sufficient fragmentation was noted in the electrogram of the left ventricular aneurysm, and perpetuation of the tachycardia was dependent upon continuous electrical activity's being present in the left ventricular aneurysm. (From Josephson and Horowitz.[40] Reproduced by permission.)

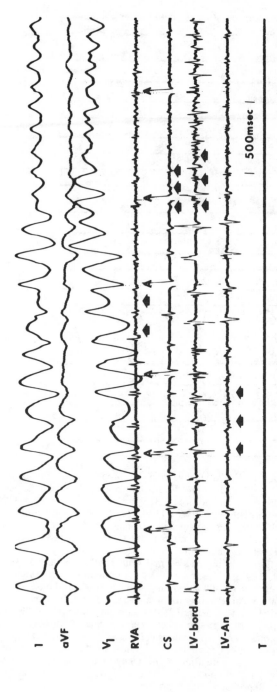

FIGURE 2 Spontaneous degeneration of ventricular tachycardia to ventricular fibrillation. Electrocardiographic leads I, AVF, and V_1 are shown with intracardiac electrograms recorded in the right ventricular apex (RVA), coronary sinus (CS), border of a left ventricular aneurysm (LV-bord), and in a left ventricular aneurysm (LV-An). Ventricular tachycardia was present on the left. There was a sudden spontaneous acceleration in the ventricular tachycardia. Fragmentation (*broad arrows*) occurred initially in the LV-An electrogram, but subsequently was seen in the other electrograms. Ventricular fibrillation was present in the electrocardiogram on the right when all electrograms showed fibrillary activity. (From Josephson *et al.*[41] Reproduced by permission.)

left ventricular stimulation in a single patient (FIG. 3). Initiation of TdP was reproducible in each patient. Neither typical, morphologically uniform, sustained ventricular tachycardia or fibrillation was inducible by programmed stimulation during the control study in these patients.

Eighty of the 87 paroxysms of TdP initiated by programmed stimulation terminated spontaneously. These episodes lasted for 6 to 34 complexes. Programmed stimulation could not be attempted during the episodes of torsade de pointes because of their brevity.

Observations During Torsade de Pointes

The individual electrograms recorded at specific sites remained discrete and did not fragment. The interelectrogram interval measured in any electrogram recording ranged from 110 to 345 msec. The activation sequences of the ventricular electrograms varied from complex to complex during TdP. The variations in QRS morphologic pattern were coincident with changes in the relationship of the left and right ventricular electrograms.

In six patients, TdP spontaneously changed to a sustained ventricular tachyarrhythmia. In three patients, TdP degenerated into VF, which was then terminated by cardioversion. In each case, progressive fragmentation of local electrograms occurred at the time of degeneration. Fragmentation proceeded in a stepwise sequence until fibrillatory activity was present in all electrograms. In three other patients, TdP spontaneously progressed into a sustained morphologically uniform ventricular flutter (cycle length, 170–205 msec) (FIG. 4). These episodes required cardioversion for termination. During the ventricular flutter the activation sequence of the ventricular electrograms was stable. The morphologic and electrophysiologic characteristics of the paroxysm of TdP that resulted in a sustained tachyarrhythmia did not differ from those of the episodes that terminated spontaneously.

In six patients, the administration of procainamide (three patients) or quinidine (three patients) converted the TdP into a morphologically uniform sustained ventricular tachycardia (FIG. 5). Although only TdP was inducible in these patients during control studies, the same stimulation protocol initiated typical VT after drug administration. The VT cycle lengths ranged from 250 to 420 msec, and in four patients the ventricular tachycardia could be terminated by extrastimuli or ventricular pacing. The electrophysiologic characteristics of these ventricular tachycardias were identical to those in the group of patients in whom sustained morphologically uniform VT was inducible during the control studies (see above).

Ventricular Fibrillation: Initiation and Termination

Ventricular fibrillation was initiated by programmed ventricular stimulation in seven patients (FIG. 6). The electrocardiogram at the time of resuscitation showed ventricular fibrillation in six of these patients. In one patient, no electrocardiogram was available for review. Ventricular fibrillation was induced by two ventricular premature depolarizations in each case. Left ventricular stimulation was required in one patient.

In six patients some or all of the episodes of VF required termination by cardioversion. In two patients, VF terminated spontaneously on at least one occasion (FIG. 7).

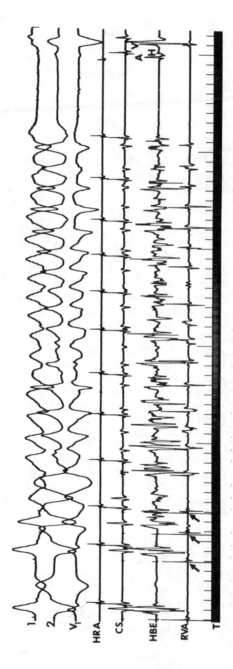

FIGURE 3. Initiation of torsade de pointes by programmed stimulation. Electrocardiographic leads I, II and V_1 are shown on electrograms recorded in the high right atrium (HRA), coronary sinus (CS), His bundle area (HBE), and right ventricular apex (RVA).
During right ventricular pacing, two premature extrastimuli were introduced and a paroxysm of typical torsade de pointes was initiated. The paroxysm lasted 18 complexes and had a typical varying QRS pattern. (From Horowitz et al.[5] Reproduced by permission.)

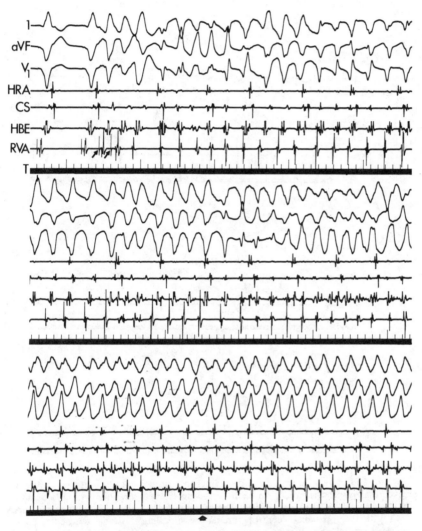

FIGURE 4. Spontaneous conversion of torsade de pointes into sustained, morphologically uniform ventricular flutter. In each of these continuous panels, electrocardiographic leads I, aVF, and V_1 are shown with electrograms recorded in the high right atrium (HRA), coronary sinus (CS), His bundle area (HBE), and right ventricular apex (RVA). During right ventricular pacing, two premature stimuli were delivered and a typical episode of torsade de pointes was initiated. It was a prolonged episode which in the bottom panel evolved into a uniform morphology ventricular flutter. At the *solid arrow*, note that the ventricular electrograms became uniform in sequence coincident with a stabilization of the QRS pattern. (From Horowitz et al.[5] Reproduced by permission.)

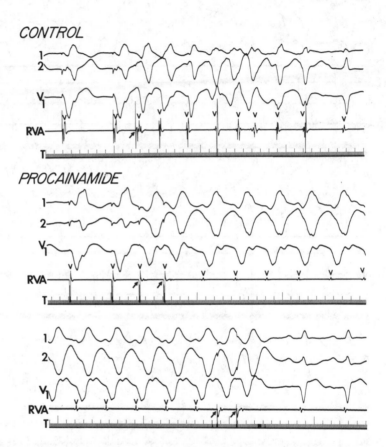

FIGURE 5. Conversion of torsade de pointes to morphologically uniform ventricular tachycardia by procainamide. In each panel, electrocardiographic leads I, II, and V_1 are shown with a ventricular electrogram recorded at the right ventricular apex (RVA). In the top panel (control) premature stimulation during ventricular pacing induced a typical paroxysm of torsade de pointes. Episodes of varying duration were induced in this patient; however, morphologically uniform ventricular tachycardia and ventricular fibrillation were not induced during control studies. After the administration of procainamide (in the middle panel), programmed stimulation induced typical morphologically uniform ventricular tachycardia. This tachycardia could be terminated by programmed extrastimuli, as seen in the bottom panel. (From Horowitz et al.[5] Reproduced by permission.)

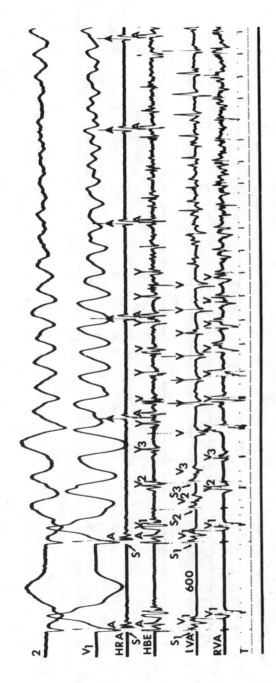

FIGURE 6. Initiation of ventricular fibrillation by programmed stimulation. Electrocardiographic leads II and V_1 are shown with electrograms recorded in the high right atrium (HRA), His bundle area (HBE), left ventricular apex (LVA), and right ventricular apex (RVA). During left ventricular pacing at a cycle length of 600 msec, two premature extrastimuli were delivered to the left ventricular apex and ventricular fibrillation was initiated. Note that in the right ventricular apical electrogram, progressive fragmentation occurred in the first seven electrograms after the premature stimuli until fibrillary activity occurred. (From Josephson *et al.*[42] Reproduced by permission.)

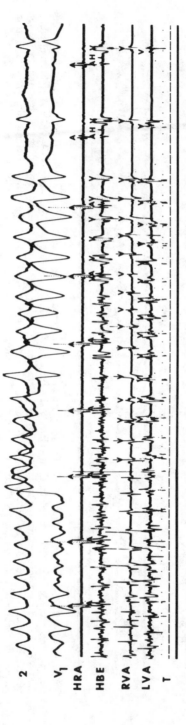

FIGURE 7. Spontaneous termination of ventricular fibrillation. Electrocardiographic leads II and V₁ are shown with electrograms recorded in the high right atrium (HRA), His bundle area (HBE), right ventricular apex (RVA), and left ventricular apex (LVA). Ventricular fibrillation was present on the left. Note that fibrillary activity was present in each of the ventricular electrograms. Electrical activity spontaneously became regular and the electrograms became discrete, first in the right and then in the left ventricular apical recordings and finally in the His bundle recording. When all electrograms were discrete and relatively regular, ventricular fibrillation spontaneously stopped and normal sinus rhythm was present, as seen on the right. (From Josephson et al.[41] Reproduced by permission.)

Observations During Ventricular Fibrillation

In each patient, local fibrillatory activity occurred after a sequence of progressively shortening interrelectrogram intervals. In two patients, the earliest degeneration to fibrillatory activity in any ventricular electrogram occurred after the second extrastimulus, which had been introduced at a shorter interval than the coupling interval of the first extrastimulus. In the other patients, the onset of local fibrillary activity occurred after a sequence of accelerating ventricular responses in the electrogram which showed the earliest degeneration to to fibrillary pattern. Frequently, during this accelerating pattern, the initially discrete ventricular electrogram fragmented progressively prior to the onset of the fibrillatory activity (FIG. 6).

Noninducible Arrhythmias

In 19 patients, no ventricular tachyarrhythmia was inducible. Nine of these patients had coronary artery disease (48%) compared with 34 of 40 patients (85%) in whom arrhythmias were inducible. In addition, prior myocardial infarction was more common in the patients with inducible arrhythmias. Left ventricular dysfunction was also more common and more severe than in patients in whom no arrhythmia was inducible. Finally, in the group of patients in whom no arrhythmia was inducible, the electrocardiogram recorded at the time of resuscitation showed VF in 17 patients and VT in 2 patients. Except perhaps for differences in demographic factors, no electrophysiologic reason for noninducibility of the tachyarrhythmia potentially responsible for cardiac arrest was found.

DISCUSSION

Ventricular tachycardia and ventricular fibrillation are the arrhythmias generally considered to be the cause of cardiac arrest [1-4]; however, the mechanisms of their initiation and the arrhythmogenic substrates are only partially characterized. In the present study, ventricular tachyarrhythmias that could be responsible for cardiovascular collapse were induced by programmed stimulation in 40 of 59 patients who had been resuscitated from out-of-hospital cardiac arrest. In many of these patients, the same tachyarrhythmia had been documented electrocardiographically at the time of resuscitation. Electrophysiologic evaluation allowed an analysis of the mechanism of initiation of these arrhythmias.

Reproducible initiation and termination of a ventricular arrhythmia has been considered the prime evidence that the underlying mechanism was reentry.[6, 7] The recent development of the concept of triggered automaticity, however, has cast some uncertainty on this criterion.[8-10] And, although the clinical relevance of triggered automaticity has not been proven, other support for the reentrant mechanism of VT is still necessary.

The classic prerequisite for a reentrant process has been electrophysiologic heterogeneity of depolarization and recovery and slow conduction. The demonstration of fragmented electrograms that increase in duration with pacing or premature stimuli, has been considered evidence for slow conduction through electrophysiologically heterogeneous tissue in the diseased human ventricle.[11] The initiation of VT in many patients in this study was dependent upon slow, fragmented activity's becoming continuous at the onset of the arrhythmia, and perpetuation of ventricular tachycardia was dependent upon the continuation of this fragmented activity. Similar demonstration of continuous fragmented activity has been recorded in experimental models of ventricular tachycardia.[12-14]

Considerable evidence supports the concept that the reentrant pathway responsible for recurrent sustained VT is localized to a relatively small circumscribed and protected area in the ventricles.[15, 16] The proximal His-Purkinje system has not been shown necessary for initiation or maintenance of the ventricular tachycardia. Furthermore, the majority of the ventricles can be depolarized prematurely by programmed stimulation without affecting the tachycardia. Atrial pacing can capture the ventricles, producing a QRS morphologic pattern indistinguishable from that of normal sinus rhythm, without interrupting the ventricular tachycardia.[15, 16] This suggests that the majority of the ventricle is not necessary for maintenance of the ventricular tachycardia. Data obtained during intraoperative mapping studies of ventricular tachycardia also support the concept of a reentrant mechanism localized to a relatively small area.[17]

Torsade de pointes is also a frequently induced tachyarrhythmia in patients who have survived cardiac arrest. Our observations suggest that TdP occurring in otherwise stable patients is also a reentrant arrhythmia. In a series of patients with TdP not related to transient pharmacologic or metabolic abnormalities, the arrhythmia was induced by programmed stimulation in 19 of 21 patients.[5] Others have reported confirmatory data.[18, 19]

The close relationship between TdP and both VT and VF is emphasized by our data. Torsade de pointes spontaneously evolved into a ventricular tachyarrhythmia with a morphologically uniform QRS pattern or was converted to typical sustained VT by antiarrhythmic drugs in eight patients. These morphologically uniform ventricular tachycardias responded to programmed stimulation in a fashion typical of reentrant VT.[15, 16] Again, others have made similar observations.[20] Torsade de pointes can also precede the onset of VF. The short cycle lengths and varying interelectrogram intervals during TdP produce the ideal electrophysiologic substrate for degeneration. Ventricular activation becomes progressively more chaotic as depolarization wavefronts encounter areas of differing refractoriness and conductivity until multiple wavelets responsible for VF are produced.

We have suggested that torsade de pointes may actually be a very rapid and regular VT that appears electrocardiographically as an irregular ventricular tachycardia because of variable patterns of ventricular activation.[5] This variable activation could be due to continuous variation of exit sites from the area of origin of the VT or local conduction block due to the rapidly formed activation wavefronts encountering areas of varying refractoriness or both. Findings in experimental models with chronic myocardial infarction provide further support for this hypothesis. Ideker et al.[21] have shown that the variable summation of depolarization wavefronts from a rapid VT can produce a pattern of TdP. Other observations have confirmed that varying exit sites from a rapid ventricular tachycardia can produce this pattern.[22] Thus, substantial evidence exists to support the hypothesis that TdP is indeed a variant VT closely related to typical sustained VT. Furthermore, the close relationship between TdP and VF may be indicative of the role torsade de pointes plays as a transition between VT and VF.

Although most studies have supported reentry as a mechanism of the perpetuation of VF, the initiation of this tachyarrhythmia could be based on reentry or enhanced automaticity.[23, 24] In our study, VF was induced by programmed stimulation directly in seven patients and via an intermediate VT form in seven other patients. The present observations at the onset of VF are consistent with the dependence of initiation on shortening of refractoriness and inhomogeneity of activation and recovery. The initiation of VF was preceded by rapidly accelerating discrete local electrical activity which degenerated to fibrillation. Progressive fragmentation of electrograms coincident with the accelerating rhythm provides evidence of the substrate of slow and intermittent conduction and short refractory periods in which VF occurs. These data are consistent with other observations of the initiation of VF in experimental animals by myocardial ischemia or electrical stimuli.[23-26] Furthermore, our observations during VF support the hypothesis based on experimental studies [27] that a reentrant mechanism is responsible for maintenance of ventricular fibrillation.

In the 40 patients in this study in whom reproducible initiation of a ventricular tachyarrhythmia was achieved, there was no evidence during the electrophysiologic study of a transient perturbation that could serve as a substrate for the arrhythmia. Although most patients had stable structural heart disease with presumably fixed pathologic abnormalities, we could not implicate acute ischemia in the initiation of the arrhythmia in any patient. This observation suggests that in these patients the substrate for initiation of the arrhythmia is always present and can be activated by the appropriate trigger. This continuing presence of the arrhythmogenic milieu explains the high incidence of the recurrence of cardiac arrest in such patients.

The observations (1) that the arrhythmia responsible for cardiac arrest can be induced by programmed stimulation, (2) that the mechanism is apparently reentrant, and (3) that vulnerability to these arrhythmias persists for relatively long periods of time, have considerable therapeutic implications. Programmed stimulation may be useful in evaluating patients at high risk for cardiac arrest as determined by risk stratification techniques in patients who have had myocardial infarctions.[28, 29] Although it would be difficult to perform electrophysiologic studies in all patients potentially at risk of cardiac arrest, such definitive study may be justified in particular subgroups of patients who are at very high risk. Furthermore, programmed stimulation has been used to define prospectively the efficacy of therapeutic interventions for reentrant supraventricular tachycardia [30] and ventricular tachycardia.[31-33] More recently, these techniques have been applied with encouraging results to the therapy of patients who have survived cardiac arrest.[34, 35] The ability to identify the cause of the tachyarrhythmia in patients who have been resuscitated from cardiac arrest should allow an objective evaluation of the available therapeutic modalities, including drugs, pacemakers and surgery.

In 19 patients, no ventricular tachyarrhythmia was inducible by programmed stimulation. Certain demographic factors were qualitatively different in these patients as compared with those in whom the arrhythmia was inducible. Also, the former group had less severe structural cardiac abnormalities and thus may have had a less persistent substrate for arrhythmogenesis. Although the VF threshold is substantially lowered by severe coronary arterial stenosis,[36, 37] the precipitation of the VF may require reversible perturbations (such as neural or metabolic ones) not present during electrophysiologic studies in these patients. It is also possible that a more sophisticated or aggressive stimulation protocol would have induced ventricular tachycardia or fibrillation. We have used techniques that are known to produce only rarely ventricular tachyarrhythmias in patients in whom they have not been previously documented to occur spontaneously.[38, 39] More aggressive stimulation techniques may not have the same specificity and thus have not been employed. Furthermore, enhanced automaticity may have been the initiating mechanism of the tachyarrhythmias in these patients. Electrophysiologic study would not be expected to elicit such arrhythmias due to enhanced automaticity.

In conclusion, in 68% of patients who have been resuscitated from cardiac arrest, a ventricular tachyarrhythmia responsible for this clinical event can be induced by programmed stimulation. This and other data suggest that the arrhythmia responsible for cardiac arrest is reentrant in the many of these patients. Furthermore, newly developed electrophysiologic techniques can be employed to develop therapy for these patients.

References

1. PANTRIDGE, J. F. & A. A. J. ADGEY. 1969. Pre-hospital coronary care. The mobile coronary care unit. Am. J. Cardiol. **24:** 266–273.
2. LIBERTHSON, R. R., E. L. NAGEL, J. C. HIRSCHMAN, S. R. NUSSENFELD, B. D. BLACKBOURNE & J. H. DAVID. 1974. Pathophysiologic observations in pre-hospital ventricular fibrillation and sudden cardiac death. Circulation **49:** 790–798.
3. BAUM, R. S., H. ALVAREZ & L. A. COBB. 1974. Survival after resuscitation from out-of-hospital ventricular fibrillation. Circulation **50:** 1231–1235.
4. SCHAEFFR, W. A. & L. A. COBB. 1975. Recurrent ventricular fibrillation and modes of death in survivors of out-of-hospital ventricular fibrillation. N. Engl. J. Med. **293:** 259–262.
5. HOROWITZ, L. N., A. M. GREENSPAN, S. R. SPIELMAN & M. E. JOSEPHSON. 1981. Torsade de pointes: Electrophysiologic studies in patients without transient pharmacologic or metabolic abnormalities. Circulation **63:** 1120–1128.
6. WELLENS, H. J. J. 1977. Electrical Stimulation of the Heart in the Study and Treatment of Tachycardias. University Park Press. Baltimore, MD.
7. CURRY, P. V. L. 1975. Fundamentals of arrhythmias: Modern method of investigation. *In* Cardiac Arrhythmias: The modern electrophysiologic approach. D. M. Krickler and J. F. Goodwin, Eds.: 65–76. W. B. Saunders Co. London.
8. CRANFIELD, P. F. & R. S. ARONSON. 1974. Initiation of sustained rhythmic activity by single propagated action potentials in canine cardiac Purkinje fibers exposed to sodium-free solution or to ouabain. Circ. Res. **34:** 477–481.
9. FERRIER, G. R., J. H. SAUNDERS & C. MENDZ. 1973. A cellular mechanism for the generation of ventricular arrhythmias by acetylstrophanthidin. Circ. Res. **32:** 600–609.
10. WIT, A. L. & P. F. CRANEFIELD. 1976. Triggered activity in cardiac muscle fibers of the simian mitral valve. Circ. Res. **38:** 85–98.
11. JOSEPHSON, M. E., L. N. HOROWITZ & A. FARSHIDI. 1978. Continuous local electrical activity: A mechanism of recurrent ventricular tachycardia. Circulation **57:** 659–665.
12. BOINEAU, J. P. & J. L. COX. 1973. Slow ventricular activation in acute myocardial infarction: A source of reentrant premature ventricular contractions. Circulation **48:** 702–713.

13. WALDO, A. L. & G. A. KAISER. 1973. A study of ventricular arrhythmias associated with acute myocardial infarction in the canine heart. Circulation **47:** 1222–1228.
14. EL-SHERIF, N., R. R. HOPE, B. J. SCHERLAG & R. LAZARRA. 1977. Reentrant arrhythmias in the late myocardial infarction period: 2. Pattern of initiation and termination. Circulation **55:** 702–719.
15. JOSEPHSON, M. E., L. N. HOROWITZ, A. FARSHIDI & J. A. KASTOR. 1978. Recurrent sustained ventricular tachycardia: 1. Mechanisms. Circulation **57:** 431–439.
16. JOSEPHSON, M. E., L. N. HOROWITZ, A. FARSHIDI, S. R. SPIELMAN, E. L. MICHELSON & A. M. GREENSPAN. 1978. Sustained ventricular tachycardia: Evidence for protected localized reentry. Am. J. Cardiol. **42:** 416–424.
17. HOROWITZ, L. N., M. E. JOSEPHSON & A. H. HARKEN. 1980. Epicardial and endocardial activation during sustained ventricular tachycardia in man. Circulation **61:** 1227–1238.
18. EVANS, T. R., P. V. L. CURRY, D. H. FITCHETT & D. M. KRICKLER. 1976. "Torsade de pointes" initiated by electrical ventricular stimulation. J. Electrocardiography. **9:** 255–258.
19. FONTAINE, G. H., R. FRANK, J. J. WELTI & Y. GROSGOGEAT. 1979. Electrophysiology of torsade de pointes. *In* Proceedings of the world Symposium on Cardiac Pacing. C. Meere, Ed. Chapt. **6:**3.
20. REDDY, C. P. & M. R. McVAY. 1981. Induction of torsade de pointes in patients with recurrent sustained ventricular tachycardia and its abolition and modification by procainamide. Clin. Res. **29:** 234A.
21. IDEKER, R. E., L. HARRISON, W. M. SMITH, J. KASELL & W. M. SMITH. 1979. Epicardial mapping of the transition to ventricular fibrillation induced by acute ischemia in the dog. Circulation **60**(Suppl 2)**:** II–110.
22. NHON, N., R. R. HOPE, G. KABELL, B. J. SCHERLAG & R. LAZARRA. 1980. Torsade de pointes: Electrophysiology of atypical ventricular tachycardia. Am. J. Cardiol. **45:** 494.
23. WIGGERS, C. J. 1940. The mechanism and nature of ventricular fibrillation. Am. Heart J. **20:** 399–412.
24. MOE, G. K., A. S. HARRIS & C. J. WIGGERS. 1941. Analysis of the initiation of fibrillation by electrographic studies. Am. J. Physiol. **134:** 473–492.
25. HARRIS, A. S. & A. G. ROJAS. 1943. The initiation of ventricular fibrillation due to coronary occlusion. Exp. Med. Surg. **1:** 105–122.
26. ZIPES, D. P. 1975. Electrophysiological mechanisms involved in ventricular fibrillation. Circulation **52**(Suppl. 3)**:** 120–130.
27. MOE, G. K. 1962. On the multiple wavelet hypothesis of atrial fibrillation. Arch. Int. Pharmacodyn. Ther. **140:** 183–188.
28. BIGGER, J. T., C. A. HELLER, T. L. WENGER & F. M. WELD. 1978. Risk stratification after acute myocardial infarction. Am. J. Cardiol. **42:** 202–209.
29. MOSS, A. J., D. T. HENRY, J. DeCAMILLA & L. W. BAYER. 1979. Ventricular ectopic beats and their relation to sudden and nonsudden cardiac death after myocardial infarction. Circulation **60:** 998–1003.
30. WU, D., C. R. WYNDHAM, P. DENES *et al.* 1977. Chronic electrophysiological study in patients with recurrent paroxysmal tachycardia: A new method for developing successful oral antiarrhythmic therapy. *In* Reentrant Arrthythmias. H. E. Kulbertus, Ed.: 294–311. University Park Press. Baltimore, MD.
31. HOROWITZ, L. N., M. E. JOSEPHSON, A. FARSHIDI, S. R. SPIELMAN, E. L. MICHELSON & A. M. GREENSPAN. 1978. Recurrent sustained ventricular tachycardia. III. Role of electrophysiologic study in the selection of antiarrhythmic regimens. Circulation **58:** 986–997.
32. HOROWITZ, L. N., M. E. JOSEPHSON & J. A. KASTOR. 1980. Intracardiac electrophysiologic studies as a method for the optimization of drug therapy in chronic ventricular arrhythmia. Prog. Cardiovasc. Dis. **23:** 81–98.

33. MASON, J. W. & R. A. WINKLE. 1978. Electrode-catheter arrhythmia induction in the selection and assessment of antiarrthythmic drug therapy for recurrent véntricular tachycardia. Circulation **58**: 971–985.
34. HOROWITZ, L. N., S. R. SPIELMAN, A. M. GREENSPAN & M. E. JOSEPHSON. 1981. The role of programmed stimulation in assessing vulnerability to ventricular arrhythmias in man. Am. Heart J. In press.
35. RUSKIN, J. N., J. P. DiMARCO & H. GARAN. 1980. Out-of-hospital cardiac arrest. N. Engl. J. Med. **303**: 607–613.
36. HOROWITZ, L. N., J. F. SPEAR, M. E. JOSEPHSON, J. A. KASTOR & E. N. MOORE. 1979. The effects of coronary artery disease on the ventricular fibrillation threshold in man. Circulation **60**: 792–797.
37. KRALIOS, A. C., W. J. BUGNI, M. A. McDONNELL, T. J. BAGARIS & H. KUIDA. 1981. Dependence of ventricular fibrillation propensity on coronary blood flow without myocardial ischemia. Am. Heart J. **101**: 440–449.
38. SPIELMAN, S. R., A. FARSHIDI, L. N. HOROWITZ & M. E. JOSEPHSON. 1978. Ventricular fibrillation during programmed ventricular stimulation: Incidence and clinical implications. Am. J. Cardiol. **42**: 913–918.
39. VANDEPOL, C. J., A. FARSHIDI, S. R. SPIELMAN, A. M. GREENSPAN, L. N. HOROWITZ & M. E. JOSEPHSON. 1980. The incidence and clinical significance of induced ventricular tachycardia. Am. J. Cardiol. **45**: 725–731.
40. JOSEPHSON, M. E. & L. N. HOROWITZ. 1979. Recurrent ventricular tachycardia: An electrophysiologic approach. Med. Clin. N. Amer. **63**: 53.
41. JOSEPHSON, M. E., S. R. SPIELMAN, A. M. GREENSPAN & L. N. HOROWITZ. 1979. Mechanism of ventricular fibrillation in man. Am. J. Cardiol. **44**: 623.
42. JOSEPHSON, M. E., S. R. SPIELMAN, A. M. GREENSPAN & L. N. HOROWITZ. 1980. Electrophysiologic observations on ventricular fibrillation in the human heart. *In* Sudden Death. H. E. Kulbertus & H. J. J. Wellens, Eds. Martinus Nijhoff. The Hague.

DISCUSSION

DR. KASTOR: These data have caught the interest of everyone who has followed them. One is impressed by the fact that the information that turns up in these studies is somewhat at variance with that found when the ambulance gets to the bedside or the street; how do you explain that?

DR. HOROWITZ: The electrocardiographic recordings obtained at the time of resuscitation are usually several minutes, if not 10 or 20 minutes, into the episode.

In a few patients morphologically uniform ventricular tachycardias can be recorded at the time of cardiac arrest, but I would say that 80% or more of these patients have ventricular fibrillation recorded. In some patients the mechanism initiated is VT which then degenerates into VF. You must remember that in the laboratory one doesn't wait quite as long as one must during spontaneous cardiac arrest to see degeneration of the rhythm.

DR. KUPERSMITH: I have some questions about the torsade de pointes arrhythmias. First, were they preceded by a prolonged Q-T interval as is supposed to occur frequently in torsade de pointes? Second, did you examine whether there was any particular increase or other sensitivity to the preceding R-R interval, that is, the pacing cycle, compared with that of the other arrhythmias? Third, did you try any of the lidocaine-like drugs on these arrhythmias?

DR. HOROWITZ: The patients with torsade de pointes did not uniformly have a long Q-T interval during normal sinus rhythm; only about a third of them did. In some patients induction could be carried out during normal sinus rhythm; in others it could only be accomplished during ventricular pacing. We did not find a particular pattern with respect to requiring either very long or very short cycle lengths for induction.

We did use lidocaine in some of these patients, but it tended to have less of an effect. That is, fewer patients responded to it and it was not given to all the patients. In the development of the therapeutic regimen it was projected as being one of the drugs that was going to be least successful. Since many of these patients required cardioversion, we used procainamide and quinidine in all of them. If those drugs worked, then we did not need to use lidocaine.

DR. KUPERSMITH: Did patients with a prolonged Q-T interval also respond to quinidine or procainamide?

DR. HOROWITZ: Some did. These are not persons in whom either hereditary abnormalities or drug toxicity were producing prolonged Q-T intervals. Some had long Q-T intervals, but they were all very minimally prolonged. Some of them did respond to quinidine or procainamide and some of them didn't, but the pattern of response was not different from that in patients who had normal Q-T intervals to begin with.

DR. KASTOR: There is a slight semantic difference here with respect to torsade de pointes. When the arrhythmia was described initially, it was in a small group of patients with rather odd and unusual disorders. The term is now being used by some of us, at least in a broader sense, to describe something that looks like what was described for the smaller group but which is now applied to a larger group of patients with coronary disease.

DR. MARCUS: I am wondering about the need for left ventricular stimulation. Can you identify patients beforehand in terms of location of dyskinesia or akinesia in the left ventricle in such a way that you can predict that you may have to use left ventricular stimulation?

DR. HOROWITZ: Unfortunately, no.

DR. MARCUS: Can ventricular arrhythmias be induced in patients who have no structural heart disease?

DR. HOROWITZ: There were only five patients in our group who fell into that category, and ventricular fibrillation was induced in only one of them. As a group these persons are less likely to have successful induction of a sustained tachyarrhythmia, but it can be induced in some of them. The vast majority of the patients referred to us for this problem have structural heart disease; in fact, most of them have coronary heart disease.

We *can* say that the group of patients in whom tachyarrhythmias cannot be induced tend to have fewer structural abnormalities, less severe coronary disease, fewer ventricular aneurysms, or previous infarctions. But there are clearly some in whom the arrhythmias cannot be induced who nevertheless have infarctions and aneurysms, and conversely there are others who have perfectly normal hearts, with the exception of some electrical problems, in whom the tachyarrhythmias can be induced. Because the group without structural disease is relatively small it will take some time before we can understand what is going on.

DR. LOZNER: How do you treat patients who still have a lot of ventricular premature beats after cardiac arrest? Is it safe to take them off their drugs before the study?

DR. HOROWITZ: We like to study the majority of patients in the baseline state so that we know what we are dealing with. Many patients have spontaneous and often frequent and complex ventricular ectopy which is asymptomatic. We have been perfectly content to discontinue medication in that situation and watch the patients. Not infrequently those patients are made worse by the drug anyway.

There is, of course, the occasional patient who is just having an episode of fibrillation or tachycardia several times a day, and then your hand is forced. One potential approach in such a case is to find something that works empirically on spontaneous episodes and then study these patients after their condition has stabilized. The drawback, of course, is that you don't know what happened in the control state. Noninducibility does not have as good a prognostic implication as it would if we knew what the control state was. The majority of these patients are not having fibrillation, or tachycardia even daily or weekly so that you can stop the drugs in preparation for the study.

DR. BIGGER: Apropos of the normal group with the long Q-T interval: they all had cardiac arrest, did they not?

DR. HOROWITZ: That is correct.

DR. BIGGER: Weren't the vast majority of these caused by coronary disease?

DR. HOROWITZ: Eighty percent had coronary disease.

DR. BIGGER: And did you perform angiography in the other patients and exclude coronary disease?

DR. HOROWITZ: Yes, we showed normalcy in these patients by routine noninvasive tests as well as by angiography.

DR. CRAMPTON: Your data implied that in some of the patients their arrhythmia terminated spontaneously and that termination could be brought about in some others by a bit of gentle burst pacing, and I think that a few required direct current countershock for synchronized cardioversion. Your data also imply that sometimes you can get ventricular fibrillation to stop on your own and that sometimes you can get it to stop with very little electricity. What amount of energy or current did you lay on the chest wall for your synchronized or unsynchronized shocks for ventricular fibrillation?

DR. HOROWITZ: In our laboratory generally when we are anticipating the induction of an arrhythmia that is going to require cardioversion we charge the defibrillator to 50 watt-seconds. In persons who have cardiac arrest and have induction of ventricular tachycardia, it is not infrequent for the ventricular tachycardia to have no isoelectric baseline. Even though the defibrillator is in the cardiovert mode, the energy may be delivered at any point in the R-R interval. This will produce conversion to normal sinus rhythm in half of the patients and may induce ventricular fibrillation in the remainder. Although ventricular tachycardia can frequently be terminated by low-energy cardioversion, when it is very rapid, the synchronization doesn't work particularly well, not because the machine is malfunctioning, but just because it is not set up to do it that way. For ventricular fibrillation we generally try to achieve cardioversion at full energy, although it possibly does not require so much. You must understand the psychology of the electrophysiologist who has just induced ventricular tachycardia or fibrillation that causes cardiovascular collapse: He or she is not going to do experiments on the way out of the arrhythmia as well as on the way in. So we generally go to full energy very quickly.

DR. CRAMPTON: It is interesting that while a 50-joule countershock has worked on some patients with ventricular fibrillation you jump from 50 to

400 without an interval sample for which there can be a 95 to 98% conversion rate. There are data that indicate that the higher amount may not help the heart even though the ventricular fibrillation is terminated.

DR. HOROWITZ: I completely agree.

DR. CRAMPTON: I was interested because you have the opportunity to examine this as you are attempting to defibrillate the heart. We have not done any programmed electrical stimulation, but we have badly synchronized DC countershocks in supraventricular arrythmias and we have defibrillated VF that we induced with a 20-joule countershock. This might be an interesting area to look at.

DR. HOROWITZ: Again, with a cycle time of about 9 seconds on the machine and the knowledge that we have just induced an arrhythmia, I would find it difficult to do, although intellectually I can sit back and agree with you. In fact I could agree with you *practically*, but I prefer someone else do that study!

DR. KASTOR: Dr. Crampton, why do we call it countershock?

DR. CRAMPTON: I believe the term honors Dr. Wiggers, who in 1940 described the induction of ventricular fibrillation by delivery of a shock to the ventricle in the vulnerable period followed by a countershock—a second shock, which terminated the ventricular fibrillation. But I was just making a plea for keeping the electricity bill down and the cardiac damage at a minimum by using a lower level of energy!

DR. HERLING: In the patients in whom the arrhythmias were not inducible, did any receive stimulation with isoproterenol? How do you explain the non-inducibility?

DR. HOROWITZ: Some of those patients did, and in none could tachyarrhythmias be induced by stimulation with isoproterenol. Noninducibility can be explained by a number of factors which are all hypotheses: there are no data for this. The most obvious explanation is that in those patients some transient perturbation, such as acute ischemia, was necessary for the cardiac arrest, and that condition was not created or was not present in the laboratory.

The other possibility is that we were not aggressive enough with the stimulation protocol. This is not a criticism that many people would level at us, but it is possible. And finally, the tachyarrhythmia may have started from a rapid automatically firing focus, which then degenerated to ventricular fibrillation, and, of course, we wouldn't be expected to induce that either. Any or all or a combination of those three factors could explain noninducibility in any particular patient and there are no data to suggest which of those is the most likely.

THE ROLE OF INTRAVENTRICULAR CONDUCTION DISORDERS IN PRECIPITATING SUDDEN DEATH

Hein J. J. Wellens,* Pedro Brugada, and Frits W. H. M. Bär

Department of Cardiology
University of Limburg
Annadal Hospital
Maastricht, The Netherlands

The estimation of risk for development of complete heart block, a condition which can result in sudden death, in patients with bundle branch block is a common clinical problem. Because this subject has been reviewed extensively in recent articles,[1, 2] we intend to address ourselves to this problem in a short and practical way.

When confronted with a patient showing bundle branch block, the first step is to place that patient into one of the following four categories:

(1) Patients with bundle branch block resulting from acute myocardial infarction;

(2) Patients in whom bundle branch block precedes acute myocardial infarction;

(3) Patients with bundle branch block without acute myocardial infarction;

(4) Asymptomic persons in whom bundle branch block was discovered on screening.

Such a classification will facilitate the discussion on risk of sudden death in patients with bundle branch block.

DISCUSSION

1. Acquired Bundle Branch Block in Acute Myocardial Infarction

When the intraventricular conduction defect occurs acutely subsequent to myocardial infarction, mortality is primarily determined by the extent of myocardial damage.[3] The typical intraventricular conduction defect is right bundle branch block with or without left-sided hemiblock developing in the setting of an acute extensive anteroseptal infarction. As shown in TABLE 1, mortality is high and primarily the result of pump failure because of the inadequate amount of surviving myocardium. Complete heart block and asystole are characteristically preceded by right bundle branch block followed by left-sided hemiblock.[3]

Candidates for such an event can therefore be identified by monitoring several electrocardiographic leads simultaneously. They can also be recognized by measuring the H-V interval.[3] Because of the extent of myocardial damage, the benefit of cardiac pacing is marginal. Only a rare patient in whom com-

* Address for correspondence: Hein J. J. Wellens, M.D., Department of Cardiology, University of Limburg, Annadal Hospital, Maastricht, The Netherlands.

0077–8923/82/0382–0136 $01.75/0 © 1982, NYAS

TABLE 1

CHARACTERISTICS OF PATIENTS IN WHOM BUNDLE BRANCH BLOCK DEVELOPS AFTER
ACUTE MYOCARDIAL INFARCTION

1. There is extensive anteroseptal infarction.
2. There is usually right bundle branch block with or without hemiblock.
3. Prognosis is poor (40 to 70% mortality).
4. Death in acute phase is usually the result of pump failure.

plete heart block develops can be saved by prophylactic insertion of a temporary pacemaker. TABLE 2 shows that one-third of the patients with bundle
branch block who survive the first week of infarction develop life-threatening
ventricular tachyarrhythmias in the next 5 weeks.[4] Only three of our 86 patients
with acquired right bundle branch block with or without hemiblock and 1 to 1
atrioventricular conduction who survived for more than 1 week after infarction
and who were continuously monitored showed the development of transient
complete atrioventricular block. This suggests that progression to complete
atrioventricular block during this period is rare. The incidence of complete
subnodal block occurring more than 6 weeks after an anteroseptal infarction
complicated by acquired bundle branch block is not known (TABLE 3). Therefore, although advocated by some investigators,[5-8] the value of implantation
of a permanent pacemaker remains uncertain. Because sudden death in these
patients may be the result of ventricular fibrillation,[4] more data on the natural
history of patients with bundle branch block subsequent to acute myocardial
infarction are needed. In our hospital all patients with acquired bundle branch
block surviving the acute episode are prospectively analyzed by H-V interval
measurements, study of arrhythmia induction, and documentation of hemodynamic and angiographic characteristics during the sixth week after the onset
of infarction. These data are required to evaluate the value of prophylactic
permanent pacing, antiarrhythmic therapy, and surgical treatment[9] in these
patients.

2. Preexistent Bundle Branch Block and Myocardial Infarction

Patients with preexistent bundle branch block have a higher mean age than
that of patients with acquired bundle branch block. They show no predilection
for site of infarction.[3] Because preexistent block is frequently in the left bundle

TABLE 2

FINDINGS IN PATIENTS WITH ACQUIRED BUNDLE BRANCH BLOCK IN THE SUBACUTE
PHASE * OF MYOCARDIAL INFARCTION

1. One-third of the patients develop ventricular tachycardia or ventricular
tachycardia and ventricular fibrillation within 2 to 6 weeks after onset of
acute myocardial infarction.
2. Persistent pump failure is common.
3. Incidence of complete heart block is rare.

* Weeks 2 through 6.

TABLE 3

PROBLEMS IN THE CHRONIC PHASE * OF ACQUIRED BUNDLE BRANCH BLOCK

1. Incidence of complete heart block is not known.
2. Risk of ventricular tachycardia and ventricular fibrillation is not known.
3. Prospective studies on H-V interval and induction of ventricular arrhythmia are required.
4. Role of prophylactic pacemaker insertion, arrhythmia prophylaxis, and surgery are presently not known.

* More than 6 weeks after myocardial infarction.

branch, the site of infarction can often not be determined. Progression to complete infranodal block is rare and therefore seldom a cause of sudden death. Temporary pacing is only indicated when preexistent bundle branch block is complicated by high-degree atrioventricular nodal block and possibly when left anterior hemiblock develops in the presence of preexistent right bundle branch block. Permanent pacing is required in the rare patient who develops complete infranodal block.

3. Patients with Bundle Branch Block without Acute Myocardial Infarction

Prospective data from in-hospital patients with chronic intraventricular conduction defects reveal a high incidence of sudden death. McAnulty et al.[10] reported on a prospective study in 257 patients with either left or right bundle branch block and axis deviation. Actuarial analysis showed an overall mortality rate of $19 \pm 2.6\%$ at 2 years with a sudden death rate of $10.2 \pm 2.6\%$.

Dhingra et al.[12] described a 4-year cumulative mortality of 75% with a sudden death mortality of 60% in 102 patients with chronic left bundle branch block. In a series of 452 patients with chronic bifascicular block, these same investigators reported a sudden death rate of $20 \pm 2.3\%$ after 4 years.[12] In these patients mortality from complete heart block was rare.

Prognosis depended upon the underlying disease, being worst in patients with coronary artery disease. The most likely mechanism of death was the occurrence of ventricular tachyarrhythmias. The value of measuring the H-V interval in hospitalized patients with chronic bifascicular block to identify a subgroup of patients at high risk for sudden death remains controversial.[11, 13–15] Rosen et al.[16] described a prospective study in 515 patients with chronic bifascicular block. The mean follow-up period was 3.9 ± 0.06 years. In 324 patients the H-V interval was equal to or less than 55 msec, in 191 patients the H-V interval was longer than 55 msec. Angina, congestive heart failure, cardiomegaly, premature ventricular contractions, and organic heart disease were significantly higher ($p < 0.05$) in patients with an H-V interval of more than 55 msec. The 5-year cumulative mortality and the 5-year sudden death mortality were 38 and 17%, respectively, in the patients with an H-V interval equal to or less than 55 msec, and 54 and 28%, respectively, in the patients with a prolonged H-V interval. There was a slight but definite difference in the development of complete heart block between the two groups (0.6% versus 4.7%). At the present time permanent pacing is required in patients with bundle branch block in whom bradycardia is documented. Prophylactic permanent pacing seems indicated in those patients who have syncope and no documentation of bradycardia (in whom other causes of syncope can be excluded) and who have a prolonged H-V interval (≥ 70 msec) or who develop a high-degree atrioventricular block during atrial pacing.

4. Asymptomatic Persons with Bundle Branch Block Discovered on Screening

In the asymptomatic, out-of-hospital population the prognosis of intraventricular conduction defects is different. Rose et al.[17] showed a low risk of cardiovascular death in 325 asymptomatic subjects with intraventricular conduction defects prospectively followed for 5 years. Similar findings were obtained by Kulbertus et al.[18] As shown in TABLE 4, there was no difference in cardiac death rate or incidence of sudden death in subjects with right bundle branch block, left bundle branch block, or right bundle branch block with left anterior hemiblock as compared with those in controls. Sudden death and progression towards complete heart block appears to be uncommon among asymptomic subjects with bundle branch block. Even in the group with right bundle branch block and left anterior hemiblock the annual risk of developing Adams-Stokes attacks is not more than 1 to 2%.[19] Because of the large number of asymptomatic persons showing this electrocardiographic pattern and because of their low risk of sudden death, systematic His bundle recordings do not seem to be indicated in this population.

CONCLUSION

In considering the contribution of intraventricular conduction disorders to sudden death it is helpful to divide the patients with bundle branch block into four subgroups. In only a selected group of patients can sudden death be prevented by cardiac pacing. Our present attitude towards cardiac pacing in patients with bundle branch block is shown in TABLE 5.

TABLE 4

COMPARISON BETWEEN ASYMPTOMATIC PATIENTS WITH BUNDLE BRANCH BLOCK AND CONTROL PATIENTS *

	No. of Patients	Mean Age (yr)	Period Follow-Up (mo)	No. of Cardiac Deaths	No. of Sudden Deaths
RBBB	161	61.78 ± 11.71	39.21 ± 16.03	2	–
Control	293	60.49 ± 10.98	38.90 ± 15.78	3	4
LBBB	57	62.79 ± 11.81	41.22 ± 15.72	–	2
Control	105	60.80 ± 9.92	40.95 ± 16.24	–	1
RBBB + LAH	45	67.04 ± 9.00	45.88 ± 15.86	1	–
Control	82	66.29 ± 8.88	45.99 ± 15.88	–	1

ABBREVIATIONS: LAH = left anterior hemiblock; LBBB = left bundle branch block; RBBB = right bundle branch block.
* From Kulbertus et al.[18]

TABLE 5

USES OF PACING IN BUNDLE BRANCH BLOCK

1. *Persons with acquired bundle branch block in acute myocardial infarction*
   Temporary pacing when acquired right bundle branch block progresses to bifascicular block or H-V interval is greater than 55 msec
   Permanent pacing only in recurrent or persistent high-degree atrioventricular block
2. *Persons with preexistent bundle branch block in acute myocardial infarction*
   Temporary pacing in high-degree atrioventricular nodal block in inferior infarction
   Temporary pacing when preexistent right bundle branch block progresses to bifascicular block
   Permanent pacing only in recurrent or persistent high-degree atrioventricular block
3. *Persons with bundle branch block without acute myocardial infarction*
   Permanent pacing in patients with documented bradycardia
   Prophylactic permanent pacing in patients with syncope having no documentation of bradycardia after exclusion of other causes of syncope when H-V interval is prolonged ($\geq$ 70 msec) or high-degree atriventricular block can be induced by atrial pacing
4. *Asymptomatic persons with bundle branch block on screening*
   No indication for prophylactic permanent pacing or measurement of H-V interval

REFERENCES

1. FISCH, G. R., D. P. ZIPES & C. FISCH. 1980. Bundle branch block and sudden death. Prog. Cardiovasc. Dis. **23:** 187–224.
2. ROSS, D. L. 1981. Approach to the patient with bundle branch block. *In* What is New in Electrocardiography. H. J. J. Wellens & H. E. Kulbertus, Eds.: 110–129. Nijhoff. The Hague.
3. LIE, K. I., H. J. J. WELLENS & R. M. SCHUILENBURG. 1976. Bundle branch block and acute myocardial infarction. *In* The Conduction System of the Heart. H. J. J. Mellens, K. I. Lie & M. J. Janse, Eds.:670. Stenfert Kroese. Leiden.
4. LIE, K. I., R. M. SCHUILENBURG, G. K DAVID & D. DURRER. 1978. A 5½ year retrospective and prospective study on early identification of candidates developing late in-hospital ventricular fibrillation. Am. J. Cardiol. **41:** 674–679.
5. ATKINS, J. M., S. J. LESHIN & G. BLOMQVIST. 1973. Ventricular conduction blocks and sudden death in acute myocardial infarction. N. Engl. J. Med. **288:** 281–285.
6. SCANLON, P. J., R. PRYOR & S. G. BLOUNT. 1970. Right bundle branch block associated with left superior or inferior intraventicular block associated with acute myocardial infarction. Circulation **42:** 1135–1141.
7. GODMAN, M. J., B. W. LASSERS & D. G. JULIAN. 1970. Complete bundle branch block complicating acute myocardial infarction. N. Engl. J. Med. **282:** 237–241.
8. WAUGH, R. A., G. S. WAGNER & T. L. HANEY. 1973. Immediate and remote prognostic significance of fascicular block during acute myocardial infarction. Circulation **47:** 765–771.
9. JOSEPHSON, M. E., A. E. HARKEN & L. N. HOROWITZ. 1979. Endocardial re-

section: A new surgical technique for the treatment of recurrent ventricular tachycardia. Circulation **65:** 1430–1441.

10. McAnulty, J. H., S. H. Rahimtoola, E. S. Murphy, S. Kauffman, L. W. Ritzmann, P. Kanarek & H. De Mots. 1978. A prospective study of sudden death in "high-risk" bundle branch block. N. Engl. J. Med. **299:** 209–215.

11. Dinghra, R. C., F. Amat-Y-Leon, C. Wyndham, S. S. Sridhar, D. Wu, P. Denes & K. M. Rosen. 1978. Significance of left axis deviation in patients with chronic bifascicular block. Circulation **59:** 238–246.

12. Dinghra, R. C., C. Wyndham, F. Amat-Y-Leon, P. Denes, D. Wu, S. S. Sridhar, A. G. Bustin & K. M. Rosen. 1979. Incidence and site of atrioventricular block in patients with chronic bifascicular block. Circulation **59:** 238–246.

13. Narula, O. 1979. Intraventicular conduction defects. *In* Cardiac Arrhythmias. O. Narula, Ed.: 114–139. Williams & Wilkins. Baltimore, MD.

14. Scheinman, M., A. Weiss & F. Kunkel. 1973. His bundle recordings in patients with bundle branch block and transient neurologic symptoms. Circulation **48:** 322–330.

15. Dinghra, R. C., P. Denes, D. Wu, C. R. Wyndham, F. Amat-Y-Leon, W. D. Twone & K. M. Rosen. 1976. Prospective observations in patients with chronic bundle branch block and marked HV prolongation. Circulation **53:** 600–604.

16. Rosen, K. M., R. C. Dinghra, C. R. Wyndham, P. Deedwania, E. Palileo, R. A. Bauernfeind & S. Swiryn. 1980. Significance of HV interval in 515 patients with chronic bifascicular block. Am. J. Cardiol. **45:** 405.

17. Rose, G., P. J. Baxter, D. Reid & P. McCartney. 1978. Prevalence and prognosis of electrocardiographic findings in middle-aged man. Brit. Heart J. **40:** 636–643.

18. Kulbertus, H. E., E. De Leval-Rutten, A. Albert, M. Dubois & J. M. Petit. Electrocardiographic changes occurring with advancing age. *In* What is New in Electrocardiography. H. J. J. Wellens & H. E. Kulbertus, Eds.: 299–315. Nijhoff. The Hague.

19. Kulbertus, H. E., F. De Leval-Rutten, M. Dubois & J. M. Petit. 1980. Sudden death in subjects with intraventricular conduction defects. *In* Sudden Death. H. E. Kulbertus & H. J. J. Wellens, Eds.: 379–392. Nijhoff. The Hague.

<hr>

Discussion

Dr. Kastor: The problem often comes up with the Federal Aviation Administration of an asymptomatic commercial pilot with right bundle branch block. Do we have any information on what a pilot or someone under a great deal of stress with right bundle branch block might show? What does KLM [Royal Dutch Airlines] do?

Dr. Brugada: As we have said, our present data suggest that you shouldn't do anything. But of course a pilot has an enormous responsibility. I might inquire why you cited a pilot and not just a normal worker.

Looking at the incidence of sudden death in these patients and at the more extensive data that we have, one should not be worried because an asymptomatic person has a right bundle branch block. The incidence of sudden death in these persons is no greater than that of the normal population, so we should handle this problem exactly the same as if the electrocardiogram is normal.

DR. KASTOR: Well we can't get away with it that easily; what about left branch bundle block picked up on a screening electrocardiogram?

DR. BRUGADA: Left bundle branch block had the same rates as right bundle branch block as far as sudden death and sudden cardiac death are concerned. It is important to stress that this group of patients is very special in that persons with heart disease were discouraged from participating in this epidemiologic survey. This yielded a population which was completely asymptomatic. So these subjects really don't have heart disease as far as we can assess with our present methods.

DR. JOSEPHSON: I would like to point out that all the sudden death that you see in these groups is not due to heart block; it is also due to the causes of sudden death that Dr. Horowitz has already mentioned. A number of studies have shown that if you don't just measure the H-V interval, but also carry out programmed stimulation, you can induce these malignant arrhythmias, and that those are the probable cause of sudden death. Pacemakers don't really prevent that.

DR. ZIPES: I would like to ask Dr. Josephson or Dr. Brugada what he would do with a patient in whom there was no history to suggest arrhythmia, but a left bundle branch block and H-V interval prolongation and in whom a sustained ventricular tachyarrythmia had been induced? A question that I am raising and that I don't think has been adequately addressed in the literature is the appropriate control group of patients.

DR. KASTOR: How did this patient come to get an H-V interval measured?

DR ZIPES: He wanted to fly an airplane!

DR. BRUGADA: I agree that we don't have control groups and nobody has the data to answer these questions.

DR. KASTOR: It looks like we have to have a study of totally normal people. Any volunteers?

CENTRAL NERVOUS SYSTEM RISK FACTORS FOR SUDDEN CARDIAC DEATH *

Regis A. DeSilva †

Cardiovascular Laboratory, Department of Nutrition
Harvard School of Public Health
Boston, Massachusetts 02115

Cardiovascular Division
Department of Medicine
Brigham and Women's Hospital, Boston, Massachusetts 02115

INTRODUCTION

Experimental studies to verify the long-postulated connection between acute emotional perturbations and sudden death have been initiated only relatively recently. William Harvey, from whom we date the modern era in cardiology, had already commented on this association when he wrote: "Every passion of the mind which troubles men's spirits, either with grief, joy, hope or anxiety and gets access to the heart, there makes it to change from its natural constitution, by distemperament, pulsation and the rest. . . ." [1]

Sudden death is most often due to ventricular fibrillation occurring in the setting of coronary heart disease. Epidemiologic studies suggest that psychosocial risk factors exist for the development of both coronary heart disease and sudden cardiac death. While it is likely that both conditions share the same standard and some behavioral and environmental risk factors, the sudden onset of ventricular fibrillation in a heart that has been long-diseased requires the operation of additional factors. Gairdner, who is cited by McWilliam, observed a century ago that "it is plainly out of the question to suppose that a chronic and by its very nature, gradually advancing lesion like fatty degeneration or disease of the coronary vessels, is the direct and immediate cause of a death which occurs in a moment." [2] McWilliam, who also first suggested that sudden death was due to ventricular fibrillation, boldly advanced the view that sympathetic discharge may be an important factor in inciting this fatal arrhythmia. [3, 4] Since early this century, several experimental and clinical studies have attempted to demonstrate that the activity of the central nervous system contributes to the onset of ventricular arrhythmias and sudden death.

INVOLVEMENT OF THE CENTRAL NERVOUS SYSTEM

Indictment of higher nervous activity in sudden death is suggested by a number of observations. Epidemiologists have associated certain indices of

* This work was supported in part by Grants HL–07776 from the National Heart, Lung and Blood Institute and MH–21384 from the National Institutes of Mental Health, United States Public Health Service, Bethesda, Maryland.

† Address for correspondence: Dr. Regis A. DeSilva, Cardiovascular Laboratory, Harvard School of Public Health, 665 Huntington Avenue, Boston, Massachusetts 02115.

143

psychosocial distress such as low-socioeconomic status,[9] bereavement,[10] lack of education,[11] and various types of emotional stress with high mortality rates from cardiovascular disease. While these studies do not, and cannot establish causality, they suggest that psychological mechanisms may contribute to the premature onset of death.

A number of considerations suggest that neither hemodynamic factors nor acute myocardial damage accounts for the majority of cases of ventricular fibrillation. Although hemodynamically induced changes during heavy physical exertion may sometimes provoke ventricular fibrillation, the victim is most often at rest when death occurs. In resuscitated victims, acute myocardial injury is absent in two-thirds or more of cases.[5] Thus, although underlying coronary artery disease is often present, acute structural damage of the heart is not a prerequisite for the occurrence of ventricular fibrillation. Furthermore, the fact that ventricular fibrillation can be terminated instantaneously even during coronary arterial occlusion, and without immediate recurrence, suggests that irreversible compromise of coronary arterial flow is not the exclusive precipitant of sudden death. These observations indicate that ventricular fibrillation may be due to transient factors which momentarily disorganize cardiac electrical activity. The ensuing arrhythmia can therefore be regarded as an "electrophysiologic accident," which, although almost always fatal when untreated, is frequently reversible by defibrillation.

On the basis of these and other considerations, Lown [6-8] has hypothesized the operation of *transient risk factors*. These factors are momentary inputs to the heart which may trigger electrically unstable myocardium into ventricular fibrillation. While definitive proof that these factors operate in man awaits further study, evidence is accumulating for the central nervous system as a source of transient risk for ventricular fibrillation.

Another hypothesis relating to the onset of sudden death deserves comment. Albutt had suggested that sudden death was related to reflex vagal inhibition of the heart.[12] Richter's experimental investigations greatly influenced thinking in that direction.[13] Rats made to swim in water tanks died from bradycardia and asystole, rather than from drowning. In Richter's view, "voodoo" death in primitive societies possibly results from such vagally mediated cardiac slowing and asystole. This hypothesis was promoted by Wolf, who suggested that vagal slowing of the heart was part of a complex patterned reaction related to the "dive reflex," an atavistic reflex in man that is elicited by facial exposure to cold.[14] A review of the literature on this subject fails to reveal any electrocardiographically documented deaths attributable to this reflex, although short periods of asystole, heart block, and ventricular arrhythmias may occur. Our own investigations on the "dive" reflex conducted on patients with ventricular arrhythmias have failed to support this hypothesis.[15]

Clinical experience also indicates that vagally-induced cessation of cardiac action is not an important mechanism of sudden death in man. It is true that episodic first- and second-degree heart block or brief asystole can result from fear or anxiety, but these do not result in sustained cardiac arrest. MacWilliam had already noted a half century ago that when sinus node activity is suppressed, escape pacemakers invariably take over to reestablish cardiac activity.[3] Inferior wall infarction is usually associated with a good prognosis when it is accompanied by enhanced vagal tone and mild bradycardia. In this setting only occasionally does severe bradycardia or asystole due to marked increase in vagal tone lead to death. Severe bradycardia, or asystole directly preceding death, without intervening ventricular arrhythmia, is usually seen in the presence of extensive myocardial damage and shock. These sequences occur in the hemodynamically compromised heart during acute myocardial infarction and are unrelated to psychological factors.

BIOBEHAVIORAL MODELS FOR THE STUDY OF SUDDEN CARDIAC DEATH

Investigators have utilized a variety of models to study the onset of psychologically-induced sudden death in animals and in man. These studies are summarized in TABLE 1. Cannon considered one prototype of this form of fatality as having its roots in so-called "voodoo" deaths resulting from tribal castigation or from superstitious beliefs and fears relating to the occult.[16] He postulated a sympathoadrenal mechanism in its genesis. Although he did not implicate a cardiac arrhythmia, he noted that such individuals were in a state of shock and manifested a rapid, thready pulse terminally. Cannon did not actually study victims of voodoo death, but rather used this model as a theoretical basis for the discussion of psychological risk factors for the onset of sudden death.

Animal Investigations

Persuasive evidence that transient risk factors originate, in part at least, from the central nervous system has been demonstrated in animal studies. These investigations have been reviewed in detail previously.[6-8, 17] Direct stimulation of the central nervous system using chemicals, drugs, and electrical probes evokes a variety of ventricular arrhythmias including ventricular fibrillation.[18, 19] Stimulation or ablation of neural structures demonstrates that the efferent pathway arises in the midbrain and quadrigeminal bodies, traverses the reticular formation, and is finally channelled to the heart via the stellate ganglia and the cardiac sympathetic nerves. In the presence of a normal myocardium it is difficult to provoke ventricular fibrillation, even with potent nonphysiological stimuli. In contrast, stimulation of the midbrain in dogs after the induction of ischemia by coronary arterial occlusion results in an incidence of ventricular fibrillation that is ten times that occurring in the absence of such stimulation.[20] This study demonstrates the powerful co-action between inputs from the central nervous system and the myocardium rendered electrophysiologically unstable by ischemia.

Studies utilizing various methods of inducing stress have indicated that psychological stress in monkeys,[21] electric shock in pigs,[22] and heat, cold, and noise stress in rats[23] lead to myocardial degeneration and sudden death. The cardiac arrhythmias preceding death have been defined in some of these studies. Corley et al., studying yoked monkeys, showed that electric shock led to the development of bradyarrhythmias and death in asystole, probably as a consequence of myocardial damage.[21] Studies in pigs by Johansson et al. on the other hand have shown that ventricular arrhythmias, including ventricular tachycardia and fibrillation, were more likely to occur than asystole.[22] As originally proposed by Raab, cardiac damage induced by psychological stress is assumed to result from catecholamine release. The myocardial lesions, consisting of necrosis and subepicardial hemorrhage, resemble those seen in patients with prolonged catecholamine infusion or in those dying from pheochromocytoma.[24] Haft *et al.* noted intravascular aggregations of platelets with subepicardial areas of hemorrhage in rats subjected to noise and thermal stress.[23] It is also likely that psychological stresses release substances such as thrombin, thromboxane, and ADP, which enhance platelet aggregation, alter the rheologic properties of blood, and change both coronary blood flow and electrical properties of the heart.

TABLE 1

MODELS USED TO STUDY CENTRAL NERVOUS SYSTEM FACTORS IN SUDDEN DEATH

Investigators	Year	Biological Model	Proposed Mechanism of Death
Cannon [16]	1942	"Voodoo death"	Sympatho-adrenal activation
Richter [13]	1957	Swimming rats	Vagally mediated asystole
Raab [24]	1964	Stress in rats	Catecholamine release and myofibrillar damage
Wolf [14]	1967	"Dive reflex" in man	Vagally induced acystole
Lown et al.[27]	1973	Stress in dogs	Transient risk factors for ventricular fibrillation
Haft et al.[23]	1974	Stress in rats	Platelet microthrombi and myocardial necrosis
Corley et al.[21]	1974	Stress in monkeys	Asystole due to mycardial degeneration
Johansson et al.[22]	1974	Stress in pigs	Ventricular arrhythmia and myocardial necrosis
Lown and DeSilva [15]	1978	Potential or resuscitated sudden death victims	Transient risk factors for ventricular fibrillation
Cebelin and Hirsch [48]	1980	Autopsy cases	Stress-induced myocardial necrosis and ventricular fibrillation
Reich et al.[49]	1981	Potential or resuscitated sudden cardiac death victims	Transient risk factors for ventricular fibrillation

We have utilized the conscious dog as the principal model for study. Since the nonischemic myocardium is unlikely to manifest ventricular arrhythmia during aversive conditioning, an alternate method of evaluating ventricular electrical stability was developed. Ventricular fibrillation threshold, the classical end-point generally used, is unsuitable for studying the psychologically stressed conscious animal because the experiment automatically terminates once this end-point is attained. Traumatic resuscitative procedures, including electrical defibrillation preclude meaningful serial observations of the effects of psychological stress on ventricular fibrillation.

The alternate method for assessing electrical stability was based on the observation that the delivery of stimuli of increasing intensity during the vulnerable period of the myocardium results in the evocation of repetitive extrasystoles and finally ventricular fibrillation. The threshold for the elicitation of repetitive extrasystoles has been shown to bear a fixed relationship to the threshold current requirements for provocation of ventricular fibrillation in both conscious and anesthetized animals. A repetitive extrasystole is elicited by two-thirds of the current requirements for the induction of ventricular fibrillation.[25, 26] Since the animal is unaware of repetitive extrasystoles, rapid, serial measurements can be made and vulnerability to ventricular fibrillation during stress-induction can be readily tracked. Using this method, rapidly occurring decreases in the repetitive extrasystole threshold amounting to 30 to 50% below control values are demonstrable in aversive situations induced by shock-conditioning in a Pavlovian sling or using a Sidman shock-avoidance protocol.[27-29] These studies illustrate the important effects the central nervous system exerts on electrical stability of normal myocardium. Corbalan et al. additionally showed that in the presence of ischemia after myocardial infarction, repeated exposure of dogs to an aversive environment produced sinus tachycardia and ventricular arrhythmias.[30] Removal of the animal from the aversive to a calm environment consistently abolished these arrhythmias. These observations are supplemented by those of Skinner et al.,[31] who demonstrated a higher incidence of ventricular fibrillation in conscious pigs when coronary arterial occlusion was performed in an unfamiliar environment as compared with one to which the animals had been previously acclimatized. In Skinner's model, it is inferential that the unfamiliar environment was more stressful than the familiar one. Verrier and Lown[31] provided direct evidence that psychological stress has a marked synergistic effect with ischemia in dogs. During coronary arterial occlusion, the incidence of ventricular fibrillation was three times greater in a Pavlovian sling, where the animals had previously undergone shock-conditioning, as compared with a nonstressful environment, where they were relaxed.

The precise mechanisms whereby experimentally-induced psychological stress activates the central nervous system and produces a state of arousal sufficient to disrupt electrical stability of the heart and cause ventricular fibrillation remain to be defined. A number of disparate mechanisms are probably involved. The psychologically stressed animal shows numerous biochemical and hemodynamic changes in addition to enhancement of vulnerability to fibrillation. For example, circulating catecholamines as well as the epinephrine/norepinephrine ratio are increased. Additionally, coronary vascular resistance and coronary sinus blood flow are reduced. Vagal tone is also noted to be diminished during psychological stress.[32, 33] Increased vagal activity protects against vulnerability to ventricular fibrillation in both ischemic and nonischemic myocardium. Thus, vagal withdrawal during aversive conditioning may be an important factor in increasing myocardial susceptibility to ventricular fibrillation during psychological stress.

Protection from neurally or psychologically induced ventricular arrhythmias or electrical instability has been attained by a number of methods.

Various pharmacologic and neurochemical interventions can be performed to protect the myocardium against ventricular fibrillation. In the anesthetized dog, reduction in sympathetic neural tone is achieved by cholinergic stimulation. Administration of methacholine or direct vagal stimulation both increase the electrical threshold for ventricular fibrillation. The mechanism of protection derives from antagonism of sympathetic neural tone on the heart.[35, 36] Similarly, administration of morphine to the anesthetized dog increases vagal tone on the heart and increases the electrical stability of the myocardium.[37] Decrease in sympathetic neural outflow is attained by increasing central stores of neurotransmitters by administration of their precursors. In animals given tryptophan (the precursor of serotonin) and tyrosine (the precursor of epinephrine, norepinephrine, and dopamine), significant increases occur in ventricular electrical stability, as measured by the repetitive extrasystole threshold.[38-40] That dopaminergic receptors may also be involved in modulating ventricular electrical stability is demonstrated by the protection afforded by bromocriptine, a dopamine agonist.[41]

Pharmacologic interventions have also been performed in conscious animal models. As in the anesthetized dog, administration of morphine to the conscious dog results in cholinergic stimulation and protects against decreases in the repetitive extrasystole threshold induced by psychological stress.[34] In dogs exposed to a Sidman shock-avoidance protocol, decreases in the repetitive extrasystole threshold are annulled by the beta-adrenergic blocking agent, tolamolol.[42] The aforementioned studies were conducted in dogs with normal hearts exposed to psychological stress. In the ischemic heart there appear to be conflicting data in regard to the effects of beta-adrenergic blockade. Skinner et al.[31] found no effect of propranolol on the emergence of ventricular fibrillation after coronary occlusion in conscious pigs undergoing psychological stress. In contrast, Rosenfeld et al.[43] showed in dogs that beta-adrenergic blockade with the cardioselective agent, tolamolol, provided significant protection against malignant ventricular arrhythmias occurring during acute coronary occlusion in conjunction with psychological stress. Differences in animal species, experimental protocols, and pharmacologic agents used may account for the disparity in results.

Certain environmental conditions appear to be protective against ventricular arrhythmias. Placing an animal in a psychologically stressful environment after experimentally-induced myocardial infarction results in the appearance of malignant ventricular arrhythmias. Removal of the animal to a nonthreatening environment consistently abolishes these arrhythmias.[30] Similarly, removal of an animal from the stress-provoking environment results in an increase in ventricular electrical stability, as demonstrated by electrophysiologic testing.[34] Ventricular fibrillation is also less likely to occur after induction of acute myocardial ischemia in a laboratory environment familiar to the experimental animal than in a strange surrounding.[31] The complex behavioral adaptations that must accompany exposure to different environments and their attendant neural and humoral changes have hitherto not been studied. Nonetheless, these experimental observations suggest that sensory input from the environment is an important determinant of ventricular electrical stability and the emergence of ventricular arrhythmias. Protection of patients at risk of developing malignant ventricular arrhythmias, especially after myocardial infarction, must take into account these considerations.

These experimental studies provide evidence for the thesis that psychological and neural factors alter ventricular electrical stability of the heart and increase the propensity of the heart to fibrillate. Furthermore, these studies indicate that it is possible to prevent neural traffic to the heart and protect vulnerable myocardium from ventricular fibrillation. Such studies provide a theoretical scaffolding for exploring the neural and psychological variables that may precipitate ventricular fibrillation in man.

Human Investigations

Study of psychological and emotional factors as related to sudden death in man is fraught with numerous difficult problems. First, it is nearly impossible to accurately replicate and quantify emotional and psychological stimuli in the laboratory. Second, these stimuli are highly unique to the individual and are frequently not evident to either investigator or to the subject being studied. Third, the fatal arrhythmia, which is ventricular fibrillation, is a singular event and is not amenable to ready investigation or clinical replication. Despite these difficulties, some studies shed light on the role of the central nervous system in provoking sudden cardiac death in man.

Psychological Stress and Sudden Death

Studies by Rahe et al.,[44] utilizing the method of weighing of life-events, showed that accumulation of various types of psychological stresses due to life change, such as divorce, bereavement and job loss, had an increased association with onset of sudden cardiac death. These data were obtained indirectly by interviewing the spouse or next-of-kin of the decedent, but are nonetheless important because they provide an initial approach to the attempt to quantify stressful events occurring before death. Several investigators have independently confirmed that death of a close person often precedes mortality from coronary heart disease.[10, 80] Such deaths are especially likely to occur among bereaved spouses.[10] Cottington et al.[80] found in a careful case-control study that among the numerous life changes they evaluated, the death of a close person was the only significant factor affecting mortality from coronary heart disease among 81 sudden death victims. These victims were six times as likely to have experienced the death of a close person within the preceding 6 months as compared with controls. Other major life events, such as financial, legal, family or work-related problems, did not have the same impact on mortality.

Sampling of clinical populations or autopsy cases has provided information on the psychological setting in which sudden death occurs.[45–49, 57] Some of these studies are summarized in TABLE 2. Greene et al.[45] interviewed the next-of-kin of 25 men who died suddenly, and they estimated that "at least 50%" of these patients had ongoing psychological and social stresses at the time of death. Many of the stresses described were acute in nature and frequently involved interaction of two or more situations deemed as psychologically stressful. These workers surmised that a combination of depressive and arousal states coexisted at the time of sudden death. Myers and Dewar found that acute psychological stress was a significant variable among 100 men dying suddenly from coronary heart disease.[46] Among these men, 23 experienced intense stress in the 30 minutes preceding death, and 40 men experienced such stresses within the preceding 24 hours. These stresses varied widely and included attendance at a surgical clinic, an attack by dogs, fights over games, involvement in a nontraumatic motor accident, notification of divorce, and so forth. Moderate physical activity, a recent meal, especially with alcoholic beverages, the time of day and day of the week were significantly related to mortality, while chronic psychological stress, strenuous exercise, season of year and environmental temperature were unrelated to onset of sudden death.

Rissanen et al. evaluated the circumstances surrounding sudden death in Helsinki by interviewing next-of-kin.[47] The prevalence of acute and chronic stress, chest pain, heaviness of the arms, dyspnea, fatigue, sweating and nervous-

TABLE 2

PREVALENCE OF ACUTE PSYCHOLOGICAL STRESS PRECEDING SUDDEN DEATH

Investigators	Population Sample	Time Frame *	Total No. of Cases	No. of Cases with Acute Stress	Prevalence of Acute Stress
Myers and Dewar [46]	Postmortem	30 min	100	23	23%
		24 hr	100	40	40%
Rissanen et al. [47]	Postmortem	2 hr	118	23	19%
Reich et al. [49]	Clinical	24 hr	117	25	21%

* Refers to time period during which acute stresses occurred.

ness was evaluated. Prodromal symptoms were common in patients who had attacks lasting longer than 2 hours. Unusual fatigue, observed in 32% of cases, was the most common antecedent. "Chronic" stress occurred in 25% and "acute" stress in 19% of patients. In patients experiencing "acute" stress, death was rapid and resulted within 2 hours; myocardial infarction was unusual in this group of 23 patients, of whom 14 (16%) died instantaneously. Acute myocardial infarction was more common in patients with long-standing stress than in patients with acute stress preceding death. These results suggest that in patients with coronary artery disease, acute psychological stress is more likely to result in instantaneous or rapid death from ventricular fibrillation without the evolution of acute myocardial infarction. In patients with chronic stress, or with no evident stress factors, symptoms were of prolonged duration prior to death and changes of acute infarction were more common.

Cebelin and Hirsch [48] reviewed 497 deaths due to homicidal assault in Cuyahoga County, Ohio, and found 15 victims in whom there was no evidence for trauma as the unequivocal cause of death. In all cases, the victims were beaten or assaulted by relatives, spouses, strangers, or others. Although external injuries were present, there was no internal damage or blood loss to account for death. In 10 cases, arguments or fights had preceded death. Cardiac microscopic studies showed that in 11 of the 15 victims, myofibrillar degeneration was present, usually in the subendocardium. Such changes were absent in the hearts of 15 victims of traffic accidents used as controls. The authors surmised that the psychological stress of the homicidal attack, with forcible restraint in some cases, produced an acute-stress cardiomyopathy with the subsequent development of ventricular fibrillation and sudden death.

The studies just cited deal with the circumstances of death in deceased victims of sudden cardiac death. We utilized another approach and studied the onset of malignant arrhythmias, defined as symptomatic ventricular tachycardia and ventricular fibrillation, in a high-risk group of patients.[49] Of the total group of 117 patients, 53% had been resuscitated from ventricular fibrillation. This group thus constituted victims or potential victims of sudden cardiac death who could provide direct knowledgeable testimony of the emotional events immediately preceding the arrhythmic event. Possible emotional precipitants for malignant arrhythmia in the preceding 24 hours were identified in separate clinical interviews by a cardiologist and a psychiatrist. In 25 (21%) of the 117 patients such triggers for malignant arrhythmia were identified. These emotional triggers included intense emotions, such as anger, fear and excitement, which were provoked by situations such as marital- and job-related stresses and bereavement. Of the total study population 66% had coronary heart disease, but only 48% patients with putative psychophysiologic "triggers" for ventricular tachycardia or ventricular fibrillation had ischemic heart disease. Of the patients without demonstrable structural heart disease 44% demonstrated psychological triggers for ventricular tachycardia or ventricular fibrillation. Our estimate of 21% is somewhat lower than that of Myers and Dewar [46] and of Rissanen et al., who reported death following such stresses.[47] However, we were careful to exclude equivocal cases, and it is likely that our estimate may be overly conservative.

Psychological Stress and Ventricular Arrhythmias

Ventricular premature beats (VPBs) occurring in patients with coronary heart disease are associated with an increased risk for sudden cardiac death.[50]

Quantification of VPBs can therefore be used as a somatic target to evaluate the effects of psychological stress on the heart. A number of studies relate the occurrence of VPBs to biobehavioral factors. These studies, though largely uncontrolled, show that emotional states resulting from recall of traumatic events, anxiety, fear, excitement, and deliberate induction of stressful states result in electrocardiographic alterations including S-T segment and T wave abnormalities and emergence of VPBs. For example, stresses as disparate as those caused by public speaking, motor car racing or driving, loud sounds, and clinical interviews relating to previous or ongoing emotional trauma have evoked VPBs in patients with and without heart disease.[51-55] We have shown in a controlled study of 19 patients, among whom 8 had been resuscitated from ventricular fibrillation, that psychological stress testing yielded a two-fold increase in VPBs. In one of these patients malignant ventricular tachycardia was induced when the patient wept while describing his fear of death. This arrhythmia, which had progressed on previous occasions to ventricular fibrillation, was completely suppressed by reassurance alone, without resort to drug treatment.[15]

As mentioned earlier, lack of education has an impact on the occurrence of premature death. Kitagawa and Hauser have shown an inverse relationship between cardiovascular mortality and educational level.[56] Recognizing that the level of education has an important psychosocial significance, Weinblatt et al. stratified 1739 male survivors of myocardial infarction into categories defined by years of schooling.[11] When these men were electrocardiographically monitored for 1 hour, men with 8 years or less of schooling, exhibited three times the risk of sudden cardiac death if complex ventricular arrhythmias were present. In contrast, better-educated men with the same type of arrhythmia had a significantly lower mortality rate. The cumulative mortality rates were 33% and 9%, respectively, for the two groups, and neither standard risk factors nor a variety of clinical characteristics accounted for these differences. This landmark study showed for the first time a significant relationship between a putative index of psychosocial distress, ventricular arrhythmias, and sudden cardiac death.

The physiological mechanisms whereby induced or naturally occurring stresses cause ventricular arrhythmias have been inadequately studied. Taggart et al. have shown that catecholamine levels are elevated when VPBs occur during psychological stress resulting from public speaking, car-racing, or driving in traffic.[51, 52] They were able to abolish stress-induced VPBs with the beta-adrenergic antagonist, oxprenolol. The contributory role of catecholamines in the genesis of malignant ventricular arrhythmias was also demonstrated by Coumel et al.[58] They described four children without organic heart disease in whom ventricular tachycardia with syncope was triggered by effort or emotion. Electrical endocavitary stimulation could not initiate the arrhythmia, but infusion with the beta-adrenergic agonist, isoproterenol, did so consistently. Treatment with beta-adrenergic antagonists alone or in combination with other drugs was helpful in suppressing these arrhythmias.

The most striking and convincing evidence that sympathetic neural inputs are important in provoking malignant ventricular arrhythmias is demonstrated by the series of disorders of ventricular repolarization known collectively as the long Q-T syndrome. A variety of sensory inputs, ranging from emotionally stressful events to noise and exertion, may trigger ventricular tachycardia or ventricular fibrillation. Early demise is the rule in such patients, although structural heart disease is invariably absent. An imbalance in sympathetic neural input to the heart between the right and the left stellate ganglia has been postulated.[59] Protection after surgical ablation of these structures or pharmacologic blockade with beta-adrenergic antagonists provides further evidence for the role of sympathetic neural inputs in the genesis of these arrhythmias.

Although these studies indicate an important role for adrenergic mechanisms in the emergence of ventricular tachycardia and ventricular fibrillation in both animals and in man, it should not be assumed that the sympathetic nervous system is the exclusive conduit for the destabilizing effects of the central nervous system on the heart. Additional neural and humoral interactions may exist that have yet to be elucidated. Neural mechanisms for the provocation of ventricular arrhythmias in particular have not been adequately studied in man. Since neural outflow to the heart is governed by the autonomic nervous system, we examined the contributing role of autonomic neural reflexes to the occurrence of ventricular arrhythmias. In a small group of patients, some of whom were resuscitated from ventricular fibrillation, we were able to increase the frequency of VPBs by means of psychological stress testing. In these patients, activation of sympathetic and parasympathetic reflexes in the absence of stress did not provoke ventricular arrhythmias.[15] In particular, elicitation of the "dive reflex" by exposure of the face to an ice-pack did not provoke significant arrhythmia, except in one patient who became emotionally distraught during the test procedure. She was a 45-year-old woman without structural heart disease who had had recurrent ventricular fibrillation in situations of emotional conflict. From these observations, it appears that the passive evocation of autonomic reflexes is not a sufficient trigger for the occurrence of ventricular arrhythmias.

Behavioral Studies

If we assume that certain individuals have a proclivity for psychophysiologically induced arrhythmias, it is logical to examine whether certain behavioral or psychological characteristics predispose to the development of ventricular arrhythmias and sudden cardiac death. Such an approach has already been applied to a variety of other disease states. Thomas, for example, prospectively evaluated healthy medical students and found that certain features such as nervous tension, anxiety, anger under stress, insomnia, smoking, and alcohol intake were associated with a higher rate of premature death and disease.[60] These precursors were evaluated in relation to the development of suicide, cancer, hypertension, myocardial infarction, and mental illness. Mean depression scores were twice as high in those developing myocardial infarction as in controls.

Depression has also been ascribed importance in relation to sudden death by some workers. Greene et al. reported in a study where the next-of-kin were interviewed that victims of sudden cardiac death had a high prevalence of depression and agitation prior to death.[45] Since the decedents' relatives provided the information, direct assessment of psychological and behavioral characteristics was not possible. A prospective study by Bruhn et al.[61] in patients with myocardial infarction indicated that elevated depression scores, a pattern of "joyless striving" at work, and Type A behavior characteristics correlated with the occurrence of sudden cardiac death. Orth-Gomer [62] attempted to correlate in a group of men the occurrence and grade of ventricular arrhythmia with psychological characteristics, as gauged by the Emotions Profile Index and a structured interview for Type A behavior pattern. No correlation was found between depression and complex ventricular arrhythmias in men with coronary heart disease or in men with risk factors for coronary heart disease. Neither was Type A behavior pattern correlated with complex ventricular arrhythmias. In our own studies, where we identified 25 of 117 patients with putative psychophysiologic triggers for ventricular tachycardia and ventricular fibrillation, we performed a variety of psychometric tests in an attempt to distinguish patients from controls.[49] No specific psychological characteristics were readily apparent, except for exceptionally high depression scores. It must be noted, however, that since such patients were studied after referral for life-threatening arrhythmias, the presence of depression may have been the consequence of their illness.

Studies designed to characterize patients psychologically and behaviorally in order to characterize or predict potential victims of a disease process are conceptually attractive. However, as noted by Aiken,[63] such studies are difficult to conduct because of current methodologic deficiencies in psychosomatic research, including the difficulty in measuring psychological variables, problems with controlling observations, fallacies in deduction of causality, proper case identification, and sampling error.

Reduction in Sympathetic Tone and Ventricular Arrhythmias

Since neural activation from psychological stress may be associated with increases in heart rate, blood pressure, and ventricular premature beat frequency, the effects of withdrawal of sympathetic tone on the heart can be expected to have the opposite effect. Sleep represents a phase during the day when there is a marked shift in consciousness and a reduction in cardiovascular hemodynamic activity. The declines in heart rate and blood pressure have been attributed to withdrawal of sympathetic tone and an increase in vagal tone. Some observers have noted that during sleep VPBs are not affected, while others have provided evidence that most patients show sleep-suppression of ventricular arrhythmias.[64-72] These disparate observations may be due to small sample sizes, or because patients were often studied in the medicated state or in the coronary care unit.

In studies involving large sample sizes, the results almost invariably indicate that sleep suppresses VPBs.[67-72] Lown *et al.* observed during Holter monitoring of 54 subjects in their own homes, that in 22 VPBs were reduced at least 50% during sleep, while 13 subjects showed 25–50% suppression.[69] The grade of VPBs was also lowered from a mean of 2.75 while awake to 1.78 during sleep. In a number of these patients, antiarrhythmic drugs were less effective than sleep in reducing the grade and frequency of VPBs. These studies were extended to include simultaneous electrocardiographic and electroencephalographic recordings and it was found that sleep suppression of VPBs in 30 patients occurred during all sleep stages except REM sleep.[70] Slow wave sleep (stages 3 and 4) had the most significant effect on VPB suppression. These results contrast with the observations of Rosenblatt *et al.*, who found emergence of arrhythmias during these stages of sleep.[64] The results we obtained were not due to alterations in heart rate, because no significant changes in rate occurred between the various sleep stages. Frequency of VPBs during awake and REM periods were similar, suggesting that the electrical properties of the heart during these two periods may also be similar. Pickering et al. reported that in 26% of 31 patients they monitored, VPBs were suppressed almost completely during sleep, while in 71% the reduction in VPBs was partial.[67] Multiform and repetitive VPBs were also decreased during sleep. These observations are important because it has been noted that sudden death is unusual during sleep.[46, 73] Although there is no direct evidence, it is very likely that a lessening of sympathetic neural and humoral activity during sleep is protective against sudden cardiac death. We have observed ventricular tachycardia or ventricular fibrillation in association with violent or frightening dreams in two cases.[49, 54] It is still inferential that when sudden death occurs during sleep it does so during the stage of REM sleep. In summary, present evidence indicates that non-REM sleep, which decreases sympathetic neural outflow, results in increased electrical myocardial stability with decrease in ventricular arrhythmias. During REM sleep, electrical instability may be provoked as a consequence of increased sympathetic neural drive on the heart and malignant ventricular arrhythmias may emerge.

Conscious modulation of sympathetic neural input to the heart may be accomplished by a variety of biofeedback and meditation techniques. Weiss and Engel[74] and Pickering and Miller[75] have shown that VPBs can be suppressed by increasing heart rate with biofeedback. Abolition of VPBs is probably secondary to overdrive suppression of an ectopic focus by acceleration in heart rate. Meditation and relaxation techniques have also been utilized to suppress VPBs. The essential cardiovascular effect of cultic and noncultic forms of meditation is reduction in heart rate and blood pressure, probably secondary to decreased sympathetic neural outflow. Eleven patients with coronary heart disease were taught by Benson et al. to elicit the relaxation response over a period of 4 weeks.[76] Although VPBs were modestly suppressed during both awake and sleep periods, this effect was significant only during the latter period. Hence the results observed by these workers may have been the result of sleep rather than meditation. Heart rate was not significantly affected by the procedure. Voukydis and Forwand[77] found that VPBs were suppressed by a similar technique in some patients while in others, arrhythmia was unaffected or actually increased.[60] In our own experience, the results of meditation on VPBs have been very variable. In an occasional patient, marked suppression of VPBs or even termination of ventricular tachycardia is possible. Objective evidence that the observed cardiovascular effects of this noncultic form of meditation are due to decreased sympathetic tone is sparse. Heart rate decreases in individual subjects were directly correlated with plasma norepinephrine changes during relaxation therapy by Davidson et al.[78] However, group means for heart rate did not change significantly between control and relaxation periods. These observations, together with the frequently variable response of VPBs, suggest that the effects of meditation and relaxation on cardiovascular function are modest in many subjects. Nonetheless, when marked effects are observed on heart rate and ventricular arrhythmias in individual subjects, they provide further evidence that neural and psychological influences have the capacity to affect electrical activity of the heart and modulate the emergence and suppression of arrhythmias.

CONCLUSION

Despite the lack of conclusive evidence as to causality, we cannot afford to ignore the clinical and experimental evidence that indicates that neural and psychological mechanisms modulate electrical properties of the heart and provoke sudden cardiac death. Each year about 450,000 victims succumb to sudden cardiac death, and this number constitutes by far the single most important cause of death in the United States. Current estimates indicate that such deaths may be preceded by acute psychological disturbances in 20 to 40% of cases. Thus, analysis of risk factors for sudden cardiac death must perforce include not only characterization of the nature and extent of heart disease, but also behavioral and psychophysiologic features and the psychosocial setting of the potential victim. Exploration of intermediary mechanisms will permit the introduction of innovative forms of treatment, including neurochemical interventions designed to prevent the psychophysiologic triggers for sudden cardiac death. Although definitive studies in this area will be long in the making, the integrative role of the central nervous system in determining the time of death should be more fully appreciated. Such an awareness will provide a basis for closer attention to psychological factors in the clinical management of patients at high risk for sudden death.[79]

ACKNOWLEDGMENT

I wish to acknowledge my deep indebtedness to Dr. Bernard Lown, who not only outlined the concepts set forth here, but also initiated and directed many of the animal and human studies described in this paper. His helpful comments and criticisms are also appreciated.

REFERENCES

1. HARVEY, W. Exercitatio Anatomic de Motu Cordis et Sanguinus in Animalibus. Francofurti Edition of 1628 (Keynes English Translation of 1928). 94.: The Classics of Medicine Library. Birmingham, Ala.
2. McWILLIAM, J. A. 1889. Cardiac failure and sudden death. Br. Med. J. 1: 6.
3. McWILLIAM, J. A. 1923. Ventricular fibrillation and sudden death. Br. Med. J. 2: 215.
4. McWILLIAM, J. A. 1923. Blood pressure and heart action in sleep and dreams: Their relation to hemorrhages, angina and sudden death. Br. Med. J. 2: 1196.
5. COBB, L. A., R. S. BAUM, H. A. ALVAREZ, III, et al. 1975. Resuscitation from out-of-hospital ventricular fibrillation: 4 years follow-up. Circulation 51 & 52 (Suppl III): III-3.
6. LOWN, B. & R. L. VERRIER. 1976. Neural activity and ventricular fibrillation. N. Engl. J. Med. 294: 1165–1170.
7. LOWN, B., R. L. VERRIER & S. H. RABINOWITZ. 1977. Neural and psychologic mechanisms and the problem of sudden cardiac death. Am. J. Cardiol. 39: 890–902.
8. DESILVA, R. A. & B. LOWN. 1978. Ventricular premature beats, stress and sudden death. Psychosomatics 19: 649–659.
9. HRUBEC, Z. & W. J. ZUKEL. 1971. Socioeconomic differentials in prognosis following episodes of coronary heart disease. J. Chron. Dis. 23: 881.

10. JACOBS, S. & A. OSTFIELD. 1977. An epidemiologic review of mortality of bereavement. Psychosom. Med. **39:** 344–357.
11. WEINBLATT, E., W. RUBERMAN, J. D. GOLDBERG, et al. 1978. Relation of education to sudden death after myocardial infarction. N. Engl. J. Med. **299:** 60.
12. ALBUTT, C. 1915. Diseases of the Heart Including Angina Pectoris. II. MacMillan. London.
13. RICHTER, C. P. 1957. On the phenomenon of sudden death in animals and man. Psychosom. Med. **19:** 91.
14. WOLF, S. 1967. The bradycardia of the dive reflex—a possible mechanism of sudden death. Cond. Reflex **2:** 89.
15. LOWN, B. & R. A. DESILVA. 1978. Roles of psychologic stress and autonomic nervous system changes in provocation of ventricular premature complexes. Am. J. Cardiol. **41:** 979–985.
16. CANNON, W. B. 1957. "Voodoo" death. Psychosom. Med. **19:** 182.
17. LOWN, B., R. A. DESILVA, P. REICH & B. J. MURAWSKI. 1980. Psychophysiologic factors in sudden cardiac death. Am. J. Psych. **137:** 1325–1335.
18. LEVY, A. G. 1913. The exciting causes of ventricular fibrillation in animals under chloroform anesthesia. Heart **4:** 319–378.
19. KORTEWEG, G. C. J., J. TH.F. BOELES & J. TENCATE. 1957. Influences of stimulation of some subcortical areas on the electrocardiogram. J. Neurophysiol. **20:** 100–107.
20. J. SATINSKY, B. KOSOWSKY & B. LOWN. 1971. Ventricular fibrillation induced by hypothalamic stimulation during coronary occlusion (abstract). Circulation (Suppl II): II–60.
21. CORLEY, K. C., H. P. MAUCK & F. O. M. SHIEL. 1975. Cardiac responses associated with "yoked-chair" shock avoidance. Psychophysiology **12:** 439.
22. JOHANSSON, G., L. JOHNSSON, N. LANNEK, et al. 1974. Severe stress-cardiopathy in pigs. Am. Heart J. **87:** 451.
23. HAFT, J. I. 1979. Role of platelets in coronary artery disease. Am. J. Cardiol. **43:** 1197–1206.
24. RABB, W. 1966. Emotional and sensory stress factors in myocardial pathology. Am. Heart J. **72:** 538.
25. MATTA, R. J., R. L. VERRIER & B. LOWN. 1976. The repetitive extrasystole threshold as an index of vulnerability to ventricular fibrillation. Am. J. Physiol. **230:** 1469–1473.
26. DESILVA, R. A., R. L. VERRIER & B. LOWN. 1979. Repetitive extrasystole threshold as an index of vulnerability to ventricular fibrillation during psychologic stress (abstract). Clin. Res. **27:** 562A.
27. LOWN, B., R. L. VERRIER & R. CORBALAN. 1973. Psychologic stress and threshold for repetitive ventricular response. Science **182:** 834–836.
28. MATTA, R. L., J. E. LAWLER & B. LOWN. 1976. Ventricular electrical instability in the conscious dog: Effects of psychologic stress and beta-adrenergic blockade. Am. J. Cardiol. **34:** 594–598.
29. DESILVA, R. A., R. L. VERRIER & B. LOWN. 1978. Effects of psychological stress and vagal stimulation with morphine on vulnerability to ventricular fibrillation (VF) in the conscious dog. Am. J. Cardiol. **34:** 692–696.
30. CORBALAN, R., R. L. VERRIER & B. LOWN. 1974. Psychologic stress and ventricular arrhythmia during myocardial infarction in the conscious dog. Am. J. Cardiol. **34:** 692–696.
31. SKINNER, J. E., J. T. LIE & M. L. ENTMAN. 1975. Modification of ventricular fibrillation latency following coronary artery occlusion in the conscious pig: The effects of psychological stress and beta-adrenergic blockade. Circulation **51:** 656–667.
32. VERRIER, R. L. & B. LOWN. The role of the nervous system in ventricular arrhythmias. Acta Med. Scand. In press.

33. LIANG, B., R. L. VERRIER, J. MELMAN & B. LOWN. 1979. Correlation between circulating catecholamine levels and ventricular vulnerability during psychological stress in conscious dogs. Proc. Soc. Exper. Biol. **161**: 266–269.
34. DESILVA, R. A., R. L. VERRIER & B. LOWN. 1978. Effects of psychologic stress and vagal stimulation on vulnerability to ventricular fibrillation in the conscious dog. Am. Heart J. **95**: 197–203.
35. KOLMAN, B. S., R. L. VERRIER & B. LOWN. 1975. The effect of vagal nerve stimulation upon vulnerability of the canine ventricle; role of sympathetic parasympathetic interventions. Circulation **52**: 578–585.
36. RABINOWITZ, S. H., R. L. VERRIER & B. LOWN. 1976. Muscarinic effects of vagosympathetic trunk stimulation on the repetitive extrasystole threshold. Circulation **53**: 622–672.
37. DESILVA, R. A., R. L. VERRIER & B. LOWN. 1976. Protective effect of the vagotonic effect of morphine sulphate on vulnerability to ventricular fibrillation. Cardiovasc. Res. **12**: 161–172.
38. RABINOWITZ, S. H. & B. LOWN. 1978. Central neurochemical factors related to serotonin metabolism and cardiac ventricular vulnerability for repetitive electrical activity. Am. J. Cardiol. **41**: 516–522.
39. BLATT, C. M., S. H. RABINOWITZ & B. LOWN. 1979. Central serotonergic agents raise the repetitive extrasystole threshold of the vulnerable period of the canine ventricular myocardium. Circ. Res. **44**: 723–630.
40. SCOTT, N. A., R. A. DESILVA, B. LOWN & R. J. WURTMAN. 1981. Tyrosine administration decreases vulnerability to ventricular fibrillation in the normal canine heart. Science **211**: 727–729.
41. FALK, R. H., R. A. DESILVA & B. LOWN. 1981. Reduction in vulnerability to ventricular fibrillation by bromocriptine, a dopamine agonist. Cardiovasc. Res. **15**: 175–180.
42. MATTA, R. J., J. E. LAWLER & B. LOWN. 1974. Ventricular electrical instability in the conscious dog. Effects of psychologic stress and beta-adrenergic blockade. Am. J. Cardiol. **34**: 692.
43. ROSENFELD, J., M. R. ROSEN & B. F. HOFFMAN. 1978. Pharmacologic and behavioral effects of arrhythmias that immediately follow abrupt coronary occlusion: A canine model of sudden coronary death. Am. J. Cardiol. **41**: 1075.
44. RAHE, R. H., M. ROMO, L. BENNETT & P. SILTANEN. 1974. Recent life changes, myocardial infarction and abrupt coronary death. Arch. Intern. Med. **133**: 221.
45. GREENE, W. A., S. GOLDSTEIN & A. J. MOSS. 1972. Psychosocial aspects of sudden death. Arch. Intern. Med. **129**: 725.
46. MYERS, A. & H. A. DEWAR. 1975. Circumstances attending 100 sudden deaths from coronary artery disease with coroners' necropsies. Br. Heart J. **37**: 1133.
47. RISSANEN, V., M. ROMO & P. SILTANEN. 1978. Premonitory symptoms and stress factors preceding sudden death from ischemic heart disease. Acta Med. Scand. **204**: 389.
48. CEBELIN, M. S. & C. S. HIRSCH. 1980. Human stress cardiomyopathy. Hum. Pathol. **11**: 123–132.
49. REICH, P., R. A. DESILVA, B. LOWN & B. J. MURAWSKI. 1981. Acute psychological disturbances preceding life-threatening ventricular arrhythmias. J. Amer. Med. Assoc. **246**: 233–235.
50. CORONARY DRUG PROJECT RESEARCH GROUP. 1973. Prognostic importance of premature beats following myocardial infarction: Experience in the coronary drug project. J. Amer. Med. Assoc. **223**: 1116–1124.
51. TAGGART, P., M. CARRUTHERS & W. SOMERVILLE. Electrocardiogram, plasma catecholamines and lipids and their modification by oxprenolol when speaking before an audience. Lancet **2**: 341–346.
52. TAGGART, P., D. GIBBONS & W. SOMERVILLE. 1969. Some effects of motor car driving on the normal and abnormal heart. Br. Med. J. **4**: 130–134.

53. WELLENS, H. J. J., A. VERMEULEN & D. DURREN. 1972. Ventricular fibrillation occurring on arousal from sleep by auditory stimuli. Circulation 46: 661–665.
54. LOWN, B., J. V. TEMTE, P. REICH, et al. 1976. Basis for recurring ventricular fibrillation in the absence of coronary artery disease and its management. N. Engl. J. Med. 294: 623.
55. SIGLER, L. H. 1961. Abnormalities in the electrocardiogram induced by emotional strain. Am. J. Cardiol. 8: 807.
56. KITAGAWA, F. M. & P. M. HAUSER. 1973. Differential Mortality in the United States. A Study in Socioeconomic Epidemiology.: 11–33, 78–79. Harvard University Press.
57. ENGEL, G. L. 1971. Sudden and rapid death during psychological stress. Folklore or folk wisdom? Ann. Intern. Med. 74: 771–772.
58. COUMEL, P., J. FIDELLE, V. LUCET et al. 1978. Catecholamine-induced severe ventricular arrhythmias with Adams-Stokes syndrome in children. Report of four cases. Br. Heart J. 40 (Suppl): 28–37.
59. SCHWARTZ, P. J. 1976. Cardiac sympathetic innervation and the sudden infant death syndrome. Am. J. Med. 60: 167–172.
60. THOMAS, C. B. 1976. Precursors of premature disease and death. Ann. Intern. Med. 85: 653–658.
61. BRUHN, J. G., A. PAREDES, C. A. ADSETT & S. WOLF. Psychological predictors of sudden death in myocardial infarction. J. Psychosom. Res. 18: 187–191.
62. ORTH-GOMER, K., M. E. EDWARDS, M. E. ERHARDT, et al. 1980. Relation between ventricular arrhythmias and psychologic profile. Acta Med. Scand. 207: 31–36.
63. AIKEN, R. C. B. 1972. Methodology of research in psychosomatic medicine. Br. Med. J. 4: 285–287.
64. ROSENBLATT, G., G. ZWILLING & E. HARTMAN. 1969. Electrocardiographic changes during sleep in patients with cardiac abnormality (abstract). Psychophysiology 6: 233.
65. SMITH, R., L. JOHNSON, D. ROTHFELD, et al. 1972. Sleep and cardiac arrhythmias. Arch. Intern. Med. 130: 751.
66. MONTI, J., L. E. FOLLE, C. PELUFFO, et al. 1975. The incidence of premature contractions in coronary patients during the sleep-awake cycle. Cardiology 60: 257.
67. PICKERING, T. G., L. GOULDING & B. A. COBERN. 1977. Diurnal variations in ventricular ectopic beats and heart rate. Cardiovasc. Med. 2: 1013.
68. PICKERING, T. G., J. JOHNSTON & A. J. HONOUR. 1978. Comparison of effects of sleep, exercise and autonomic drugs on ventricular extrasystoles, using ambulatory monitoring of electrocardiogram and electroencephalogram. Am. J. Med. 65: 575.
69. LOWN, B., M. TYKOCINSKI, A. GARFEIN, et al. 1973. Sleep and ventricular premature beats. Circulation 48: 691–701.
70. DESILVA, R. A., Q. R. REGESTEIN & B. LOWN. Unpublished observations.
71. WINKLE, R. A., M. G. LOPES, J. W. FITZGERALD, et al. 1975. Arrhythmias in patients with mitral valve prolapse. Circulation 52: 73.
72. BRODSKY, M., D. WU, P. DENES, et al. 1977. Arrhythmias documented by 24 hour continuous electrocardiographic monitoring in 50 male medical students. Am. J. Cardiol. 39: 390.
73. FRIEDMAN, M., J. H. MANWARING, R. H. ROSENMAN, et al. 1973. Instantaneous and sudden deaths. J. Amer. Med. Assoc. 225: 1319–1328.
74. WEISS, T. & B. T. ENGEL. 1971. Operant conditioning of the heart in patients with premature ventricular contractions. Psychosom. Med. 33: 301.
75. PICKERING, T. G. & N. E. MILLER. 1977. Learned voluntary control of heart rate and rhythm in two subjects with premature ventricular contractions. Br. Heart J. 39: 152.

76. BENSON, H., S. ALEXANDER & C. L. FELDMAN. 1975. Decreased premature ventricular contractions through the use of the relaxation response in patients with stable ischemic heart disease. Lancet **2**: 380.
77. VOUKYDIS, P. C. & S. A. FORWAND. 1977. The effect of elicitation of the relaxation response in patients with intractable ventricular arrhythmias. Circulation 55 & 56 (Suppl III): 111–157.
78. DAVIDSON, D. M., M. A. WINCHESTER, C. B. TAYLOR, et al. 1979. Effects of relaxation therapy on cardiac performance and sympathetic activity in patients with organic heart disease. Psychosom. Med. **41**: 303–309.
79. LOWN, B. 1979. Sudden cardiac death: The major challenge confronting contemporary cardiology. Am. J. Cardiol. **41**: 313–328.
80. COTTINGTON, E. M., K. A. MATTHEWS, E. TALBOTT & L. H. KULLER. 1980. Environmental events preceding sudden death in women. Psychosom. Med. **42**: 567–574.

DISCUSSION

DR. KASTOR: It seems that the notion of the Type A or Type B personality or the stress versus nonstress theory represents much too simple a point of view. Can you draw any conclusions about basic underlying personality types or characteristics that are applicable in this kind of work?

DR. DESILVA: We have viewed the Type A–Type B dichotomy as being an extremely simple one, but one that has some validity. Osler and several others since then have all observed that the man in a hurry tends to be more prone to a coronary. In the last 5 or 6 years we've been doing psychometric assessment using standard psychiatric profiles. Patients with sudden cardiac death are not easily distinguished from those suffering nonfatal myocardial infarctions.

DR. HERMAN: What type of meditation did your patients use? Did the people who were resuscitated have experiences in common?

DR. DESILVA: The meditation process, which really should not be called meditation, is Jacobsen's form of muscular relaxation. It consists of sitting with the eyes closed followed by a verbal induction of muscular relaxation starting with the scalp, down to the eyes, jaw and feet. The second part consists of a breathing exercise during which the patients concentrate on breathing. The third part consists of concentration on expiration and saying the word "Breathe" to themselves. This is continued for 15 to 20 minutes.

To answer the second part of your question, about whether there were common experiences in these patients: I have interviewed about a hundred patients about the entire death experience, and about two-thirds to three-quarters of them do not recollect anything of significance other than passing out. They report themselves to be sucked into a black void or a tube or through a black window. These patients are unmedicated and are normal in other respects, except that they've had ventricular fibrillation. I cannot agree with Elizabeth Kübler-Ross or with Raymond Moody and their findings. I suspect that their observations, while valid, are probably in other disease conditions and in people with prolonged and debilitating illnesses, such as cancer, or in people who were probably on psychotropic or mind-altering drugs at the time.

UNIDENTIFIED SPEAKER: Are you making any attempt at the chronic reduction of stress?

DR. DESILVA: The chronic reduction of stress is very difficult because we believe that it is extremely difficult to change the personality; furthermore, it is extremely difficult to change life patterns, and we have not attempted to do that. But implicit in our management of patients is the fact that they get a lot of reassuring support, as I'm sure most of you give. Unless there's a very good reason for not sending them back to a productive life, we do not tell them to give up their jobs. This applies as well to our patients who have had cardiac arrest.

THE ROLE OF THE AUTONOMIC NERVOUS SYSTEM IN SUDDEN CORONARY DEATH *

Peter J. Schwartz † and H. Lowell Stone

Arrhythmia Research Center
Institute of Clinical Physiology
Cardiovascolari C.N.R.
Università di Milano
Milano, Italy

Department of Physiology and Biophysics
University of Oklahoma School of Medicine
Oklahoma City, Oklahoma 73190

INTRODUCTION

The question of the role of the autonomic nervous system in sudden death is of paramount importance because, if fully elucidated, it may give critical insights into the basic mechanisms that lead to ventricular fibrillation and may provide the rationale for prevention.

This article does not intend to review the entire question of the relationship between the autonomic nervous system and sudden coronary death since this subject or part of it has been largely dealt with in recent reviews; [1-5] rather, it aims at providing updated information on recent progress in this area with particular reference to the role of cardiac sympathetic nerves and to the development of appropriate animal models specifically designed for the study of neurally mediated life-threatening arrhythmias.

The cardiovascular effects of autonomic nerves are often studied by using the technique of electrical stimulation, which, although valuable in identifying neural circuits, is limited because it shows the artificial effect of massive activation of all nerve fibers present in the stimulated nerves, a very unlikely event in a system characterized by an extreme degree of specificity.[6] We believe that the importance of the autonomic nervous system in relationship to pathophysiologic events which occur in real life situations, such as sudden coronary death, can be best studied by the use of selective denervation. In this way the resultant effects are due to the absence of the tonic sympathetic or vagal activity physiologically present in the nerves under investigation and it is possible to meaningfully compare what happens when the nerves are present and when they are absent.

An attempt to understand the role of the autonomic nervous system in sudden coronary death requires a knowledge of the neural events associated with acute myocardial ischemia, of the effects of neural activity on coronary blood flow, and of the autonomic effects on cardiac electrical stability in ischemic and nonischemic hearts. It requires also the potential of developing relevant animal models in which adequate manipulations of the autonomic

* This work was supported in part by Grant HL-18798 from the National Institutes of Health, Bethesda, Maryland.

† Address for correspondence: Peter J. Schwartz, M.D., Istituto di Clinica Medica IV dell'Università di Milano, Via F. Sforza 35, 20122 Milano, Italy.

nervous system can be performed in order to acquire new information, to test hypotheses, and to develop strategies for prevention.

NEURAL EVENTS ASSOCIATED WITH ACUTE MYOCARDIAL ISCHEMIA

Myocardial ischemia excites both vagal [7, 8] and sympathetic afferent fibers of cardiac origin eliciting a variety of reflex responses. For an extensive analysis of this problem the interested reader is referred to the recent reviews by Brown [9] and by Bishop, Malliani, and Thoren.[10] Here, only those basic aspects potentially more relevant to the problem of sudden coronary death will be briefly reviewed; for this reason the sympathetic component will be discussed in greater detail.

The cardiac sympathetic sensory endings [11, 12] are mechanoreceptors normally excited by mechanical events, but their activity can be further enhanced by chemical substances, like bradykinin,[13] which are known to be released in the ischemic heart. This activation elicits an excitatory cardiocardiac reflex [14] (FIG. 1). This reflex, which takes place within a few seconds of ischemia, plays an important role in the genesis of the early ventricular arrhythmias as shown by the fact that the interruption of its afferent limb by a section of dorsal roots from the eight cervical segment to the fifth thoracic segment is capable of reducing to a major extent the arrhythmias associated with short-lasting coronary occlusion [15] (FIG. 2).

The excitation of cardiac sympathetic afferents not only leads to an increase in efferent cardiac sympathetic activity, but can also reflexly and selectively inhibit the activity of efferent cardiac vagal fibers [16] (FIG. 3). This sympathovagal reflex has the potential of impairing the vagally-mediated maintenance of an optimal heart rate,[17] thus facilitating the occurrence of a dangerous tachycardia.

It is noteworthy that the afferent limbs of most cardiocardiac sympathetic reflexes seem to be preferentially distributed through left-sided nerves, which makes these reflexes dependent to a major extent on an intact left stellate ganglion.

The effects of sympathetic discharges relevant to sudden coronary death are mostly those affecting the electrophysiologic properties of the heart, the coronary circulation, and the level of heart rate.

The observation that in the majority of patients seen within 30 minutes after the onset of acute myocardial infarction there were signs of "autonomic disturbance," namely signs of sympathetic hyperactivity mostly in patients with anterior infarction and signs of vagal hyperactivity mostly in patients with inferior infarction, not only represented a major contribution,[18, 19] but also provided a necessary link between experimental studies and clinical reality.

The relationship between acute myocardial ischemia and sympathetic reflexes has just been discussed. Also vagal reflexes have been observed experimentally after myocardial ischemia, particularly of the posterior wall of the left ventricle.[8, 20, 21]

The role of vagal reflexes during acute myocardial ischemia is still controversial,[3, 15, 22] and both protective and detrimental effects have been claimed. Verrier and Lown have provided ample evidence that the protective result of increased vagal activity is mostly due to an indirect effect obtained by opposing the arrhythmogenic influence of adrenergic activity.[23] In uncontrolled situa-

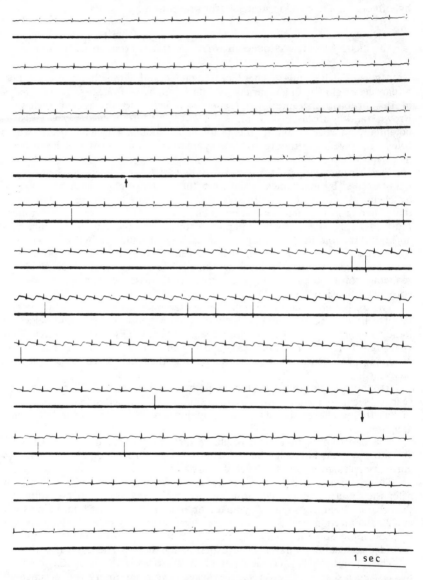

1 sec

FIGURE 1. Continuous recording of electrocardiogram (*upper trace*) and of sympathetic activity (*lower trace*) in an anesthetized cat. Sympathetic activity was recorded
from the left third thoracic ramus communicans (T3) and the Figure shows a single
preganglionic sympathetic fiber, spontaneously silent, excited by coronary arterial
occlusion. The two *arrows* indicate beginning and end of occlusion. (From Malliani
et al.[14] Reproduced by permission.)

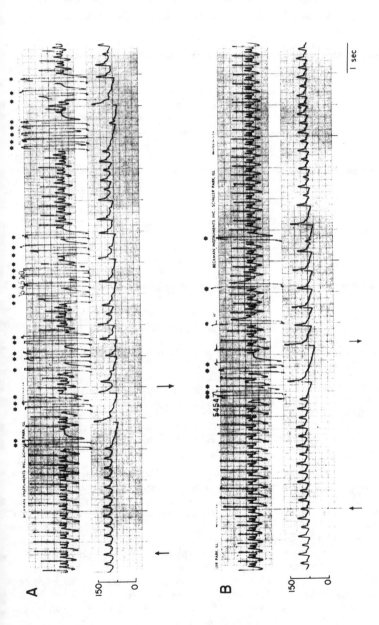

FIGURE 2. Electrocardiogram (*upper trace*) and aortic blood pressure (mm Hg) (*lower trace*) in a vagotomized dog. *Arrows* indicate a 5-sec occlusion of the left descending coronary artery. (A) Coronary arterial occlusion during control conditions produces a large number of premature ventricular beats (marked by asterisks), which result in runs of ventricular tachycardia. (B) same occlusion after dorsal root section produces only a few ectopic beats. (From Schwartz *et al.*[15] Reproduced by permission.)

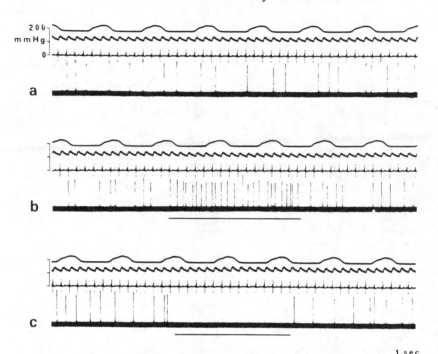

FIGURE 3. Effects of electrical stimulation on the neural discharge of a single right efferent cardiac vagal fiber in a decerebrate, anesthetized cat. (a) Spontaneous activity. (b) Electrical stimulation (5 volts, 1.5 msec, 30 Hz) of the cut central end of the left cervical vagus (afferent stimulation). (c) Electrical stimulation (10 volts, 1.5 msec, 30 Hz) of the cut central end of the left inferior cardiac nerve. The tracings in each section show from *top to bottom:* respiration (positive-pressure inflation is an upward deflection), systemic arterial blood pressure, electrocardiogram, and neural activity. The figure shows that while afferent vagal stimulation reflexly increases efferent cardiac vagal activity, activation of cardiac sympathetic afferent fibers has the opposite effect. (From Schwartz *et al.*[36] Reproduced by permission.)

tions, a major determinant of the effects of vagal reflexes is represented by the attendant changes in heart rate, which makes it difficult to interpret correctly those studies in which the change, or lack of change, in heart rate is not accounted for. As an example, the suppression induced by phenylephrine of ventricular arrhythmias has been initially interpreted [24] as due to the reflex increase in vagal activity, while a subsequent study [25] which in addition employed atrial pacing has shown that the antiarrhythmic effect of phenylephrine is mostly due to the attendant slowing in heart rate.

Some enhancement in vagal tone is beneficial inasmuch as it prevents excessive increases in heart rate, thus preserving underperfused tissue from impending ischemia. However, when the increase in vagal activity is excessive, it may produce hypotension and further reduce coronary flow to the ischemic areas, eventually resulting in either asystole or in ventricular fibrillation, as it can be observed in experimental animals.[26] Why such an overwhelming vagal activity may occur is still unclear. The critical factor may be the existing level of sympathetic activity. If sympathetic activity is high enough, the vagal reflex may prevent unduly high heart rates without the detrimental effects that may occur if the increased vagal activity is left completely unopposed. The balance between sympathetic and vagal efferent activity may be a key to survival during acute myocardial ischemia.

NEURAL CONTROL OF CORONARY BLOOD FLOW

It has been generally accepted that the major factor controlling coronary blood flow is the metabolic demand of the myocardial tissue [27] and the ability of the coronary vessels to autoregulate to meet these demands. The ability of the sympathetic nervous system to cause coronary vasoconstriction was reported by Feigl [28] in 1967, and subsequently coronary vasoconstriction was reflexly elicited through carotid sinus activation.[29, 30] The reflex activation of coronary vasoconstriction, dependent upon the sympathetic nervous system, was shown to be blocked by alpha-adrenergic antagonists and enhanced by beta-adrenergic antagonists. The relationship between the metabolic and neurogenic components of the control of coronary blood flow to the left ventricle was examined specifically and a sympathetic vasoconstriction could be demonstrated when the metabolic demand of the myocardium was elevated in the anesthetized dog.[31] However, the importance and the extent of this mechanism in physiologic conditions in the nonanesthetized animal remained elusive.

Subsequently, in the conscious dog, using the coronary flow response to 10-second occlusions, we found that removal of the left stellate ganglion would increase the reactive hyperemic payback [32] and this result could be mimicked by alpha-adrenergic blockade (FIG. 4). This study clearly showed, for the first time, that a tonic vasoconstrictor tone was present on the coronary vessels and

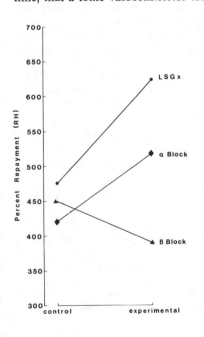

FIGURE 4. Reactive hyperemia in conscious dogs before and after left stellectomy (LSGx), phentolamine (α-block), and propranolol (β-block). The data points represent the means of 130 trials in 16 dogs. They indicate that left stellectomy and alpha-adrenergic blockade increase reactive hyperemia, a variable that relates to the capability of the coronary bed to dilate, whereas beta-adrenergic blockade has an opposite effect. The same kind of responses were found when heart rate was kept constant by pacing. (After Schwartz and Stone.[32])

that at least brief periods of ischemia were not sufficient to cause a withdrawal of the vasoconstrictor tone despite a significant metabolic alteration as a result of the occlusion. Removal of the left stellate ganglion eliminates the adrenergic fibers that travel down the major left coronary arteries [33] and would be expected to interrupt the tonic vasoconstrictor tone and improve coronary blood flow.

In a further attempt to characterize the role of the sympathetic nervous system in controlling coronary flow in physiologic and clinically relevant conditions, we examined the effect of left stellectomy during submaximal exercise. Left stellate ganglion removal increased coronary flow during exercise and indicated that a tonic sympathetic vasoconstrictor tone can limit coronary blood flow even during the physiologic stress of exercise.[34] Coronary blood flow during submaximal [35, 36] and maximal [37] exercise could also be increased by alpha-adrenergic blockade independent of changes in myocardial oxygen consumption.

It has been recently shown that cyclical changes in coronary blood flow resulting from spontaneous disaggregation of aggregate platelets, at the site of coronary arterial stenosis, were abolished by stellectomy and were enhanced by stimulation of the stellate ganglion.[38] These results probably depend on a catecholamine-mediated fluctuation in platelet aggregability, potentially a phenomenon of high clinical relevance.

In human subjects, Mudge et al.[39] measured the reflex coronary vasoconstriction as a result of a cold pressor test and suggested that the vasoconstriction may contribute to the manifestation of ischemic heart disease. If myocardial ischemia or reduced blood flow resulting in tissue hypoxia causes an increase in coronary flow through a purely metabolic mechanism, then coronary stenosis would be expected to result in coronary vasodilation and withdrawal of the tonic vasoconstrictor tone. Recent evidence would suggest that this does not occur and that the ability to constrict the coronary vessels still exists.[40]

A reflex reduction in coronary blood flow can occur, as evidenced by the foregoing discussion, despite an increase in the metabolic demand of the tissue. During myocardial ischemia and with the activation of cardiocardiac sympathetic reflexes, a reduction in coronary blood flow to the marginally ischemic tissue can occur and may be a major factor in the concomitant arrhythmias. The marginally ischemic zone would receive coronary flow from adjacent coronary vessels and from collateral coronary vessels. It appears that the sympathetic nervous system can exert control not only on these adjacent coronary vessels, but also over some of the collateral vessels,[41, 42] which would further increase the extent of ischemia and exacerbate the potential for arrhythmias. This may also explain why infarct size is significantly reduced by left stellectomy.[43]

AUTONOMIC NERVOUS SYSTEM AND LIFE-THREATENING ARRHYTHMIAS

Vagal efferent activity has, in most instances, a protective effect and antiadrenergic interventions, including bilateral stellectomy, also decreases vulnerability to ventricular fibrillation. These topics have been recently discussed in detail.[1-5, 26] This section will only deal with the recent evidence of the effects on arrhythmias of an imbalance in cardiac sympathetic innervation.

Since the pioneering work by Hunt in 1899,[44] many investigators have shown differential effects of right and left cardiac sympathetic nerves on various aspects of cardiac performance, such as heart rate, ventricular contractility, and ventricular repolarization. In regard to cardiac arrhythmias, the assumption had been made that, since bilateral stellectomy and beta-adrenergic blockade have an antiarrhythmic effect, to remove one part of the sympathetic innervation would at most confer partial protection. Actually, the situation is quite different and while unilateral left stellectomy has indeed a major protective effect, right stellectomy is attended by a paradoxical arrhythmogenic effect.

Our first investigations in this area were the result of our interest in a congenital disease, the idiopathic long Q-T syndrome, which is associated with a high incidence of sudden death and which seems to depend upon a specific imbalance in cardiac sympathetic innervation, namely a lower-than-normal right cardiac sympathetic activity which reflexly results in a higher-than-normal left cardiac sympathetic activity.[45-47]

The first model to be explored was that of coronary arterial occlusion in the dog because it has been studied widely and because it has been clearly shown by many, including Harris in his careful study,[48] that bilateral stellectomy prevents the arrhythmias elicited in that setting. By using a reversible cold blockade, we were able to compare in the same animal the responses to a brief coronary occlusion in control conditions and during functional absence of either right or left stellate ganglion.[49] We found that left stellate ganglion blockade had a protective effect, but that the incidence of arrhythmias was actually augmented by right stellate ganglion blockade. This finding was completely unexpected on the basis of the current knowledge, but has subsequently been confirmed in a variety of different experimental preparations. The next logical step was to investigate whether or not these effects of unilateral stellectomy were present also in nonischemic hearts, and the first study involved examination of ventricular vulnerability to fibrillation. We found that left stellectomy produced a major increase in ventricular fibrillation threshold, while right stellectomy had the opposite effect.[50] The clinical implications of the possibility of decreasing vulnerability to ventricular fibrillation by left stellectomy have been recently discussed.[26] Although these experiments confirmed the opposite effects of right and left stellectomy, they did not illuminate the causes of these differences. Progress was made when, in a study aimed at ascertaining the tonic sympathetic influence on ventricular refractoriness,[51] it was observed that the paradoxical effect of right stellectomy was dependent upon an intact left stellate ganglion. A reflex activation of the quantitatively dominant left stellate ganglion, induced by right stellectomy, is the most likely explanation, as has been discussed elsewhere.[34]

All these experiments had the limitation of having been performed in open chest animals. The effect of unilateral stellectomy was therefore approached in a more physiologic condition, that is, observing the effect of chronic unilateral denervation on arrhythmias induced by exercise.[34] This study was performed in chronically instrumented dogs, and exercise-induced ventricular arrhythmias were found in 8% of the control animals, in 11% of the dogs with left stellectomy, and in 86% of the dogs with right stellectomy. This observation seemed decisive for the acceptance of these strikingly different effects of unilateral stellectomy, but another question had to be answered: are these effects present also in man? In order to reply adequately, in 75 patients stellectomized as a treatment for the Raynaud syndrome (all without cardiac involvement), the incidence of arrhythmias induced by an exercise stress test was compared with that in 25 healthy subjects. The incidence of ventricular arrhythmias was

3% in the control subjects, 5% in the group with left stellectomy, and 21% in the group with right stellectomy.[52] It has to be noted that stellectomy in man produces only a partial denervation, which is at variance with the case in most experimental animals; therefore, our results have actually underestimated the effects of unilateral sympathetic denervation. To achieve in man results similar to those obtained in animals, it is necessary to perform a high thoracic sympathectomy, removing the first four to five thoracic ganglia.[5]

The arrhythmogenic effect of right stellectomy was also found in cats presented with emotional stimuli;[53] under these circumstances both left stellectomy and propranolol had a protective effect. The latter point is of interest because three studies involving stressful stimuli and cardiac arrhythmias yielded somewhat conflicting results about the effectiveness of beta-adrenergic blockade. In these studies different kinds of stressful stimulation were employed (cats wildly attacked by another cat,[53] pigs subjected to coronary occlusion in an unfamiliar environment,[54] dogs shifted from a quiet to a stressful environment,[55] and dogs stressed acoustically with a gun shot[56]); thus, the possibility should not be completely discounted that qualitatively and/or quantitatively different autonomic responses might be elicited under these different circumstances.

Finally, the studies mentioned in this section have demonstrated another aspect of the autonomic nervous system, previously not fully appreciated and quite relevant to the problem of sudden coronary death, namely the major arrhythmogenic potential of left-sided cardiac sympathetic nerves. This concept has already been substantiated by several different investigators[57-61] and is now generally accepted. Examples of ventricular tachyarrhythmias induced by stimulation of left stellate ganglion are represented in FIGURES 5 and 6. Of particular interest is FIGURE 6, which shows ventricular premature beats elicited by just touching with a blunt instrument the left stellate ganglion of a patient who suffered an anterior myocardial infarction 50 days earlier. This observation was made just prior to performing a high thoracic left sympathectomy; the patient is participating in a multicenter clinical trial in which survivors of an anterior myocardial infarction complicated by ventricular fibrillation are randomly assigned treatment with either placebo, beta-adrenergic blockade with propranolol, or high thoracic left sympathectomy.

ANIMAL MODELS FOR SUDDEN CORONARY DEATH

The choice of an appropriate model for sudden coronary death is critical for an attempt to understand the mechanisms involved and for a meaningful assessment of antiarrhythmic interventions. Too often, drugs are claimed to have a major antiarrhythmic effect on the basis of results obtained in conditions far different from those relevant to the clinical problem. The question of animal models for sudden death has been widely discussed.[26, 62, 63]

Two models currently in use in our laboratories will be presented here. They have different objectives and different characteristics. The first aims at providing the opportunity for a preliminary but specific evaluation of antiarrhythmic drugs with an internal control preparation that avoids group comparisons and deals specifically with acute myocardial ischemia and sympathetic hyperactivity. The second is designed in such a way to allow an in-depth analysis of the role of the autonomic nervous system in sudden coronary death taking

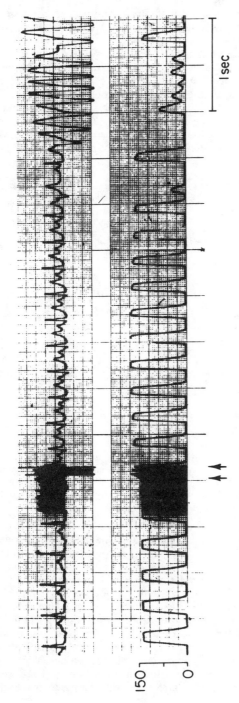

FIGURE 5. Electrocardiographic (*top*) and left ventricular pressure tracings (*bottom*) in an anesthetized dog. The *arrows* indicate the electrical stimulation of the left stellate ganglion, which results in an episode of ventricular tachycardia. After stimulation, the T wave becomes positive and the Q-T interval lengthens. (From Schwartz.[67] Reproduced by permission.)

into account also the association with stress, and a final evaluation, prior to a clinical trial, of an antiarrhythmic intervention already tested in simpler conditions.

The first model involves anesthetized cats in which the left anterior descending coronary artery is occluded for 2 minutes while the left stellate ganglion is electrically stimulated for 30 seconds, starting 1 minute after the beginning of occlusion (FIG. 7). The timing of the two stimuli is such that it is possible to discriminate between arrhythmias induced by ischemia, by ischemia plus sympathetic stimulation, and by reperfusion. In about 65% of experiments the same degree of arrhythmias may be elicited for six to seven consecutive trials; this reproducibility is always evident within the first three trials. If the results are

A.B. 50 YEARS - DURING ANESTHESIA

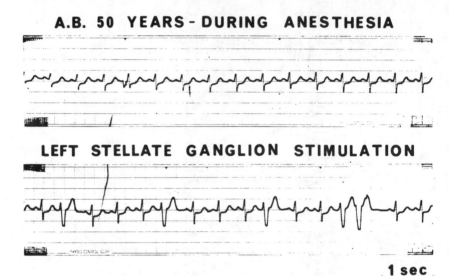

LEFT STELLATE GANGLION STIMULATION

1 sec

FIGURE 6. Electrocardiographic tracing in an anesthetized man 50 days after occurrence of an anterior myocardial infarction complicated by ventricular fibrillation. The patient was in sinus rhythm until the left stellate ganglion was mechanically stimulated, leading to frequent premature ventricular beats and couplets. Details are given in the text.

consistent they will be reproducibly elicited in the next three to four trials. This allows internal control analysis because if a consistent arrhythmic response is elicited for three consecutive trials, the drug under study may be administered and three additional trials may be repeated. In approximately 45 to 50% of animals, ventricular fibrillation is constantly produced; in the remaining animals, frequent premature ventricular beats or ventricular tachycardia is the usual response. It has to be stressed that once an animal, during the first three trials, responds with a given type of arrhythmia, this response will remain constant throughout the experiment. Preliminary data indicate a major protective effect induced by either verapamil [64] or by creatinine phosphate, while lidocaine and mexiletine do not seem to provide sufficient protection. A likely reason for the reproducibility of life-threatening arrhythmias in this model is the fact that these

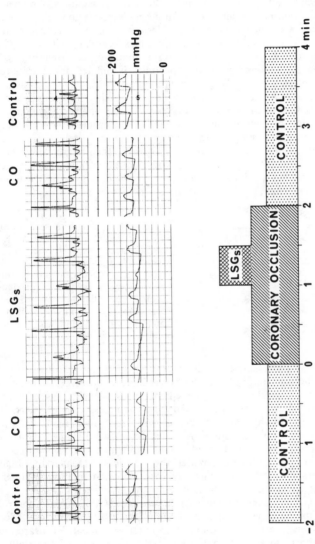

FIGURE 7. Diagram of experimental model with an example of electrocardiographic and blood pressure changes. The *second panel* shows the changes occurring after 1 minute of coronary occlusion (CO) just prior to sympathetic stimulation: blood pressure is lower and classic ischemic changes are obvious. In the *third panel*, electrical stimulation of the left stellate ganglion (LSGs) induced the occurrence of premature ventricular beats and a slight increase in blood pressure; stimulation artifacts are visible in the electrocardiographic tracing. In the *fourth panel*, after cessation of sympathetic stimulation while coronary occlusion is still maintained ventricular premature beats are still present. In the *fifth panel*, a few seconds after release of occlusion both the electrocardiogram and pressure have returned to normal. (From Schwartz and Vanoli.[83] Reproduced by permission.)

ventricular tachyarrhythmias are specifically dependent on the interaction between acute myocardial ischemia and sudden increases in cardiac sympathetic
activity. This model seems particularly well suited for the preliminary evaluation, before the study in conscious animals, of drugs potentially protective
against the malignant arrhythmias associated with acute myocardial ischemia.

The second animal model involves the interaction of a few clinically relevant
factors in conscious animals. Briefly, dogs undergo implantation for chronic
measurement of various hemodynamic variables and balloon occluders are
placed around the left descending and left circumflex coronary arteries. The
dogs are subjected to submaximal exercise on a motor-driven treadmill for
18 minutes. At the 17th minute a balloon occluder is inflated for 2 minutes
and acute myocardial ischemia is produced (FIG. 8). Thus, this short-lasting
ischemic episode affects the last minute of exercise and the first minute after
exercise, and this sequence of events allows separation between arrhythmias
dependent on cessation of exercise or on release of occlusion. This protocol
begins 3 weeks after initial surgery and is repeated after production of an
anterior or inferior myocardial infarction.[65] Grossly, this model resembles
what may happen to a patient with a prior myocardial infarction who engages
in physical activity and has a brief reduction in coronary flow (spasm?) leading
to acute myocardial ischemia, cardiac pain, and arrest of exercise.

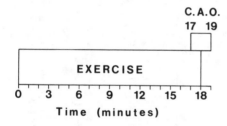

FIGURE 8. Experimental protocol. At the 17th minute of an exercise stress test performed on a
treadmill, a balloon occluder previously positioned around one coronary artery is inflated to produce
acute myocardial ischemia. Exercise stops after 1 minute of ischemia, which is maintained for an
additional minute.

A critical point is represented by the fact that such a brief myocardial
ischemia does not induce ventricular arrhythmias at rest; however, when it is
coupled with exercise, it results in a high incidence of life-threatening arrhythmias, which are particularly frequent immediately after cessation of exercise.
This represents a step forward in comparison with our previous study,[26] in
which conscious dogs with a prior myocardial infarction were subjected, while
resting, to a 10-minute coronary arterial occlusion, which certainly affected
left ventricular function. In this new model, the ventricular tachyarrhythmias
depend on the interaction between acute myocardial ischemia, level of heart
rate, exercise and its cessation, and vagal and sympathetic reflexes.

Using this protocol, ventricular tachyarrhythmias occurred in 8 of 15 control
dogs (53%), culminating in ventricular fibrillation in 6 (40%) (FIG. 9). Ten
dogs were studied 3 weeks after production of an anterior myocardial infarction
and in this group the incidence of ventricular arrhythmias and of ventricular
fibrillation was higher (70% and 60%, respectively). It is noteworthy that
most instances of ventricular fibrillation occurred immediately after cessation
of exercise. The underlying mechanism for this still unexplained specific temporal relationship is under investigation; in any case, it bears a striking similarity
with what happens in most sudden deaths in athletes. Do autonomic interven-

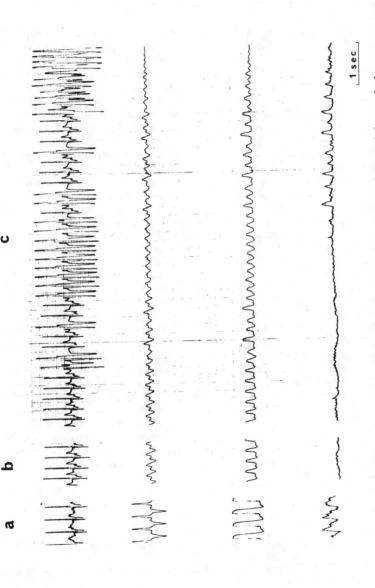

FIGURE 9. Tracings from *top to bottom* are: electrocardiogram, left ventricular pressure, and circumflex coronary flow. (a) After 17 minutes of exercise; (b) after 1 minute of occlusion of the left anterior descending coronary artery, as treadmill has stopped; (c) 15 seconds later onset of ventricular tachycardia that degenerates into ventricular fibrillation. The large decrease in blood pressure within 1 minute of coronary arterial occlusion is an uncommon event in this model.

tions affect the susceptibility to ventricular fibrillation in this setting? Preliminary data suggest an affirmative answer, because in 8 dogs with an anterior myocardial infarction that were studied after left stellectomy, ventricular arrhythmias occurred in only two cases (25%) and ventricular fibrillation in none, despite the fact that heart rate was even higher compared with that of control animals.

The possibility of studying these dogs before they would actually be exposed to a high-risk situation has prompted us to search for possible clues for the identification of subgroups of dogs at higher risk of dying suddenly during the exercise plus ischemia trial. Since autonomic reflexes clearly play a major role in that setting and since some of our preliminary observations in the first group of dogs suggested that vagal reflexes may be protective, we have decided to evaluate in nine dogs with an anterior myocardial infarction the propensity for vagal or sympathetic responses. This was achieved by baroreceptive testing.[66] Blood pressure was increased or lowered by using intravenous infusions of phenylephrine and nitroprusside while heart rate changes were recorded together with changes in aortic blood pressure. The relationship between R-R intervals and the different levels of blood pressure was expressed by a linear regression line, the slope of which would allow distinction between "hypervagal" and "hypersympathetic" responses. Nine animals with prior anterior myocardial infarction were studied: four dogs did not show arrhythmias during the exercise plus ischemia test, while four of the remaining five had ventricular fibrillation and one had ventricular tachycardia. The baroreflex slope was compared between these two groups and was found to be significantly higher (9.3 ± 2.2 versus 4.3 ± 1.6 msec/mm Hg) in the group that showed no arrhythmias. The difference was mostly due to a greater reduction in heart rate in response to phenylephrine; this indicates that the dogs that survived had a greater tendency for powerful vagal reflexes. This finding strongly suggests a protective effect of vagal reflexes when conscious animals undergo an episode of acute myocardial ischemia. If these data are confirmed in a larger series of animals, this finding may have important clinical implications. Baroreceptor testing is a safe, non-invasive procedure that may be performed in patients with a recent myocardial infarction before discharge from the hospital. A prospective study in these patients would reveal whether baroreceptor testing has prognostic implications in man. The early identification of subgroups of patients with ischemic heart disease at higher risk for sudden death remains a critical but still elusive problem. Should the analysis of autonomic responses be found to have significant prognostic value, new and important insights with several therapeutic implications might be gained on the role of the autonomic nervous system in sudden coronary death.

References

1. LOWN, B. 1979. Sudden cardiac death: The major challenge confronting contemporary cardiology. Am. J. Cardiol. **43:** 313–328.
2. LOWN, B. & R. L. VERRIER. 1976. Neural activity and ventricular fibrillation. N. Engl. J. Med. **294:** 1165–1170.
3. VERRIER, R. L. 1980. Neural factors and ventricular electrical instability. In Sudden Death. H. E. Kulbertus & H. J. J. Wellens, Eds.: 137. Nijhoff. The Hague.
4. SCHWARTZ, P. J., A. M. BROWN, A. MALLIANI & A. ZANCHETTI. 1978. Neural Mechanisms in Cardiac Arrhythmias.: 442. Raven Press. New York, NY.

5. MALLIANI, A., P. J. SCHWARTZ & A. ZANCHETTI. 1980. Neural mechanisms in life-threatening arrhythmias. Am. Heart. J. **100**: 705–715.
6. PAGANI, M., P. J. SCHWARTZ, R. BANKS, F. LOMBARDI & A. MALLIANI. 1974. Reflex responses of sympathetic preganglionic neurones initiated by different cardiovascular receptors in spinal animals. Brain Res. **68**: 215–225.
7. RECORDATI, G., P. J. SCHWARTZ, M. PAGANI, A. MALLIANI & A. M. BROWN. 1971. Activation of cardiac vagal receptors during myocardial ischemia. Experientia **27**: 1423–1424.
8. THOREN, P. 1978. Vagal reflexes elicited by left ventricular C-fibers during myocardial ischemia in cats. In Neural Mechanisms in Cardiac Arrhythmias. P. J. Schwartz, A. M. Brown, A. Malliani & A. Zanchetti, Eds.: 179. Raven Press. New York, NY.
9. BROWN, A. M. 1979. Cardiac reflexes. In Handbook of Physiology, Section 2, The Cardiovascular System, Vol. 1. R. M. Berne, Ed.: 677. American Physiological Society. Bethesda, MD.
10. BISHOP, V. S., A. MALLIANI & P. THOREN. 1981. Cardiac mechanoreceptors. In Handbook of Physiology, Section 2, The Cardiovascular System. J. T. Shepherd & F. M. Abboud, Eds.: American Physiological Society. Bethesda, MD. In press.
11. MALLIANI, A., G. RECORDATI & P. J. SCHWARTZ. 1973. Nervous activity of afferent cardiac sympathetic fibers with atrial and ventricular endings. J. Physiol. **229**: 457–469.
12. CASATI, R., F. LOMBARDI & A. MALLIANI. 1979. Afferent sympathetic unmyelinated fibers with left ventricular ending in cats. J. Physiol. **292**: 135–148.
13. LOMBARDI, F., P. DELLA BELLA, R. CASATI & A. MALLIANI. 1981. Effects of intracoronary administration of bradykinin on the impulse activity of afferent sympathetic unmyelinated fibers with left ventricular endings in the cat. Circ. Res. **48**: 69–75.
14. MALLIANI, A., P. J. SCHWARTZ & A. ZANCHETTI. 1969. A sympathetic reflex elicited by experimental coronary occlusion. Am. J. Physiol. **217**: 703–709.
15. SCHWARTZ, P. J., R. D. FOREMAN, H. L. STONE & A. M. BROWN. 1976. Effect of dorsal root section on the arrhythmias associated with coronary occlusion. Am. J. Physiol. **231**: 923–928.
16. SCHWARTZ, P. J., M. PAGANI, F. LOMBARDI, A. MALLIANI & A. M. BROWN. 1973. A cardiocardiac sympatho-vagal reflex in the cat. Circ. Res. **32**: 215–220.
17. CHADDA, K. D., V. S. BANKA & R. H. HELFANT. 1974. Rate dependent ventricular ectopia following acute coronary occlusion. Circulation **49**: 654–658.
18. WEBB, S. W., A. A. J. ADGEY & J. F. PANTRIDGE. 1972. Autonomic disturbance at onset of acute myocardial infarction. Br. Med. J. **3**: 89–92.
19. PANTRIDGE, J. F. 1978. Autonomic disturbance at the onset of acute myocardial infarction. In Neural Mechanisms in Cardiac Arrhythmias. P. J. Schwartz, A. M. Brown, A. Malliani & A. Zanchetti, Eds.: 7. Raven Press. New York, NY.
20. GILLIS, R. A. 1971. Role of the nervous system in the arrhythmias produced by coronary occlusion in the cat. Am. Heart J. **81**: 677–684.
21. THAMES, M. D., H. S. KLOPFENSTEIN, F. M. ABBOUD, A. L. MARK & J. L. WALKER. 1978. Preferential distribution of inhibitory cardiac receptors with vagal afferents to the inferoposterior wall of the left ventricle activated during coronary occlusion in the dog. Circ. Res. **43**: 512–519.
22. CORR, P. B. & R. A. GILLIS. 1978. Autonomic neural influences on the dysrhythmias resulting from myocardial infarction. Circ. Res. **43**: 1–9.
23. VERRIER, R. L. & B. LOWN. 1981. Autonomic nervous system and malignant cardiac arrhythmias. In Brain Behaviour and Bodily Disease. H. Wiener, M. A. Hofer & A. J. Stunkard, Eds.: 273. Raven Press. New York, NY.
24. WAXMAN, M. B. & R. W. WALD. 1977. Termination of ventricular tachycardia by increase in cardiac vagal drive. Circulation **56**: 385–301.

25. WEISS, T., G. MANCIA, A. DEL BO, D. CAVORETTO, S. GRAZI, L. PRETI & P. J. SCHWARTZ. 1979. The role of heart rate in the phenylephrine-induced suppression of premature ventricular beats. Europ. J. Clin. Invest. 9: 39.
26. SCHWARTZ, P. J. & H. L. STONE. 1980. Left stellectomy in the prevention of ventricular fibrillation caused by acute myocardial ischemia in conscious dogs with anterior myocardial infarction. Circulation 62: 1256–1265.
27. BERNE, R. M. & R. RUBIO. 1979. Coronary circulation. In Handbook of Physiology, Vol. 1.: 873. American Physiological Society. Bethesda, MD.
28. FEIGL, E. O. 1967. Sympathetic control of coronary circulation. Circ. Res. 20: 262–271.
29. FEIGL, E. O. 1968. Carotid sinus reflex control of coronary blood flow. Circ. Res. 23: 223–237.
30. VATNER, S. F., D. FRANKLIN, R. L. VAN CITTEN & E. BRAUNWALD. 1970. Effects of carotid sinus nerve stimulation on the coronary circulation of the conscious dog. Circ. Res. 27: 11–21.
31. MOHRMAN, D. E. & E. O. FEIGL. 1978. Competition between sympathetic vasoconstriction and metabolic vasodilation in the canine coronary circulation. Circ. Res. 42: 79–86.
32. SCHWARTZ, P. J. & H. L. STONE. 1977. Tonic influence of the sympathetic nervous system on myocardial reactive hyperemia and on coronary blood flow distribution. Circ. Res. 41: 51–58.
33. DENN, M. J. & H. L. STONE. 1976. Autonomic innervation of dog coronary arteries. J. Appl. Physiol. 41: 30–35.
34. SCHWARTZ, P. J. & H. L. STONE. 1979. Effects of unilateral stellectomy upon cardiac performance during exercise in dogs. Circ. Res. 44: 637–645.
35. GWIRTZ, P. A., P. J. SCHWARTZ & H. L. STONE. 1980. Alpha-adrenergic blockade during exercise in dogs with myocardial infarction and left stellate ganglionectomy. Physiologist 23: 256.
36. GWIRTZ, P. A. & H. L. STONE. 1981. Coronary blood flow and myocardial oxygen consumption following alpha-adrenergic blockade during submaximal exercise. J. Pharmacol. Exp. Ther. 217: 92–98.
37. MURRAY, P. A. & S. F. VATNER. 1979. Alpha-adrenoreceptor attenuation of the coronary vascular responses to severe exercise in the conscious dog. Circ. Res. 45: 654–660.
38. RAEDER, E. A., R. L. VERRIER & B. LOWN. 1981. Influence of adrenergic tone on cyclical coronary blood flow changes induced by partial stenosis. Fed. Proc. 40: 564A.
39. MUDGE, G. H., W. OROSSMAN, R. M. MILLS, JR., M. LESCH & E. BRAUNWALD. 1976. Reflex increase in coronary vascular resistance in patients with ischemic heart disease. N. Engl. J. Med. 295: 1333–1337.
40. BUFFINTEN, C. W. & E. O. FEIGL. 1981. Adrenergic coronary vasoconstriction in the presence of coronary stenosis in the dog. Circ. Res. 48: 416–423.
41. JUHASZ-NAGY, A. & M. SZENTIVANYI. 1974. Effect of adrenergic activation on collateral coronary blood flow. Jap. Heart J. 15: 289–298.
42. JONES, C. E. & K. W. SCHEEL. 1980. Reduced coronary collateral resistance after chronic ventricular sympathectomy. Am. J. Physiol. 238: H196–201.
43. VANOLI, E., A. ZAZA, G. ZUANETTI, M. PAPPALETTERA & P. J. SCHWARTZ. Reduction in infarct size produced by left stellectomy. Submitted for publication.
44. HUNT, R. 1899. Direct and reflex acceleration of the mammalian heart with some observation on the relationship of the inhibitory and accelerator nerves. Am. J. Physiol. 2: 395–470.
45. SCHWARTZ, P. J., M. PERITI & A. L. MALLIANI. 1975. The long Q-T syndrome. Am. Heart J. 89: 378–390.
46. MOSS, A. J. & P. J. SCHWARTZ. 1979. Sudden death and the idiopathic long Q-T syndrome. Am. J. Med. 66: 6–7.

47. SCHWARTZ, P. J. 1981. The sudden infant death syndrome. *In* Reviews in Perinatal Medicine, Vol. 4. E. M. Scarpelli & E. V. Cosmi, Eds.: 475–524. Raven Press, NY.

48. HARRIS, A. S., A. ESTANDIA & R. F. TILLOTSON. 1951. Ventricular ectopic rhythm and ventricular fibrillation following cardiac sympathectomy and coronary occlusion. Am. J. Physiol. **165:** 505–512.

49. SCHWARTZ, P. J., H. L. STONE & A. M. BROWN. 1976. Effects of unilateral stellate ganglion blockade on the arrhythmias associated with coronary occlusion. Am. Heart J. **92:** 589–599.

50. SCHWARTZ, P. J., N. G. SNEBOLD & A. M. BROWN. 1976. Effects of unilateral cardiac sympathetic denervation on the ventricular fibrillation threshold. Am. J. Cardiol. **37:** 1034–1040.

51. SCHWARTZ, P. J., R. L. VERRIER & B. LOWN. 1977. Effect of stellectomy and vagotomy on ventricular refractoriness. Circ. Res. **40:** 536–540.

52. AUSTONI, P., R. ROSATI, L. GREGORINI, E. BIANCHI, E. BORTOLANI & P. J. SCHWARTZ. 1979. Stellectomy and exercise in man. Am. J. Cardiol. **43:** 399.

53. SCHWARTZ, P. J. 1978. Experimental reproduction of the long Q-T syndrome. Am. J. Cardiol. **41:** 374.

54. SKINNER, J. E., J. T. LIE & M. L. ENTMAN. 1975. Modification of ventricular fibrillation latency following coronary artery occlusion in the conscious pig: The effects of psychological stress and beta-adrenergic blockade. Circulation **51:** 656–667.

55. MATTA, R. J., J. E. LAWLER & B. LOWN. 1976. Ventricular electrical instability in the conscious dog. Effects of psychologic stress and beta-adrenergic blockade. Am. J. Cardiol. **38:** 594–598.

56. ROSENFELD, J., M. R. ROSEN & B. F. HOFFMAN. 1978. Pharmacologic and behavioral effects of arrhythmias which immediately follow abrupt coronary occlusion: A canine model of sudden coronary death. Am. J. Cardiol. **41:** 1075–1082.

57. HAGEMAN, G. R., J. M. GOLDBERG, J. A. ARMOUR & W. C. RANDALL. 1973. Cardiac dysrhythmias induced by autonomic nerve stimulation. Am. J. Cardiol. **32:** 823–830.

58. RANDALL, W. C., J. X. THOMAS, D. E. EULER & G. J. ROZANSKI. 1978. Cardiac dysrhythmias associated with autonomic nervous system imbalance in the conscious dog. *In* Neural Mechanisms in Cardiac Arrhythmias. P. J. Schwartz, A. M. Brown, A. Malliani & A. Zanchetti, Eds.: 123–138. Raven Press. New York, NY.

59. ZIPES, D., V. ELHARRAR, A. M. WATANABE, W. E. GAUM & H. R. BESCH. 1977. Induction of ventricular fibrillation in probucol-treated dogs. Clin. Res. **25:** 459A.

60. COYER, B. H., R. PRYOR, W. M. KIRSCH & S. J. BLOUNT, JR. 1978. Left stellectomy in the long QT syndrome. Chest **74:** 584–586.

61. CRAMPTON, R. S. 1979. Preeminence of the left stellate ganglion in the long Q-T syndrome. Circulation **59:** 769–778.

62. FOZZARD, H. A. 1975. Validity of myocardial infarction models. Circulation **51–52**(Suppl. 3): 131–146.

63. SCHWARTZ, P. J. & E. VANOLI. 1981. A new experimental model for the study of cardiac arrhythmias dependent on the interaction between acute myocardial ischemia and sympathetic hyperactivity. J. Cardiovasc. Pharmacol. **3:** 1251–1259.

64. SCHWARTZ, P. J., E. VANOLI & A. ZAZA. 1981. The prevention of cardiac arrhythmias associated with myocardial ischemia and dependent upon increases in sympathetic activity. *In* Calcium Antagonism in Cardiovascular Therapy. Experiences with Verapamil. A. Zanchetti, Ed.: 314–325. Excerpta Medica. Amsterdam.

65. SCHWARTZ, P. J., G. E. BILLMAN & H. L. STONE.   1981.   Autonomic interventions in a new animal model for sudden death. Circulation **64** (Suppl. IV): 289.

66. BILLMAN, G. E., P. J. SCHWARTZ & H. L. STONE.   1981.   Circulation **64:** (Suppl. IV): 156.

67. SCHWARTZ, P. J.   1976.   Cardiac sympathetic innervation and the sudden infant death syndrome. Am. J. Med. **60:** 167.

IN PRAISE OF SUDDEN DEATH *

Henry Greenberg

Department of Medicine
St. Luke's-Roosevelt Hospital Center
New York, New York 10019
Department of Medicine
Columbia University
College of Physicians & Surgeons
New York, New York 10032

As you know, this Conference on Sudden Coronary Death grew out of the deliberations of the executive committee of a multicenter study of patients with myocardial infarction. This executive committee is composed of independent and innovative investigators, all of whom have different opinions on nearly every topic under consideration. The committee has been functioning for more than three years now, and everyone is still talking to everyone else, friendships endure, and productive collaboration continues. It is clear that much of our success is due to the skill, patience, and charm of our leader, and I would here like to thank Arthur Moss of the University of Rochester who has filled this role so uniquely and admirably.

As cochairman and organizer of this conference, as a practicing cardiologist, and as director of a coronary care unit, I think that I have established my credentials as a physician committed to the fight against premature death from coronary disease. Notwithstanding this effort devoted to preventing sudden coronary death, I would like to say a few words on its behalf. While this may represent a chronic tendency to root for the underdog, I believe that it would be a grievous error to spend three days condemning sudden death and not to offer five minutes of praise.

In a short, uncontrolled series, I sampled the opinions of a variety of physicians, their friends and spouses, and not one wished anything but a sudden, unexpected exit while in the pink of health. There were not even any votes for a classic deathbed scene, with the family gathered at the last great congress before death, sadly but resignedly helping to prepare for the final journey. When we think of the long and noble tradition such an ingathering has had, its eclipse is even more startling. Perhaps this is another example of the breakdown of the extended family or of the computer age mentality which desires every transition from one state to another as an instantaneous event. It is possible that my findings are due to bias introduced by restricting the survey to physicians and their families. However, less formal inquiries of medically unsophisticated colleagues support the original observations.

There was another characteristic of the vote that should be mentioned: The minimum age suggested for shuffling off this mortal coil was at least fourscore and some years. Obviously, sudden death at 85 years of age is far preferable to a grizzly carcinoma at age 40. I asked some respondents about the reciprocal, namely, a grizzly carcinoma at 85 years of age versus sudden

---

* Remarks delivered after a dinner held for certain members of the New York Academy of Sciences, the Conference Committee, and the conference participants.

death at 40. This produced a pause, often followed by more silence and finally by a nonverbal indication that the age of 40 was simply unacceptable. Death at such a childlike age had little appeal, confirming that the desire for sudden death is not a death wish, but in fact a life wish blended with a comprehension of one's own mortality and an understanding of the real world. There is little enthusiasm for sentimentality to be a component of last chapters and an assumption that preparations have been made in advance. We all want to live to the fullest extent of our capacity as a sapient being capable of joy and delight, but at the proper time life can be quickly and gently rounded with a sleep.

What if we are fully successful in the purpose of our gathering? What if we find the proper elixir? What if, for example, a super pill composed of nifedipine, timolol, amiodarone, and a baby aspirin eliminates sudden death altogether? Will we devoutly wish for a new risk factor to call into play as we see memory slipping as our dotage arrives? Will we fear that our friends and neighbors will not heed our Medalert bracelets which will read "do not resuscitate"? Will we avoid physicians and hospitals for routine ailments because we are afraid that unacceptable illnesses will be prolonged interminably by a well-meaning system that too easily cannot let us go? These questions are, of course, rhetorical, but the major reason that they are rhetorical is that none of us expects that this conference or even the immediate future will find a cure or prevention for sudden coronary death. It does remain, however, a theoretical possibility that such a condition might come to pass. Then we shall have a real problem, and perhaps we can all reassemble for another conference, again under the auspices of the New York Academy of Sciences, to look at sudden death from the opposite point of view. I would again consider myself privileged to address this group and to discuss the contrary point of view.

REGULATION OF CALCIUM
IN CARDIAC MUSCLE

Arnold Schwartz

Department of Pharmacology and Cell Biophysics
University of Cincinnati Medical Center
College of Medicine
Cincinnati, Ohio 45267

If acute myocardial infarction is related to sudden death, the Ca^{2+} antagonists of Ca^{2+}-channel blockers offer a unique combination of potential beneficial actions on the cardiovascular system. Verapamil, nifedipine, and diltiazem are the most frequently used (FIG. 1). These agents differ widely in chemical structure and include both lipophilic and hydrophilic moieties. Their cardiac and vascular actions appear to be mediated at least partly by the inhibition of Ca^{2+} influx, which accompanies a voltage-dependent process. The diminution of Ca^{2+} can cause depressed myocardial contractile force, decreased heart rate, shortened action potential duration, and coronary vasodilation. This combination of effects predicts a therapeutic approach that diminishes myocardial metabolic demand, decreases systematic blood pressure, and improves myocardial blood flow to margins of the ischemic myocardium.

In order to understand how these drugs work in the setting of acute and chronic coronary insufficiency, we must have an understanding of the biochemical and morphologic aspects of excitation, contraction, and relaxation in cardiac muscle.

FIGURE 2 shows models of cardiac and skeletal muscle cells. There are certain interesting and significant differences in the geometry of cellular inclusions between cardiac and skeletal muscle. The T-system is much wider in cardiac muscle than in fast skeletal muscle; cardiac muscle is approximately 30–40% mitochondria, whereas skeletal muscle is sparse in mitochondrial content. The inner membrane system that is responsible for relaxation, the sarcoplasmic reticulum (SR), is divided into three areas: (1) free SR, (2) the junctional SR, or lateral cisterna, which is quite prominent in skeletal muscle but not so in cardiac muscle, and (3) junctional "feet" or projections. There are peripheral couplings and interior couplings with the plasma membrane of the cell surface and of transverse tubules, respectively, with the junctional SR (JSR). Two couplings make a triad, which is prominent in skeletal muscle, and one coupling makes a dyad, which is prominent in heart muscle. Note also that there are subsarcolemmal cisternae (SSC) quite prominent in cardiac muscle; this structure may be of importance in facilitating calcium movement from the outside of the cell to the interior. It is well known that cardiac muscle, unlike fast skeletal muscle, requires a constant source of external calcium. The current thought on excitation–contraction coupling with respect to calcium in both skeletal and cardiac muscle arises chiefly from the research of Endo *et al.*[3] and that of the Fabiatos.[4] Depolarization at the cell membrane of skeletal muscle probably traverses the T-system and somehow changes the

183

0077–8923/82/0382–0183 $01.75/0 © 1982, NYAS

permeability of the JSR so that calcium is released and interacts with troponin C. Calcium is sequestered during the relaxation event by the free SR. In cardiac muscle, it appears that a small amount of calcium accompanies the action potential via a "slow channel," and then a release of a large amount of calcium occurs probably from the SR region closest to the T-system and/or from the subsarcolemmal cisternae. The sequestration process, if, as is probable, the same as that of skeletal muscle, and the subsequent handling of calcium are thought to be similar in both muscle types. The exact mechanism by which calcium efflux occurs to remove calcium from the muscle is still unknown. There is some evidence that a sodium–calcium electroneutral or electrogenic

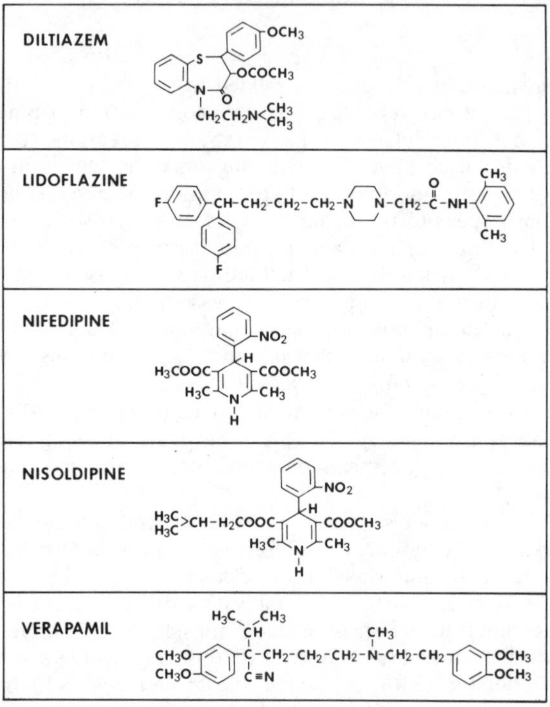

FIGURE 1. Structural formulas of certain Ca^{2+}-channel blockers. (From Schwartz et al.[1] Reprinted by permission.)

exchange system exists in the cell membrane which may be involved in the removal of calcium.[5, 6]

It is believed that the Na,K-ATPase is part of the cell membrane and is responsible for the maintenance of Na^+ and K^+ gradients. The Na,K-ATPase is inhibited by low, therapeutic concentrations of digitalis, which interact with the enzyme in a highly specific manner. Cardiac glycosides produce a positive inotropic effect that is significant in all mammals except in the rat heart, where the effect is minimal. I believe that this enzyme system is the pharmacologic receptor.

The electrical events taking place before the contractile process in the heart

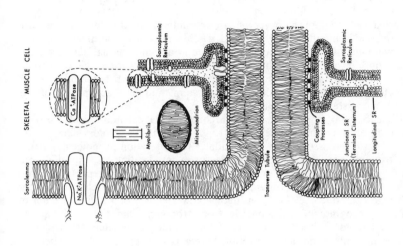

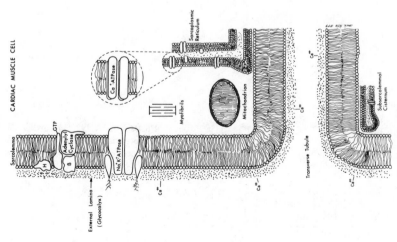

FIGURE 2. Diagrammatic representation of cardiac (*left*) and skeletal (*right*) muscle cells. (From Schwartz and Adams.[2] Reprinted by permission.)

are important. It is well known that the electrocardiogram represents depolarization and repolarization, as well as recovery associated with contraction changes. It is of interest that an action potential obtained by the insertion of a microelectrode into a segment of ventricular myocardium coincides with the QRS complex and appears as indicated in FIGURE 3. The rising phase of the action potential is a "sodium current" and is due to a rapid change in permeability to external sodium, with very small amounts of sodium entering the cell. The overshoot is manifested by a rapid decline in sodium permeability. The well known plateau or phase II of the ventricular action potential, characteristic of heart muscle, is probably due in part to a slow, inward calcium current, through a "slow channel." The recovery phase of the action potential involves active cation transport of sodium and potassium, and the "activation" of the Na,K-ATPase system.

The basic unit of contraction is the sarcomere. The calcium receptor protein at the molecular contractile level is troponin, and this protein changes its conformation when associated with calcium. The alteration in molecular structure of troponin causes a cascading series of events leading to a specific conformational change in charge in tropomyosin, which then "derepresses relaxation" by "revealing" specific binding sites on actin to which the elements of the cross-bridge can attach. Relaxation involves the removal of about 100 μmol of calcium per kilogram of heart muscle from troponin primarily to the sarcoplasmic reticulum. Mitochondria cannot be excluded completely from playing some role in contraction and relaxation (other than supplying ATP), because the average cardiac muscle cell contains from 20 to 50% mitochondria, and it is well known that these organelles can accumulate large amounts of calcium. Mitochondria also transports potassium and protons. A typical excitation–contraction–relaxation event is depicted in FIGURE 4. It is apparent that calcium represents the most important controlling cation in modulating cardiac function. It is believed that the intracellular concentration of "activator" calcium varies from 10^{-7} to 10^{-5} M during contraction and relaxation. Because the cardiac

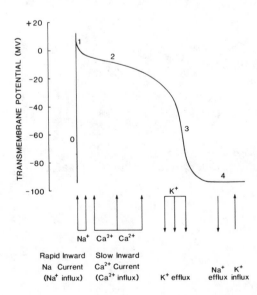

FIGURE 3. A typical cardiac action potential. (From Naylor and Merrillees.[7] Reprinted by permission.)

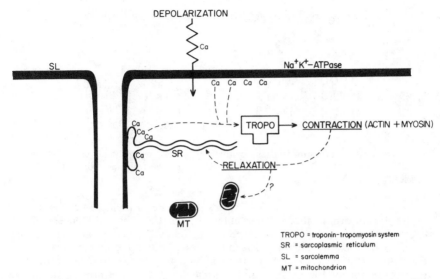

FIGURE 4. A typical excitation–contraction–relaxation event. (From Schwartz.[8] Reprinted by permission.)

muscle cell is extremely heterogeneous, it is difficult at this time to be certain of the concentrations, although the range listed above seems logical.

We have been studying the sarcoplasmic reticulum (SR) from cardiac muscle. This fraction, sometimes referred to as microsomal vesicles, is labile in cardiac muscle, less so in skeletal muscle. Using a rapid procedure for preparation, we have collected a membrane fraction that is active. We have concluded that this membrane fraction does indeed possess both the rate and capacity characteristics to effect relaxation of heart muscle *in vivo*. This membrane fraction seems to show very few contaminating enzymatic activities present from other membrane systems of the cardiac muscle cell, and it is relatively unresponsive to a variety of drugs, including digitalis, and only to high concentrations of calcium blocking agents.

The SR may be quite labile and subject to alterations in intracellular environment during various pathologic conditions. For example, it is well known that in myocardial ischemia there is an intracellular acidosis that occurs quite rapidly after the insult. In a variety of *in vitro* experiments, we have shown that the cardiac relaxing system is sensitive to pH changes. Once calcium is bound to the sarcoplasmic reticulum, for example, at pH 6.8, an abrupt increase in pH causes an immediate release of calcium from the sarcoplasmic reticulum, and a drop in pH to as low as 5.99 produces a rebinding of calcium and an inhibition of release. Using a variety of severely failing human and animal hearts, we found a defect in the sarcoplasmic reticulum. The SR isolated from these hearts showed a diminution of binding and a retardation of calcium release. Consequently, it seems that an early biochemical lesion in all types of failing heart preparations studied to date is found in the sarcoplasmic reticulum. In terms of the calcium blockers, we have shown that diltiazem has a protective effect on experimentally induced myocardial ischemia, preventing the damage

Before Ca²⁺ Blocker   **After Ca²⁺ Blocker**

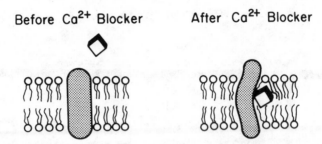

FIGURE 5. Conformational changes involving lipids and proteins caused by interactions of membranes and Ca²⁺ blockers. (From Schwartz et al.[1] Reprinted by permission.)

to jeopardized cardiac tissue. This seems to be due to multiple actions unique to the class of drugs called calcium antagonists or Ca²⁺-channel blockers. Their effects include potent coronary vasodilation, inhibition of certain currents that describe the action potential, in some cases a slight negative inotropic and chronotropic influence, a drop in afterload, and a very interesting and protective effect on mitochondria. It is possible, although certainly not proven, that some aspects of this therapeutically beneficial array involve interaction with membranes containing calmodulin, which leads to modification of important enzyme systems. I like to think of the agents, which are lipophilic, as interacting with membranes causing perturbations and conformational changes (FIG. 5).

REFERENCES

1. SCHWARTZ, A., et al. 1981. In New Perspectives on Calcium Antagonists. G. B. Weiss, Ed.: 191–210. Williams & Wilkins. Baltimore, MD.
2. SCHWARTZ, A. & R. J. ADAMS. 1980. Studies on the digitalis receptor. Circ. Res. 46:
3. ENDO, M., M. TUNAKA & Y. OGAWA. 1970. Ca⁺⁺-induced release of Ca⁺⁺ from the sarcoplasmic reticulum of skinned skeletal muscle fibers. Nature 228: 34–36.
4. FABIATO, A. & F. FABIATO. 1977. Calcium release from sarcoplasmic reticulum: A brief review. Circ. Res. 40: 119–129.
5. REUTER, H. 1974. Exchange of calcium ions in the mammalian myocardium. Circ. Res. 34: 559–605.
6. LANGER, G. 1978. The structure and function of the myocardial cell surface. Am. J. Physiol. 235: H461–H468.
7. NAYLOR, W. G. & N. C. R. MERRILLEES. 1971. In Calcium and the Heart. P. Harris and L. H. Opie, Eds.: 36. Academic Press. New York, NY.
8. SCHWARTZ, A. 1973. Subcellular calcium transport mechanism in the normal and failing heart. In The Paul D. White Symposium on Cardiovascular Disease: Major Advances in Cardiovascular Therapy. H. I. Russek, Ed.: 17–26. Williams & Wilkins. Baltimore, MD.

DISCUSSION

DR. LOCKHART: What is the effect of phenothiazines on calmodulin?

DR. SCHWARTZ: Trifluoperizine (TFP) has been called a calmodulin blocker and is active at a concentration of about 10^{-5} or 10^{-6} molar.

Chlorpromazine is less active than trifluoperizine. We, and I imagine others, are beginning to examine TFP and other tricyclic antidepressants as protecting against the ischemic event.

THE ROLE OF PLATELETS IN THE GENESIS OF ISCHEMIA *

Robert W. Colman

Thrombosis Research Center
Temple University School of Medicine
Philadelphia, Pennsylvania 19140

INTRODUCTION

Sudden cardiac death occurring without symptoms or with symptoms of less than an hour's duration is widely accepted to be due to myocardial ischemia leading to a fatal arrhythmia. Although there is general agreement that the underlying disease is atherosclerotic disease of the coronary arteries, the relationship of this pathologic abnormality to genesis of ischemia—supply versus demand—is the subject of debate. For many years conventional wisdom [1] has focused on the change in myocardial oxygen demand. Increased oxygen consumption of the cardiac muscle was assumed to lead to ischemia because it was superimposed on coronary thrombosis, acute or chronic. An alternate hypothesis suggests that reductions in oxygen supply to the myocardium may result from spasm of the coronary artery. Maseri and coworkers [2] have presented arteriographic evidence of such spasm during unstable angina, and presumably a similar mechanism could operate during sudden death. Braunwald [3] has emphasized that therapy aimed at lowering oxygen demand, such as treatment with propanolol, may even be deleterious because it blocks the vasodilation caused by stimulation of beta-2-adrenegic receptors. Choice of appropriate drugs depends not only on whether one aims to decrease the demand or increase the supply of oxygen, but also on the mechanism responsible for coronary spasm or transient obstruction of a coronary artery.

This paper will focus on the possible central role of the platelet not only in the genesis of myocardial ischemia, but also in coronary thrombosis and atherosclerosis. Two direct pathways involving platelets in the pathogenesis of myocardial ischemia will be described. Platelets that are activated form aggregates which can directly occlude vessels supplying the myocardium. Activated platelets also release thromboxane A_2, a coronary vasconstrictor which further decreases the diameter of the arterial lumen. In addition, the way in which risk factors for coronary artery atherosclerosis, such as stress, hyperlipoproteinemia and smoking, could act in part through platelets will be discussed. Among other mechanisms, the release of platelet growth factor, which stimulates vascular smooth muscle, is considered. This presentation will deal only with the possible pathophysiologic relations between platelets and myocardial ischemia. However, it is hoped that this paper will provide the mechanistic underpinning for the paper by Dr. Jack Hirsh on the role of antiplatelet drugs in preventing sudden coronary death which will appear later in this volume.

* This paper was supported by SCOR Grant HL 14217 from The National Institutes of Health.

0077–8923/82/0382–0190 $1.75/0 © 1982, NYAS

RESULTS AND DISCUSSION

Chronic endothelial injury experimentally leads to atherosclerosis.[4] The earliest changes observed after mechanical denudation of the endothelial linings of vessels are adhesion of platelets' to the subintimal basement membrane. Adhesion of platelets requires the presence in the plasma of the von Willebrand protein, which interacts with its receptor glycoprotein I on the platelet surface membrane.[5] The importance of this reaction for the pathogenesis of atherosclerosis is dramatized by the decrease of the incidence of atheromas in pigs lacking the von Willebrand factor.

After adhesion, platelets change shape from discs to speculated spheres. With soluble activators, this reaction appears in the absence of adhesion concomitant with binding of the agonist. Usually, platelet aggregation follows change in shape. There is a plethora of potential platelet agonists that may be responsible for the platelet aggregation in this situation. Collagen is a prominent component of the basement membrane and collagen is a potent platelet-aggregating agent.[7] The physical form of the collagen is critical to its role as a platelet agonist. We have shown that [8] the ability of collagen to initiate platelet shape change is proportional to the concentration of collagen multimers present (FIG. 1). A similar requirement for collagen multimer formation exists with respect to platelet aggregation.[9] Type IV collagen, which predominates in basement membrane, does not appear to exist in a fibrillar form, and its ability to produce platelet aggregation *in vivo* is not known.

An even more potent aggregator of platelets which is produced after endothelial injury is thrombin. Endothelial cells contain a potent activator [10] which converts factor XII (Hageman factor) to an activated enzyme. Alternatively, the subendothelial basement membrane may act as a surface to activate factor XII. The intrinsic coagulation cascade is thus triggered with the activation of factor XI. Since calcium is present *in vivo*, activation of factors IX and X occurs, with the eventual conversion of prothrombin to thrombin.

Another possibility is that the abnormal surface of the atheromatous plaque is itself capable of triggering platelet aggregation. A clinical situation in which foreign surfaces activate platelets is provided by extracorporeal cardiopulmonary bypass. We have demonstrated that exposure of platelets to two different types of silicone rubber surfaces in an isolated extracorporeal circuit is sufficient to cause thrombocytopenia due to platelet adhesion to two different foreign surfaces.[11] A decrease in platelet counts of only 10% occurred in both standard silicone rubber (SSR) and filler-free silicone rubber (FFSR) circuits of surface area of 0.1 m², while a decrease of 80% was detected in both circuits of 0.9 m² (FIG. 2). The scanning electron microscope has revealed platelets adherent to the surface. Perhaps other foreign surfaces act in the same way.

Adenosine diphosphate (ADP) arising from injured endothelial cells, red cells or other platelets can aggregate platelets. The action of ADP on platelets appears to be mediated by a classic agonist-receptor interaction since the reaction is rapid and surface-oriented, results in recruitment of further cellular response (release reaction, prostaglandin synthesis), and is stimulus–response-coupled. The ADP affinity label 5' fluorosulfonylbenzyl adenosine (5'FSBA) was found to incorporate into a single membrane protein ($M_r = 100,000$) in intact platelets in plasma [12] (FIG. 3A) or in platelets isolated by gel filtration (FIG. 3B).[13] Incorporation of 5'FSBA into the 100,000-dalton external membrane protein was prevented by ADP or adenosine triphosphate (ATP) and

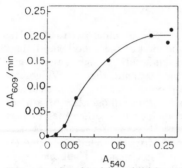

FIGURE 1. Effect of the concentration of multimeric collagen on platelet shape change activity. For each collagen incubation interval, the response rate of platelet shape change (Δ A_{609}/min) is plotted against concentration of collagen multimer (A_{540}). (From Brown et al.[8] Reproduced by permission.)

was associated with inhibition of platelet shape changes, aggregation, and exposure of fibrinogen binding sites. Thus, our studies indicate that ADP may bind to a surface receptor of molecular weight 100,000 as a first step in initiating platelet shape change [12] and platelet aggregation. In contrast, when platelets are washed by multiple centrifugations (FIG. 3C) or when isolated platelet membranes (FIG. 3D) are prepared, 5'FSBA labels four proteins, including actin and myosin, which are attached to the internal or intracellular aspect of the plasma membrane.

Two naturally occurring aromatic amines, epinephrine and serotonin, also can induce human platelet aggregation. Usually, supraphysiologic concentrations are required of these hormones, and aggregation, if it occurs with lower concentrations, is usually reversible. Even ADP, in the presence of plasma calcium concentration, may only produce reversible aggregation. Since an increased incidence of platelet aggregates and an increased number of mural thrombi were found in the coronary microcirculation of patients with coronary artery disease dying suddenly,[14] it is appropriate to inquire what mechanism could transform the reversible platelet aggregates into irreversible plugs. To understand this conversion, it is necessary to consider one of the major mechanisms of recruitment, the platelet-release reaction.

Weak agonists, such as ADP and epinephrine, produce a release reaction which depends on prior aggregation. The platelet compounds released by ADP are contained in two different granules, each with a distinct morphologic appearance and unique content. Dense bodies are visualized by transmission electron microscopy filled with electron-dense material containing a non-

FIGURE 2. Mean changes in platelet count during recirculation in each circuit. Platelet counts are plotted as a percentage of the platelet count of blood drawn directly from donors. O—O, 0.1-m² standard silicone rubber (SSR) circuit; O - - - - O, 0.1-m² filler-free silicone rubber (FFSR) circuit; ●—●, 0.9-m² SSR circuit; ● - - - - ●, 0.9-m² FFSR circuit. Each point is mean of three platelet counts. Point i indicates 2 minutes of recirculation in this and subsequent figures. (From Hennesey et al.[11] Reproduced by permission.)

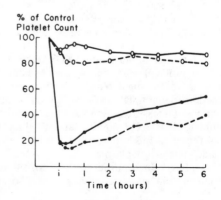

metabolic pool of adenine nucleotides (ADP, ATP, serotonin, pyrophosphate, catecholamines) and a characteristic cation, which in human platelets is calcium. The secretion of the contents of the dense bodies markedly amplified aggregation and further release. Several of the dense granule contents, such as ADP, calcium, serotonin, and epinephrine, can themselves cause aggregation. In addition, certain aggregating agents potentiate each other. Thus, a mixture of subthreshold concentrations of ADP and epinephrine can produce aggregation where neither component could initiate aggregation separately.

The alpha-granule contents include coagulant proteins, such as fibrinogen, factor V, and factor VIII (the von Willebrand factor). Each of these can augment the aggregation process. Fibrinogen is required for aggregation, and

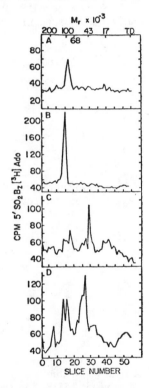

FIGURE 3. Incorporation of 5'FSBA into intact platelets and isolated platelet membranes. In these experiments the effect of various methods of platelet preparation on the pattern of 5'FSBA incorporation into intact platelets was compared with the pattern of label incorporation into isolated platelet membranes. Intact platelets or isolated membranes were incubated with 100 μM [^{3}H]-5'FSBA for 10 minutes at 37° C without stirring. The labelled intact platelets were washed and lysed and the labeled membrane fraction was isolated. The labeled membranes were then dissolved in SDS, dithiothreitol, and urea, and dialyzed to remove unincorporated [^{3}H]-5'FSBA. Labeled membrane polypeptides were separated by 0.1% SDS-5% polyacrylamide disc gel electrophoresis. Pyronin Y was used on the tracking dye (T.D.). (A) Intact platelets in platelet-rich plasma; (B) intact gel-filtered platelets; (C) intact multiply-centrifuged washed platelets; (D) isolated platelet membranes. (From Bennett *et al.*[13] Reproduced by permission.)

both ADP and epinephrine alter the platelet surface to reveal latent receptors.[15] We have demonstrated[16] that factor V is a component of the alpha-granules since it fractionates similarly to low-affinity platelet factor 4 (LA-PF$_4$), a known alpha-granule protein (FIG. 4). Factor V is released from platelets by collagen[16] or thrombin.[17] Factor V is then in turn required for binding of factor Xa.[18] The presence of factor Xa and calcium in association with platelets containing factor V allows for a rapid conversion of prothrombin to thrombin,[19] resulting in further platelet aggregation. The role of von Willebrand factor has already been described. Thus, both alpha-granule and dense-body release augment aggregation and positively reinforce the release reaction. Thrombin, in addition to releasing the contents of dense bodies and alpha-granules, can stimulate lysosomal granule release of acid hydrolases. The role of these enzymes is not clear, but elastase may participate in the disruption of vascular elastin known to occur in atherosclerosis. Another product of the release reaction that may play a role in the pathogenesis of atherosclerosis is the platelet-derived growth factor (PDGF). The peptide released from alpha-granules of platelets adhering to injured vessels stimulates smooth-muscle cell proliferation [20] and could be important in causing the intimal thickening of atherosclerotic lesions.

Having summarized changes accompanying aggregation and release, we will now consider the regulation of these responses. We have already considered positive feedback, as demonstrated in terms of the augmentation of extracellular ADP by released ADP. In addition to ADP release, two more processes occur intracellularly, one of which is the formation of stimulatory prostaglandin

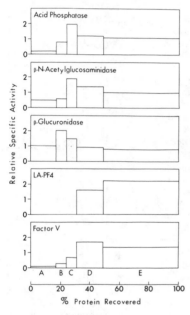

FIGURE 4. Relative specific activities of acid phosphatase (membrane marker), β-N-acetyl-glucosaminidase and β-glucuronidase (lysosomal markers), LA-PF$_4$ (alpha-granule marker), and factor V in platelet fractions obtained when the 12,000 g pellet from disrupted platelets was resuspended and subfractionated by ultrafugation on a sucrose gradient. Fraction A represents the top and Fraction E the bottom of the gradient. (From Chesney et al.[16] Reproduced by permission.)

derivatives within the platelet. Thrombin, collagen, and to a lesser extent epinephrine, ADP, and serotonin are able to trigger platelet responses in part by the production of potent intracellular messengers. These compounds are derived from the oxidation products of arachidonic acid, in particular the endoperoxide derivatives of prostaglandins and thromboxane A$_2$.[21] The formation of these compounds is a multi-step enzymatic process. The exact mechanisms by which the aggregating and releasing agents stimulate the pathway are not clear at the present time. Arachidonic acid, a 20-carbon fatty acid containing four double bonds, is present esterified to the glyceride backbone of membrane phospholipids. Phospholipase A$_2$ is able to hydrolyze the ester bond and liberate arachidonic acid from the second carbon atom of glycerol.[22] Alternatively, phospholipase C hydrolyzes the base from the 3-position and by the action of the diglyceride lipase, arachidonic acid is released.[23] The result of either reaction is to deliver free arachidonic acid to the initial intracellular enzyme in the pathway cyclooxygenase located in the internal platelet membranes. This enzyme is capable, in the presence of molecular oxygen, of introducing oxygen into the molecule to produce the cyclic endoperoxides, PGG_2 and PGH_2. Both of these compounds are able to stimulate platelet aggregation and release, but the half-life is about 5 minutes in plasma. They are rapidly transformed by thromboxane synthetase to thromboxane A_2, a potent platelet stimulatory compound with an even shorter half-life of 30 seconds. Thromboxane A_2 is a potent coronary vasoconstrictor and may be responsible for myocardial ischemia by inducing coronary arterial vasospasm.[24] The formation of thromboxane A_2 and the cyclic endoperoxides is critical for the action of other aggregating agents. Inhibition of cyclooxygenase with aspirin can block the irreversible phase of the platelet aggregation as well as platelet release by epinephrine, ADP, and serotonin. However, the primary response, the initial phase of reversible aggregation, still occurs. In addition, collagen action is not fully inhibited by aspirin at a high concentration of collagen. Both the inhibition of the formation of thromboxane A_2 and as well as the depletion of extracellular ADP are required to completely inhibit collagen-induced platelet aggregation.[25]

For thrombin the situation is still more complicated. High doses of thrombin will cause platelet release and aggregation even in the presence of both aspirin and ADP-depleting enzymes. There must be a third stimulatory pathway, although the nature of this pathway is still not clear. It appears that one of the important mediators is intracellular calcium. Translocation of intracellular calcium from its membrane-bound position to free form in the cytosol may allow mediation of aggregation and release. All of these three regulatory pathways involving intracellular calcium, arachidonic acid derivatives, and ADP apparently work in concert with each other and account for the potentiation of one stimulus by another.

Finally, it is important to consider the inhibitory regulation of these pathways. The antagonism to the agonist may occur at the receptor level. Each of these compounds probably binds to an individual protein or lipid on the external plasma membrane of the platelets. Antagonism of this action could prevent platelet activation. For example, ATP apparently can compete with ADP for its receptor site. We have shown that compounds such as 5'-fluorosulfonylbenzyladenosine appeared to mimic ATP and bind to an ADP receptor of molecular weight 100,000 (FIG. 2). However, the binding is covalent since this is an affinity label and the effect is to prevent all platelet reactions including the earliest reaction of platelet shape change.[12] Another example of this kind of inhibition is typified by epinephrine antagonists. The stimulation of platelets by epinephrine involves alpha receptors since it is inhibited by alpha antagonists, such as dihydroergocriptine and phentolamine, rather than by beta antagonists, such as propanolol.[26]

The inhibition may involve the subsequent stimulus-response coupling rather than binding to a receptor. The most important inhibitory regulator is the level of intracellular cyclic adenosine monophosphate (cAMP). Cyclic AMP is formed from ATP by the action of adenylate cyclase and is degraded by a specific phosphodiesterase to AMP. Prostaglandins, which are inhibitory to platelets, and in particular the prostaglandins, PGD_2, PGE_1, and PGI_2 (prostacyclin), appear to act by stimulating adenylate cyclase, thereby increasing intracellular concentration of cyclic AMP. The increased levels of cyclic AMP formed inhibit all platelet responses, including adhesion, shape change, and aggregation and release, and antagonize most platelet agonists. Alternatively, platelet cyclic AMP can be elevated by inhibitors of the degrading enzyme, phosphodiesterase. Inhibitors such as caffeine, theophylline, and dipyridamole may act in this fashion. Although the site of the action of cyclic AMP is unknown, there is evidence that various steps of the prostaglandin synthesis pathway are inhibited. However, inhibition of these enzymes cannot be the only effect of cyclic AMP since the inhibition of prostaglandin synthesis by aspirin does not block shape change or even primary aggregation by the agonists.

Levels of cyclic AMP can also be affected by compounds that serve as platelet agonists. For example, ADP can lower PGE_1- or PGI_2-stimulated adenylate cyclase activity and thus decrease cAMP. However, this effect of ADP is probably mediated by a receptor separate from the aggregation and shape change receptor for ADP.

Thus far, the mechanisms have been described by which the platelets participate in the formation of platelet aggregates and also in the genesis of the atherosclerotic plaque through the release of platelet-derived growth factor. Now the focus will turn to how risk factors known to predispose to coronary disease might act through the platelets. Some of the known risk factors for coronary arterial disease include smoking, stress, and cholesterol. Two mechanisms appear to enhance the activation of platelets by smoking. Products that can be extracted from tobacco smoke can directly activate the zymogen coagulant factor XII to the active enzyme factor XIIa.[27] Factor XIIa can then stimulate the intrinsic coagulation cascade to eventually produce thrombin, a potent platelet agonist. Smoking also may act to stimulate the release of amines such as epinephrine, perhaps directly through the action of nicotine on the adrenal glands. Indeed, smokers have been found to have increased numbers of platelet aggregates in the circulation.[28] A second risk factor is stress. Stress may increase the concentration of epinephrine 10-fold and thereby activate platelets. A third risk factor is diabetes, which accelerates the development of atherosclerosis and its vasoocclusive complications.[29] Platelet aggregates have been observed in the retinal capillaries of some patients with diabetic retinopathy.[30] Platelet aggregation has been reported to be enhanced in diabetics,[31] especially in those with complications. Increased prostaglandin synthesis has been documented in the platelets of diabetics [32] compared with control subjects. In addition, the plasma levels of beta thromboglobulin, an alpha-granule platelet-specific protein, are increased in diabetic patients with retinopathy, suggesting *in vivo* platelet activation and release.[33] Since platelet growth factor is released concomitantly with beta-thromboglobulin from alpha-granule, elevated levels of the former would be expected to enhance the formation of atherosclerotic plaques.

It is worthwhile to demonstrate how these risk factors may interact with the various mechanisms to enhance each of the platelet aggregators in the production of intracellular prostaglandins. Epidemologic evidence points to hyperbetalipoproteinemia as an important risk factor in coronary and cerebral arterial occlusion.[29] Our laboratory has gathered clinical and experimental evidence that lipoprotein composition may influence platelet reactivity by altering the platelet lipid composition and, thus, the membrane protein function. Persons with type IIa hyperlipoproteinemia have elevated levels of low-density lipoprotein (LDL) and cholesterol. Several studies from our laboratory and others indicate that the platelets of patients with type IIa lipoproteinemia have increased membrane protein function.[34] Platelet sensitivity is defined as the lowest concentration of an aggregating agent capable of producing irreversible aggregation in the platelet-rich plasma. In Carvalho's study, 17 patients with type IIa hyperlipoproteinemia had a platelet sensitivity to epinephrine that was 140-fold greater than normal (Fig. 5).[34] In another eight patients studied by Mielke[35] platelet sensitivity was 200 times greater than normal. The platelets from the former patients were also more sensitive to ADP. Studies from Dr. Carvalho's laboratory[36] also indicate that the platelets from patients with hyperbetalipoproteinemia stimulate increased amounts of thromboxane A_2 after exposure to aggregating agents. Normally, *in vivo* the concentrations of epinephrine are insufficient to activate platelets to aggregate and release. How-

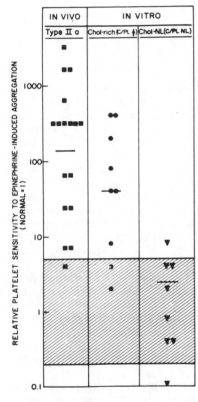

FIGURE 5. The relative sensitivity of platelets to epinephrine-induced aggregation. Sensitivity is defined as the lowest concentration of epinephrine producing complete "second wave" aggregation at 37° C in an aggregometer. It is expressed relative to the sensitivity of normal platelets **(shaded area)** obtained from asymptomatic persons with normal plasma lipids. In the *left column*, platelets from persons with type IIa hyperlipoproteinemia were a mean 140-fold more sensitive than normal.[34] In the *center column*, platelets incubated with cholesterolrich lipid dispersions gained cholesterol, resulting in an increase in the ratio of cholesterol to phospholipids (C/PL), and became a mean 35-fold more sensitive than normal. In contrast, in the *right column*, when platelets were incubated with lipid dispersions similar in lipid composition to normal low-density lipoprotein, they neither gained cholesterol nor became hypersensitive to epinephrine.[38] (From Shattil and Colman.[44] Reproduced by permission.)

ever, cholesterol incorporation sensitizes the platelets so that they respond to concentrations of epinephrine which may be secreted during stress. This finding is a graphic demonstration of risk factors interacting through the platelets.

Searching for a chemical correlate of the heightened response, we have compared the lipid composition of subcellular fraction in normal and type IIa patients (Fig. 6). The ratio of cholesterol to phospholipids (C/PL) is increased 8% over normal[37] when measured in the whole platelet of type IIa patients compared with that of normal subjects. However, when the increase was examined in platelet membrane fractions, it was found that the cholesterol/phospholipid ratio is increased 20% in the type IIa patients' membranes over

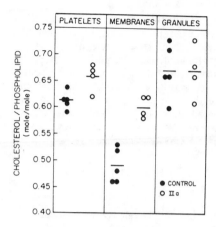

FIGURE 6. The cholesterol to phospholipid ratio is shown in whole platelets, platelet membranes, and platelet granules for normal and type IIa platelets. (From Shattil et al.[37] Reproduced by permission.)

that of normal membranes, while no significant changes in the C/PL were found in the platelet granule fractions. The assay of the composition of type IIa low-density lipoprotein showed an increase in the cholesterol to phospholipid ratio when compared with the norm and a reasonable correlation between the cholesterol to phospholipid ratio in low-density lipoprotein with that in platelets. These studies suggest that the cholesterol may be transferred *in vivo*. In order to clarify the mechanism of platelet hypersensitivity in type IIa patients, the relationship between the platelet lipid composition and function and the lipid composition of plasma was examined in an *in vitro* model.[38] The normal platelets were incubated in plasma in which the free cholesterol/phospholipid ratio of the lipoproteins was varied by the addition of cholesterol-phospholipid dispersions. The sensitivity of the platelet-aggregating agents was found to be increased in those plasmas in which cholesterol could be transferred to platelets, especially to the membranes, resulting in a bulk increase of cholesterol and an increase in platelet cholesterol/phospholipid ratio of 39%. This was associated with a 35-fold increase of sensitivity to epinephrine-induced aggregation (FIG. 5), as determined by both the platelet aggregation threshold and the measure of the release reaction. This experimental procedure can produce platelets similar in structure and function to those in type II patients. *In vivo* platelets cannot synthesize cholesterol. Thus, another possible source of the excess cholesterol in type IIa platelets is from their progenitor, megakarocytes, which have the capacity to synthesize cholesterol.

These platelets were then useful in indicating the action of drugs and other regulatory inhibitors, such as cyclic AMP, on platelets. Of special importance is the interaction of cholesterol enrichment of platelet membranes with the cyclic AMP system known to inhibit platelet function. We have demonstrated that basal cyclic AMP concentration of platelets incubated with cholesterol-enriched dispersions increases with time, closely correlating with the increase in cholesterol.[39] In 5 hours the platelet cholesterol has increased 56% and basal adenylate cyclase activity was 2.5-fold higher than in the control platelet. However, this basal cyclic AMP level may not be the important regulatory factor. It has been suggested that the increase of cyclic AMP through the action of inhibitory prostaglandins, such as PGE_1 on PGD and PGI_2 on adenylate cyclase levels, may influence function. Platelets after cholesterol incorporation were found to be five- to ten-fold less sensitive to inhibitory prostaglandin than they were in normal platelets (FIG. 7). This response was found to be due to the failure of the adenylate cyclase of cholesterol-enriched platelets to respond when stimulated with PGE_1. This in turn may be due to the cholesterol inhibiting the interaction of membrane phospholipid and adenylate cyclase by inhibiting the enzyme-lipid interaction, since phospholipids are known to be necessary for hormonal stimulation of adenylate cyclase. Alternatively, cholesterol may restrict the fluidity of the phospholipid fatty acid and thus impair the transmembrane event necessary for hormonal stimulation of the enzyme. Increased sensitivity of cholesterol-enriched platelets to aggregating agents and their increased resistance to inhibitory prostaglandins would render these platelets more sensitive.

Platelets also make valuable models for studying the effects of drugs on platelets. For example, we have demonstrated that clofibrate [40] and halofenate [41] both are able to restore the more sensitive platelets back to normal reactivity. Both are able to reduce the sensitivity of normal platelets to aggregating agents and can reverse experimental platelet hypersensitivity. All these drugs are limited by their side effects. We have shown that a series of amantadine derivatives, drugs known to alter viral and CNS lipids, can inhibit platelet activation. [42] These drugs also produce phase transition in artificial lipid membranes, as seen by differential scanning calorimetry. The technique measures the ability of drugs to alter lipid interactions and produce a different environment in the platelet membrane. The ability to induce a phase transition in a model membrane is correlated ($r = 0.70$) with the ability to inhibit platelets. Similar effects have been found in our laboratory for local anesthetics as well as for phenothiazine derivatives. [43] Thus, cholesterol incorporation in blood platelets increased the microviscosity of the platelet membrane, resulting in an increase of sensitivity to platelet ADP and epinephrine and resistance to inhibitory prostaglandins. Conversely, a drug-induced increased fluidity of the membrane may lead to decreased platelet aggregation. It also appears that the changes in membrane lipids can alter the membrane proteins, including both the externally

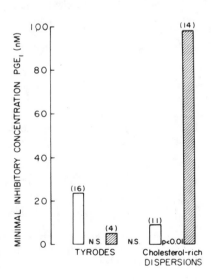

FIGURE 7. Effect of cholesterol on the inhibitory potency of PGE_1 on epinephrine-induced platelet aggregation. The height of the bars represents the geometric mean. *Open bars* represent incubated platelets, whereas *hatched bars* represent platelets incubated for 5 hours at 37°. The number in parentheses above each bar indicates the number of experiments performed. The significance of the difference between the means was calculated by Student's *t* test. (From Sinha *et al* [39] Reproduced by permission.)

oriented receptors, which are receiving environmental stimuli, and the internally oriented regulatory proteins, such as adenylate cyclase. Certain lipid-soluble drugs may have unique applications for disorders such as type IIa hypolipoproteinemia.

This paper has reviewed the clinical and laboratory evidence that platelets may play a role in the sudden death due to coronary artery disease. This role may be at two levels. First, platelets undergoing the release reaction in the neighborhood of endothelial cells may release destructive enzymes which can injure these vessels or growth factors which stimulate smooth muscle proliferation characterizing the atherosclerotic lesion. Second, in the presence of risk factors known to favor coronary artery disease, such as stress, smoking and hypolipoproteinemia, platelets may become intrinsically more sensitive to environmental stimuli. The environmental stimuli then may trigger platelet aggregates which obstruct the microcirculation, producing myocardial ischemia. Alternatively, the platelets may release thromboxane A_2, a potent vasoconstrictor of coronary vessels, which would result in coronary arterial spasm. Trials of antiplatelet agents such as sulfapyrazone indicate that they are capable of preventing sudden death in myocardial infarction. Agents such as aspirin appear to have an effect in the prevention of transient ischemic attacks. Problems exist in the interpretation of the epidemiologic evidence for the efficacy of these drugs. However, the studies have identified enough important trends to indicate that further studies of antiplatelet drugs in modifying the sudden death syndrome may be useful.

We lack precise knowledge of the *in vivo* events, including those in the coronary vessels, of sudden death and whether these events correlate with the findings of the *in vitro* studies I have reviewed. The mechanisms are important to design new drugs or in the trial of existing drugs. For example, aspirin will prevent release and irreversible aggregation with stimuli such as ADP or epinephrine, but not with thrombin. Promising drugs, such as stable derivatives of the inhibitory prostaglandin, which can prevent all platelet actions, including shape change and primary aggregation, might have greater efficacy than existing agents. Further study of the role of platelets in this syndrome is clearly indicated, both in the laboratory in experimental animals and finally in patients. In particular, the interactions of platelets with risk factors and the influence of platelets on the formation of the atherosclerotic plaque seem particularly exciting areas for further research.

ACKNOWLEDGMENTS

I wish to thank Ms. Deborah Morinelli for typing this manuscript and Drs. Roberta F. Colman and Paul Schick for helpful discussion.

REFERENCES

1. FRIEDBERG, C. K. 1966. Diseases of the Heart, 3rd ed.: 796–797. W. B. Saunders. Philadelphia, PA.
2. MASERI, A., A. L'ABBATE & G. BAROLDI, et al. 1978. Coronary vasospasm as a possible cause of myocardial infarction: A conclusion derived from a study of "preinfarction" angina. N. Engl. J. Med. 299: 1271–1277.

3. BRAUNWALD, E. 1978. Coronary spasm and acute myocardial infarction: New possibility for treatment and prevention. N. Engl. J. Med. **299:** 1301–1303.
4. ROSS, R. & J. GLOMSET. 1976. The pathogenesis of atherosclerosis. New Engl. J. Med. **295:** 369–377.
5. JENKINS, C. S. P., D. R. PHILLIPS, K. S. CLEMETSON, D. MEYER, M. S. LARRIEU & E. F. LUSCHER. 1976. Platelet membrane glycoproteins implanted in ristocetin-induced aggregation. J. Clin. Invest. **57:** 117–124.
6. FUSTER, V. & E. J. W. BOWIE. 1978. The von Willebrand pig as a model for atherosclerosis research. Thromb. Haemostas. **39:** 322–327.
7. CHESNEY, C., E. HARPER & R. W. COLMAN. 1972. Critical role of carbohydrate side chain of collagen in platelet aggregation. J. Clin. Invest. **51:** 2693–2701.
8. BROWN, J., S. JIMINEZ & R. W. COLMAN. 1980. Collagen-induced shape change: The role of collagen quarternary structure. J. Lab. Clin. Med. **95:** 90–98.
9. SIMONS, E. R., C. M. CHESNEY, R. W. COLMAN, E. HARPER & E. SAMBERG. 1975. The effect of the conformation of collagen on its ability to aggregate platelets. Thromb. Res. **7:** 123–139.
10. WIGGINS, R. C., D. J. LOSKUTOFF, C. G. COCHRANE, J. H. GRIFFIN & T. S. EDGINGTON. 1980. Activation of rabbit Hageman factor by homogenates of cultural rabbit endothelial cells. J. Clin. Invest. **65:** 197.
11. HENNESEY, V., R. HICKS, S. NIEWIAROWSKI, L. H. EDMUNDS, JR. & R. W. COLMAN. 1977. Effects of surface area and composition on the function of human platelets during extracorporeal circulation. Am. J. Physiol. **232:** H622.
12. BENNETT, J., R. F. COLMAN & R. W. COLMAN. 1978. Identification of adenine nucleotide binding proteins in human platelet membranes by affinity labelling with 5'-p-fluorosulfonyladenonine. J. Biol. Chem. **253:** 7346–7354.
13. BENNETT, J. S., G. VILAIRE, R. F. COLMAN & R. W. COLMAN. 1981. Localization of human platelet membrane-asociated actomyosin using the affinity label 5'-p-fluorosulfonylbenzoyl adenosine. J. Biol. Chem. **256:** 1185–1190.
14. HAEREM, J. 1972. Platelet aggregates in intramyocardial vessels of patients dying suddenly and unexpectedly of sudden coronary disease. Atherosclerosis **15:** 529–554.
15. BENNETT, J. S. & G. VILAIRE. 1979. Exposure of platelet fibrinogen receptors by ADP and epinephrine. J. Clin. Invest. **64:** 1343.
16. CHESNEY, C. M., D. D. PIFER & R. W. COLMAN. 1981. Subcellular localization and secretion of factor V human platelets. Proc. Natl. Acad. Sci. USA **78:** 5180.
17. KANE, W. H., M. J. LINDHOUT, C. M. JACKSON & P. W. MAJERUS. 1980. Factor Va-dependent binding of factor Xa to human platelets. J. Biol. Chem. **255:** 1170–1174.
18. MILETICH, J. P., C. M. JACKSON & P. W. MAJERUS. 1978. J. Biol. Chem. **253:** 6908–6916.
19. CHESNEY, C. M., D. D. PIFER & R. W. COLMAN. 1978. Factor V coagulant activity of human platelets generated by collagen. Circulation **58:** 208.
20. ROSS, R., J. GLOMSET, B. KARIYA & L. A. HARBER. 1974. A platelet-dependent serum factor that stimulates the proliferation of arterial smooth-muscle cells *in vitro*. Proc. Natl. Acad. Sci. USA **71:** 1207–1210.
21. HAMBERG, M., J. SVENSSON & B. SAMUELSON. 1974. Prostaglandin endoperoxides. A new concept concerning the modification and release of prostaglandins. Proc. Natl. Acad. Sci. USA **71:** 3824–3828.
22. BILLS, T. K., J. B. SMITH & M. J. SILVER. 1977. Selective release of arachidonic acid from the phospholipids of human platelets in response to thrombin. J. Clin. Invest. **60:** 1–6.
23. RITTENHOUSE-SIMMONS, S. 1979. Production of diglyceride from phosphatidylinositol in activated human platelets. J. Clin. Invest. **63:** 580–587.

24. BORER, J. S. 1980. Unstable angina: A lethal gun with an invisible trigger. N. Engl. J. Med. **302:** 1200–1201.
25. PACKHAM, M. A., M. A. GUCCIONE, J. P. GREENBERG, R. L. KINLOUGH-RATHBONE & J. F. MUSTARD. 1977. Release of ^{14}C-serotonin during initial platelet changes induced by collagen, thrombin and A23187. J. Lab. Clin. Med. **90:** 707–719.
26. ALEXANDER, R. W., B. COOPER & R. I. HANDIEN. 1978. Characterization of the human platelet α-adrenegic receptor. Correlation of ^{8}H-dihydroergocryptine binding with aggregation and adenylate cyclic inhibition. J. Clin. Inv. **62:** 1136–1144.
27. BECKER, C. G. & T. DUBIN. 1977. Activation of Factor XII by tobacco glycoprotein. J. Exp. Med. **146:** 457–467.
28. DAVIS, J. W. & R. W. DAVIS. 1979. Acute effect of tobacco cigarette smoking on the platelet aggregative ratio. Am. J. Med. Sci. **278:** 139–143.
29. KANNEL, W. B., W. P. CASTILLI, T. GORDON & P. M. MCNAMARA. 1971. Cholesterol, lipoproteins and the risk of coronary heart disease. The Framingham Study. Ann. Intern. Med. **74:** 1–12.
30. BLOODWORTH, J. M. B. & D. L. MOLITOR. 1965. Ultrastructural studies of human and canine diabetic retinopathy. Invest. Ophthal. **4:** 1037–1048.
31. KWANN, H. C., J. A. COLWELL, S. CRUZ, N. SAWANWELA & J. C. DOBBIE. 1972. Increased platelet aggregation in diabetes mellitus. J. Lab. Clin. Med. **80:** 236–246.
32. GENSINI, G. F., R. ABBATE, S. FAVILLA & G. G. NERI SERNERI. 1979. Changes of platelet function and blood clotting in diabetes mellitus. Thromb. Haemostas. **42:** 983–993.
33. ZAHAVI, J., J. A. G. JONES, D. J. BETTERIDGE, J. LEYTON, D. J. GALTON & J. E. CLARK. 1979. Platelet factor 4, β-thromboglobulin, malondialdehyde formation and blood lipids in patients with diabetes mellitus. Thromb. Haemostas. **42:** 334.
34. CARVALHO, A. C. A., R. W. COLMAN & R. S. LEES. 1974. Platelet function in hyperbetalipoproteinemia. N. Engl. J. Med. **290:** 434–438.
35. COLMAN, R. W. 1978. Platelet function in hyperbetalipoproteinemia. Thromb. Haemostas. **39:** 284–293.
36. BIZIOS, R., L. K. WONG, R. VAILLANCOURT, R. S. LEES & A. C. CARVALHO. 1977. Platelet prostaglandins endoperoxides formation in hyperlyemias. Thromb. Haemostas. **38:** 228.
37. SHATTIL, S. J., J. S. BENNETT, R. W. COLMAN & R. A. COOPER. 1977. Abnormalities of cholesterol-phospholipid composition in platelets and low-density lipoproteins of human hyperbetalipoproteinemia. J. Lab. Clin. Med. **89:** 341–353.
38. SHATTIL, S. J., R. ANAYA-GALINDO, J. BENNETT, R. W. COLMAN & R. A. COOPER. 1975. Platelet hypersensitivity induced by cholesterol incorporation. J. Clin. Invest. **55:** 636–643.
39. SINHA, A. K., S. J. SHATTIL & R. W. COLMAN. 1977. Cyclic AMP metabolism in cholesterol-rich platelets. J. Biol. Chem. **252:** 3310–3314.
40. CARVALHO, A. C. A., R. W. COLMAN & R. S. LEES. 1974. Clofibrate reversal of platelet hypersensitivity in hyperbetalipoproteinemia. Circulation **50:** 570–574.
41. COLMAN, R. W., J. S. BENNETT, J. F. SHERIDAN, R. A. COOPER & S. J. SHATTIL. 1976. Halfenate: A potent inhibitor of normal and hypersensitive platelets. J. Lab. Clin. Med. **88:** 282–291.
42. COLMAN, R. W., J. KUCHIBHOLTA, M. K. JAIN & R. K. MURRARY. 1977. Phase separation in lecithin biolayers as a prediction of inhibition of blood platelet aggregation by amantadines. Biochem. Biophys. Acta **467:** 273–279.
43. JAIN, M. K., E. ESKOW, J. KUCHIBHOLTA & R. W. COLMAN. 1978. Correlation

of inhibition of platelet aggregation by phenothiazines and local anesthetics and their effects on a lipid bilayer. Thromb. Res. **13:** 1007–1075.

44. SHATTIL, S. & R. W. COLMAN. 1976. Plasma lipoprotein-platelet interactions. *In* Current Cardiovascular Topics, Vol. 2. E. Dunoso & J. I. Haft, Eds.: 110–121. Stratton Intercontinental Medical Book Corp. New York, NY.

DISCUSSION

DR. BIGGER: I was intrigued with the high-cholesterol platelet model and I wonder if you might expand on it a little.

DR. COLMAN: Patients with type IIa hyperlipidemia have enhanced platelet sensitivity to ADP and epinephrine. These platelets show an 8% overall increase in cholesterol to phospholipid ratio. What is more striking is that there is a 20% increase when the membrane fraction of the platelets is isolated. These same changes can be produced experimentally with normal platelets.

DR. BIGGER: Was this reversible?

DR. COLMAN: Yes. If cholesterol is removed from normal platelets, they become hyporesponsive.

DR. BIGGER: But if the patient's serum cholesterol was lowered by other means, would the platelet defect reverse?

DR. COLMAN: That is not known.

ROLE OF CORONARY ARTERIAL SPASM IN SUDDEN CORONARY ISCHEMIC DEATH

Attilio Maseri,* Silva Severi, and Paolo Marzullo

Institute of Clinical Physiology, C.N.R.
Pisa, Italy

Cardiovascular Research Unit, R.P.M.S.
Hammersmith Hospital
London, England

Sudden coronary death together with myocardial infarction and angina pectoris represent the clinical manifestation of ischemic heart disease. Interventions for the prevention of sudden death ought to be based on a clear and rational understanding of the underlying pathogenetic mechanisms. However, this syndrome has been so variably defined in the epidemiologic literature that the term "sudden death" has come to encompass many different types of events with different underlying pathogenetic mechanisms, each of which would require a specific preventive approach.

A PROVISIONAL PATHOGENETIC CLASSIFICATION OF SUDDEN CARDIAC DEATH

Clinical and pathophysiologic experience with sudden death prompts the need for a pathogenetic classification of this syndrome which, together with the assessment of the relative incidence of the various pathogenetic mechanisms in population studies, should point the way toward a rational basis for preventive trials.

Usually the term "coronary" is introduced to define a specific subset of deaths which are supposedly caused by coronary atherosclerosis. Indeed, the lack of an independent yardstick *a posteriori* tends to cause the inclusion by definition in this category of only those patients in whom coronary atherosclerosis is found at postmortem examination.[1] Thus, even if only a single raised lesion is found at post mortem, it is usually interpreted as the culprit, and the possibility that it could be only an "innocent bystander" or a generically predisposing factor is not considered. Conversely, if normal coronary arteries are found, the diagnosis of coronary death is excluded. Indeed, the severity of coronary atherosclerosis found in patients who die suddenly shows a remarkable variability from patient to patient, suggesting that other factors superimposed on a variable degree of atherosclerosis may substantially contribute to this variance. Furthermore, the presence of atherosclerosis does not explain *per se* the mechanism that actually triggered sudden death, except for the minority of patients in whom a fresh thrombus is found at autopsy.

Therefore, it would seem appropriate to specify "ischemic" coronary death,

* Present address: Sir John McMichael Professor of Cardiovascular Medicine, Director, Cardiovascular Research Unit, Royal Postgraduate Medical School, Hammersmith Hospital, Ducane Road, London W12 OHS, England.

0077-8923/82/0382-0204 $1.75/0 © 1982, NYAS

because ischemia of the myocardium is, by itself, potentially responsible for the fatal event, whereas the anatomic lesions of the coronary arteries may only favor or predispose, but not necessarily cause, the development of ischemia.[2]

We will, therefore, define *sudden coronary ischemic death* as death occurring suddenly as a consequence of events resulting from an episode of acute myocardial ischemia, which can occur in the presence of extremely variable degrees of coronary atherosclerosis. Even with this restricted meaning, the prevailing triggering mechanisms leading to sudden ischemic death may be different in the early minutes after the onset of ischemia, in the immediate reperfusion phase, and in the established myocardial infarction (early, middle and late phase), and would hence require specific preventive measures (TABLE 1). For example, the mechanism of death in a patient dying suddenly who is found to have a large, fresh infarction may be different from that of a patient who has minimal coronary atherosclerosis and no myocardial lesions. The failure of the attempts to reduce sudden death in epidemiologic studies may be related to the underlying

TABLE 1

PATHOGENETIC CLASSIFICATION OF SUDDEN CARDIAC DEATH

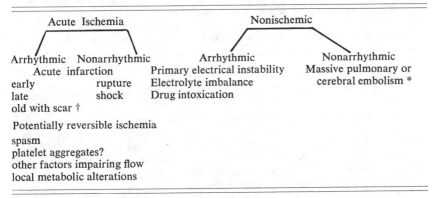

Acute Ischemia		Nonischemic	
Arrhythmic	Nonarrhythmic	Arrhythmic	Nonarrhythmic
	Acute infarction	Primary electrical instability	Massive pulmonary or
early	rupture	Electrolyte imbalance	cerebral embolism *
late	shock	Drug intoxication	
old with scar †			
Potentially reversible ischemia			
spasm			
platelet aggregates?			
other factors impairing flow			
local metabolic alterations			

* May be secondary to myocardial infarction.
† May cause arrhythmias independently of acute ischemia.

assumption that the mechanism responsible for sudden death was practically unique in the populations studied and that it was effectively counteracted by the intervention.

In this presentation we will concentrate on a specific subset of cases of sudden ischemic death caused by coronary spasm. We will examine the incidence and prognostic significance of potentially fatal arrhythmias occurring during transient episodes of acute but *potentially reversible* myocardial ischemia caused by coronary arterial spasm. We became interested in this particular aspect of sudden ischemic death because potentially fatal arrhythmias are frequent in acute transient vasospastic myocardial ischemia and because these arrhythmias can be prevented by specific antivasospastic treatment rather than by antiarrhythmic drugs.

Coronary Spasm

Historical Notes

The hypothesis of spasm as a possible cause of death is ancient. The first case of sudden ischemic death during a typical anginal attack attributed to coronary spasm was reported by Galli in 1908 as "vasospasm with fatal outcome (true angina pectoris without coronary lesion)" in a patient who died suddenly during a severe anginal attack which occurred at the very end of a close, but successful chess game.[3] Subsequently, Leary in 1935 hypothesized "coronary spasm as a possible factor in producing sudden death."[4] However, even earlier, several accurate reports by famous clinicians have described death during a paroxysm of angina pectoris with coronary arteries that appeared normal at postmortem examination.[5, 6] In particular, Gallavardin in 1925 recognized that patients with angina at rest usually had normal coronary arteries at autopsy and he proposed that their symptoms were caused by coronary spasm. He therefore recognized that people with angina and normal coronary arteries could indeed die suddenly during an attack as a result of spasm.[7]

These isolated personal conclusions were based on careful clinical observations and postmortem studies made by the same person, who therefore could be confident of both his clinical diagnosis and of his postmortem findings. However, a dichotomy began to grow between the clinician and the pathologist, so that findings that did not fit with the preconceived ideas of either the pathologist or of the clinician were reciprocally distrusted and hence disregarded.

The Revival of Spasm as a Clinical Entity

Prompted by the work of Prinzmetal et al.,[8] coronary spasm became a proven hypothesis not only for "variant" angina,[9] but also for angina with S-T segment depression, infarction, and sudden death.[10] Figures 1, 2, and 3 show a typical case of coronary spasm causing ventricular fibrillation in a patient without critical coronary arterial narrowings; this patient subsequently died suddenly soon after the onset of chest pain.

Salient features of this revival of the notion of spasm as a cause of ischemia are three: (1) Spasm can be observed both in angiographically normal vessels and in vessels with severe coronary lesions; thus, critical coronary atherosclerotic narrowings are not a prerequisite for the development of spasm.[11] (2) Acute myocardial ischemia secondary to spasm can occur in the absence of anginal pain in spite of a documented decrease of coronary sinus oxygen saturation and lactate production.[12–15] (3) Coronary spasm and platelet aggregation are closely associated because spasm favors platelet adhesion and aggregation to the arterial wall; on the other hand, substances released by platelets stimulate smooth muscle constriction.[16]

The Current Diagnostic Problem

Now that the possible role of coronary spasm in acute myocardial ischemia has been seen, a reasonably practical diagnosis of potentially fatal arrhythmias caused by coronary spasm is needed. So far a practical diagnosis of acute vaso-

spastic ischemia can only be based on the assumption that variant angina represents an acceptably reliable, easily identifiable hallmark of acute transient
ischemia caused by spasm.[17] Although variant angina appears to represent only
the most easily recognizable extreme of a continuous spectrum of ischemia
caused by spasm,[18] it appears to be the type of ischemia in which arrhythmias
are more frequent, probably because the ischemia is transmural rather than
predominantly subendocardial.[19] Thus, we selected variant angina, not only

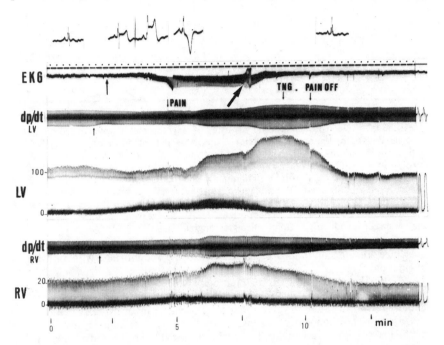

FIGURE 1. Time course of events during a typical episode of variant angina.
Low-speed playback of an ischemic episode recorded in a patient with normal
coronary arteries (electrocardiographic lead III; LV and RV=left and right ventricular pressure tracings, respectively). *Arrows* indicate beginning of changes of
various measurements, as determined on high-speed tracings. At *top,* superimposed
are electrocardiographic alterations visible on high-speed tracing during various
phases of attack. Pain appears more than 2 minutes after onset of S-T segment
elevation, which is followed by long period of very deep negative T waves and by
marked increase of ventricular pressure. A burst of ventricular ectopic beats is
seen at *large arrow* under the electrocardiographic tracing. TNG=sublingual administration of nitroglycerin.

because it is an easily recognizable form of vasospastic ischemia, but also
because it appears to be the form of transient acute vasospastic ischemia in which
potentially fatal arrhythmias are more frequent.

The diagnosis of arrhythmias or of sudden ischemic death secondary to
spasm can be considered:

(1) practically certain when arrhythmias are recorded a few minutes after
the onset of S-T segment elevation or during the waning phase of the episode

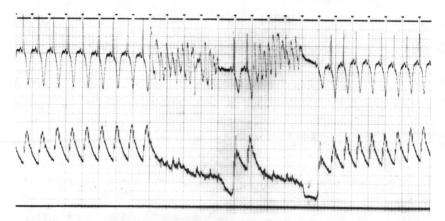

FIGURE 2. Electrocardiographic tracing of asymptomatic myocardial ischemia associated with malignant arrhythmia in the same patient as in FIGURE 1. He had a history of fainting during chest pain; ventricular fibrillation was repeatedly documented in the CCU Coronary care unit when S-T segment elevation was followed by deep negative T waves, with or without anginal pain. This low-speed playback of electrocardiographic lead III and aortic pressure tracing shows two transient bouts of ventricular fibrillation (VF), which spontaneously reverted to sinus rhythm at the end of an asymptomatic ischemic episode. Three years after these observations, the patient died suddenly at home during an anginal attack.

(detected during continuous electrocardiographic monitoring, with or without anginal pain);

    (2) highly probable when palpitations, paroxysmal tachycardia, syncope, or sudden death occur a few minutes after the onset of typical anginal pain in a patient known to suffer from episodes of vasospastic myocardial ischemia;

    (3) possible when syncope, ventricular tachycardia, or sudden, instantaneous death (even without anginal pain) occurs in a patient with known episodes of vasospastic myocardial ischemia (because pain can be a late phenomenon and may be absent altogether during acute myocardial ischemia [12-15]).

FINDINGS IN VARIANT ANGINA

    In order to evaluate only patients in whom spasm can be considered practically certain, we shall confine our analysis to hospital studies and long term follow-up on a group of 187 consecutive patients with documented "variant" angina who were observed by us between 1970 and 1979. Among these 187 patients, 32 presented on one or more occasions with episodes of ventricular tachycardia, fibrillation, or severe arrhythmias (Group 1) during hospitalization in our institutions. The characteristics of these patients as well as their short- and long-term prognosis are compared with those of the remaining 155 patients (Group 2).

    Females constituted less than 10% in both groups and the mean age was not statistically different (53 and 52 years). The history of old myocardial infarction was similar in the two groups (37% and 34%); and coronary arteriographic findings were not statistically different (for 0-, single-, double-, and triple-vessel disease the figures were 17%, 43%, 13%, and 27%, respectively, in Group 1, and 9%, 33%, 34%, 24%, respectively in Group 2). S-T segment elevation was predominantly anterior in 60% and inferior in 40% in Group 1, and predominantly anterior in 70% and inferior in 30% in Group 2. Spasm was demonstrated in 10 of the patients in Group 1 and in 35 of the patients in Group 2 (lately, provocative tests have not been performed when the diagnosis of variant angina was documented). Electrocardiographic stress testing was positive in 56% of the patients in Group 1 and in 70% of those in Group 2. Therefore, no significant differences emerged between Groups 1 and 2 with respect to the variables already mentioned. The differences between the two groups became apparent in the history, in the findings on continuous electrocardiographic monitoring in the coronary care unit, and in the mortality rate.

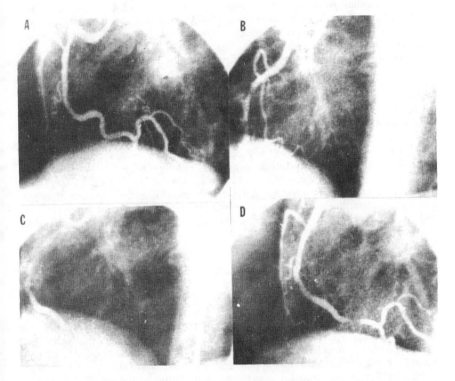

FIGURE 3. Right coronary arteriography in the same patient as in FIGURES 1 and 2 showing injection (A) in absence of electrocardiographic abnormalities and subjective symptoms. (B) frame obtained 5 seconds after beginning of contrast injection into right coronary artery during S-T segment elevation in leads II, III, and aVF accompanied by angina. No dye progression occurs beyond the middle third of the artery, which appears diffusely narrowed. (C) frame obtained 10 seconds after frame illustrated in (B). Dye persists in distal part of middle third of right coronary artery, but no dye is filling the distal third. (D) injection performed after nitroglycerin administration during appearance of deep negative T waves. Persistent severe narrowing is observed at the point that was previously occluded, but no filling or runoff delay was observed.

History

In Group 1, five patients reported syncope (preceded by angina in three), and in eight patients ventricular tachycardia, fibrillation, and complete atrioventricular block were documented in other hospitals. In Group 2, only six patients reported syncope, and three episodes of ventricular tachycardia or fibrillation were documented in other hospitals.

Continuous Electrocardiographic Monitoring

Group 1. Patients were monitored for an average period of 28 days per patient (range, 7 to 196 days per patient). A total of 2490 transient episodes of acute myocardial ischemia (documented by typical transient electrocardiographic changes) were observed (from 1 to 376 episodes per patient).

During transient ischemic episodes, single ectopic beats and bigeminy were quite frequent, and 92 episodes (3.7%) of the total were accompanied by severe rhythm disturbances: 66 by ventricular tachycardia (22 during asymptomatic episodes); 9 by ventricular fibrillation; 8 by complete atrioventricular block (2 followed by cardiac arrest); 6 by sinus block with severe bradycardia; and 3 by fatal arrhythmias (see later).

Seventeen patients had more than one episode of arrhythmia, and six had more than one type of arrhythmia. In the 46 episodes in which recording of the entire episode was obtained, severe bradyarrhythmias occurred always during the episode, whereas ventricular tachycardia occurred during the episode in 15 and at the moment of its resolution (reperfusion phase) in 21.

Group 2. Patients were monitored for an average period of 14 days per patient (range, 1 to 80 days per patient). A total of 5109 episodes of acute transient myocardial ischemia were observed (from 1 to 290 episodes per patient). According to the criteria of inclusion, no severe arrhythmia was observed in this group.

Mortality

In-hospital Death Rate

Group 1. Three of the 92 episodes of arrhythmias were fatal: one patient had unexpected syncope while in the toilet during a quiescent phase of his disease (terminal irreversible ventricular fibrillation was documented); in (2) patients cardiac standstill developed followed by complete atrioventricular block and electromechanical dissociation. One additional patient died of pump failure after acute myocardial infarction. All four patients had triple-vessel disease.

Group 2. Three patients died after acute myocardial infarction. All had one or more previous infarctions.

Follow-up Mortality

Group 1. Of the 28 surviving patients, 2 died during the first year; one died suddenly 8 months after a successful bypass operation for an isolated left anterior descending lesion and the other died during an episode of chest pain. A third patient died in the third year of follow-up study soon after the onset of chest pain (he had only minimal irregularities in his coronary arteries and documented spasm of the right coronary artery). No patients died in the second and fourth years of follow-up study.

Group 2. Of the 152 surviving patients, 2 died of noncardiac causes (neoplasm, hepatitis); 2 died in the first year (one suddenly and one after acute myocardial infarction); 3 died during the second year (two during prolonged episodes of chest pain, and one during an attack of acute pulmonary edema); 2 died during the third year (during a prolonged episode of chest pain); and one died during the fifth year (suddenly). Five of the eight patients dying had an old myocardial infarction; coronary arteriography was performed in five of the eight and showed single-vessel disease in one patient and double- or triple-vessel disease in the other four.

DISCUSSION

It is established that transient acute myocardial ischemia caused by coronary arterial spasm may trigger potentially fatal arrhythmias. The common feature of these arrhythmias is their causal relation with an episode of acute ischemia that is potentially reversible or preventable by antiischaemic rather than antiarrhythmic therapy. It is also proven that potentially fatal arrhythmias can occur during transient ischemic episodes caused by a sudden reduction in coronary blood supply and that these episodes are completely asymptomatic (associated only with transient ischemic electrocardiographic changes and with transient impairment of left ventricular function), thus representing the only clinical manifestation of acute ischemia.

Severe Arrhythmias Caused by Coronary Arterial Spasm

Taking variant angina as a hallmark of ischemia caused by coronary spasm, we can examine the incidence of arrhythmias in this syndrome as well as the available information on the characteristics of the patients and of the ischemic episodes.

Incidence of Arrhythmias in Variant Angina

The reported incidence of severe arrhythmias in the largest series of patients with variant angina, although variable, is quite high. Kerin *et al.* observed severe arrhythmias in 12 of 26 patients with variant angina (ventricular fibrillation and tachycardia were found in 4), but they were unable to identify characteristic features of the patients who presented with arrhythmias.[20] Commonly, arrhythmias tend to recur in the same patient and to be consistently absent in others. In the series reviewed in this report, severe arrhythmias were present in 18% of the patients, but occurred only in 3.6% of the electrocardiographic ischemic episodes recorded in the Coronary Care Unit in this group of patients. Therefore, severe arrhythmias appear to be a rather rare event during episodes of vasospastic ischemia, even in the patients who appear to be more prone to the development of arrhythmias. Tachyiarrhythmias are considerably more common than bradyarrhythmias, and in about 30% of the cases they appear to occur during the resolution of the transient ischemic episode, compatible with a reperfusion phenomenon.[21, 22] In agreement with Kerin et al.,[20] we were unable to identify characteristic features of the patients who had the tendency to develop arrhythmias during or at the end of the ischemic episode relative to those who never showed arrhythmias. About 15% of patients with severe arrhythmias had no critical lesions, 35% had single-vessel disease, and 50% double- or triple-vessel disease. Moreover, during continuous hemodynamic monitoring [12-14] we were unable to detect appreciable differences in the hemodynamic variables between episodes with and without arrhythmias in the same patient.

Sudden Death in Variant Angina

In a previous article [18] we reported successful defibrillation and/or resuscitation in 16 patients during or at the end of episodes of variant angina. Three patients died minutes after the onset of an acute ischemic episode, one of irreversible ventricular fibrillation detected too late and the other two of electromechanical dissociation. Conti et al.[23] reported five episodes of cardiac arrest (two successfully defibrillated) in 36 patients with proven spasm; 4 of the 5 patients also had organic coronary stenoses. More information is available for overall cardiac death, which also includes death from acute myocardial infarction. McAlpin reviewed the literature and found a 15% incidence of death within the first 3 months of symptoms.[24]

In all series, the majority, but not all, of the patients who die have severe coronary atherosclerosis, and usually, but not invariably, die during the waxing of symptoms. After the acute phase, mortality decreases considerably and, on the average, appears related to the underlying severity of coronary atherosclerosis and of alterations in ventricular function.

More recently, investigators of larger series have reported a much lower hospital and long-term mortality. Schroeder et al.[25] in a study of 42 medically treated patients with variant angina reported only two hospital deaths and a late death during an average follow-up period of 24 months. Severi et al. reported a 3.6% hospital mortality and an overall mortality of 1.7% per year (0.7% for patients with no critical organic stenosis or with single-vessel disease, and 2.7% for patients with double- or triple-vessel disease) during a complete follow-up period of 2 to 4 years on medical therapy.[26]

Thus, it appears that mortality in our group of patients with variant angina, which is the largest series on medical therapy with prospective long and complete follow-up study, is lower than that reported in the Framingham Study for complicated and for uncomplicated angina pectoris.[27] Moreover, it should be considered that in our series about one-third of the patients had a documented old myocardial infarction and about 60% had double- or triple-vessel disease (mean age, 55 years). Even considering only the group with double- or triple-vessel disease, mortality was only 2.7% per year in spite of the fact that these patients had an incidence of old myocardial infarction that was greater than 45%. This favorable prognosis, the low incidence of reinfarction (0.8% per year), and the progressive amelioration of symptoms might be related to therapy with slow channel blocking agents and high doses of nitrates,[28, 29] which could have helped to prevent vasospasm.

Coronary Spasm and Sudden Death in the General Population

The incidence of coronary spasm in the genesis of clinical manifestation of ischemic heart disease is only speculative. A number of clues suggests that it may be much more common than generally thought.[10] Also, the role of coronary arterial spasm in the genesis of sudden ischemic coronary death in the general population may be not negligible if we consider the findings in the rather large series of persons resuscitated from sudden death.

In survivors of sudden death, electrocardiographic evidence of acute myocardial infarction was found only in 19% of 305 patients in the Seattle series [30] and in 44% of 142 patients in the Ohio-Michigan series [31] (in this later series strict selective criteria for "coronary" death were adopted). Enzymatic changes suggestive of acute myocardial cell damage were found in 19% and 34% of the patients, respectively, and no persistent electrocardiographic changes or elevated enzyme levels were detected in the remaining survivors. While it seems reasonable to infer that in the patients with acute myocardial infarction cardiac arrest was the result of infarction, for the others different mechanisms must be postulated. A transient ischemic episode too short to evolve into transmural infarction can be assumed for patients with minor degrees of myocardial damage, and a transient completely reversible, ischemic episode or a primary arrhythmia can be assumed for the remaining patients. Coronary arterial spasm should be considered among the possible causes of acute transient ischemia, and its role may be even greater if it represents one of the possible initiating events of acute infarction.[10]

The role of spasm in sudden death is strongly supported by the findings in patients who died during ambulatory monitoring shortly after the onset of S-T segment elevation [32, 33] or depression, which was likely reciprocal of S-T elevation in other leads.[34] These recordings also prove that the arrhythmia can begin without any previous S-T segment changes [34, 35] or can follow the onset of S-T segment depression [35, 36] which may or may not have been caused by changes in vasomotor tone.

Finally, the epidemiologic criteria for defining sudden coronary ischemic death should be updated because fatal arrhythmias may occur during transient ischemic episodes in the absence of anginal pain in patients with normal coronary arteries at post mortem examination,[37] as is illustrated in FIGURES 1, 2, and 3. Therefore, neither the absence of organic coronary stenotic lesions nor the absence of chest pain allows us to rule out the possibility of sudden coronary ischemic death.

Possibilities of Prevention

The Framingham Study indicates that the first manifestation of ischemic heart disease is sudden death in about 10 to 13% of cases. These figures might have been considerably lower when we consider that in this study the diagnosis of angina was rejected in patients in whom "substernal distress . . . radiating into the arms or neck also occurred as often at rest (as during exertion or excitement)." [27]

Therefore, prevention of sudden death might be attempted with reasonable hope of success in symptomatic patients, provided that the degree of risk can be stratified and that prevailing pathogenetic mechanisms in different subsets can be identified and rationally treated. The information available so far indicates that patients are at the greatest risk at the very onset of anginal symptoms and during the period when the symptoms of angina wax.

The remarkably low incidence of sudden death as well as of other manifestations of ischemic heart disease in our group of patients treated medically with drugs known to prevent vasospasm suggest the potential reward of new lines of research. Long-term treatment with slow channel blockers and nitrates, which appear highly effective in the acute phase of the disease,[28, 29, 40–42] should be tried in other centers. If our results are confirmed, an additional preventive approach for sudden death and for the clinical manifestations of heart disease in general might emerge, and large-scale trials with slow channel blockers and nitrates may be considered in patients with recent onset angina or with "crescendo" angina and in other subsets of patients who are identified as being at high risk.

SUMMARY

Sudden coronary death is a syndrome caused by different mechanisms, all of which should be separately considered with respect to preventive measures. Ventricular fibrillation, tachycardia, and complete atrioventricular block were repeatedly observed during ischemic episodes caused by spasm in both the presence and absence of anginal pain. Spasm is, therefore, a potential cause of sudden coronary death.

In "variant" angina, which is a reasonably reliable indicator of coronary spasm, arrhythmias occur in about 25% of patients and tend to recur in the same patient. The severity of coronary atherosclerosis in patients who develop severe arrhythmias is quite variable and not dissimilar from patients who do not. Mortality is considerably higher in patients with severe disease, but fibrillation and death can occur also in patients with angiographically normal arteries. In these patients acute and long-term treatment with nitrates and slow channel blockers appears to give remarkable results. Prevention of arrhythmias in patients in whom arrhythmias are secondary to acute ischemic episodes caused by vasospasm should be attempted by preventing vasospasm.

REFERENCES

1. GOLDSTEIN, S. 1974. Sudden Death and Coronary Heart Disease. Futura Publishing Co. Mount Kisco, NY.
2. MASERI, A. 1980. Pathogenetic mechanisms of angina pectoris: expanding views. Br. Heart J. **43:** 648–60.
3. GALLI, G. 1908. Vasospasmo con esito letale (angina pectoris vera senza lesione coronaria). Gazz. Osp. Clin. **29:** 137–138.
4. LEARY, T. 1935. Coronary spasm as a possible factor in producing sudden death. Am. Heart J. **10:** 338–344.
5. LATHAM, P. M. 1876–78. Collected Works (2 vols.), vol. 1: 461.
6. OSLER, W. 1910. The Lumleian lectures on angina pectoris. II. Lancet **i:** 839–844.
7. GALLAVARDIN, L. 1925. Les Angines de Poitrine. Paris.: 130–132.
8. PRINZMETAL, M., R. KENNAMAR, R. MERLISS, T. WADA & N. BOR. 1959. Angina pectoris. 1. A variant form of angina pectoris. Am. J. Med. **27:** 375–388.

9. MELLER, J., A. PICHARD & S. DACK. 1976. Coronary arterial spasm in Prinzmetal's angina: A proven hypothesis. Am. J. Cardiol. **37:** 938–940.

10. MASERI, A., S. CHIERCHIA & A. L'ABBATE. 1980. Pathogenetic mechanisms underlying the clinical events associated with atherosclerotic heart disease. Circulation **62** (Suppl): 3–13.

11. MASERI, A., A. L'ABBATE, A. PESOLA, A. M. BALLESTRA, M. MARZILLI, S. SEVERI, G. MALTINTI, M. DE NES O. PARODI & A. BIAGINI. 1977. Coronary vasospasm in angina pectoris. Lancet **1:** 713–717.

12. MASERI, A., R. MIMMO, S. CHIERCHIA, C. MARCHESI, A. PESOLA & A. L'ABBATE. 1975. Coronary artery spasm as a cause of acute myocardial ischemia in man. Chest **68:** 625–633.

13. CHIERCHIA, S., M. LAZZARI, M., I. SIMONETTI & A. MASERI. 1980. Haemodynamic monitoring in angina at rest. Herz **5:** 189–197.

14. CHIERCHIA, S., C. BRUNELLI, I. SIMONETTI, M. LAZZARI & A. MASERI. 1980. Sequence of events in angina at rest: Primary reduction in coronary flow. Circulation **61:** 759–768.

15. CHIERCHIA, S., M. LAZZARI & A. MASERI. 1981. Hemodynamic monitoring in painless myocardial ischemia. Am. J. Cardiol. **47:** 446.

16. ELLIS, E. F., O. OELZ, L. J. ROBERTS, II, N. A. PRYNE, B. J. SWEETMAN, A. S. NIES & A. OATES. 1976. Coronary arterial smooth muscle contraction by a substance released from platelets: evidence that it is thromboxane A2. Science **193:** 1135–1137.

17. MASERI, A. 1981. The revival of coronary spasm. Am. J. Med. **70:** 752–754.

18. MASERI, A., S. SEVERI, M. DE NES, A. L'ABBATE, S. CHIERCHIA, M. MARZILLI, A. M. BALLESTRA, O. PARODI, A. BIAGINI & A. DISTANTE. 1978. "Variant" angina: One aspect of a continuous spectrum of vasospastic myocardial ischemia. Pathogenetic mechanisms, estimated incidence and clinical and coronary arteriographic findings in 138 patients. Am. J. Cardiol. **42:** 1019–1035.

19. MASERI, A., O. PARODI, S. SEVERI & A. PESOLA. 1976. Transient transmural reduction of myocardial blood flow, demonstrated by thallium-201 scintigraphy, as a cause of variant angina. Circulation **54:** 280–288.

20. KERIN, N. Z., M. RUBENFIRE, M. NAINI, W. WAJSZCZUK, A. PAMATMAT & P. N. CASCADE. 1979. Arrhythmias in variant angina pectoris. Relationship of arrhythmias to ST-segment elevation and R-wave changes. Circulation **60:** 1343–1350.

21. BATTLE, W. E., S. NAIMI, B. AVITALL, A. H. BRILLA, J. S. BANAS, JR., J. M. BETE & H. J. LEVINE. 1974. Distinctive time course of ventricular vulnerability to fibrillation during and after release of coronary ligation. Am. J. Cardiol. **34:** 42.

22. CORBALAN, R., R. L. VERRIER & B. LOWN. 1976. Differing mechanisms for ventricular vulnerability during coronary artery occlusion and release. Am. Heart J. **92:** 223.

23. CONTI, C. R., C. J. PEPINE & R. C. CURRY JR. 1979. Coronary artery spasm: An important mechanism in the pathophysiology of ischemic heart disease. *In* Current Problems in Cardiology. W. Proctor Harvey, Ed. Vol. IV: 1. Year Book Medical Publishers. Chicago & London.

24. MACALPIN, R., A. KATTUS & A. ALVARO. 1973. Angina pectoris at rest with preservation of exercise capacity. Prinzmetal's variant angina. Circulation **47:** 946–958.

25. SCHROEDER, J. S., R. O. RUSSELL, JR., L. RESNEKOV, M. WOLK, A. M. HUTTER, JR., R. A. ROSATI, C. R. CONTI, L. C. BECKER, T. BIDDLE, E. M. KAPLAN, J. P. GILBERT & M. B. MOCK. 1978. Unstable angina pectoris—national randomized study of surgical vs. medical therapy: Results in Prinzmetal type angina (abstr). Am. J. Cardiol. **41:** 397–405.

26. SEVERI, S., G. J. DAVIES, A. MASERI, P. MARZULLO & A. L'ABBATE. 1980.

216   Annals New York Academy of Sciences

Long-term prognosis of "variant" angina with medical treatment. Am. J. Cardiol. **46:** 226–232.
27. KANNEL, W. B. & M. FEINLEIB. 1972. Natural history of angina pectoris in the Framingham study. Am. J. Cardiol. **29:** 154–163.
28. DISTANTE, A., A. MASERI, S. SEVERI, A. BIAGINI & S. CHIERCHIA. 1979. Management of vasospastic angina at rest with continuous infusion of isosorbide dinitrate. Am. J. Cardiol. **44:** 533–539.
29. PARODI, O., A. MASERI & I. SIMONETTI. 1978. Management of unstable angina by verapamil. A double-blind crossover study in CCU. Br. Heart J. **41:** 167–174.
30. COBB, L. A., J. A. WERNER & G. B. TROBAUGH. 1980. Sudden cardiac death. 1. A decade's experience with out-of-hospital resuscitation. Mod. Concepts Cardiovasc. Dis. **XLIX:** 31–36.
31. GOLDSTEIN, S., J. R. LANDIS, R. LEIGHTON, G. RITTER, C. M. VASU, A. LANTIS & R. SEROKMAN. 1981. Characteristics of the resuscitated sudden death victim with coronary heart disease. Circulation. In press.
32. BLEIFER, S. B., D. J. BLEIFER, D. R. HANSMANN, J. J. SHEPPARD & H. L. KARPMAN. 1974. Diagnosis of occult arrhythmias by Holter electrocardiography. Prog. Cardiovasc. Dis. **XVI:** 569–599.
33. DELEBARRE, PH., P. FOUILLAND, E. HANSEN, M. LEFEVRE, J. LEMONNIER, CH. CAPRONNIER & J. CRAMER. 1980. Syndrome du clic mésosystolique, spasme coronaire et mort subite. Revue générale à propos d'un tracé terminal de type Prinzmetal, enregistré par la méthode de Holter. Arch. Mal. Coeur. **73:** 1145–1152.
34. LAHIRI, A., V. BALASUBRAMANIAN & E. B. RAFTERY. 1979. Sudden death during ambulatory monitoring. Br. Med. J. **1:** 1676–1678.
35. POOL, J., K. KUNST & J. L. VAN WERMESKERKEN. 1978. Two monitored cases of sudden death outside hospital. Br. Heart J. **40:** 627–629.
36. GRADMAN, A. H., P. A. BELL & R. F. DEBUSK. 1977. Sudden death during ambulatory monitoring: Clinical and electrocardiographic correlations. Report of a case. Circulation **55:** 210–211.
37. AUZÉPY, F., M. BLONDEAU & F. ALBESSARD. 1974. Aspects electrocardiographiques suggestifs d'un angor de Prinzmetal avec artéres coronaires normales à autopsie. Arch. Mal. Coeur. **9:** 1107–1113.
38. LASSER, R. T. & N. S. DE LA PAZ. 1973. Repetitive transient myocardial ischemia, Prinzmetal's type, without angina pectoris, presenting with Stokes-Adams attacks. Chest **64:** 350–352.
39. PREHKOV, V. K., S. MOOKHERGEE, W. M. SCHEISS & A. I. OBEID. 1974. Variant anginal syndrome, coronary arterial spasm and ventricular fibrillation in absence of chest pain. Ann. Int. Med. **81:** 858.
40. MULLER, J. E. & S. J. GUNTHER. 1978. Nifedipine therapy for Prinzmetal's angina. Circulation **57:** 137–139.
41. PREVITALI, M., J. A. SALERNO, L. TAVAZZI, M. RAY, A. MEDICI, M. CHIMIENTI, G. SPECCHIA & P. BOBBA. 1980. Treatment of angina at rest with nifedipine: A short-term controlled study. Am. J. Cardiol. **45:** 825–830.
42. SCHROEDER, J. S., S. ROSENTHAL, R. GINSBURG & I. LAMB. 1980. Medical therapy of Prinzmetal's variant angina. Chest **78:** 231–233.

DISCUSSION

DR. R. CASE: Do you find any relationship between the severity of response in terms of arrhythmias or ventricular fibrillation in a patient with repeated spasms?

DR. MASERI: No. We found no relationship between duration of S-T segment elevation and arrhythmias.

DR. HIRSH: During your studies have you been able to use fairly specific pharmacologic agents to come to grips with the cause of the spasm?

DR. MASERI: We have tried, but the problem is that the agents we think are specific probably have multiple effects.

DR. HIRSH: Has anything worked?

DR. PITT: A controversy exists over whether thromboxane plays a primary or a secondary role in ischemic spasm. The bulk of the evidence that is accumulating suggests that thromboxane release is secondary to ischemia and is not the primary event. Some of your studies and those of others show that regardless of the mechanism of ischemia platelets release thromboxane, and interfering with this mechanism does not seem to be a very important strategy.

DR. MASERI: I can agree with this, but with caution, because the mechanism of spasm is different in different patients, and there may be some patients in whom this mechanism could be active.

DR. S. SCHERLIS (*Baltimore, Maryland*): Have you any comments with regard to small vessel as opposed to large vessel spasm?

DR. MASERI: There is no way that you can document this by angiography, but I would not rule out the possibility of small vessel spasm. There are a number of patients in whom angina is not caused by the traditionally ascribed mechanism and who do not respond to ergonovine or who respond in a very peculiar way. Spasm of small vessels might exist in these patients; I would not be surprised.

DR. A. Moss (*Rochester, New York*): Have you tried stellate ganglion block to see whether it modulates or alters the frequency and severity of the episodes of the coronary spasm, particularly in patients who have clearly repetitive episodes?

DR. MASERI: No we haven't.

DR. COBB (*Seattle, Washington*): Do you have any evidence whether your Group 1 patients with ventricular ectopic activity are adversely affected by the administration of beta blocking drugs? It has been speculated that beta adrenergic blocking agents might make the situation worse.

DR. MASERI: While I concur that reports are appearing about the dangers of beta blockade in these patients, we have not found definite evidence of this phenomenon.

SUDDEN CARDIAC DEATH:
ROLE OF LEFT VENTRICULAR DYSFUNCTION

Bertram Pitt

Division of Cardiology
Department of Internal Medicine
University of Michigan Medical Center
Ann Arbor, Michigan 48109

Early studies from the Coronary Drug Project of sudden cardiac death in patients surviving an episode of myocardial infarction called attention to the importance of ventricular ectopic beats.[1] In that study, complex ventricular ectopic beats recorded on a 12-hour Holter electrocardiogram were found to be associated with an excessive risk of sudden cardiac death. When the relationship was examined between complex ventricular ectopic beats and other risk factors, such as age, number of prior infarctions, angina pectoris, hypertension, serum cholesterol, glucose intolerance, cardiomegaly seen on chest X-ray films, and cigarette-smoking, complex ventricular ectopic beats were found to be independent risk factors with respect to sudden cardiac death. The importance of ventricular ectopic beats as a predictor of sudden cardiac death during the convalescent or late hospital phase of acute myocardial infarction in this and other studies has led to the use of prophylactic antiarrhythmic therapy in an attempt to prevent or reduce these ectopic beats and hence to prevent sudden cardiac death.

In a subsequent study by Schulze *et al.* patients surviving an episode of acute myocardial infarction underwent 24-hour Holter electrocardiographic recording and gated radionuclide left ventricular angiography prior to discharge from the hospital.[2] Several important findings emerged from this study: It was noted that 26 of 29 (90%) patients with complex ventricular arrhythmias (Lown Class III–V) on Holter electrocardiographic recording had a left ventricular ejection fraction of <40% compared with only 19 of 52 (37%) without complex ventricular arrhythmias. During a mean follow-up period of 7 months, eight patients had documented ventricular fibrillation. All eight patients who suffered sudden death were in the subset of patients with complex late hospital phase ventricular arrhythmias and a left ventricular ejection fraction of <40%. This study was one of the first to call attention to the role of ventricular dysfunction in patients with sudden cardiac death after an episode of acute myocardial infarction. The failure of left ventricular dysfunction to be recognized as an important predictor of sudden death after myocardial infarction in the Coronary Drug Project and in other previous studies may be related to the use of the cardiothoracic (CT) ratio on chest X-ray film as an index of left ventricular function. Subsequent studies have pointed out that the CT ratio is a poor index of left ventricular function and that the correlation between the CT ratio and left ventricular ejection fraction is poor. Schulze *et al.* also found that the left ventricular ejection fraction and the percent of left ventricular akinesia on gated blood pool imaging were significantly better predictors of subsequent sudden cardiac death than was peak creatine phosphokinase (CPK) determined during the episode of acute infarction. Patients who subsequently died suddenly had

218

0077–8923/82/0382–0218 $1.75/0 © 1982, NYAS

a higher peak CPK than those who survived, but this difference was not significant. In contrast, those who died suddenly had a significantly lower left ventricular ejection fraction and a greater percentage of left ventricular akinesia than those who survived. The failure of peak CPK to adequately predict those at risk for subsequent sudden death is due to the fact that it is the total myocardial damage that appears to be of importance rather than just the acute damage, which is reflected by the rise in CPK. Left ventricular ejection fraction and the percent of left ventricular akinesia reflect total myocardial damage due to previous infarction as well as acute infarction and therefore appear to be better predictors.

The importance of ventricular dysfunction as a predictor of subsequent sudden cardiac death after myocardial infarction can also be seen in a study by Ruberman et al.[3] In that study of 1739 patients with prior myocardial infarction who underwent a 1-hour electrocardiographic recording and were followed for a mean of 24.4 months, complex ventricular ectopic beats were again found to be an important predictor of subsequent sudden and nonsudden cardiac death. However, the combination of complex ventricular ectopic activity on the 1-hour electrocardiographic recording and a history of congestive heart failure showed the highest relative risk for subsequent death, both sudden and nonsudden.[3]

In subsequent studies by Schulze et al. it was noted that patients with complex late hospital phase ventricular ectopic beats on 24-hour Holter electrocardiographic recording prior to discharge from the hospital after an episode of acute myocardial infarction had a significantly greater incidence of multivessel coronary artery disease than did those without complex ventricular arrhythmias, as well as a significantly greater incidence of abnormally contracting myocardial segments and a lower left ventricular ejection fraction on contrast left ventriculography.[4] The more extensive coronary artery disease and left ventricular dysfunction and hence increased risk of myocardial ischemia in patients with complex ventricular arrhythmias after myocardial infarction were thought to help explain the relative refractoriness of many of the arrhythmias in these patients to standard antiarrhythmic therapy.

In a study of 106 patients surviving an episode of acute myocardial infarction who underwent 24-hour Holter electrocardiographic recording and coronary angiography prior to hospital dischage, Taylor et al., using univariate analysis, also noted that a low left ventricular ejection fraction, proximal left anterior descending coronary artery disease, and significant triple-vessel disease were associated with a high risk of subsequent sudden cardiac death.[5] Multivariate analysis of 30 clinical and laboratory values identified previous myocardial infarction and a left ventricular ejection fraction of <40% as the best predictor of mortality. In this analysis the presence of complex late hospital phase ventricular arrhythmias did not provide additional prognostic information as to subsequent sudden death once the information as to previous infarction and ejection fraction was considered. In a recent study in which 10-hour Holter electrocardiographic recordings were made on 289 survivors of an episode of acute myocardial infarction Klieger et al. also found that the occurrence of ventricular runs on electrocardiographic recording was related to left ventricular dysfunction.[6] However, analysis of the data led the authors to conclude that the presence of ventricular runs on electrocardiographic recording was a marker of severe cardiac disease rather than an independent risk factor for predicting subsequent sudden cardiac death.

On the basis of these and other studies, it appears that complex ventricular arrhythmias and left ventricular dysfunction are important predictors of death after myocardial infarction, both sudden and nonsudden. The complex ventricular arrhythmias seen during the late hospital phase of acute myocardial infarction, however, may be "innocent bystanders" and merely markers of left ventricular dysfunction rather than independent risk factors for subsequent sudden cardiac death. Indirect support for this hypothesis can be found from an analysis of several recent therapeutic trials. Attempts to reduce sudden cardiac death by prophylactic antiarrhythmic therapy or by suppressing complex ventricular ectopic activity after myocardial infarction have not been successful. For example, in a recent study of mexiletine in the postinfarction period it was found that complex ventricular ectopic beats could be successfully suppressed.[7] Nevertheless, the incidence of sudden cardiac death was not reduced. In fact, there was a slightly higher incidence of death in those receiving mexiletine. Previous and ongoing trials of antiarrhythmic agents given to prevent sudden cardiac death after myocardial infarction have also failed, and although one could argue that such failure to reduce the incidence of sudden cardiac death after myocardial infarction may be due to the inadequacies of either the trial design or of currently available antiarrhythmic agents, it could equally be argued that the concept of prophylactic or suppressive antiarrhythmic therapy to prevent sudden death is inadequate and that new approaches to this problem are needed. Further support for the hypothesis that complex ventricular arrhythmias after myocardial infarction are merely incidental and not critical to the subsequent development of sudden cardiac death comes from the recent Norwegian trial of timolol in patients recovering from an episode of acute myocardial infarction.[8] In this study timolol was shown to significantly reduce the incidence of both sudden and nonsudden death after infarction. However, the reduction in incidence of sudden cardiac death by timolol was not reported to be associated with any significant reduction in complex ventricular ectopic activity.

If complex ventricular ectopic beats during the late hospital phase of acute myocardial infarction are merely "innocent bystanders" and markers of ventricular dysfunction and/or extensive ischemic heart disease rather than primary etiologic factors for subsequent sudden death, how can we explain the importance of ventricular dysfunction as a risk factor and what is its implication for the prevention of subsequent sudden cardiac death after infarction? Our current hypothesis, based upon our previous experience [2, 4, 5] and that of others, is that extensive myocardial damage makes the ventricle vulnerable to what might otherwise be subthreshold stimuli. These stimuli may cause heterogeneous repolarization and electrical disorganization, resulting in ventricular fibrillation and sudden death. For example, a patient with extensive myocardial damage and multivessel coronary artery disease may develop ventricular fibrillation after administration of relatively small concentrations of catecholamines. Similar catecholamine concentrations in a patient wtih a normal ventricle without coronary artery disease would not cause ventricular fibrillation or sudden cardiac death. Thus, timolol could have prevented sudden cardiac death by blocking the effects of catecholamines in patients with extensive myocardial damage or coronary arterial narowing, or both. Other subthreshold humoral or neural humoral factors or both may also be of impotance and precipitate ventricular fibrillation in patients with extensive myocardial dysfunction. Recent studies in our laboratory suggest that intracerebral opiate administration can cause profound systemic and coronary vasoconstriction,[9] and in the presence of extensive myocardial damage, it is possible that intracerebral endogenous opioid release could result in myocardial ischemia, ventricular fibrillation, and sudden cardiac death.

In the foregoing discussion it has been emphasized that left ventricular dysfunction and extensive coronary artery disease are important factors in the occurrence of sudden cardiac death. This, of course, is true only for those with ischemic heart disease. A relatively large percentage of patients who die suddenly do not have ischemic heart disease or ventricular dysfunction. Sudden cardiac death in these patients without known cardiac disease may be due to threshold rather than subthreshold stimuli. For example, a release of high concentrations of catecholamines and/or other neural or humoral factors may be required to cause inhomogeneity in ventricular conduction and to precipitate sudden death in the normal ventricle. The incidence of sudden death in those without myocardial damage and ischemic heart disease is relatively low since it is relatively uncommon that these neural or humoral factors reach threshold levels. On the other hand, in the patient with extensive myocardial dysfunction and ischemic heart disease, catecholamine levels in the coronary sinus are relatively high. The presence of left ventricular dysfunction and an increased vulnerability to ventricular fibrillation may in conjunction with other neural or humoral factors lead to sudden death. If this hypothesis is correct, the approach to the prophylaxis of sudden cardiac death will depend upon a better understanding of the neural and humoral stimuli, both subthreshold and threshold, which result in ventricular fibrillation. If these stimuli can be identified and the factors that control their release and mechanisms of action understood, it is possible that appropriate prophylactic strategies for the prevention of sudden cardiac death could be developed. Development of new antiarrhythmic agents, the use of extensive Holter electrocardiographic recording, and the application of electrophysiologic techniques may be of benefit to the patient with symptomatic ventricular tachycardia and/or recurrent ventricular fibrillation, but these techniques have not and probably will not be of benefit in developing an effective prophylactic approach to the overall problem of sudden cardiac death or to the particular subset of patients surviving an episode of acute myocardial infarction with extensive left ventricular dysfunction.

REFERENCES

1. KOTLER, M. N., B. TABATZNIK, M. M. MOWER & S. TOMINAGA. 1973. Prognostic significance of ventricular ectopic beats with respect to sudden death in the late postinfarction period. Circulation 47: 959–966.
2. SCHULZE, R. A., H. W. STRAUSS & B. PITT. 1977. Sudden death in the year following myocardial infarction. Relation to ventricular premature contractions in the late hospital phase and left ventricular ejection fraction. Am. J. Med. 62: 192–199.
3. RUBERMAN, W., E. WEINBLATT, J. GOLDBERG, C. FRANK & S. SHAPIRO. 1977. Ventricular premature beats and mortality after myocardial infarction. N. Engl. J. Med. 297: 750.
4. SCHULZE, K. A., J. O. HUMPHRIES, L. S. C. GRIFFITH, H. DUCCI, S. ACHUFF, M. G. BAIRD, E. D. MELLITS & B. PITT. 1977. Left ventricular and coronary angiographic anatomy. Relationship to ventricular irritability in the late hospital phase of acute myocardial infarction. Circulation 55: 839–843.
5. TAYLOR, G. J., J. O. HUMPHRIES, E. D. MELLITS, B. PITT, R. A. SCHULZE,

L. S. C. GRIFFITH & S. C. ACHUFF. 1980. Predictors of clinical course, coronary anatomy and left ventricular function after recovery from acute myocardial infarction. Circulation **62:** 960–970.
6. KLEIGER, R. E., J. P. MILLER, S. THANAVARO, M. A. PROVINCE, T. F. MARTIN & G. C. OLIVER. 1981. Relationship between clinical features of acute myocardial infarction and ventricular runs 2 weeks to 1 year after infarction. Circulation **63:** 64–70.
7. CHAMBERLAIN, D. A., D. E. JEWITT, D. G. JULIAN, R. W. F. CAMPBELL, D. M. C. BOYLE, R. G. SHANKS, *et al.* 1980. Oral-mexiletine in high-risk patients after myocardial infarction. Lancet **2:** 8208–8209.
8. NORWEGIAN MULTICENTER STUDY GROUP. 1981. Timolol-induced reduction in mortality and reinfarction in patients surviving acute myocardial infarction. N. Engl. J. Med. **304:** 801–807.
9. PASYK, S., J. A. WALTON & B. PITT. 1981. Central opioid mediated coronary and systemic vasoconstriction in the conscious dog. Circulation **64** (Suppl. IV): IV–41.

DISCUSSION

R. BAIGRIE (*Toronto, Ontario, Canada*): Dr. Pitt could you tell me what percentage of sudden deaths in North America each year are postinfarction sudden deaths?

DR. PITT: Perhaps Dr. Cobb would be better prepared to answer that.

DR. COBB: It is difficult to answer with certainty, but this question is very important. Of the patients that we see after resuscitation from out-of-hospital ventricular fibrillation due to coronary disease, 60% have no history of prior myocardial infarction, and 40% do. About 15% of the patients appear to have had a myocardial infarction within the preceding 6 months to a year. So while they do not represent an enormous part of the sudden death population, this subset is obviously very important.

DR. P. GALLERSTEIN (*New York, New York*): We have noticed that in a lot of the patients coming to our coronary care unit with very poor left ventricular function and complex arrhythmias, the arrhythmias have actually subsided as we have sought to improve left ventricular function by the very aggressive use of both pre- and afterload agents. Have you looked at this?

DR. PITT: We haven't examined this directly, but the few data that I am familiar with seem to indicate that although ventricular function can be altered by afterload-reducing agents, the overall mortality has not changed. Perhaps these premature ventricular contractions are really markers, but not necessarily the event that triggers death.

DR. HERLING: You appropriately negate the role of empirical antiarrhythmic therapy in preventing sudden death in the high-risk subgroup, but how do you regard the role of programmed electrical stimulation in the electrophysiology laboratory to identify those high-risk subsets who may sustain recurrent ventricular tachycardia?

DR. PITT: This will be discussed later by others.

EFFECT OF INFARCT SIZE LIMITATION BY PROPRANOLOL ON VENTRICULAR ARRHYTHMIAS AFTER MYOCARDIAL INFARCTION

James R. Stewart,* John K. Gibson,† and
Benedict R. Lucchesi †

*Departments of Internal Medicine * and Pharmacology †
University of Michigan Medical Center
Ann Arbor, Michigan 48109*

Pharmacologic interventions designed to preserve ischemic myocardium have been the subject of extensive basic and clinical investigation over the past 10 years.[1-3] Whereas most of these studies have been concerned with the concept of feasibility of reduction of infarct size by a variety of means, none has looked systematically at the long-term sequelae of such interventions, particularly with regard to late-phase arrhythmias and sudden death. The purpose of this paper is to briefly review the rationale behind infarct size reduction and then to present some experimental data which question the advisability of widespread use of pharmacologic reduction of infarct size as an isolated clinical strategy.

Without attempting an exhaustive review of literature, I have chosen a few clinical studies that I believe are either *pro* or *con* the concept of infarct size reduction. Although these studies are not necessarily intended as such, they form the background for our investigations.

The rationale for preserving ischemic myocardium stems from both pathologic [4, 5] and clinical [6] studies that show a direct relationship between infarct size and subsequent clinical course with respect to the development of congestive heart failure and cardiogenic shock and also with respect to prognosis. Work by Roberts *et al.*[7] and Cox *et al.*[8] has shown a direct relationship between infarct size as determined by creatine phosphokinase (CPK) measurements and the frequency of ventricular arrhythmias in the first 20 hours after acute myocardial infarction. These studies suggest that the frequency of early ventricular arrhythmias after acute myocardial infarction reflects the extent of myocardial injury.

Schulze *et al.*[9] have investigated the relationship of complex ventricular arrhythmias (Lown Class III–V) 10 to 21 days post infarction to left ventricular dysfunction using Holter monitor recordings and gated blood pool scans. Patients with these late-phase complex ventricular arrhythmias were found to have significantly lower ejection fractions and presumably larger infarcts than did patients without complex ventricular arrhythmias. The overall survival in the group with complex arrhythmias was less than 50%, despite standard anti-arrhythmic therapy.

On the basis of these studies, one could postulate that reduction of infarct size should reduce the incidence of postinfarction arrhythmias, both early and late, and subsequently reduce the tendency to the development of ventricular fibrillation and sudden death.

These studies are just a few of the many investigations that have provided the basis for attempts to limit infarct size.

0077-8923/82/0382-0223 $1.75/0 © 1982, NYAS

Recent studies suggest, however, that in addition to infarct size, areas of jeopardized myocardium play an important role in the etiology of post-infarction arrhythmias. Schaeffer and Cobb [10] have reported the Seattle experience with survivors of out-of-hospital ventricular fibrillation. They found that recurrent ventricular fibrillation or sudden death developed primarily in those patients whose initial episode was not associated with myocardial infarction. Despite lack of evidence of myocardial necrosis, this group of patients remains at a high risk for the development of malignant ventricular arrhythmias. This suggests that these patients have an area of myocardium at risk for the development of ischemia-related changes in myocardial activation and repolarization with resultant malignant arrhythmias. In contrast, those patients who have evidence of a completed infarction after resuscitation do not have an area of jeopardized myocardium at risk for subsequent ischemia and malignant arrhythmias.

Recent angiographic studies by Taylor et al.[11] have identified groups of patients at different degrees of risk for sudden death after infarction. Those patients at low risk for the development of sudden death were those with an occluded vessel leading to an akinetic myocardial segment with all other areas of ventricle showing normal wall motion. The patients at highest risk were those with an occluded or partially narrowed vessel supplying the hypokinetic myocardial segment. This suggests that patients with a completed infarct who do not have an area of jeopardized myocardium fare better from the standpoint of sudden death than do those patients with a segment of myocardium at risk for subsequent ischemia.

Finally, population studies [12, 13] have shown that patients surviving an episode of subendocardial infarction have a risk of recurrent infarction and sudden death equal to or greater than that of patients with transmural infarction. This again suggests that despite a smaller area of myocardial necrosis, patients with subendocardial infarction have an area of jeopardized myocardium which may lead to recurrent infarction and sudden death.

Thus, on the basis of these studies, one can postulate that reduction of infarct size by pharmacologic intervention, by salvaging viable yet jeopardized myocardium, may increase the risk for the development of malignant arrhythmias and sudden death.

While many pharmacologic agents have been shown to limit the extent of myocardial necrosis resulting from coronary occlusion, propranolol has been consistently effective in reducing infarct size in a variety of animal models [14] and in two clinical studies. In one clinical study, Norris et al.[15] gave intravenous propranolol, 0.1 mg/kg, to patients with acute myocardial infarction within 4 hours of the onset of symptoms and this was followed by oral propranolol for several days. These investigators were able to show a decrease in the number of completed (Q wave) infarcts and lower peak CPK values in the propranolol-treated patients than in control patients. So from this study it appears that the concept of infarct size reduction in the clinical setting is feasible.

With this background in mind, we undertook a series of experiments designed to test the hypothesis that pharmacologic reduction of infarct size may be detrimental to electrophysiologic stability after acue myocardial infarction. In choosing an experimental model, we wanted to be able to achieve several goals. First, we wanted to achieve maximal infarct size reduction. Second, most of the earlier experiments that studied the relationship between ventricular arrhythmias and infarct size reduction used anesthetized animals.

Since anesthesia may have a profound effect on arrhythmia development, we wanted to be able to monitor for arrhythmias in the conscious, unsedated animal. Third, in addition to looking at spontaneous ventricular arrhythmias, we wanted to have another measure of electrical stability in the conscious animal. In order to do this, we wanted a model in which we could attempt to induce ventricular tachycardia by means of programmed electrical stimulation in the conscious dog after myocardial infarction.

In order to achieve maximal infarct size reduction, we performed a 90-minute proximal occlusion of the left anterior descending (LAD) artery, followed by reperfusion through a critical stenosis in anesthetized male mongrel dogs weighing between 10 and 20 kg. Group I animals received pretreatment with intravenous propranolol, 1 mg/kg, 30 minutes before LAD occlusion. Group II animals received an equal volume of saline solution 30 minutes before occlusion and served as controls, and Group III animals were sham-operated controls who underwent thoracotomy and electrode placement only. All animals were monitored continuously intraoperatively for determination of electrocardiographic rhythm and blood pressure. The number and complexity of ventricular arrhythmias during the 90-minute period of LAD occlusion and for 30 minutes after LAD reperfusion were quantitated. After 30 minutes of reperfusion, bipolar electrodes were attached to the left atrium and right ventricular outflow tract to be used for subsequent recording and programmed stimulation studies. The animals were then allowed to recover and subsequently were monitored daily while standing in a sling, unsedated, for a period of 1 hour until the disappearance of spontaneous ventricular arrhythmias. Significant ventricular arrhythmias were arbitrarily defined as being equal to or greater than 10 premature ventricular depolarizations per minute. This enabled us to assess the time course of spontaneous ventricular ectopy in the conscious animal after myocardial infarction. On the first day in which no significant ventricular ectopy was recorded, the animals underwent programmed electrical stimulation studies using the indwelling electrodes. The stimulation protocol consisted of both atrial and ventricular pacing with the introduction of single and double ventricular extrastimuli as well as short bursts of rapid ventricular pacing to a maximal rate of 250 per minute. The animals were then sacrificed and infarct size determined by triphenyl tetrazolium staining and direct gravimetric analysis and expressed as percent of left ventricular mass.

Animals that were pretreated with propranolol developed an infarct that was on the average 20% of the left ventricular mass and this was significantly smaller ($p < 0.005$) than the infarct size in the control animals, which averaged 30% of left ventricular mass. However, despite significant infarct size reduction, the time course of spontaneous ventricular arrhythmias after infarction was prolonged in the propranolol-treated animals compared with the control group. Thus, by 72 hours after occlusion, half of the propranolol-treated animals still had significant ventricular ectopy, whereas none of the control animals continued to display significant arrhythmias by this time. By 96 hours after occlusion, both groups of animals were quiescent from the standpoint of spontaneous ventricular ectopy. Despite this difference between the two groups in the time course of spontaneous ventricular arrhythmias, there was no difference in the ability to induce ventricular tachycardia by means of programmed stimulation between the two groups.

Of interest, none of the sham-operated control animals exhibited any spontaneous ventricular ectopy nor did they exhibit induced ventricular tachycardia, and none had any evidence of infarction by our staining techniques.

SUMMARY

These experiments show that pretreatment with propranolol was able to achieve significant infarct size reduction in this particular animal model of LAD occlusion followed by reperfusion through a critical stenosis. Despite infarct size reduction, the propranolol pretreatment prolonged the time course of spontaneous ventricular arrhythmias after acute myocardial infarction in the conscious dog. In contrast to this, propranolol pretreatment did not appear to protect against inducible ventricular arrhythmias in the late postinfarction period in the conscious dog.

While it is, of course, impossible to extrapolate the results of animal studies to the clinical situation, future clinical studies designed to limit infarct size by pharmacologic intervention should specifically address the question of electrophysiologic instability after myocardial infarction, both in the early and late phases. The possibility exists that pharmacologic limitation of infarct size may preserve viable but potentially jeopardized areas of myocardium, leaving the risk of subsequent malignant arrhythmias and sudden death.

REFERENCES

1. GILLESPIE, T. A. & B. E. SOBEL. 1977. A rationale for therapy of acute myocardial infarction. Limitation of infarct size. Advan. Intern. Med. **22:** 319–353.
2. CORDAY, E., ED. 1976. Symposium on the management of jeopardized ischemic myocardium. Am. J. Cardiol. **37:** 461–605.
3. BRAUNWALD, E., Ed. 1976. Protection of the Ischemic Myocardium. American Heart Association Monograph 48.
4. AMSTERDAM, E. A. 1973. Function of the hypoxic myocardium. Am. J. Cardiol. **32:** 461–471.
5. HARNARYAN, C., M. A. BENNETT, B. L. PENTECOST, et al. 1970. Quantitative study of infarcted myocardium in cardiogenic shock. Br. Heart J. **32:** 728–732.
6. SOBEL, B. E., G. F. BRESHNAHAN, W. E. SHELL, et al. 1972. Estimation of infarct size in man and its relationship to prognosis. Circulation **46:** 640–648.
7. ROBERTS, R., A. HUSAIN, H. D. AMBOS, et al. 1975. Relation between infarct size and ventricular arrhythmia. Br. Heart J. **37:** 1169–1175.
8. COX, J. R., R. ROBERTS, H. D. AMBOS, et al. 1976. Relations between enzymatically estimated myocardial infarct size and early ventricular dysrhythmia. Circulation **50:** I-150–155.
9. SCHULZE, R. A., H. W. STRAUSS & B. PITT. 1977. Sudden death in the year following myocardial infarction: Relation to late hospital phase VPC's and left ventricular ejection fraction. Am. J. Med. **62:** 192–199.
10. SCHAFFER, W. A. & L. A. COBB. 1975. Recurrent ventricular fibrillation and modes of death in survivors of out-of-hospital ventricular fibrillation. N. Engl. J. Med. **293:** 259–262.
11. TAYLOR, G., J. O. HUMPHRIES, L. GRIFFITH, et al. 1977. Prognosis after acute infarction: A function of angiographically identified myocardial risk segments (abstract). Circulation **56:** 562.
12. CANNOM, D. S., W. LEVY & L. S. COHEN. 1976. The short and long term prognosis of patients with transmural and nontransmural myocardial infarction. Am. J. Med. **61:** 452–458.
13. SCHEINMAN, M. M. & J. A. ABBOTT. 1973. Clinical significance of transmural

versus nontransmural electrocardiographic changes in patients with acute myocardial infarction. Am. J. Med. **55:** 602–607.

14. MAROKO, P. R., J. K. KJEKSHUS, B. E. SOBEL, *et al.* 1971. Factors influencing infarct size following coronary artery occlusion. Circulation **43:** 67–82.

15. NORRIS, R. M., N. L. SAMMEL, *et al.* 1978. Protective effect of propranolol in threatened myocardial infarction. Lancet: 907–909.

DISCUSSION

DR. BIGGER: I would like to discuss your remark concerning persons with nontransmural myocardial infarction who are now recognized as being at risk of early reinfarction or death. You attribute this risk to the possibility of the occurrence of arrhythmias, but it seems to me that the risk is just as likely to occur through ischemia or left ventricular dysfunction.

DR. STEWART: I didn't mean to imply a primary arrhythmic etiology, but I did mean to imply that without a transmural infarction, there is an area of myocardium presumably in jeopardy for ischemia-related reinfarction or ischemia-related arrhythmic changes.

DR. BIGGER: Do all beta adrenergic blocking agents have the same effects as those you showed with propranolol? Or is it possible that they are not all the same?

DR. STEWART: There is no way I can answer that since we did not investigate other beta blockers in our study.

DR. SCHWARTZ: As to the higher incidence of arrhythmias at 72 hours: Is there any difference in heart rate between the two groups? A lower heart rate with propanalol might have favored the appearance of arrhythmias. Also I am concerned about your way of inducing infarction. Reperfusion is very nice, but I wonder whether you are not somehow changing the situation, which may be far different from what happens with complete stenosis. Before extrapolations are made from your studies, it would be good to repeat the study with a more traditional method of coronary arterial occlusion.

DR. STEWART: Your points are well taken. In the clinical situation both effects are probably operative. Certainly, infarctions are due to complete occlusion, but recent angiographic studies of infarcts have shown reperfusion in patients within hours after acute infarction.

DR. MASERI: I want to make two points. First, you were very careful to point out that you were describing the results in your model in terms of reducing infarct size. What happens in daily life with patients may be slightly different from what happens to an experimental animal whose artery is occluded and perhaps released.

Second, it is very important, when looking at sudden death after myocardial infarction, to determine whether these sudden deaths are related to arrhythmias *per se* or to a new episode of ischemia, because if they are related to a new episode of ischemia, then we must strive to prevent such an occurrence. Conversely, if they are related to primarily electrical instability, then anti-arrhythmic drugs may have a place. The distinction between causes must be made.

DR. STEWART: I agree with you completely. The main emphasis should be placed on preventing subsequent ischemia.

DR. LOZNER: Dr. Pitt's earlier review made the point that survival after myocardial infarction really depends on how much damage has been done to the ventricle. The cumulative effects of multiple infarctions identify the patients who do not do well. Nobody has mentioned yet that we have an exciting clinical tool on the horizon for limiting infarct size by lysing coronary thrombi within hours of the infarction. Although those patients may be at early risk of arrhythmias, especially at the time of reperfusion, a patient whose infarct has been markedly limited by that technique is going to do better over the long term than will someone who just sits and hopes for one of the "good" kinds of infarction, which is a nice neat package with no ischemic area.

DR. STEWART: I have two comments on that: First, the streptokinase studies may be more relevant to our reperfusion models. Second, patients who receive streptokinase will continue to have a high-grade stenosis in the vessel that was initially responsible for the infarction. If nothing is done about the residual high-grade stenosis, the person is again at a high risk of subsequent infarction.

PART IV. PREVENTION OF SUDDEN CORONARY DEATH: PHARMACOLOGIC STUDIES

DRUGS AND SUDDEN CARDIAC DEATH

J. Thomas Bigger, Jr. and Francis M. Weld

Departments of Medicine and Pharmacology
College of Physicians & Surgeons
Columbia University
New York, New York 10032

In this section of the volume we will discuss the role of drugs in sudden coronary death. After a brief consideration of drug-induced sudden death, the discussion will focus on the use of drugs for the secondary prevention of coronary death. Drug trials for secondary prevention are complex. Good design requires an adequate control group, random assignment to treatment and, if possible, a double-blind study. Every drug has a dose–response relationship, and individualized dose adjustment should improve the chance of efficacy in a trial. However, individualization of dosage presents substantial logistic difficulties in drug trials. A major intervention trial should have a rationale and test a well-defined hypothesis. The latter consideration implies careful selection of the study group on the basis of likelihood of beneficial or adverse effects. The statistical and pharmacologic principles of drug intervention trials will be discussed thoroughly in the following papers. Drugs that show promise for secondary prevention trials or those that have been used already have been selected for discussion.

SUDDEN CARDIAC DEATH CAUSED BY DRUGS

Along with their potential for benefit, drugs have very significant potential for adverse effects, including sudden death. Adverse effects may result from simple overdosage or from interactions between the drug and diseased human hearts, electrolyte abnormalities, or other drugs. We intend to discuss a few examples here to indicate the potential impact of toxic drug effects on the problem of sudden coronary death in the population of the United States. The examples we have selected are K^+-lowering drugs or diets, digitalis, quinidine, and tricyclic antidepressants.

Potassium-Lowering Drugs

Clinical Considerations

Hypokalemia can cause severe ventricular arrhythmias and death. Although there are many causes of hypokalemia, most instances are iatrogenic, caused by diuretic therapy or dietary aberrations. The widespread use of potent diuretics as the first-line treatment for hypertension exposes a very large group of patients to the potential hazard of hypokalemia and lethal ventricular arrhythmias. Many diuretics, such as the thiazides, have a short duration of action relative to the customary once-a-day dosage. This relationship between dosing interval

0077–8923/82/0382–0229 $1.75/0 © 1982, NYAS

and duration of action permits the kidney to conserve K+ between doses and to restore K+ balance, if there is adequate K+ in the diet. Diuretics with a very long duration of action, such as chlorthalidone, are more prone to produce hypokalemia because of their incessant action.[1] The use of diuretics to treat the edema of congestive heart failure often results in hypokalemia, probably because diuretic dosing is often titrated against edema or loss of body weight and treatment is more aggressive than in hypertension. In heart failure, the danger of potentially lethal ventricular arrhythmias is great when hypokalemia occurs in digitalized patients (see later). Occasionally, unusual dietary habits, such as fad reducing diets, will cause hypokalemia, ventricular arrhythmias, and sudden death. The rash of sudden deaths associated with liquid protein diets in recent years may be caused by lethal hypokalemic arrhythmias.[2-6] However, the causes of death with liquid protein diets are probably more complex than just hypokalemia. Patients with normal serum K+ may develop prolonged Q-T intervals and malignant ventricular arrhythmias on liquid protein diets.

Cellular Mechanisms

Normal automaticity in cardiac fibers is due to spontaneous phase 4 depolarization in pacemaker cells.[7] Clinical arrhythmias associated with hypokalemia may be due, in part, to its ability to to enhance "normal" automaticity by increasing the rate and magnitude of spontaneous phase 4 depolarization in the His-Purkinje system (FIG. 1). At plasma potassium concentrations less than 3 mM, membrane potassium conductance falls and outward current during phase 4 decreases; both of these effects promote accelerated phase 4 depolarization.[8, 9] Enhanced phase 4 depolarization induces an increased firing rate for spontaneously active fibers and initiates spontaneous firing in previously quiescent cells (latent pacemakers). At very low potassium concentrations (less than 2 mM), cardiac cells may fail to repolarize fully and instead either rest at a partially depolarized voltage (near −40 mV) or exhibit repetitive firing of "slow" action potentials (early afterdepolarizations) in the plateau voltage range (FIG. 1). Not only can these early afterdepolarizations initiate arrhythmias per se, but also such areas of partially depolarized cells in the His-Purkinje system can cause decremental conduction and blockage of normally propagating action potentials. Thus, hypokalemia may cause ventricular arrhythmias because of several of its effects in the His-Purkinje system: (1) enhanced normal automaticity; (2) abnormal automaticity due to early afterdepolarizations; and (3) depressed conduction.

Digitalis

Clinical Considerations

Digitalis ranks among the top ten prescription drugs in the United States. The most commonly used digitalis glycoside in this country is digoxin. It is commonly used to treat cardiac failure and supraventricular arrhythmias. Digitalis toxicity most frequently occurs in the context of its therapeutic use; about 25 per cent of hospitalized patients taking digitalis show signs of toxicity.[10] Also, about one-third of the patients who develop toxicity will die during the same hospitalization period. It is important to stress the potentiating effect of hypokalemia on arrhythmias induced by digitalis toxicity. Since the advent of potent diuretics which promote urinary K^+ loss, the increase in the incidence of digitalis toxicity has been striking.[10] The reasons for this pharmacodynamic interaction are discussed in the next subsection, entitled *Cellular Mechanisms*. Other abnormalities of electrolyte or acid–base balance, such as hypercalcemia, hypomagnesemia, and alkalosis, promote digitalis toxicity. Most of the other factors that promote digitalis toxicity can be attributed either to increased intake or decreased elimination. Recently, an interaction between quinidine and digoxin has been described.[11, 12] When quinidine is given to patients with stable serum digoxin concentrations, the serum concentration of digoxin increases. There is some evidence that this interaction can provoke potentially lethal cardiac arrhythmias.[11]

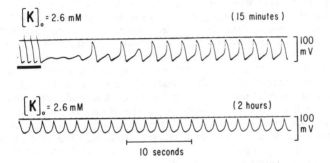

FIGURE 1. Effect of hypokalemia on calf Purkinje fiber action potentials. The *horizontal line* in each panel is a zero voltage reference. During stimulation with external electrodes (*heavy bar* below trace), "fast-response" action potentials were obtained. After cessation of external stimulation, the resting membrane developed spontaneous oscillations which attained threshold and led to automatic firing at 25/min. Prolonged hypokalemia (*bottom panel*) produced a depolarized maximal diastolic voltage (plateau voltage range) and automatic firing of "slow potentials"; the fiber was refractory to external stimuli. Then the fiber was repolarized by increasing $[K]_o$ to 6.0 mM. When the fiber was exposed to $[K]_o = 2.6$ mM again, findings similar to those in the top panel were obtained again.

Serious digitalis toxicity is nearly always associated with significant cardiac arrhythmias. In persons with normal hearts, digitalis toxicity usually produces marked sinus bradycardia or atrioventricular nodal block, or both. In patients with coronary heart disease, digitalis toxicity is more likely to manifest itself as severe ventricular arrhythmias or nonparoxysmal atrioventricular junctional tachycardia. Toxicity due to massive overdose causes malignant hyperkalemia associated with sinoatrial and atrioventricular block, severe ventricular arrhythmias, and finally asystole or ventricular fibrillation.[14] Until the advent of treatment with Fab fragments of digoxin-specific antibodies, the syndrome of malignant hyperkalemia in digitalis toxicity was uniformly fatal.[14] Several retrospective studies have implicated digitalis as a cause of cardiac death in patients with a recent myocardial infarction.[15–17]

Cellular Mechanisms

Low concentrations of digitalis slow the spontaneous sinus rate in intact animals, but high concentrations may accelerate the sinus pacemaker.[18] At toxic concentrations, digitalis depresses conduction in the atrioventricular node and accelerates the spontaneous firing rate of atrioventricular junctional cells. The toxic effects of digitalis preparations causing ventricular arrhythmias are probably due to its effects on cells of the His-Purkinje system. Ouabain and acetylstrophanthidin increase the rate of spontaneous phase 4 depolarization in isolated superfused mammalian Purkinje fibers at concentrations of 2×10^{-7} M or less.[19-21] Spontaneous phase 4 depolarization induced by digitalis is enhanced either by increasing the stimulation rates or by hypokalemia. In cardiac Purkinje fibers, digitalis compounds do not increase phase 4 depolarization either by increasing the magnitude of the normal potassium pacemaker current, iK_2, or by shifting the iK_2 activation curve to more positive voltages.[22] Instead, digitalis elicits abnormal automatic firing by two separate mechanisms: First, digitalis induces a new abnormal transient inward current after membrane repolarization.[23-26] Transient inward current is carried predominantly by Na^+ ions, which cross the membrane via tetrodotoxin-insensitive channels.[25] Second, digitalis compounds block time-independent outward current caused by the electrogenic pumping of Na^+ to the extracellular compartment.[27] These actions can account for partial membrane depolarization and both early and delayed afterdepolarizations observed in isolated superfused cardiac preparations during exposure to toxic concentrations of digitalis. Although cellular uncoupling also occurs during exposure to toxic digitalis concentrations,[28] this mechanism probably does not play a major role in clinical digitalis-toxic arrhythmias except perhaps in severe overdoses.

Quinidine

Clinical Considerations

Aside from digitalis, quinidine is the oldest and most commonly used antiarrhythmic drug. Its use is attended by occasional instances of sudden cardiac death. When death occurs during treatment of malignant ventricular arrhythmias with quinidine, it is difficult to distinguish quinidine toxicity from failure to control the preexisting arrhythmia. Recently, electrophysiologically guided antiarrhythmic treatment makes it clear that quinidine aggravates sustained ventricular tachycardia in coronary heart disease in about 10% of the cases. In addition, sudden death soon after initiation of quinidine therapy for supraventricular arrhythmias in persons who have no significant compromise of mechanical performance of the heart casts suspicion on quinidine. Two important factors increase the risk of severe ventricular arrhythmias after administration of therapeutic doses of quinidine: the long Q-T syndrome,[29] and digitalis therapy.[13] Small doses of quinidine can provoke severe ventricular arrhythmias in patients who have either obvious or covert long Q-T syndromes; the Q-T interval becomes strikingly prolonged, and rapid ventricular arrhythmias with bizarre QRS morphology ensue. Since 1978, it has been suggested that many instances of "quinidine toxicity" occurring at therapeutic quinidine concentrations really represent digitalis toxicity induced by quinidine.[11] At toxic plasma quinidine concentrations or in the presence of hyperkalemia, quinidine will cause significant intraventricular conduction delays which contribute to severe ventriular arrhythmias (see later).

Cellular Mechanisms

The cellular mechanisms for lethal ventricular arrhythmias due to an idiosyncratic reaction to quinidine remain obscure. The cellular mechanisms of dose-related "quinidine-toxic" ventricular arrhythmias are better understood. Electrocardiographic evidence of quinidine toxicity includes the demonstration of intraventricular conduction delay, atrioventricular block, ventricular tachy-arrhythmias, and cardiac arrest. These abnormalities can be caused by depression of action potential phase 0 with conduction block and/or abnormal

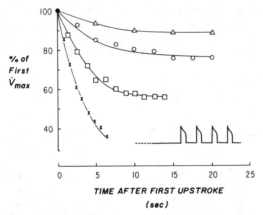

FIGURE 2. Effect of stimulation rate on quinidine-induced depression of maximal upstroke velocity. During superfusion with quinidine at 10 mg/liter, a calf Purkinje fiber was clamped at —80 mV for 30 seconds. Action potentials were obtained by opening the voltage clamp circuit for 500 msec and stimulating the membrane with external electrodes immediately after release of the clamp. The fiber was stimulated at cycle lengths of 5000 msec (*triangles*), 2500 msec (*circles*), 1250 msec (*squares*), or 800 msec (*crosses*). Quinidine-induced depression of maximal upstroke velocity was so marked at a cycle length of 800 msec that the fiber failed to follow the external stimulus with a 1:1 response before a steady-state was achieved.

automaticity. Quinidine-induced depression of conduction increases with stimulation rate [30, 31] (FIG. 2) and membrane depolarization.[32, 33] Enhanced phase 4 depolarization or afterdepolarizations rarely occur, even at quinidine concentrations as high as 10 to 50 mg per liter, in isolated superfused Purkinje fibers.[33] Thus, impaired conduction usually is responsible for quinidine toxicity. Quinidine depresses upstroke velocity by binding to and blocking Na+ channels. Quinidine dissociates very slowly from Na+ channels; dissociation is faster at more negative transmembrane voltages. These observations have important clinical implications: electrocardiography should show quinidine toxicity to be less severe as heart rate decreases, and interventions that produce a more negative transmembrane voltage, such as molar sodium lactate, will antagonize quinidine toxicity.

Tricyclic Antidepressants

Clinical Considerations

Two retrospective drug surveys have examined the association between the use of tricyclic antidepressants (TCA) and mortality. A Scottish study found a relationship between sudden cardiac death and TCA use,[34, 35] while the Boston Drug Surveillance Program failed to find such an association.[36]

We studied a group of 44 depressed patients with multiple 24-hour Holter recordings to determine whether imipramine either produced new ventricular arrhythmias or aggravated preexisting ventricular arrhythmias.[37] On the contrary, we found that therapeutic antidepressant plasma concentrations of imipramine had a potent antiarrhythmic action on ventricular arrhythmias. It is not known whether tricyclic antidepressants, like quinidine, cause arrhythmias in the long Q-T syndrome. We have searched for an interaction between imipramine and digoxin of the type produced by quinidine and have not found it. Like quinidine, tricyclic antidepressants have a potent effect on conduction in the His-Purkinje system and ventricles. At therapeutic plasma concentration, tricyclic antidepressants cause an increase in the P-R, H-V and QRS in-

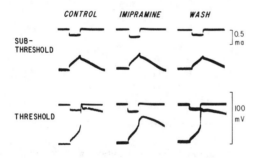

FIGURE 3. Effect of imipramine (1×10^{-6} g/ml) on threshold current and voltage. In each panel *top trace* = transmembrane current; *bottom trace* = transmembrane voltage. During superfusion with imipramine, threshold current increased from 0.18 to 0.25 mA and threshold voltage was shifted by +5 mV. (From Weld and Bigger.[42] Reproduced by permission.)

tervals.[38, 39] This effect becomes striking during accidental or suicidal overdosage from TCA.[38, 39] When intraventricular conduction becomes severely slowed during TCA overdose and particularly when hypotension coexists, malignant ventricular arrhythmias may ensue. In patients with severe preexisting bundle branch disease, TCA can induce complete atrioventricular heart block in the His-Purkinje system at therapeutic concentrations.[40, 41] This may relate to the conducting system disease and sudden death reported elsewhere in this volume.

Cellular Mechanisms

Several studies have examined the cardiac electrophysiologic effects of tricyclic antidepressants. The best studied of the tricyclic antidepressants is imipramine. At toxic concentrations, imipramine has cellular actions which can account for intraventricular conduction blocks, atrioventricular block in the His-Purkinje system, and cardiac arrest. Upstroke velocity and slowing or block of conduction occur in Purkinje and ventricular muscle fibers exposed to imipramine at 10^{-6} g/ml.[42, 43] Imipramine depresses automaticity by increasing threshold (FIG. 3).[42] Like quinidine, imipramine depresses action potential phase 0 more at faster stimulation rates; however, reactivation of the Na⁺ channel is faster during imipramine treatment.

During imipramine therapy in man, hydroxylation and demethylation produce electrophysiologically active metabolites in concentrations which may exceed the plasma concentration of imipramine. Preliminary experiments with 2-hydroxyimipramine, desmethylimipramine, and 2-hydroxydesmethylimipramine suggest that these compounds are qualitatively and quantitatively similar to imipramine in depressing action potential phase 0.[44]

REFERENCES

1. FRAZIER, H. S. & H. YAGER. 1973. The clinical use of diuretics. N. Engl. J. Med. **288:** 246–249; 455–457.
2. 1977. Medical news: Details released on deaths of ten on liquid protein diets. J. Am. Med. Assoc. **238:** 2680.
3. SINGH, B. N., T. D. GAARDER, T. KANEGAE, M. GOLDSTEIN, J. Z. MONTGOMERIE & H. MILLS. 1978. Liquid protein diets and torsade de pointes. J. Am. Med. Assoc. **240:** 115–119.
4. BROWN, J. M., J. F. YETTER, M. J. SPICER & J. D. JONES. 1978. Cardiac complications of protein-sparing modified fasting. J. Am. Med. Assoc. **240:** 120–122.
5. VAN ITALLIE, T. B. 1978. Liquid protein mayhem. J. Am. Med. Assoc. **240:** 144–145.
6. MOORE, M. J. 1979. Liquid protein diets and electrolyte deficiency. J. Am. Med. Assoc. **241:** 1464.
7. WEIDMANN, S. 1951. Effect of current flow on the membrane potential of cardiac muscle. J. Physiol. **115:** 227–236.
8. ARNSDORF, M. F. & J. T. BIGGER, JR. 1972. Effect of lidocaine hydrochloride on membrane conductance in mammalian cardiac Purkinje fibers. J. Clin. Invest. **51:** 2252–2263.
9. NOBLE, D. & R. W. TSIEN. 1968. The kinetics and rectifier properties of the slow potassium current in cardiac Purkinje fibres. J. Physiol. **195:** 185–214.
10. SMITH, T. W. 1975. Digitalis toxicity: Epidemiology and clinical use of serum concentration measurements. Am. J. Med. **58:** 470–476.
11. LEAHEY, E. B., JR., J. A. REIFFEL, R. E. DRUSIN, R. H. HEISSENBUTTEL, W. P. LOVEJOY & J. T. BIGGER, JR. 1978. A drug interaction between quinidine and digoxin. J. Am. Med. Assoc. **240:** 533–534.
12. DOERING, W. 1979. Quinidine-digoxin interaction. Pharmacokinetics, underlying mechanism and clinical implications. N. Engl. J. Med. **301:** 400–404.
13. LEAHEY, E. B., JR., J. A. REIFFEL, R. H. HEISSENBUTTEL, R. E. DRUSIN, W. P. LOVEJOY & J. T. BIGGER, JR. 1979. Enhanced cardiac effect of digoxin during quinidine treatment. Arch. Intern. Med. **139:** 519–521.
14. SMITH, T. W., E. HABER, L. YEATMAN & V. P. BUTLER, JR. 1976. Reversal of advanced digitalis toxication with Fab fragments of digoxin-specific antibodies. N. Engl. J. Med. **294:** 797–800.
15. MOSS, A. J., H. T. DAVIS, D. CONRAD, J. J. DECAMILLA & C. L. ODOROFF. 1980. Digitalis associated cardiac mortality after myocardial infarction. Circulation **62**(Suppl. III): 39.
16. BOUDOULAS, H., W. O'NEILL, Y. SOHN & A. M. WEISSLER. 1981. Digitalis therapy in patients recovered from acute myocardial infarction: An independent risk factor. Clin. Res. **29:** 179.
17. BIGGER, J. T., JR., F. M. WELD, L. M. ROLNITZKY & K. FERRICK. 1981. Is digitalis treatment harmful in the year after acute myocardial infarction? Circulation. In press.

18. HOFFMAN, B. F. & J. T. BIGGER, JR. 1980. Digitalis and allied cardiac glycosides. *In* The Pharmacological Basis of Therapeutics, 6th ed. A. G. Gilman, L. S. Goodman & A. Gilman, Eds. Macmillan. New York, NY.
19. DAVIS, L. D. 1973. Effect of changes in cycle length on diastolic depolarization produced by ouabain in canine Purkinje fibers. Circ. Res. **32**: 206–214.
20. ROSEN, M. R., H. GELBAND, C. MERKER & B. F. HOFFMAN. 1973. Mechanisms of digitalis toxicity. Effects of ouabain on phase four of canine Purkinje fiber transmembrane potentials. Circulation **47**: 681–689.
21. FERRIER, G. R., J. H. SAUNDERS & C. MENDEZ. 1973. A cellular mechanism for the generation of ventricular arrhythmias by acetylstrophanthidin. Circ. Res. **32**: 600–609.
22. ARONSON, R. S., J. M. GELLES & B. F. HOFFMAN. 1973. Effect of ouabain on the current underlying spontaneous diastolic depolarization in cardiac Purkinje fibres. Nature **243**: 118–120.
23. LEDERER, W. J. & R. W. TSIEN. 1976. Transient inward current underlying arrhythmogenic effects of cardiotonic steroids in Purkinje fibres. J. Physiol. **263**: 73–100.
24. KASS, R. S., W. J. LEDERER, R. W. TSIEN & R. WEINGART. 1978. Role of calcium ions in transient inward currents and after contractions induced by strophanthidin in cardiac Purkinje fibres. J. Physiol. **281**: 187–208.
25. KASS, R. S., R. W. TSIEN & R. WEINGART. 1978. Ionic basis of transient inward current induced by strophanthidin in cardiac Purkinje fibers. J. Physiol. **281**: 209–226.
26. ISENBERG, G. & W. TRAUTWEIN. 1974. The effect of dihydro-ouabain and lithium ions on the outward current in cardiac Purkinje fibers. Pfluegers Arch. **350**: 41–54.
27. TSIEN, R. W. & D. O. CARPENTER. 1978. Ionic mechanism of pacemaker activity in cardiac Purkinje fibers. Fed. Proc. **37**: 2127–2131.
28. WEINGART, R. 1977. The actions of ouabain on intercellular coupling and conduction velocity in mammalian ventricular muscle. J. Physiol. **264**: 341–365.
29. KOSTER, R. W. & H. J. J. WELLENS. 1976. Quinidine-induced ventricular flutter and fibrillation without digitalis therapy. Am. J. Cardiol. **38**: 519–523.
30. JOHNSON, E. A. & M. G. MCKINNON. 1957. The differential effect of quinidine and pyrilamine on the myocardial action potential at various rates of stimulation. J. Pharmacol. Exp. Ther. **120**: 460–468.
31. HEISTRACHER, P. 1971. Mechanism of action of antifibrillatory drugs. Naunyn Schmiedebergs Arch. Pharmacol. **269**: 199–212.
32. WEIDMANN, S. 1955. Effects of calcium ions and local anesthetics on electrical properties of Purkinje fibres. J. Physiol. **129**: 568–582.
33. WELD, F. M., J. N. ROTTMAN & J. T. BIGGER, JR. 1980. Quinidine toxicity: An electrophysiological evaluation in cardiac Purkinje fibers. Am. J. Cardiol. **45**: 428.
34. COULL, D. C., J. CROOKS, I. DINGWALL-FORDYCE, A. M. SCOTT & R. D. WEIR. 1970. Amitriptyline and cardiac disease. Lancet **2**: 590–591.
35. MOIR, D. C., J. CROOKS, W. B. CORNWELL, K. O'MALLEY, I. DINGWALL-FORDYCE, M. J. TURNBULL & R. D. WEIR. 1972. Cardiotoxicity of amitriptyline. Lancet **2**: 561–564.
36. BOSTON COLLABORATIVE DRUG SURVEILLANCE PROGRAM. 1972. Adverse reactions to the tricyclic antidepressant drugs. Lancet **1**: 529–531.
37. GIARDINA, E. G. V., J. T. BIGGER, JR., A. H. GLASSMAN, J. M. PEREL & S. J. KANTOR. 1979. The electrocardiographic and antiarrhythmic effects of imipramine hydrochloride at therapeutic plasma concentrations. Circulation **60**: 1045–1052.
38. VOHRA, J., G. BURROWS, D. HUNT & G. SLOMAN. 1975. The effect of toxic and therapeutic doses of tricyclic antidepressant drugs on intracardiac conduction. Eur. J. Cardiol. **3**: 219–227.

39. SMITH, R. B. & B. J. RUSBATCH. 1967. Amitriptyline and heart block. Br. Med. J. 3: 311.
40. SPIKER, D. G., A. N. WEISS, S. S. CHANG, J. E. RUWITCH & J. T. BIGGS 1975. Tricyclic antidepressant overdose: Clinical presentation and plasma levels. Clin. Pharmacol. Ther. 18: 539–546.
41. KANTOR, S. J., J. T. BIGGER, JR., A. H. GLASSMAN, D. L. MACKEN & J. M. PEREL. 1975. Imipramine-induced heart block: A longitudinal case study. J. Am. Med. Assoc. 231: 1364–1366.
42. WELD, F. M. & J. T. BIGGER, JR. 1980. Electrophysiological effects of imipramine on ovine cardiac Purkinje and ventricular muscle fibers. Circ. Res. 46: 167–175.
43. RAWLING, D. R. & H. A. FOZZARD. 1979. Effects of imipramine on cellular electrophysiological properties of cardiac Purkinje fibers. J. Pharmacol. Exp. Ther. 209: 371–375.
44. WELD, F. M., D. A. RUBIN, J. T. BIGGER, JR. & J. M. PEREL. 1978. Electrophysiological effects of 2-hydroxyimipramine on ovine cardiac Purkinje fibers and ventricular muscle. Circulation 58: 106.

PHARMACOKINETIC STUDIES: THEIR ROLE IN DETERMINING THERAPEUTIC EFFICACY OF AGENTS DESIGNED TO PREVENT SUDDEN DEATH *

David G. Shand,† Edward L.C. Pritchett, Stephen C. Hammill,
W. Wayne Stargel, and Galen S. Wagner

Divisions of Clinical Pharmacology and Cardiology
Duke University Medical Center
Durham, North Carolina 27710

Ideally, drug therapy should involve (1) a knowledge of the pathophysiology of the disease to be treated, (2) drug selection on the basis of an appropriate mechanism of action to reverse that pathophysiology, and (3) individualization of the drug regimen to produce the desired effect without toxicity. Even in the absence of the perfect marriage of pathophysiology and drug action, therapeutic efficacy can often be demonstrated by clinical trial. When this involves a definable and easily measured clinical end-point, such as blood pressure, individualization of drug dosage is a simple matter. Indeed, the success of antihypertensive therapy lies as much in our ability to individualize dose as it does in the number of antihypertensive drugs available to treat high blood pressure and its disasterous sequelae. Against this background, drug trials in the secondary prevention of sudden death in normotensive patients perhaps represent the ultimate challenge in individualization of therapy.

It is generally thought that the event terminaing in sudden death is ventricular fibrillation, but the precise mechanisms involved in the precipitation of this fatal arrhythmia are not at all clear. The current interest in drugs other than traditional antiarrhythmic agents (including beta-adrenergic blocking agents, antiplatelet drugs, and calcium antagonists) attests to our ignorance of mechanism and has led to the study of drugs chosen on the basis of other known actions. The choice of an appropriate drug regimen is confounded by the fact that therapy is prophylactic because sudden death itself is clearly not a clinical end-point that can be used to guide an individual's response. Even monitoring other, related end-points may not be easy. For example, patients may not have an arrhythmia, and if they do, assessing antiarrhythmic drug efficacy is fraught with problems. It is not at all clear whether total or partial suppression of arrhythmias would suffice or whether suppression of ventricular tachycardia, leaving single ectopic beats, would be an effective approach. Measuring antiplatelet effects is technically quite difficult and not easily applicable to large-scale studies. Similarly, monitoring coronary spasm is out of the question at the present time. Of all the methods being currently considered, beta-adrenergic blockade is the easiest to monitor pharmacodynamically by performing serial exercise tests. To date, however, this method has not been used in any of the many clinical trials of these drugs, presumably because of inconvenience and/or

* This work was supported by Grants HL/GM 26699, RR–30, HL21347, HL24920, and LM03373 from the National Institutes of Health.
† Burroughs-Wellcome Scholar in Clinical Pharmacology.

expense. Thus, for all of the published trials of drugs in the prevention of sudden death fixed-dosage regimens were utilized that were based on the "average" dose used in the treatment of other conditions. This is unfortunate, because we already know that many patients will receive inadequate therapy and others will be overtreated: who, for example, would treat all hypertensive patients with the same dose of propranolol? Thus fixed-dose trials may tell us that a drug *can* work, but they will not tell us how to use the drug optimally in order to maximize the number of patients who will benefit. It is in this area of individualization of drug therapy that pharmacokinetics can be helpful.

There are two major causes for variation in dosage requirement: pharmacodynamic and pharmacokinetic. Pharmacodynamic factors include variation in the effectiveness of a given concentration at the site of action (true receptor sensitivity) and the "severity" of the disease or the strength of the stimulus that must be overcome. Pharmacokinetic factors include variations in total plasma concentration after a given dose, variations in plasma drug-binding, and the generation of active metabolites. While pharmacodynamic variation does exist, it is relatively poorly understood. In addition, pharmacokinetic factors appear quantitatively more important and easy to measure. In particular, it is clear that a drug's effects relate better to circulating concentration than to the administered dose. Despite some uncertainties, we should like to develop the thesis that in the absence of a simple, defined clinical end-point to monitor, pharmacokinetic knowledge can be helpful in the design and implementation of secondary prevention trials in three major ways: (1) designing a drug regimen suitable for the "average" patient; (2) predicting pharmacokinetic variability when average doses are administered; and (3) monitoring circulating concentrations during prolonged drug administration.

DOSAGE REGIMENS

Acute Therapy

Taking the broad view of secondary prevention, we may wish to institute therapy as soon after infarction as possible and therefore we need to develop a method to rapidly achieve and maintain therapeutic concentrations using intravenous therapy. Several theoretical approaches are possible [1] and we shall illustrate these with reference to lidocaine. Early experience with the drug showed that the rapid injection of large doses could lead to seizures, but that the effect of smaller, nontoxic doses dissipated within about 15 minutes. This was due to the fact that concentrations fall bi-exponentially after intravenous administration and the early rapid (or α-) phase caused levels to drop below the therapeutic range. This occurs even when the injection is followed by a constant maintenance infusion and results in a "dip" below the therapeutic range that can last for 1 to 2 hours before the infusion approaches steady-state, which takes 4 to 5 half-lives. [2] Another approach involves giving a more rapid, followed by a slower, maintenance infusion. Under these circumstances, however, it takes a finite time (5 to 10 minutes) to reach therapeutic levels during the more rapid infusion. [1] We have therefore devised a regimen comprising a single (75 mg) injection followed by a further 150 mg, either as an infusion or as three (50 mg) injections over 20 minutes, followed by the maintenance infusion of 2 mg/min. Quite predictably, wider swings in plasma concentrations were seen with multiple injections than during the rapid infusion (FIG. 1). In addition minor toxicity was associated with the lidocaine injections in five of six patients, though none experienced seizures. In contrast only one of 11 patients experienced mild toxicity during the rapid infusion.

The described loading regimen for lidocaine was derived semiempirically over a period of years. In addition, it is not possible to devise a loading/ maintenance regimen for lidocaine on the basis of its kinetics after a single dose because the clearance of the drug is lower at steady-state during a prolonged infusion.[3] Fortunately, this is not always the case, and it is now a relatively simple matter to devise complex regimens on the basis of single-dose kinetics. We have recently devised an approach based on the method of separate exponentials that is simple enough to avoid the use of complex computer programs for dosage-regimen design with drugs showing multicompartmental kinetics.[4]

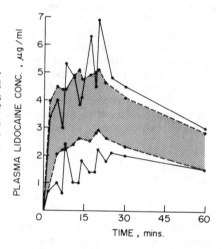

FIGURE 1. Range of plasma concentration seen after a 75-mg injection and an infusion of 150 mg over 20 minutes followed by a maintenance infusion of 2 mg/min (*shaded area*) compared with a regimen in which the 150 mg was given as three 50-ng injections (*open area*).

Chronic Therapy

Problems with the early-distribution phase do not usually arise after oral administration because distribution is usually complete during the process of drug absorption. Thus, during chronic oral therapy, we are usually only concerned with the drug's systemic availability and the terminal half-life. Systemic availability refers to the fraction of an oral dose that reaches the systemic circulation where its concentration is sampled. It may be reduced due to incomplete alimentary absorption or to elimination during its passage through the gut wall and liver (the so-called presystemic or "first-pass" effect). Very often incomplete availability can be simply overcome by giving larger doses. In the case of some drugs which undergo first-pass metabolism, problems may arise because of the production of increased quantities of metabolites which may be toxic or active. For example, the increased generation of toxic metabolites is often given as the reason for not using oral lidocaine, although this has been questioned.[5] An active metabolite of propranolol, 4-hydroxy propranolol, is generated after oral but not after intravenous administration,[6] and this results in an apparently greater effectiveness of a given plasma propranolol concentration after single oral administration of the drug compared with intravenous doses.[7] This is not so important during chronic oral therapy because the proportion of 4-hydroxy propranolol decreases so that its effects can no longer be obviously detected.[8, 9] Verapamil is another drug whose effective concentration depends on the route of administration. For example, we have recently found that a given concentration of verapamil has much fewer negative dromotropic effects after oral than after intravenous administration. The mechanism of this effect is unclear, but might involve preferential metabolism of the active *l*-isomer, or an antagonistic effect of a metabolite generated during the first pass. Thus, the oral route may be associated with either enhanced or diminished drug effectiveness. It is therefore important to define the therapeutic range of plasma concentrations according to the route of administration.

It is generally considered best to administer drugs as infrequently as possible in order to better ensure patient compliance. In choosing an appropriate dosage interval, it is well to remember that the duration of drug action depends as much on the amount of drug administered as it does on drug half-life. Thus, it may be possible to give larger doses less frequently and yet maintain minimal effective levels at the end of the dosage interval. For example, it is now recognized that beta-adrenergic blocking agents with half-lives of only 3 to 6 hours may nonetheless be given twice daily. The ability to do this depends on the therapeutic index since we want to avoid toxicity due to high peak concentrations after large doses. The optimal dosage interval therefore depends on the therapeutic index and drug half-life.

The Value of Early Kinetic Studies

In the past the investigation of new drugs was based largely on assessing its pharmacologic effects and toxicity. The drug was often administered by mouth under the false premise that this was safer than intravenous administration, and pharmacokinetic studies were often delayed and focused mainly on estimating the bioavailability of the formulation compared with that of an orally administered solution. More recently, it has been recognized that pharmacokinetics can be extremely helpful in the rational development of new drugs, particularly those likely to have a narrow therapeutic index, such as antiarrhythmic drugs. In fact, a great deal of valuable information can be obtained from a relatively small number of studies. For example, we have recently been involved in the development of a new antiarrhythmic agent, pirmenol. First a dose-ranging study was performed in ten patients using a 30-minute infusion. The last four patients responded to a 150-mg infusion and the pharmacokinetics were evaluated by measuring blood, plasma, and free pirmenol concentrations. The clearance of the drug was found to be 160 to 210 ml/min, of which about 50% was by the kidneys, as determined from the renal excretion of parent drug. Thus nonrenal (metabolic) clearance amounted to only about 100 ml/min. Were this to occur in the liver, with a blood flow of some 1500 ml/min, the hepatic extraction ratio would only be some 7%. It is the hepatic extraction ratio that determines the fraction of drug removed during the first pass, so that we could confidently predict that systemic availability would be high after oral administration, provided the drug was well absorbed. The terminal half-life of the drug was also quite long (7 to 9.4 hours). Finally, it was clear that the arrhythmia began to return in these patients at plasma concentrations of 0.8 to 1.4 μg/ml. No serious untoward effects were noted, but one patient developed QRS prolongation and showed the highest peak plasma level (3.8 μg/ml) at the end of the infusion. Thus, after a quite limited study, a good idea of the drug-effect range in plasma concentrations was obtained and the pharmacokinetic characteristics of the drug evaluated. The kinetic information was particularly valuable in designing future studies. For example, a loading maintenance regimen was designed to achieve and maintain plasma levels of about 2 μg/ml and this is being used to investigate the hemodynamic effects of the drug. Secondly, the data suggested good oral availability so we might expect the effective oral dose to be on the order of 150 mg. We have just completed an oral dose-ranging study followed by a double-blind placebo-controlled trial of the apparently effective dose. In seven patients single oral doses of 150 to 250 mg were effective compared with placebo, greater than 97% suppression of the ventricular ectopic beats being noted at peak plasma concentrations of 0.9 to 1.6 μg/ml. The drug's half-life ranged from 7 to 12 hours and 52 to 100% suppression was noted at 8 hours when plasma concentrations ranged from 0.4 to 1.2 μg/ml. In five of the patients intravenous data were available and systemic availability averaged 83%, consistent with predictions. On the basis of these data, it would appear that a twice-daily regimen may well be effective. These data serve to emphasize just how helpful early pharmacokinetic studies can be to rational and safe drug development. Indeed, failure to obtain such data may lead to the development of a suboptimal regimen. For example, it has recently been shown that the terminal half-life of dipyridamole (11 hours) is much longer than previously thought,[10] so that there is a real possibility that the drug could be given twice rather than four times a day.

PREDICTING PHARMACOKINETIC VARIATION

Having settled on an "average" dosage regimen, it is important to recognize that considerable pharmacokinetic heterogeneity exists. Some of this variability can be predicted and accounted for in a general way from a knowledge of the various factors that may influence drug disposition. A full discussion of all of the factors involved is beyond the scope of this paper, but the factors may be constitutional or acquired. While demographic factors such as weight and age can and do affect drug disposition, each factor on its own has only a small effect. The effects of disease and drug interactions are quantitatively more important. With perhaps the exception of the value of creatinine clearance in estimating renal drug elimination, it is well to remember that such dosage adjustments that can be made are only approximate and that considerable variation remains. For example, even after correction for all the factors known to influence its disposition, we have found that plasma lidocaine concentrations spanned the entire therapeutic range of 1.5 to 5.0 μg/ml. During chronic oral administration of drugs eliminated by metabolism it is not uncommon to find a five- to ten-fold range of concentrations, even in healthy young adults.

Of particular interest in the context of sudden death is the fact that myocardial infarction may also affect drug disposition, quite aside from any attendant heart failure. For example Prescott et al.[11] found that plasma lidocaine concentrations continued to rise over 48 hours during a constant infusion and they thought that this might lead to late toxicity. However, accumulation is also associated with an increase in the acute-phase reactant protein, α_1-acid glyco-protein, which is largely responsible for the plasma binding of the drug.[12] As a result, the rise in total plasma levels of the drug is not accompanied by a similar rise in free (unbound) drug, which is the presumably active form.[13] Indeed, we have seen a patient(FIG. 2) who had a plasma lidocaine concentration of 8.2 μg/ml without any evidence of toxicity, presumably because enhanced plasma binding caused the free drug concentration to remain relatively stable. Interestingly, the plasma binding of propranolol is also increased post infarction. This raises the issue of whether free, rather than total, plasma concentration should be measured routinely. While this would be ideal, and should be done whenever possible in detailed pharmacokinetic studies, the added effort to measure plasma drug binding is probably not yet justified in monitoring large-scale studies.

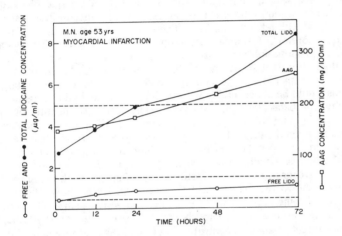

FIGURE 2. The effects of time on total and free plasma lidocaine and α_1-acid glycoprotein (AAG) concentrations during a constant infusion in a patient with a myocardial infarct.

THERAPEUTIC MONITORING

It should be clear that even after dosage adjustment for all the factors known to influence drug disposition, intrasubject variation will remain large. In view of this, it is unfortunate, although perhaps understandable, that all of the published studies on the prevention of sudden death have involved fixed doses. This raises the real possibility that some of the patients receiving the active drug may have only a subtherapeutic concentration and therefore would constitute what might be termed an "active placebo" group. This would not only tend to produce a beta error statistically, but would also require a large population to establish drug efficacy. It is unclear to what extent this problem may have influenced some of the early studies. Certainly, the early negative study of propranolol after acute myocardial infarction employed relatively low doses by present standards (60 to 120 mg daily). In the multicenter study of practolol, it was noted that heavier subjects did not benefit.[14] While this was attributed to a greater risk factor, it was also noted that the plasma concentrations of the drug were lower in these patients. These facts were known at the inception of the currently ongoing multicenter trial of propranolol (BHAT) and some effort was made to incorporate rational dosage adjustments into the protocol. In fact, propranolol provides an excellent example of the problems facing fixed-dose trials and of possible ways to avoid an "active placebo" effect. The disposition of the drug is highly variable, even in normal subjects, so that a ten-fold variation in plasma levels is seen after the same oral dose is administered. Furthermore, there is a reasonably good relationship between plasma concentration and cardiac beta-adrenergic blockade, whether this is measured by a reduction in exercise or by isoproterenol-induced tachycardia. While there has been some question about what constitutes maximal blockade and what concentrations are required to produce it, it was clear that (1) plasma levels of 50 to 100 ng/ml were associated with a high degree of cardiac beta-adrenergic blockade[7] and (2) that the variation in the effects of a given plasma concentration was less than that associated with a fixed oral dose. These concentrations were similar to those seen after abolition of ventricular ectopic beats[15] in 8 of 12 patients given intravenous propranolol. Thus, it was decided to aim for plasma concentrations greater than 50 ng/ml at the end of the dosage interval. An alternative way to overcome pharmacokinetic variability would be simply to give a large dose. While this would be unacceptable with traditional antiarrhythmic agents because of toxicity, the beta-adrenergic blocking agents demonstrate little or no dose-related toxicity in properly selected patients. This approach, however, was rejected largely on the grounds of conservatism, as it was feared that the required dosage would be much higher than that clinically acceptable at the time and would be associated with an unacceptably high incidence of dose-related side effects. In retrospect, this was a fortunate decision, for in the interim Woosley et al.[16] have shown that while plasma propranolol levels above 100 ng/ml can be effective in some patients, there is a subset in which such levels were associated with reappearance of a previously controlled ventricular arrhythmia.

After a target plasma concentration is chosen, the next problem is to achieve this safely and without destroying the double-blind nature of the study. Therapy with relatively low doses can be initiated in the hospital and a plasma sample obtained at the end of a dosage interval once steady-state is reached (2 to 3 days with propranolol). Thus, before the patient's discharge, immediate untoward effects can be detected and a plasma concentration determined on which to base subsequent dosage adjustments. Clearly, such an estimate must be performed in a central laboratory and instructions for the appropriate dosage change (either immediate or in steps) made on the basis of the ratio of the target to observed concentrations. These dosage adjustments can be made in a double-blind fashion by matching the required changes in active drug with similar, computer-generated alterations in the dose of placebo.

It is clear that attempts to ensure a certain target plasma concentration will add to the complexity of a large-scale clinical trial and will pose logistic problems. It should also be mentioned that the attainment of the target concentration cannot be guaranteed over the long term. Rather, we are offering the patients the opportunity to comply with an apparently rational regimen; whether they do so remains to be seen. Unfortunately, the results of the BHAT trial are not yet available, so that we cannot judge what influence therapeutic drug monitoring may have had. However, the design and implementation of the first double-blind, variable dose, prophylactic trial is an important experiment in itself and we await the outcome with considerable interest.

REFERENCES

1. WOOSLEY, R. L. & D. G. SHAND. 1978. Pharmacokinetics of antiarrhythmic drugs. Am. J. Cardiol. **41:** 986–995.
2. ZITO, R. A., P. R. REID & J. A. LONGSTRETH. 1977. Variability of early lidocaine levels in patients. Am. Heart J. **94:** 292–296.
3. OCHS, H. R., G. CASTENS & D. J. GREENBLATT. 1980. Reduction in lidocaine clearance during continuous infusion and by coadministration of propranolol. New Engl. J. Med. **303:** 373–376.
4. SHAND, D. G., R. E. DESJARDINS, T. D. BJORNSSON, S. C. HAMMILL & E. L. C. PRITCHETT. 1981. The method of separate exponentials: A simple aid to devise intravenous drug-loading regimens. Clin. Pharmacol. Ther. **29:** 542–547.
5. PERUCCA, E. & A. RICHENS. 1979. Reduction of oral bioavailability of lignocaine by reduction of first pass metabolism in epileptic patients. Br. J. Clin. Pharmacol **8:** 21–31.
6. PATERSON, J. W., M. E. CONOLLY, C. T. DOLLERY, A. HAYES & R. G. COOPER. 1970. The pharmacodynamics and metabolism of propranolol in man. Pharmacol. Chem. **2:** 127–133.
7. COLTART, D. J. & D. G. SHAND. 1970. Plasma propranolol levels in the quantitative assessment of β-adrenergic blockade in man. Br. Med. J. **iii:** 731–735.
8. WALLE, T., E. C. CONRADI, U. K. WALLE, T. C. FAGAN & T. C. GAFFNEY. 1980. 4-hydroxypropranolol and its glucuronide after single oral and long-term doses of propranolol. Clin. Pharmacol. Ther. **27:** 22–31.
9. CLEAVELAND, C. R. & D. G. SHAND. 1972. Effect of route of administration on the relationship between β-adrenergic blockade and plasma propranolol levels. Clin. Pharmacol. Ther. **13:** 181–185.
10. MAHONY, C., K. M. WOLFRAM, D. COCHETTO & T. D. BJORNSSON. 1981. Pharmacokinetics of dipyridamole in man. Clin. Pharmacol. Ther. **29:** 264.
11. PRESCOTT, L. C., K. K. ADJEPON-YAWOAH & R. G. TALBOT. 1976. Impaired lignocaine metabolism in patients with myocardial infarction and cardiac failure. Br. Med. J.: 939–941.
12. ROUTLEDGE, P. A., A. BARCHOWSKY, T. D. BJORNSSON, B. B. KITCHELL & D. G. SHAND. 1980. Lidocaine plasma binding. Clin. Pharmacol. Ther. **271:** 347–351.
13. ROUTLEDGE, P. A., W. W. STARGEL, G. S. WAGNER & D. G. SHAND. 1980. Increased alpha-1-acid glycoprotein and lidocaine disposition in myocardial infarction. Ann. Intern Med. **93:** 701–704.
14. MULTICENTRE INTERNATIONAL STUDY. 1975. Improvement in prognosis of myocardial infarction by long term beta-adrenoceptor blockade using practolol. Br. Med. J. **iii:** 737–740.
15. COLTART, D. J., D. G. GIBSON & D. G. SHAND. 1971. Plasma propranolol levels associated with suppression of ventricular ectopic beats. Br. Med. J. **i:** 490–491.
16. WOOSLEY, R. D., D. KORNHAUSER, R. SMITH, S. REELE, S. B. HIGGINS, A. S. NIES, D. G. SHAND & J. A. OATES. 1979. Suppression of chronic ventricular arrhythmias with propranolol. Circulation **60:** 819–827.

DISCUSSION

DR. BIGGER: What about the complexity of adjusting the dose, measuring levels, and adjusting placebos in a central laboratory? It really hasn't been tried that often in major trials. It has been difficult to get any information about the experience with ventricular fibrillation. What do you think about the practicality of the BHAT trial? Do you think the investigators regret initiating this trial?

DR. SHAND: I imagine they may be, although if the trial gives positive findings, they'll be delighted. Setting up this trial was an experiment on its own. We did not know whether a more rational approach to dosage within these trials was really going to be worth it.

DR. BIGGER: It will be interesting to watch the results because this trial involves 42 centers, and its findings will probably point our way with respect to whether to retrench or to advance.

DR. SHAND: We may find different outcomes at different centers depending on the dose. There are some countries north of the border in which large doses of propranolol are more frequently used. It will be interesting to see whether those differences between the centers will be reflected in the findings.

DR. HERLING: Would you comment on the recent literature on procainamide levels? What does the literature say is therapeutic and does it differ from what is therapeutic in the electrophysiology laboratory?

DR. SHAND: We know that there *are* differences. One of the things that we don't realize is just how little information there is and how old the information is on which we base our therapeutic range. For example, the dosage for lidocaine is apparently very well established and is based on the single study of Gianelli. Nobody else has published anything. The literature on procainamide and especially on quinidine is very old and will have to undergo revision.

DR. HJALMARSON: Beta adrenergic blocking agents present a problem in that there is a poor relationship between plasma concentration and effect. Huge differences in effect can be obtained with the same plasma concentrations. The dose should be titrated to the effect, but we don't do that now. We don't know what we are looking for when we want to protect from sudden deah. Is that protection correlated to a reduction in heart rate? I'm not sure that it is.

But there is a practical problem as well. If the BHAT study is positive, the plasma concentration of propranolol has to be measured in every patient before it can be started. So this represents a scientific advantage, but it is not very practical.

DR. SHAND: It's as practical as the physician is convinced that it's practical and does it. I might add that the variation of alprenolol is just as great and just as multifactorial and in the trial of alprenolol, at least one of which is convincingly positive, a fixed dose was also used. In these trials we're showing that the drug can be effective. The question is: is it being optimally effective in every patient? I'd rather have at least therapeutic levels than a fixed lower dose that does not really give protection.

The study will also show whether these dosage levels have been of any value at all. If they haven't, then they can be discontinued.

CLINICAL EFFICACY OF ANTIARRHYTHMIC DRUGS IN PREVENTION OF SUDDEN CORONARY DEATH

Roger A. Winkle

Cardiology Division
Stanford University Medical Center
Stanford, California 94305

Patients with coronary artery disease are at increased risk of sudden unexpected death. The greatest risk occurs during the period after acute myocardial infarction. As the clinician's ability to successfully treat acute myocardial infarction in the hospital setting increased, attention turned to the postmyocardial infarction period. A number of studies in the late 1960s and early 1970s showed that these patients had approximately a 10% mortality during the first year after myocardial infarction. At the start of the 1970s two hypotheses were put forth: (1) that it was possible to identify high-risk subsets of patients after myocardial infarction; and (2) that it was possible to intervene to prevent sudden cardiac death. Throughout the 1970s studies have documented that it is indeed possible to identify high-risk subgroups whose overall mortality is several times the average. Most studies agree that complex ventricular arrhythmias on ambulatory electrocardiographic recordings and evidence of left ventricular dysfunction identify subjects in these high-risk subsets.[1] The primary form of intervention therapy discussed at the beginning of the last decade was antiarrhythmic therapy directed against the presumed cause of cardiac death, ventricular tachycardia and fibrillation. It is clear, however, that a number of patients die of causes other than acute arrhythmias, including reinfarction and congestive heart failure. Although during the past decade investigators have generated enthusiasm for therapy with beta blocking drugs,[2-4] antiplatelet agents,[5] coronary artery bypass grafting, and vasodilator therapy, little evidence accumulated to suggest that antiarrhythmic therapy can prevent sudden cardiac death in the postinfarction period. In this paper we will examine the studies that have been performed to determine whether antiarrhythmic therapy can prevent sudden death and we will discuss the shortcomings of these studies. Discussion will focus on past, present, and future difficulties in performing such studies.

SUMMARY OF STUDIES PERFORMED

Phenytoin

The largest clinical experience with the use of an antiarrhythmic agent for the prevention of sudden death exists for phenytoin. In 1971 a nicely controlled clinical trial evaluating the effectiveness of phenytoin for preventing sudden coronary death was reported by the collaborative group from Australia.[6] Five hundred sixty-eight patients were treated with phenytoin beginning at the time of discharge from the hospital after myocardial infarction. These patients were treated with either 300 or 400 mg of phenytoin daily or 3 or 4 mg of

247

0077-8923/82/0382-0247 $1.75/0 © 1982, NYAS

phenytoin daily. The study was single-blind and continued for one year post infarction. On entry into the study the two treatment groups were well matched and the only significant differences occurring during the subsequent 1 year were an increased rate of withdrawal from the study due to side effects and a decreased incidence of palpitations in the phenytoin-treated group. Sudden death occurred at the same rate in each group despite a statistically significant decrease in ventricular ectopic beats on resting rhythm strips.

One conclusion of the original phenytoin study was that there was a wide range of variation in plasma phenytoin levels in the treatment group. It was noted in a subsequent report [7] that there were 10 deaths in 64 patients whose phenytoin plasma concentration was less than 10 μg/ml and no deaths in 32 patients whose concentration was in the therapeutic range (greater than 10 μg/ml). This publication suggested that the failure of the study to demonstrate a reduction in sudden death was due to failure to achieve therapeutic concentrations of phenytoin in the plasma in many of the subjects in the trial.

Because of the controversy over drug plasma concentrations a subsequent prospective randomized open trial [8] was performed in 150 patients (74 treated subjects, 76 control subjects) with emphasis on achievement of therapeutic phenytoin levels in the plasma. Subjects post myocardial infarction were randomly assigned to treatment with phenytoin with a goal of achieving a plasma concentration between 40 and 80 μmol per liter. Plasma drug concentrations were in the therapeutic range in between 51 and 75% of subjects on any subsequent follow-up visit. There was no significant difference in mortality between the treatment and the control group. Furthermore, deaths during treatment were not associated with the presence of a low concentration of phenytoin in the plasma.

Procainamide

Kosowsky et al.[9] examined the long-term prophylactic antiarrhythmic actions of procainamide in a group of 78 patients with a recent myocardial infarction. Patients entered the study after transfer from the coronary care unit and prior to discharge from the hospital. Those patients requiring antiarrhythmic therapy for an existing arrhythmia were excluded. Treatment consisted of administration of 500 mg of procainamide every 6 or 8 hours. Patients were studied for a period of up to 36 months. By current standards, patients in this study received a subtherapeutic dose of procainamide with average plasma concentrations falling to a low of less than 2 μg/ml by the end of the dosing interval. There was a high dropout rate because of adverse reactions from procainamide, with 23 of the 39 treatment patients forced to withdraw from the study because of side effects. Despite these shortcomings there was a suggestion, although not statistically significant, of a reduction in deaths in the procainamide treatment group. Only one of the 39 treatment patients died, whereas there were 5 deaths in the control group, 4 of which were sudden.

Aprindine

Recently the results of a double-blind randomized trial of aprindine have been reported.[10, 11] This study was carried out as a multicenter trial in the

Netherlands and Belgium. Patients were randomly assigned to treatment and placebo groups 2 weeks after the onset of myocardial infarction. The duration of treatment for 1 year, and therapy was limited to those patients thought to be at high risk because of the presence of ventricular arrhythmias on a 24-hour ambulatory electrocardiography recording. Arrhythmias qualifying a patient for inclusion in the study were those that were of peak frequency of more than 5 per minute or multifocal within 30 minutes, repetitive ventricular ectopic beats, or runs of ventricular tachycardia. The initial dose of aprindine was 100 mg and patients were studied with sequential ambulatory electrocardiographic recordings. It was possible to adjust the dose upward or downward on the basis of the electrocardiographic findings, Holter recordings, and the occurrence of side effects. The upper limit of aprindine dosage was 200 mg daily. There was a total of 153 aprindine-treated patients and 152 placebo-treated patients. At one year 60% of the patients treated with aprindine had no ventricular ectopic beats as compared with only 25% of placebo-treated patients. There were 12 deaths (7.8%) in the aprindine treatment group as opposed to 19 deaths (12.5%) in the placebo group. Ten of the deaths in the aprindine treatment group were sudden as were 13 of deaths in the placebo group. These differences were not statistically significant. It is of note that none of the sudden deaths in the aprindine treatment group occurred in those subjects who were free of ventricular irritability on ambulatory monitoring. Twenty-two percent of the patients in the aprindine treatment group dropped out of the study because of adverse effects as opposed to 13% of the patients in the placebo group.

Mexiletine

Recently a multicenter report[12] from the United Kingdom has evaluated the effects of oral mexiletine for the prevention of sudden death after myocardial infarction. Patients were selected to enter the study 6 to 14 days after myocardial infarction. Entry was limited to a high-risk group defined as those having persistent S-T segment elevation on the second or third day after infarction, pulmonary edema on a chest X-ray film during the first 48 hours, tachycardia persisting for 24 hours in the first 48 hours, and left bundle branch block. Patients were treated for only 3 months with mexiletine in a dose of 200 or 250 mg every 8 hours. Downward dose adjustment was possible if drug-related side effects occurred. Three hundred forty-four patients were entered into the study. On entry the number of ventricular ectopic beats and the occurrence of pairs, runs and other complex forms were identical in the two groups. At 1 month and 3 months there was a rise in the number of ventricular ectopic beats per hour per patient in the control group and a statistically significant reduction of ventricular ectopic beats in the treatment group compared with the control group. Overall, mexiletine had no effect on mortality. Twenty-four patients (13.2%) in the mexiletine treatment group died and 19 (11.6%) of the placebo group died. Seven of the patients dying in the mexiletine group had been withdrawn from the protocol because of side effects, as had three in the placebo treatment group. Seventy-seven percent of the deaths in both groups were thought to be due to arrhythmias with or without myocardial infarction. It is of note that mortality was considerably higher in both treatment and placebo group among those patients with complex ventricular ectopic beats greater than 30 per hour or with ventricular tachycardia or pairs. It is also noteworthy that the number of patients in this study with ventricular tachycardia or R on T beats was not significantly reduced by mexiletine treatment. Furthermore, evaluation of drug plasma concentration indicated that 29% of subjects had less than the minimal therapeutic plasma concentration (0.75 μg/ml) of drug at one month and 41% had drug levels below the therapeutic range at 3 months of therapy.

STUDY DESIGN CONSIDERATIONS

The few antiarrhythmic drug intervention trials performed to date to prevent sudden coronary death have had disappointing results. While it is possible that antiarrhythmic drugs are unable to influence the occurrence of sudden death in coronary artery disease in the period after myocardial infarction, there are also a number of study design factors that could account for the negative results observed so far.

What Is the Question Being Asked?

Studies to date have basically been designed to answer the question of whether or not an antiarrhythmic drug given either to all postinfarction subjects or to selected high-risk populations can reduce the occurrence of sudden death as compared with results when that therapy is not given. It must be recognized that this "shotgun" approach of giving all subjects the same drug in approximately the same doses and plasma concentrations differs significantly from current clinical practice with postmyocardial infarction patients at most hospitals. Current practice generally reflects the hypothesis that patients with frequent complex ventricular ectopy in the late postinfarction period are at high risk of sudden cardiac death and that *suppression of this ectopy with an antiarrhythmic drug will diminish this risk.* Patients are generally monitored continuously in the hospital and a variety of antiarrhythmic drugs in a wide range of doses are given until arrhythmia suppression is accomplished without significant toxicity. Experience in the treatment of various supraventricular arrhythmias and recurrent sustained ventricular tachycardia and fibrillation in other populations suggests that such an individualized approach to therapy may be necessary, rather than the current approach of expecting all patients to respond to a single drug. The two studies with follow-up monitoring make it clear that a single drug will not suppress ectopy in all patients. Furthermore, the absence of sudden deaths in the aprindine treatment group free of ventricular ectopy supports the concept of ventricular ectopic suppression as an endpoint of therapy. If individualized antiarrhythmic therapy is necessary to prevent sudden death, then study designs in the future will differ radically from those in the past. It may also be necessary to consider new methods for judging drug efficacy, such as invasive electrophysiologic testing in carefully selected high-risk patients.

What Is the Population Being Studied?

Early studies, such as the initial phenytoin study, attempted to include all patients with a recent myocardial infarction. Assuming antiarrhythmic therapy will result in a 50% reduction in sudden deaths, it is easy to calculate that such an approach requires extremely large patient populations to show significance in preventing sudden death. Furthermore, unnecessarily large numbers of patients would be unlikely to receive significant benefit because their overall risk of sudden death is low and yet they would be subjected to the side effects and potential dangers of the treatment. More recent studies have focused on high-risk subsets, thereby requiring fewer patients in order to show drug efficacy. It is quite possible that both the procainamide and aprindine studies would have shown a significant reduction in sudden death if slightly larger numbers of patients or an even higher-risk subgroup had been studied. However, it is important to note that at present we clearly do not have methods for distinguishing those patients in the high-risk subsets who will die of sudden arrhythmic cardiac death from those who will die of reinfarction or progressive congestive heart failure. What little data are available to assist us in identifying risk factors for *sudden* death are contaminated by definitions of sudden death which include *all* deaths within 24 hours of the onset of symptoms. Clearly, sudden deaths that might be prevented with prophylactic antiarrhythmic therapy are those where death is instantaneous or nearly so. Even among instantaneous deaths, as many as one-quarter will be due to bradyarrhythmias rather than to ventricular tachycardia or fibrillation, which might have been prevented by drug therapy. The mexiletine and the aprindine studies provide an excellent example of how widely criteria to identify a high-risk subset of patients may vary from one study to the next. The factors utilized in the mexiletine study are primarily reflections of left ventricular dysfunction whereas entry into the aprindine study was solely on the basis of ventricular irritability seen on ambulatory electrocardiographic recordings in the late infarction period. One might speculate that the group chosen for therapy in the mexiletine trial might have better been treated with vasodilating agents and that the trend towards a beneficial result for aprindine might have reached statistical significance had the study included a slightly larger number of patients. If findings on ambulatory electrocardiographic recordings are to form the entry criteria for randomized trials, it is important that feedback be rapid so that patients may be entered into the study at the earliest possible date.

Considerations for Drug Pharmacokinetics

During the past decade there has been tremendous increase in information about the clinical pharmacology of the antiarrhythmic drugs. Although it is unknown whether there is a "therapeutic plasma concentration" for prevention of sudden cardiac death, therapeutic ranges of a number of antiarrhythmic drug concentrations in the plasma have been well established for suppression of ventricular ectopic beats. Experience with the phenytoin trial indicates that even when attempts are made to adjust dosage into the therapeutic range, large numbers of patients will receive drug therapy that falls below the generally accepted therapeutic plasma concentration range. This may in part reflect poor compliance, and drugs with longer half-lives (thereby requiring less frequent administration) and fewer side effects may increase the clinician's ability to maintain continuously therapeutic plasma concentrations. The availability of several newer agents with improved pharmacokinetics may make it easier to carry out long-term drug intervention trials in the postinfarction group.

Dose Adjustments

Although it was the initial intention of the early phenytoin study to permit dosage adjustments, the lack of availability of plasma concentration measurement at all centers prohibited this goal from being achieved. The wide intersubject variation in pharmacokinetics and effective plasma concentration for many of the antiarrhythmic drugs make dose adjustment an almost mandatory feature of most future drug intervention trials. Indeed, lack of dose adjustment in the initial phenytoin trial essentially negated the ability to interpret the data from the study. A subsequent study had to be carried out in order to resolve this matter. The mexiletine intervention trial permitted some downward dose adjustments. The aprindine trial had the most sophisticated dose adjustment method based on both side effects and findings on ambulatory electrocardiographic recordings. While dose adjustments are important to optimize antiarrhythmic efficacy and to minimize the occurrence of side effects, it is important to emphasize, however, that dose adjustment alone is not necessarily an important factor in determining the outcome of the study. To be optimally valuable in contributing to the prevention of sudden death, dose adjustments must occur early in the trial. Since the highest risk from sudden death is in the first few months after myocardial infarction, the majority of dose adjustments should be possible during the first few days or weeks of therapy. In order to incorporate dose adjustment into the protocol design, it is mandatory that drug plasma concentration and/or results of ambulatory electrocardiographic recordings be available almost immediately to the physicians caring for the patients.

The Drug Being Studied

It is not surprising to most clinicians who have treated patients with cardiac arrhythmias that phenytoin was ineffective in preventing sudden cardiac death. It is apparent that phenytoin is not the most effective antiarrhythmic agent. Quinidine and procainamide are both limited by high dropout rates due to side effects and procainamide has poor pharmacokinetic characteristics which require frequent dose administration. Because of the small number of antiarrhythmic drugs available, the pharmaceutical industry has directed tremendous resources at the development of new membrane-active antiarrhythmic agents with good pharmacokinetic properties, a low incidence of side effects, and a high degree of efficacy. One of the major reasons for developing such drugs is the prevention of sudden cardiac death, which represents a very substantial potential market. If suppression of ventricular ectopic beats is necessary to prevent sudden death, an antiarrhythmic agent must be highly efficacious in the majority of subjects in order to be used as a single drug in comparison with placebo. Several new drugs appear to be capable of suppressing ventricular ectopic beats totally or nearly so in a very high percentage of patients undergoing treatment and thus seem to be candidates for large-scale intervention trials. Rather than limiting therapy to a single drug, we might want to permit the use of other drugs in those patients in whom ventricular ectopy is not suppressed or in whom side effects limit therapy with the initial drug. If a drug needs only to have an effect against ventricular tachycardia and fibrillation without necessarily suppressing ventricular ectopic beats, then perhaps drugs such as bretylium or amiodarone might be able to prevent sudden cardiac death. Dose adjustments based on plasma concentrations or ambulatory electrocardiographic recordings would be difficult for a drug such as amiodarone, which requires weeks or months to come to steady-state.

IMPLICATIONS OF OTHER THERAPY FOR ANTIARRHYTHMIC DRUG INTERVENTION TRIALS

In the late 1960s and early 1970s antiarrhythmic drug therapy seemed to be the only potential intervention to be tested for prevention of sudden cardiac death. As it became apparent that deaths were due not only to ventricular tachycardia and/or fibrillation, but also to reinfarction and progressive power failure, it became apparent that other forms of treatment might also be effective. Optimistic reports have been generated for the use of coronary artery bypass surgery, beta adrenergic blocking drugs, and antiplatelet agents in the immediate and late postinfarction period. At many hospitals in the United States it has become the standard of care for patients to undergo routine coronary arteriography several weeks after a myocardial infarction and to have all lesions bypassed. Even more recently, enthusiasm for streptokinase infusion in the first hours after a coronary occlusion to dissolve the thrombus with subsequent balloon angioplasty or early coronary bypass grafting in order to preserve myocardium suggests that the types of treatment given to patients with an acute myocardial infarction may change dramatically in the next decade. Certainly such therapy could ultimately make it completely impossible to perform an antiarrhythmic drug intervention trial in postmyocardial infarction patients, and these early interventions would eliminate our present ability to identify high-risk subgroups because they will have altered the natural history of the disease.

WHO SHOULD PAY FOR ANTIARRHYTHMIC DRUG INTERVENTION TRIALS?

One obstacle to the performance of a large number of antiarrhythmic drug intervention trials is the large number of patients who must be screened and/or treated and the enormous expense therefore involved. Although the United States government is currently sponsoring a propranolol intervention trial, there have been no other government-supported postinfarction antiarrhythmic drug intervention trials. Industry has been supportive of trials in other countries, but has not supported such a trial in the United States. While the expenses are large, the financial rewards would be enormous if any drug could be shown to prevent sudden cardiac death. It would seem only logical that each new antiarrhythmic agent undergoing clinical trial should ultimately be tested for its ability to prevent sudden cardiac death. One other potential source for funding of such studies is third-party payers. Prolongation of hospitalization for drug therapy for patients with asymptomatic ventricular arrhythmias is a common practice and undoubtedly raises the cost of postinfarction care. If antiarrhythmic therapy is not efficacious, then third-party payers are spending large amounts of money unnecessarily. It would be in their interest to assist in the funding of large-scale intervention trials to answer the question of drug efficacy in these patients.

CONCLUSIONS

During the past ten years we have failed to demonstrate the efficacy of antiarrhythmic drugs for preventing sudden death. Although the goal may be unachievable, the relatively small number of studies to date have, for a variety of reasons, been inadequate to answer the question. It is clear that we need better methods to identify subsets of patients at risk for "instantaneous" sudden death because this is the population most likely to benefit from antiarrhythmic drugs. The drugs used must be effective antiarrhythmic agents that are relatively free of side effects and they must be given in a dosage schedule that achieves continuously "therapeutic" levels. Protocol designs incorporating multiple drugs and suppression of ventricular ectopic beats as an end-point of therapy must also be considered. Electrophysiologic testing to identify high-risk patients and to monitor drug efficacy should also be evaluated. Finally, changes in the methods of therapy given during and after acute myocardial infarction may alter the disease's natural history to an extent that would severely compromise our ability to conduct controlled trials of antiarrhythmic drugs.

REFERENCES

1. WINKLE, R. A. 1980. Detection of patients at high risk for sudden death: The role of electrocardiographic monitoring. In Sudden Death. H. Kulbertus & H. J. Wellens, Eds.: 275–296. Martinus Nijhoff The Hague.
2. MULTICENTRE INTERNATIONAL STUDY. 1975. Improvement in prognosis of myocardial infarction by long-term beta-adrenoreceptor blockade using practolol. Br. Med. J. 3: 735–740.
3. WILHELMSSON, C., L. WILHELMSEN, J. A. VEDIN, G. TIBBLIN & L. WERKÖ. 1974. Reduction of sudden deaths after myocardial infarction by treatment with alprenolol. Lancet 2: 1157–1160.
4. NORWEGIAN MULTICENTER STUDY GROUP. 1981. Timolol-induced reduction in mortality and reinfarction in patients surviving acute myocardial infarction. N. Engl. J. Med. 304: 801–807.
5. ANTURANE REiNFARCTION TRIAL RESEARCH GROUP. 1980. Sulfinpyrazone in the prevention of sudden death after myocardial infarction. N. Engl. J. Med. 302: 250–256.
6. COLLABORATIVE GROUP. 1971. Phenytoin after recovery from myocardial infarction: Controlled trial in 568 patients. Lancet 2: 1055–1057.
7. VAJDA, F. J. E., R. J. PRINEAS, R. R. H. LOVELL & J. G. SLOMAN. 1973. The possible effect of long term high plasma levels of phenytoin on mortality after acute myocardial infarction. Eur. J. Clin. Pharmacol. 5: 138–144.
8. PETER, T., D. ROSS, A. DUFFIELD, M. LUXTON, R. HARPER, D. HUNT & G. SLOMAN. 1978. Effect on survival after myocardial infarction of long-term treatment with phenytoin. Br. Heart J. 40: 1356–1360.
9. KOSOWSKY, B. D., J. TAYLOR, B. LOWN & R. F. RITCHIE. 1973. Long-term use of procaine amide following acute myocardial infarction. Circulation 47: 1204–1210.
10. HAGEMEIJER, F., B. GLASER, J. P. VAN DURME & M. BOGAERT. 1977. Design of a study to evaluate drug therapy of serious ventricular rhythm disturbances after an acute myocardial infarction. Eur. J. Cardiol. 6(4): 299–310.
11. HUGENHOLTZ, P. G., F. HAGEMEIJER, J. LUBSEN, B. GLASER, J. P. VAN DURME & M. G. BOGAERT. 1978. One year follow-up in patients with persistent ventricular dysrhythmias after myocardial infarction treated with aprindine

or placebo. *In* Management of Ventricular Tachycardia: Role of Mexilitine. E. Sandøe, D. G. Julian & J. W. Bell, Eds.: 572–578. Excerpta Medica. Amsterdam.

12. CHAMERLAIN, D. A., D. G. JULIAN, D. McC. BOYLE, D. E. JEWITT, R. W. F. CAMPBELL & R. G. SHANKS. 1980. Oral mexiletine in high-risk patients after myocardial infarction. Lancet **2:** 1324–1327.

DISCUSSION

DR. CRAMPTON: Several Scandinavian studies have shown that the Q-T interval shortens on long-term therapy with metoprolol. In this group of patients a reduced late mortality is beginning to emerge. I think we have some clues as to why this happens. As you have pointed out, Dr. Winkle, we should not be worrying just about ventricular premature beats; we should be thinking of other factors as well. We may have to take a heterogeneous approach to factors that we are going to study to see whether the constellation is controllable. This approach means that we won't just look at the ventricular premature beats on the Holter tape, but that we will also study the Q-T interval on it.

DR. WINKLE: I agree. I'd like to mention that there has been a tremendous change in attitude in the last couple of years with respect to testing the hypothesis that suppression of ventricular premature beats has any value. Current thought seems to be that suppression of ventricular premature beats is not important, yet we've never really tested the hypothesis. So I want to go on record as saying that this hypothesis should be tested.

DR. BIGGER: Your point is extremely well taken, because it has become fashionable in cardiologic circles to downgrade the R on T ventricular premature beats. I know that Pantridge's group has tape-recorded quite a few of their patients in the first 30 minutes of an acute coronary event. They have not looked at the Q-T intervals, but they have examined the R on T ventricular premature beat. They've seen very few, but the peculiar thing about it is that the majority of the episodes of ventricular fibrillation that they did document were initiated by an R on T ventricular premature beat.

There are several retrospective studies that have shown that the Q-T interval lengthens immediately before the onset of ventricular tachycardia or fibrillation in ischemia. So perhaps we should be looking at more than one thing at a time.

DR. DESILVA: What do you consider to be adequate suppression of ventricular arrhythmia? I have not heard anyone define adequacy of treatment in suppression of ventricular premature beats. We are assuming that we're all talking about the same thing when we say that we have suppressed the arrhythmia. Can you define your criteria as well as the criteria for various antiarrhythmic studies now ongoing in the United States?

DR. WINKLE: I'm not aware of any ongoing studies with antiarrhythmic drug prophylaxis in which suppression of ventricular premature contractions is the end-point. Our experience is with clinical pharmacologic studies of new antiarrhythmis drugs in patients with chronic ventricular ectopic beats, which may be different from those that occur in early postmyocardial infarction patients. I don't know the end-point.

Suppression of complex forms virtually always goes in parallel with suppression of total numbers. From a practical standpoint, suppression of all isolated pairs and runs is quite difficult. Most of the scanners available can't even accurately detect isolated forms. I can't tell you what number I'd like to see, but I can say that with several of the new antiarrhythmic drugs it's not at all unreasonable to attempt to achieve nearly total suppression of ventricular ectopic beats. With these new drugs, it's really possible to suppress more than 90% of ventricular ectopic beats. So we can talk about almost complete suppression, but not total suppression.

DR. DE SILVA: One of the fundamental problems in therapy for prophylaxis against ventricular fibrillation is that we are all using disparate end-points. Our group makes the basic assumption that high grades of arrhythmia, that is, Lown grades of 4A, 4B, and 5, are significant risk factors for future sudden death. As a corollary, the target for treatment should be elimination of all arrhythmias of grades 4A, 4B, and 5. The way we have assessed this, in patients who have quantifiable amounts of ventricular ectopic activity, is to try to attempt, through drug therapy, to totally eliminate repetitive forms of arrhythmia as seen on both Holter monitoring and exercise stress testing.

In those 141 patients in whom arrhythmias of grades 4A, 4B, and 5 have been eliminated the actual mortality on follow-up study was 3.4% per year. If these types of ventricular ectopic activity are not seen to be eliminated on both Holter monitoring and maximal exercise stress testing, the actual mortality rate is 40% per year. We believe that these results substantiate the thesis that high grade arrhythmias are a significant risk factor for future sudden death and also that elimination of these grades of arrhythmia is preventive against sudden death.

DR. WINKLE: Your data are very impressive and certainly lend credence to your hypothesis.

From a practical standpoint it is very difficult to detect R on T premature beats with any sort of automatic detection system.

DR. BAIGRIE: In terms of morbidity and mortality after myocardial infarction, what is the minimum sample size needed to prove efficacy in a sudden death trial?

DR. WINKLE: The least number of patients who should be entered into a trial would be about 300 in each group. That assumes that you have a reasonable high-risk population. Dr. Bigger, do you have any thoughts on that?

DR. BIGGER: If you're going to attempt to reduce the death rate by perhaps just 25%, you would need to have at least 200 to 400 patients in each group.

DR. HERLING: We tested the hypothesis of the relationship of ventricular ectopic activity to suppression of recurrent sustained ventricular tachycardia, which we reported last year in the *American Journal of Cardiology*. We found that even if complete suppression of ventricular premature beats over a 24-hour period was achieved, there were nevertheless five patients in whom recurrence of sustained ventricular tachycardia could be induced. Conversely, many persons in whom tachycardia could not be induced after surgical therapy continued to have complex forms of ectopy. So, although I'm talking about a different patient population, I don't think that there is any constant correlation that can be made on the basis of data on suppression.

DR. WINKLE: I also don't think a direct correlation can be made because, as you said, yours is a totally different patient population. Furthermore, the inducibility of arrhythmias may not necessarily relate to long-term outcome. If you really believe that it takes a few beats to initiate an episode of ventricular tachycardia, then a drug which can virtually eliminate ventricular ectopic beats may be effective, even though you can still induce ventricular tachycardia.

I also think that your data suggest that there may be some value in looking at ventricular ectopic beat suppression. If you cannot suppress ventricular ectopic beats, then you can always induce ventricular tachycardia, whereas if you suppress ventricular ectopic beats, you can only induce ventricular tachycardia about half of the time. That suggests that there is some value in suppressing ventricular ectopic beats for predicting clinical outcome.

DR. GALLERSTEIN: Some of the most elegant studies have come out of your center, Dr. Winkle, but how does the practicing physician, who does not have all these resources, manage a postmyocardial infarction patient who is having a lot of ventricular arrhythmias? Do you think that there is any benefit in placing the patient on a drug that he will tolerate at "therapeutic levels"?

DR. WINKLE: I don't know whether there is any basis for this kind of therapeutic approach. I am very skeptical that an arbitrarily chosen drug will be effective. I see too many persons with recurrent ventricular tachycardia or those who have survived sudden death and with these patients you have to go through a whole series of drugs until you get one that actually works.

CALCIUM ANTAGONISTS AND THEIR POTENTIAL ROLE IN THE PREVENTION OF SUDDEN CORONARY DEATH *

Douglas P. Zipes† and Robert F. Gilmour, Jr.

Krannert Institute of Cardiology
Indianapolis, Indiana 46202

Department of Medicine and Pharmacology
Indiana University School of Medicine
Indianapolis, Indiana 46223

Veterans Administration Medical Center
Indianapolis, Indiana 46202

INTRODUCTION

Hodgkin and Katz [1] demonstrated that a large and relatively specific increase in the membrane permeability to sodium ions accounted for the amplitude and rate of voltage change of the depolarization phase of squid nerve action potentials. Using the voltage-clamp technique, Hodgkin and Huxley [2] analyzed the currents underlying the nerve action potential. They described two constituents —an inward sodium flow followed by an outward potassium flow—and formulated equations to describe how these currents vary with transmembrane voltage potential and time.

In the ensuing years, cardiac electrophysiologists, assuming that exclusively sodium and potassium movements were involved, applied the Hodgkin-Huxley analysis of transmembrane current flow to explain the considerably more complex waveforms of cardiac action potentials. [3] However, as early as 1956, Coraboeuf and Otsuka [4] noted that the overshoot of the ventricular action potential was rather insensitive to the extracellular sodium concentration, and in the early 1960s many investigators working independently (for reviews, see Weidmann, [5] Trautwein, [6] Reuter, [7] Cranefield, [8] and Zipes *et al.* [9]) showed that the kinetics of the inward ionic flow in cardiac fibers could not be satisfactorily described in terms of sodium ion movement alone. Neidergerke and Orkand [10] soon demonstrated a sodium-calcium competition for entry into myocardial cells, and Hagiwara and Nakajima [11] developed a very important pharmacologic tool by demonstrating that cardiac fibers possessed one current sensitive to tetrodotoxin (TTX) and another current sensitive to manganese (Mn).

In the late 1960s, Reuter [12] presented evidence for a slow component of depolarization that is not very sensitive to variations in the extracellular concentration of sodium ions, but is uniquely sensitive to the extracellular concentration of calcium ions, and is sluggish in its kinetics of activation and, espe-

* This work was supported in part by the Herman C. Krannert Fund; by Grants HL–06308, HL–07182, and HL–18795 from the National Heart, Lung and Blood Institute, National Institutes of Health; and by the American Heart Association, Indiana Affiliate, Inc.

† Address for correspondence: Douglas P. Zipes, M.D., Indiana University School of Medicine, 1100 West Michigan Street, Indianapolis, Indiana 46223.

cially, inactivation. Subsequent work established that the fast inward sodium current, responsible for the rapid upstroke of the cardiac action potential, produces a voltage change that triggers this second slower current, which is carried by calcium ions or by sodium ions (or possibly by both) and which contributes to the overshoot (of some animal species) and the plateau phase of the cardiac action potential. These two inward currents, the fast and the slow current, are probably interdependent; depolarization is undoubtedly more complex than simply a rapid component followed by a slow component. Both currents are present in specialized conducting tissues and in atrial and ventricular muscle cells. In cardiac muscle cells, the slow inward current is essential for coupling excitation of the cell membrane to activation of the contractile proteins. Although some species differences in characteristics of the slow current may eventually be found, it is now clear that this current is a fundamental physiologic property of all myocardial tissue.[5-9]

The term "calcium antagonists," catchy and likely to remain, is incorrectly used for several reasons. First, agents that block the slow inward current are a diverse lot and exhibit other properties as well. Some also affect the fast current, or outward potassium currents. Second, the slow channel does not transport calcium exclusively, and other ions, particularly sodium, also travel through it.

MANIPULATION OF INWARD CURRENTS

Both the fast and slow currents are voltage- and time-dependent, but have sufficiently different characteristics to allow them to be studied independently (TABLE 1). For example, the fast inward channel may be rendered inactive under conditions that do not interrupt the function of the slow channels. Partial loss of resting membrane potential in ventricular fibers, which ordinarily exhibit a large fast component, may allow emergence and identification of action potentials that are dependent on the slow component during depolarization. The fast channels may be inactivated by depolarizing fibers using a variety of techniques.[13, 14] Also, TTX, which has been shown to specifically block the fast sodium conductance in nerve tissue,[15] pharmacologically suppresses the rapid current in cardiac fibers without altering resting potential.[11] Under these conditions the tissue becomes inexcitable. Factors that augment transmembrane calcium flux restore regenerative, propagated action potentials to the tissue. For example, agents such as catecholamines, histamine, xanthines, and dibutyryl cyclic adenosine monophosphate, all of which increase intracellular cyclic adenosine monophosphate (cAMP) levels, directly augment the slow inward current.[16-19] Recent evidence suggests that the increase in slow inward current caused by elevated cAMP levels is responsible for the positive inotropic effects of these diverse agents. These restored responses do not occur in a calcium-free medium unless calcium is replaced by certain other divalent cations such as strontium or barium.[11, 16] The restored action potentials are characterized by a slow upstroke velocity, delayed recovery of excitability, and slow propagation through the tissue, exhibiting unidirectional block, summation, inhibition, and reentry.[20, 21]

The slow current may be selectively blocked by the cations manganese, cobalt, nickel, and lanthanum, as well as by the synthetic organic compounds verapamil and D600 (a methoxy derivative of verapamil).[22] Verapamil appears to block the slow inward current at a site distal to the beta-adrenergic receptor, and therefore allows catecholamine-induced elevation of cAMP levels without permitting an increase in calcium influx.[18, 19] More recently developed agents that block the slow inward current include nifedipine, diltiazem, and perhexiline.[23] Verapamil appears to alter the kinetics of activation and recovery from inactivation, while nifedipine may reduce the number of available slow inward channels.[23]

TABLE 1

CHARACTERISTICS OF FAST AND SLOW CURRENTS

Electrophysiologic Property	Rapid Current	Slow Current
Activation and inactivation kinetics	Rapid	Slow
Dependent on extracellular ion concentration of:	Sodium	Calcium (sodium)
Abolished by:	Tetrodotoxin	Manganese, cobalt, nickel, lanthanum, verapamil, D600, diltiazem, nifedipine
Threshold of activation	−60 to −70 mV	−30 to −40 mV
Conduction velocity	0.5–3.0 M/sec	0.01–0.1 M/sec
Overshoot	+20 to +35 mV	0 to +15 mV
Rate of rise (dV/dt) of action potential upstroke	200–1000 V/sec	1–10 V/sec
Action potential amplitude	100–130 mV	35–75 mV
Response to stimulus	All-or-none	Affected by characteristics of stimulus
Safety factor for conduction	High	Low
Recovery of excitability	Prompt; ends with repolarization	Delayed; outlasts full repolarization

SLOW INWARD CURRENT AND TACHYARRHYTHMIAS

Tachyarrhythmias result from disorders of impulse formation, impulse conduction, or combinations of both mechanisms. Since cells dependent on the slow inward current possess the properties of impulse formation and conduction,[8, 9] it is quite plausible to consider that the slow inward current may serve as an important ionic substrate in fibers responsible for, or at least participating in, the genesis or maintenance of various supraventricular and ventricular tachyarrhythmias that occur clinically. Such ionic characterization can be made on experimental preparations and ample evidence supports the role of the slow inward current in the generation of action potentials from normal and abnormal fibers in the atrium and abnormal fibers in the ventricle. For example, the data strongly indicate that the normal sinus and atrioventricular (AV) nodes are slow-channel-dependent. In addition, other atrial and ventricular fibers, some made abnormal by a variety of methods, may be slow-channel-dependent. However, our present diagnostic tools do not permit unequivocal determination of the electrophysiologic mechanisms responsible for most clinically occurring tachyarrhythmias, that is, reentry or automaticity, and certainly do not allow convincing differentiation into which arrhythmias may be slow-channel-dependent. Nevertheless, extrapolating from observations in experimental animal, from *in vitro* studies on human tissues, and from the response of arrhythmias to the clinically available slow-channel blocking agents, we will consider the evidence supporting the possible participation of the slow inward current in the genesis of supraventricular and ventricular tachycardias. We will assume that the slow inward current may play a role in the genesis or maintenance of the tachycardia if it can be established that the tachycardia (1) originates in fibers known to be slow-channel-dependent; (2) exhibits rate responses consistent with automaticity thought to be the result of the slow inward current; (3) requires such fibers as part of its conduction pathway; and/ or (4) is affected by verapamil. A brief analysis of these criteria follows:

Criteria

1. Origination of the tachycardia in fibers thought to generate slow-channel-dependent potentials: We will apply this criterion to tachycardias thought to be caused by automaticity and consider whether they originate in the sinus or atrioventricular (AV) nodes, coronary sinus, mitral or tricuspid valves, or possibly other sites that disease has rendered slow-channel-dependent.

2. Rate responses consistent with automaticity that responds differently from "normal" automaticity: In some instances, such automaticity may be due to the slow inward current. We will apply this criterion to tachycardias thought to be caused by automaticity and consider whether the tachycardias exhibit an "anomalous" response to pacing, such as triggering or overdrive acceleration. Triggering refers to initiation of sustained rhythmic activity in which a quiescent fiber is triggered to depolarize by an impulse arising elsewhere and each subsequent discharge emerges from the afterdepolarization of the preceding impulse. Such triggering can be observed in transmembrane recordings, but, as yet, not from extracellular recordings *in vivo*. Triggered activity may arise from fibers with high or low resting membrane potentials and its relationship to the slow inward current remains obscure in spite of verapamil's ability to suppress triggered activity in several preparations. Overdrive acceleration is defined as capture of the tachycardia by pacing or by a spontaneous rhythm (sinus rhythm, for example) at faster rates than the tachycardias, with persistence or emergence of the tachycardias at a faster rate after loss of capture. As with triggering, fibers that exhibit overdrive acceleration behave differently from fibers with "normal" automaticity, but the relationship to the slow inward current remains to be defined.

3. Initiation or maintenance of tachycardias resulting from conduction over fibers known to be slow-channel-dependent: We will apply this criterion to tachycardias thought to be caused and maintained by reentry, and we will

consider whether the reentry occurs within the sinus or AV nodes, or possibly over other sites that disease has rendered slow-channel-dependent.

4. Alteration of the tachycardias by verapamil: Although termination of electrical activity by verapamil cannot be used as the *sine qua non* of slow-channel dependence, it is one of the best clinical estimates we have, and we will assume that verapamil is a relatively specific slow-channel blocker, knowing that the racemic mixture, drug concentrations, and tissue types all may affect the response produced by verapamil.

SUPRAVENTRICULAR TACHYCARDIAS

Although supraventricular tachycardias (SVT) are not generally considered causally related to sudden cardiac death, in some patients a fairly rapid supraventricular tachycardia may create conditions that result in initiation of a fatal ventricular tachyarrhythmia. With this in mind, supraventricular tachycardias will be discussed briefly.

ATRIOVENTRICULAR NODAL SUPRAVENTRICULAR TACHYCARDIA

The weight of evidence implicates reentry as the mechanism responsible for initiation and maintenance of AV nodal SVTs and places the site of the anterogradely conducting pathway(s) in the AV node. The site of retrogradely conducting pathway, as well as the geometry and electrophysiology of its fibers, is still being defined and may not be the same for all patients with AV nodal reentrant SVT (FIG. 1).

Slow-channel blockers, such as manganese [24] and verapamil,[25-29] strikingly depress AV nodal propagation and lengthen AV nodal refractoriness, without significantly affecting conduction in the His-Purkinje system or ventricular or atrial muscle. Tetrodotoxin fails to inhibit AV nodal activity, while suppressing activity in the His bundle and atrial [24] and ventricular muscle. In an isolated rabbit AV nodal preparation, verapamil prevented AV nodal reentry and initiation of atrial tachycardia by causing premature atrial impulses to block rather than to conduct with the delay needed to initiate reentry.[27] By this mechanism, verapamil may terminate AV nodal reentrant SVT in man.

Verapamil, administered intravenously, has been shown repeatedly to terminate effectively episodes of AV nodal reentrant SVT in man.[28, 30-33] In a recent study, we have confirmed the fact that verapamil terminated AV nodal reentrant SVTs by causing prolongation and eventual block of anterograde AV nodal conduction.[31] We also found that verapamil only affected conduction and refractoriness in the anterogradely conducting pathway, exerting no significant effect on the pathway used for retrograde conduction during the SVT [30] (FIGS. 2 and 3). This observation lends further credence to the concept that, at least in some patients with AV nodal reentrant SVT, the retrogradely conducting pathway may not be composed of typical AV nodal fibers.[34] Verapamil may block the retrograde pathway on occasion.[35]

In conclusion, present evidence indicates that SVT involving the AV node is most probably due to reentry; that at least the anterogradely conducting pathway or pathways are composed of AV nodal tissue; and that verapamil effectively blocks conduction in this pathway to terminate the SVT. Thus we conclude that criteria 3 and 4 are applicable to AV nodal reentrant SVT, and therefore that the slow inward current plays a role in the genesis and maintenance of this SVT.

SUPRAVENTRICULAR TACHYCARDIA RELATED TO THE WOLFF-PARKINSON-WHITE SYNDROME

Reciprocating tachycardia in the Wolff-Parkinson-White (WPW) syndrome most often involves conduction over the AV node anterogradely, and thus involves slow-channel-dependent fibers in this portion of the reentrant loop.[36]

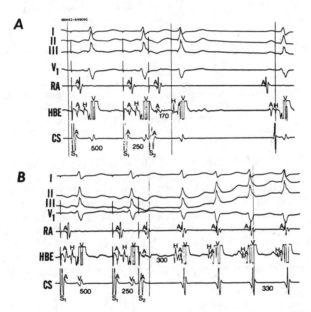

FIGURE 1. Initiation of supraventricular tachycardia in a patient with dual atrioventricular (AV) nodal pathways. Panels **A** and **B** show the last two paced beats (S_1) of a train delivered to the coronary sinus at a pacing cycle length of 500 msec. The results of premature atrial stimulation at an S_1–S_2 interval of 250 msec on two occasions are shown. In panel **A**, S_2 was conducted to the ventricle with an A-H interval of 170 msec. In panel **B**, S_2 was conducted with an A-H interval of 300 msec, followed by AV nodal reentry. RA, right atrial electrogram; HBE, His bundle electrogram; CS, coronary sinus electrogram; I, II, III, V_1, scalar electrocardiographic leads. (From Rinkenberger et al.[31] Reproduced by permission.)

The remaining fibers in the reentrant pathway, atrium, ventricle, or accessory pathway are normally fast-channel-dependent.

Verapamil exerts no significant electrophysiologic effects on the accessory pathway (FIG. 4) and terminates SVT in patients with the WPW syndrome by slowing and blocking conduction over the normal AV node.[30, 31] Thus supraventricular tachycardias in the WPW syndrome most commonly terminate after administration of verapamil during anterograde conduction. If verapamil

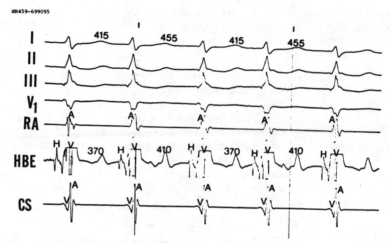

FIGURE 2. Same patient as in FIGURE 1. After intravenous verapamil, supraventricular tachycardia developed cycle length alternans of 40 msec, caused by alternation in A-H intervals. The H-A interval, H-V interval, and atrial activation sequence remain constant. (From Rinkenberger et al.[31] Reproduced by permission.)

does not produce block in the AV node during SVT, the tachycardia continues at a slower rate, resulting from prolongation of AV nodal conduction time.

Some data suggest that the AV node in patients with WPW syndrome may conduct more rapidly and exhibit a shorter refractory period than in patients with SVT.[37] We have found that verapamil prolonged AV nodal conduction time, functional and effective refractory periods of the AV node to a lesser extent in patients with WPW who had SVT than in patients who had SVT due to AV nodal reentry.[31] The reason for the reduced electrophysiologic response of the AV node to verapamil in patients with WPW syndrome is unknown.

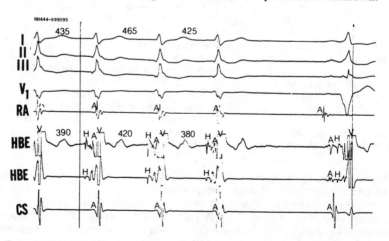

FIGURE 3. Same patient as in FIGURE 1. Supraventricular tachycardia terminated because of block of the atrial depolarization proximal to the His bundle recording site. (From Rinkenberger et al.[31] Reproduced by permission.)

The reciprocating tachycardia in patients who have WPW syndrome is slow-channel-dependent, meeting criteria 3 and 4.

SUPRAVENTRICULAR TACHYCARDIA RESULTING FROM SINUS NODAL REENTRY

The sinus node shares with the AV node several similar electrophysiologic features, such as reduced resting potential and rate of rise of phase zero, slow propagation, and the potential for dissociation of conduction.[38] In many ways, the sinus node is a prototype of a slow-channel-dependent automatic fiber, and its activity is suppressed by slow-channel blockers.[8, 9, 25-29]

Premature stimulation can produce slow propagation in the sinus node,

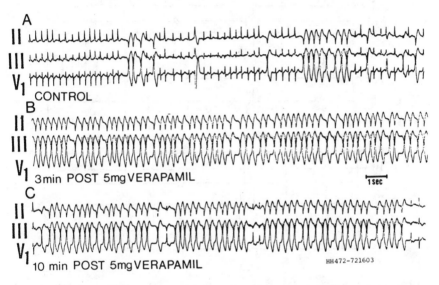

FIGURE 4. Effect of verapamil on ventricular activation during atrial fibrillation in a patient with Wolff-Parkinson-White syndrome. Tracings were recorded before and 3 and 10 minutes after verapamil administration. An increase in ventricular rate and an increased number of preexcited ventricular complexes occurred 3 minutes after verapamil administration. The effect diminished at 10 minutes. (From Rinkenberger et al.[31] Reproduced by permission.)

block in some areas, and the development of repetitive responses, most likely owing to reentry. Evidence from a number of studies in man [39-43] and animals [38, 44] supports the concept that sustained reentry in the sinus node can occur and cause SVT. Recently, Alessie and Bonke [44] showed that the reentrant circuit in the isolated rabbit preparation was located entirely within the sinus node and that the atrium was not an essential link.

Supraventricular tachycardias thought to be from sinus nodal reentry generally have a slower rate than SVTs from AV nodal reentry or rentry over an accessory pathway. P waves appear in front of the QRS complex and exhibit a contour similar to that of the P wave during sinus rhythm with the expected sequence of activation beginning in the upper right atrium and progressing caudally (FIG. 5).

The effects of verapamil in patients with SVT from sinus nodal reentry have not been investigated systematically. A recent study evaluating the effects of verapamil given intravenously in dogs suggested a possible differential response on the sinus and AV nodes.[45] Verapamil prolonged AV nodal conduction time and produced AV block at plasma concentrations that did not significantly alter the spontaneous discharge rate of the sinus node. Verapamil's effect on conduction within the sinus and AV nodes was not compared. Similar observations have been made in man.[46] When given after beta-adrenergic blockade, verapamil achieves more significant depression of sinus nodal auto-

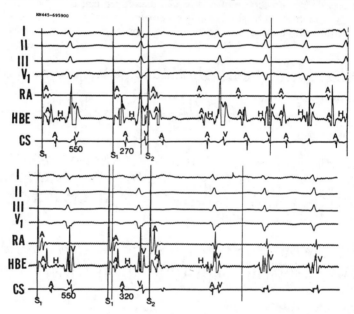

FIGURE 5. Initiation of AV nodal and sinoatrial nodal reentrant tachycardias. In the *top* panel, premature stimulation of the high right atrium at an S_1–S_2 interval of 270 msec initiated an atrial tachycardia with an activation sequence similar to that occurring during high right atrial pacing. In the *bottom* panel, premature stimulation of the right atrium at an S_1–S_2 interval of 320 msec resulted in a prolonged A-H interval and initiated AV nodal reentry. Retrograde low right atrial activation occurred before ventricular activation and was followed by the left (coronary sinus) and high right atrial activation. (From Rinkenberger *et al.*[31] Reproduced by permission.)

maticity. It is possible that reflex increased sympathetic tone prevents verapamil, when given alone intravenously, from significantly altering sinus nodal automaticity.[47]

Curry and Krikler[43] found that verapamil promptly terminated SVT from sinus nodal reentry in two patients and prevented reinitiation of the tachycardia in five. We have given verapamil in two patients with SVT from AV nodal reentry.[31] Two patients—one before and the other after verapamil administration—also exhibited an SVT from sinus nodal reentry. In both patients, the SVT from sinus nodal reentry persisted for several minutes after verapamil had terminated the AV nodal reentrant SVT. It would appear that the sinus nodal reentrant SVT resisted the suppressing effects of verapamil (10 mg intravenously) more than did the AV nodal reentrant SVT. In fact, in the second patient, verapamil may have even caused the sinus nodal reentrant SVT, which could not be produced prior to verapamil administration, by causing partial conduction delay in the sinus node.

Sinus nodal reentrant SVT meets criteria 3 and 4 and is therefore considered to be dependent on the slow inward current.

ATRIAL REENTRY

Reentry within the atrium, unrelated to the sinus node, has been shown experimentally to occur in the rabbit [48-50] and dog [51] atrium, with or without an anatomic obstacle, and may be a cause of SVT in man. Examples of SVT purported to be due to atrial reentry have been cited,[41, 52, 53] but their relative infrequency in the literature suggests that it is not a commonly recognized cause of SVT in man. Atrial reentry differs from sinus nodal reentry by a P wave morphology and atrial sequence of activation unlike that found during sinus rhythm. Distinguishing atrial tachycardia owing to automaticity from atrial tachycardia sustained by reentry over very small areas (that is, microreentry) is very difficult, and therefore conclusions regarding electrophysiologic mechanisms of this SVT on the basis of presently available information must be accepted cautiously.

One can speculate that verapamil might terminate the SVT if the latter were due to reentry over atrial fibers possibly altered by disease to be slow-channel-dependent. However, to our knowledge, no available information exists regarding the clinical effects of verapamil on SVT from atrial reentry. In experimentally induced reentrant atrial tachycardia in the rabbit, verapamil exerted no significant effects.[54]

The clinical importance of reentry in the atrium, unrelated to the sinus node, as a cause of SVT is presently unknown, as is the role of the slow channel in its initiation or maintenance.

AUTOMATIC ATRIAL TACHYCARDIA

Several types of atrial fibers possess the capacity for spontaneous diastolic depolarization.[55, 56] When enhanced, this spontaneous diastolic depolarization could be responsible for SVT in some patients. Of interest has been the demonstration that fibers in the rabbit,[57] canine,[58] simian,[59] and human [60] atrioventricular valves, and in the canine coronary sinus,[61] when superfused with norepinephrine, exhibit the capacity for triggered sustained rhythmic activity.[62] In general, the fibers exhibited delayed afterhyperpolarizations, followed by delayed afterdepolarizations that were capable of reaching threshold and triggering sustained rhythmic activity.[63] Action potentials of the mitral valve possessed less negative resting potentials and slower upstrokes than did action potentials in the coronary sinus and more clearly resembled the slow-response kind of action potential.[59] Verapamil suppressed the triggered activity in these preparations, and it is possible that the slow inward current played a role in their genesis. However, the membrane potential of these fibers, particularly those in the coronary sinus, was not sufficiently depressed to have inactivated the fast response or to have activated the slow inward current.[8, 9]

Saito et al.[64] recorded oscillatory potentials and triggered sustained rhythmic activity in fibers of the upper pectinate muscle and in the pectinate muscle along the crista terminalis in the rabbit right atrium. Norepinephrine was not necessary to trigger the activity. A train of stimuli sometimes increased the rate of discharge of the spontaneous activity rather than suppressing it.[65] The effects of slow-channel blockers were not tested. Triggered activity can also be found in diseased human atrial myocardium.[66]

In man, SVTs interpreted to be automatic by a variety of criteria have been described,[52, 67, 68] but remain incompletely characterized. Their differentiation from other forms of SVT, such as sinus nodal reentry (if the P wave of the automatic atrial tachycardia resembles the sinus-initiated P wave) or atrial reentry (particularly if caused by microreentry), may be difficult. However, in view of the experimental findings of triggered activity from a variety of atrial fibers, including human mitral valve, it is possible that such triggered activity occurs in man.

We have performed electrophysiologic studies on three patients who exhibited SVT that met the previously established criteria for automaticity.[31] Overdrive suppression after a period of rapid pacing occurred in all patients; capture of the SVT by atrial pacing was not followed by a faster SVT rate when pacing was discontinued. Premature stimulation was not followed by shorter return cycles and the return cycle was inversely, not directly, related to the premature cycle. In all three patients, the SVT could not be initiated or terminated by premature or rapid atrial pacing. The SVT originated in the lower right atrial septum in one patient and in the high right atrium in two patients. Its origin in or near the tricuspid valve or coronary sinus could not be established. Two additional patients were treated with verapamil but did not undergo electrophysiologic study.

In our group of five patients, verapamil given intravenously (10 mg to one patient, 5 mg to two patients) resulted in AV nodal block with persistence of the SVT at an unchanged rate. Administered orally (480 mg/day) to the remaining two patients, verapamil also had no significant effect on the rate of atrial discharge during the SVT (FIG. 6).

The experimental observations of triggered activity in isolated preparations of the mitral valve, coronary sinus, and normal and diseased atria, with suppression by verapamil, suggest but do not prove that the slow inward current may play a role in the genesis of this triggered activity. However, the clinical information, though meager, at present does not support that conclusion, and none of the criteria implicating the slow inward current are applicable to the clinically occurring SVTs. Further data are necessary to delineate whether automaticity figures as an important cause of clinically occurring SVTs and whether they are slow-channel-dependent.

NONPAROXYSMAL ATRIOVENTRICULAR JUNCTIONAL TACHYCARDIA

Nonparoxysmal AV junctional tachycardia (NPJT) is often due to cardiac surgery, acute rheumatic heart disease, digitalis intoxication, or myocardial infarction.[69] Sometimes no cause can be determined and the patient may be otherwise healthy. Conversely, NPJT at very rapid rates has been described in four children, and was found to be a very serious SVT that was difficult to control.[70] The mechanism responsible for NPJT is generally assumed to be enhanced automaticity of the His bundle or a contiguous structure that possesses automatic activity. It is possible that NPJT originates in atrial fibers, without recognition of the latter's role in the scalar electrocardiogram or from invasive electrophysiologic studies, unless a careful search is made.[71] Wenckebach periods may occur, but the presence of exit block has not yet been demonstrated clinically, and the block may be in the AV node, with the origin of the NPJT proximal to the site of His bundle recording. From one interesting report of accelerated junctional escape beats came the observation of shorter junctional

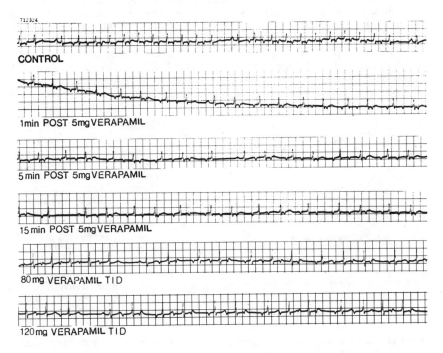

FIGURE 6. Effects of intravenous and oral verapamil in a patient who had an ectopic (presumed automatic) atrial tachycardia. Note that verapamil produced slight slowing of the discharge rate of the atrial tachycardia and caused primarily a reduction in the ventricular response.

escape intervals after premature atrial complexes, raising the possibility of overdrive acceleration in these fibers. Pacing studies and the effects of verapamil were not tested.[72]

Clinical information regarding the effects of verapamil on NPJT is negligible. Automaticity in the His bundle is generally thought to be similar to that found in Purkinje fibers and therefore not slow-channel-dependent. However, it is certainly possible that some of the interventions responsible for NPJT may create conditions in which the slow inward current is operative.

We conclude that although criterion 2 may be satisfied in one study, there are no other data at present indicating that the slow inward current plays a role in NPJT.

ATRIAL FLUTTER AND ATRIAL FIBRILLATION

Whether reentry, automaticity, or both factors are responsible for atrial fibrillation is still a debated issue.[73] Much evidence supports the role of reentry as a cause of atrial flutter,[74] but abnormal automaticity cannot be excluded (for review, see Boineau et al.).[51] Since sustained atrial flutter or atrial fibrillation occurs uncommonly in patients without heart disease, it is possible that the atria in these patients manifest abnormal electrophysiologic characteristics, some of which may be consistent with slow-channel-dependent action potentials.[66] At present, however, insufficient data prevent any definite conclusions.

Verapamil reportedly converts to sinus rhythm approximately 30% of episodes of atrial flutter and 16% of episodes of atrial fibrillation.[75] These may be optimistic figures. In our own series of 12 patients with atrial fibrillation, two developed sinus rhythm at a time (2 and 5 hours, respectively, after drug administration) beyond intravenous verapamil's peak drug effect, raising questions about causality. The two patients with atrial flutter whom we treated with verapamil developed atrial fibrillation, and one patient transiently had

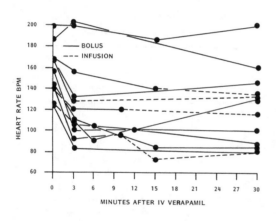

FIGURE 7. Response of atrial fibrillation after intravenous verapamil. The heart rate in beats/minute (ordinate) is plotted against time in minutes (abscissa). *Solid lines* indicate response after bolus injection and *dashes* indicate intravenous infusion. The mean ventricular response was reduced to 81.6% of control rate at 3 minutes ($p < 0.01$). After maximal response, the ventricular rate tends to increase slightly. (From Rinkenberger et al.[31] Reproduced by permission.)

sinus rhythm. The consistent effect of verapamil in patients with atrial flutter or atrial fibrillation was a prompt decrease in the ventricular response, lasting at least 30 minutes [31] (FIG. 7).

In some patients with atrial flutter or atrial fibrillation, the slow response may play a role in the genesis and maintenance of the arrhythmias. However, that conclusion is based on consideration of *in vitro* observations of transmembrane potentials recorded from diseased human atrial fibers.[66] No clinical information is available to support the importance of the slow inward current in these SVTs and none of the four criteria can be satisfied at present.

VENTRICULAR TACHYCARDIA

Experimental Observations

Electrical activity due to the slow inward current has been demonstrated in a variety of experimental preparations of ventricular and cardiac Purkinje fibers in which the rapid inward current is blocked or absent. Such conditions can be produced by perfusing or superfusing the preparation with solutions that contain elevated external potassium concentration or tetrodotoxin, or solutions that have no sodium or by reducing the resting potential of the fiber with current passage. Also, measures that increase the slow inward current, such as elevation of extracellular calcium concentration, addition of catecholamines, histamine, xanthine derivatives, or fluoride, or measures that decrease the outward current, such as the use of tetraethylammonium chloride or chloride-free media, contribute to the development of potentials that are slow-channel-dependent.[76, 77]

The slow inward current can also be responsible for pacemaker activity in cardiac Purkinje or ventricular muscle fibers by depolarizing the fibers with current passage, by inhibiting or blocking the sodium electrogenic pump, or by applying external solutions containing low potassium concentration, low pH, barium, tetraethylammonium, or cesium. The oscillations maintained at reduced potentials are suppressed by slow-channel blockers, but not by tetrodotoxin or lidocaine.[76-78] Similar oscillatory activity has been noted recently in the subendocardium of rodents studied 24 hours after receiving 3 mg/kg epinephrine subcutaneously (FIG. 8).[79]

Afterdepolarizations and triggered activity have been found at high resting potentials in a variety of preparations, including those treated with digitalis glycosides (FIGS. 9 and 10).[80] The relationships of these afterdepolarizations to the slow inward current are not entirely clear. It may be that digitalis inhibition of sodium–potassium exchange results in an intracellular accumulation of sodium that is responsible for an increase in intracellular calcium. The latter may then increase the conductance of the channel responsible for the afterdepolarization, which appears to be carried mostly by sodium.[81]

The electrophysiologic consequences of myocardial ischemia have been studied for many years.[82] Because ischemia results in a large increase in extracellular potassium concentration, as well as a release of catecholamines, it was hypothesized that these conditions could result in electrical activity due to the slow response.[8] To test the hypothesis, we administered verapamil to dogs prior to coronary arterial occlusion and found that the extent of ischemia-induced conduction delay (FIG. 11) and prevalence of cardiac arrhythmias were reduced.[83] This was an unexpected finding, considering that verapamil should have suppressed activity due to the slow response and possibly increased the extent of ischemia-induced conduction delay or suppressed entirely conduction in the ischemic zone. Depending on the degree of depressed conduction, the prevalence of ventricular arrhythmias could increase or decrease. Protection against ischemia-induced ventricular fibrillation has been found in other studies as well.[84-87] Of interest, the (−) isomer of verapamil appeared to be more effective than the (+) isomer.[86]

Conflicting data have been reported. In one study, verapamil given *after* coronary arterial occlusion resulted in increased conduction delay.[88] In that study, however, it cannot be established whether verapamil reached the ischemic zone in physiologic concentrations, since drugs given after coronary arterial occlusion reach a low concentration in the ischemic zone.[89]

Verapamil has been shown to mitigate ischemic-induced conduction delay and fragmentation of electrograms recorded with composite electrodes in dogs several days after coronary arterial occlusion. Tetrodotoxin produced marked suppression of depressed cells recorded in ventricular epicardium removed from

FIGURE 8A. Patterns of initiation of spontaneously occurring sustained irregular rhythmic activity in rat myocardium 24 hours after epinephrine injection. The bursts in panels A–F are depicted sequentially and occurred over approximately 2 hours; they were separated by periods of quiescence. Note regularization of initial action potential with time. (From Gilmour and Zipes.[79] Reproduced by permission.)

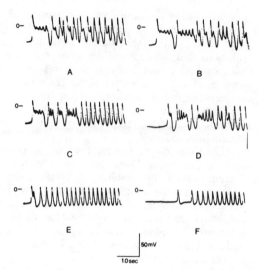

dogs several days after coronary arterial occlusion. In contrast, D600 improved electrical activity in these cells.[90]

Recently, we[91] studied transmembrane electrophysiologic properties of blood-perfused pieces of neonatal hamster atrial and ventricular myocardium transplanted to the adult hamster cheek pouch. Interrupting blood flow to spontaneously beating transplants reduced diastolic depolarization and suppressed automaticity. After automaticity ceased, the transplants were paced using a bipolar electrode or intracellular microelectrode. Action potential amplitude, resting potential, and dV/dt_{max} decreased during ischemia. Action potential duration and the intracellular current threshold for excitation increased initially, subsequently decreased to values less than control, and increased again prior to the onset of inexcitability. Conduction delay and block occurred during the later stages of ischemia. Depressed action potentials recorded during

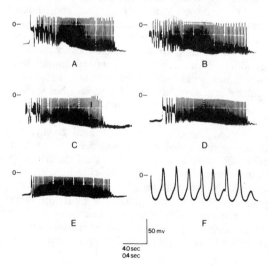

FIGURE 8B. Patterns of termination of spontaneously occurring sustained irregular rhythmic activity in rat myocardium 24 hours after epinephrine injection. Format is the same as in FIGURE 8A except that the terminating sequence of burst F has been omitted. Panel F illustrates, at an increased sweep speed, the terminating sequence of burst A. (From Gilmour and Zipes.[79] Reproduced by permission.)

ischemia were suppressed by tetrodotoxin (10^{-5} M) but not by verapamil (2×10^{-6} M). These data indicate that ischemia suppresses transplant automaticity, and that action potentials generated during ischemia appear to be depressed fast responses, rather than slow responses.

All of these experimental data suggest at present that the depressed fast response is responsible for the slow conduction that characterizes acute and subacute myocardial infarction. No data exist to support the role of the slow response in producing these early changes. Indeed, many of the metabolic alterations accompanying ischemia might be expected to suppress electrical activity due to the slow inward current.

Spear et al.[92] studied subendocardial specimens of human ventricular aneurysms resected from patients at the time of cardiac surgery. Both muscle and Purkinje fibers displayed automatic activity (at fairly slow rates), and the majority of the fibers exhibited characteristics consistent with the slow response.

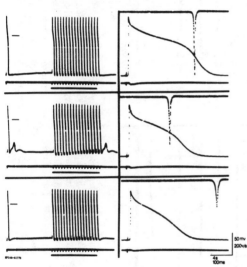

FIGURE 9. Effect of aprindine (3×10^{-6} M) on transient depolarizations induced by acetylstrophanthidin (1.7×10^{-7} M). From *top to bottom*, the traces of each panel in the **left** column represent the transmembrane action potential, the bipolar electrogram, and the stimulation period (8 seconds) at a cycle length of 500 msec. In the **right** column, the traces represent (from *top to bottom*) the dV/dt of the upstroke, the transmembrane action potential, and the bipolar electrogram. *Upper panel:* control recording. *Middle panel:* after 32 minutes of superfusion with acetylstrophanthidin. *Lower panel:* 9 minutes after superfusion with aprindine. All recordings were obtained from the same impalement. (From Elharrar et al.[120] Reproduced by permission.)

Some action potentials could be suppressed by verapamil and enhanced by increasing extracellular calcium concentration and were not suppressed by tetrodotoxin. Triggered activity was not seen in any preparation. Marked heterogeneity of electrical characteristics was noted and could provide an appropriate substrate for arrhythmias to develop. However, from these studies, the authors could not establish that the slow response recorded *in vitro* played any role in the genesis of ventricular tachyarrhythmias in these patients.

Clinical Observations

While it is quite clear from the foregoing data that the slow response can be created and demonstrated in a variety of experimental preparations of ventricular fibers, it is not at all clear whether the slow response can be related

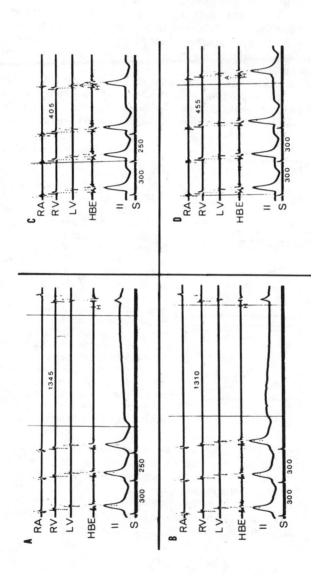

FIGURE 10. Ouabain-induced repetitive ventricular responses. Panels **A** and **B**, control; panels **C** and **D**, after ouabain administration. Stimuli delivered to right atrium and ventricle simultaneously. Basic cycle length, 300 msec; premature stimulus interval, 250 msec. Last three stimuli for each period of pacing are depicted. In panels **A** and **C**, the heart was paced for 8 cycles at 300 msec and then a premature stimulus was introduced at 250 msec. In panels **B** and **D**, the heart was paced for 8 cycles at 300 msec with sudden termination of pacing. In the control state, a supraventricular escape beat initiated by discharge in or near the His bundle followed cessation of pacing (H-V interval 35 msec). After ouabain administration, a repetitive ventricular response followed termination of pacing (His activation begins after onset of ventricular activation). (From Foster *et al.*[12] Reproduced by permission.)

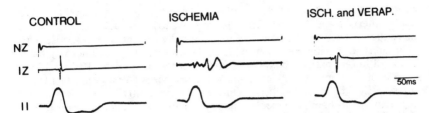

FIGURE 11A. Effect of verapamil on the fractionation of the epicardial electrogram recorded in the ischemic zone after 5 minutes of occlusion of the left anterior descending coronary artery during pacing at a cycle length of 500 msec. *Left panel,* before coronary occlusion; *center and right* panels, 5 minutes after coronary occlusion, before (*center*) and 11 minutes after (*right*) administration of verapamil. Note that verapamil (*right*) prevented the fractionation recorded from the ischemic zone (*center*). (From Elharrar et al.[53] Reproduced by permission.)

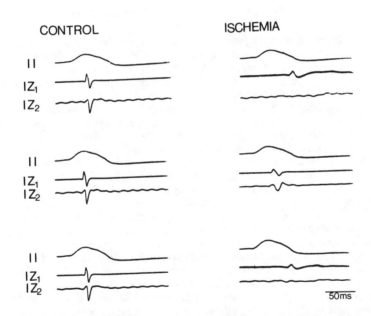

FIGURE 11B. Effects of verapamil on ischemia-induced conduction delay. IZ_1 and IZ_2 are two epicardial bipolar electrograms obtained from the ischemic zone during pacing at the base of the right ventricle at a cycle length of 500 msec. The *left* and *right* panels were obtained before 5 minutes after coronary occlusion (A), before, (B) 11 minutes after, and (C) 47 minutes after administration of verapamil (0.2 mg/kg). Note that 11 minutes after administration of verapamil, the extent of conduction delay at IZ_1 and IZ_2 was less than either before or 47 minutes after verapamil administration. (From Elharrar et al.[53] Reproduced by permission.)

causally to the genesis of ventricular tachyarrhythmias in man. One cannot apply criteria 1 and 3, cited earlier for supraventricular tachyarrhythmias, since there are no fibers in the ventricle that normally exhibit slow response activity. A response to pacing consistent with the behavior of triggered activity has been reported in one patient, possibly satisfying criterion 2 (FIGS. 12 and 13).[93]

Finally, we are left with criterion 4, the response of ventricular tachyarrhythmias to slow-channel blockers. Only a few noncontrolled studies have been reported on a small number of patients, and the data are inconclusive.[94-98] Generally, verapamil has not been very effective in terminating ventricular tachycardia. In an electrophysiologic study of ventricular tachycardia, Wellens[99] demonstrated recently that verapamil terminated ventricular tachycardia that was initiated by programmed stimulation in only one of eight patients tested.

Thus, preliminary data suggest that the slow response may not be important in the genesis of ventricular tachyarrhythmias in man and that the slow-channel blockers may not be as effective in treating ventricular tachyarrhythmias as they are in treating supraventricular tachyarrhythmias. If this is so, how then, can slow-channel blockers affect sudden cardiac death that is, in most instances, the result of ventricular fibrillation?

PREVENTION OF SUDDEN CARDIAC DEATH

Although death rates from ischemic heart disease appear to be decreasing for unknown reasons in some parts of the world, sudden cardiac death remains the most pressing contemporary health problem facing modern industrialized nations. Three-fourths of survivors of ventricular fibrillation have significant coronary arterial obstruction, implicating myocardial ischemia as a cause.[100] Sudden cardiac death also occurs in association with congestive and hypertrophic cardiomyopathies, mitral valve prolapse, long Q-T syndrome, valvular disease, bundle branch block, and Wolff-Parkinson-White syndrome. Some patients who die suddenly have no evidence of organic heart disease.

Several recent reviews have examined this multifaceted problem. The weight of evidence incriminates ventricular fibrillation as the mechanism[101] responsible for most sudden cardiac deaths. Experimentally, ventricular fibrillation may result after coronary arterial occlusion, as well as on release of the occlusion. In man, it is possible that relaxation of coronary spasm, lysis of thrombus, dispersion of platelet thrombi, or other events that restore coronary flow may result in ventricular fibrillation without myocardial infarction.

Assuming that the patient at risk of developing sudden cardiac death can be identified, by one means or another, what therapeutic measures can be used to prevent ventricular fibrillation from occurring?[102] Since most of these patients have complex ventricular arrhythmias and since ventricular fibrillation is the most likely cause of sudden death, the most obvious approach has been to treat susceptible patients with antiarrhythmic drugs. In this regard, procainamide, phenytoin, and aprindine have been tried and have been found not to reduce the incidence of sudden death, although aprindine decreased the prevalence of ventricular arrhythmias in the treated group.[103] The beta-adrenergic blocking agents, practolol and alprenolol, and the platelet inhibitor, sulfinpyrazone, have been reported to reduce the incidence of sudden death after acute myocardial infarction. However, practolol has been withdrawn

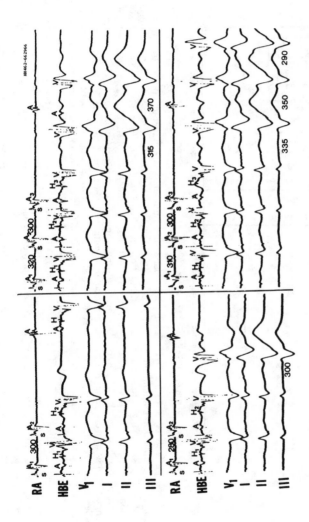

FIGURE 12. Initiation of premature ventricular complexes by premature atrial stimulation. Only the last stimulus of a train at a basic cycle length of 450 msec is displayed. Premature atrial stimulation with a single stimulus at an A_1–A_2 interval of 300 msec resulted in an H_1–H_2 interval of 330 msec and was not followed by a premature ventricular complex (*top left*). Premature atrial stimulation at an A_1–A_2 interval of 280 msec resulted in an H_1–H_2 interval of 320 msec and was followed by a single premature ventricular complex (*bottom left*). Premature atrial stimulation at an A_1–A_2 interval of 320 msec and an A_2–A_3 interval of 300 msec resulted in an H_1–H_2 interval of 340 msec and an H_2–H_3 interval of 315 msec and was followed by two premature ventricular complexes (*top right*). Premature stimulation at an A_1–A_2 interval of 310 msec and an A_2–A_3 interval of 300 msec resulted in an H_1–H_2 interval of 330 msec and an H_2–H_3 interval of 315 msec and was followed by three premature ventricular complexes (*bottom right*). (From Zipes *et al.*[93] Reproduced by permission.)

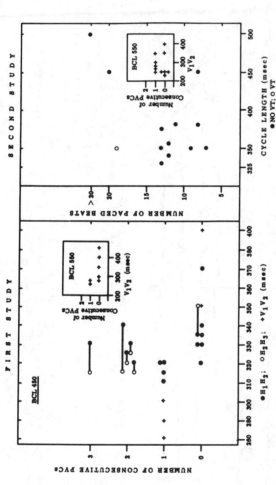

FIGURE 13. Same patient as in FIGURE 12. In the **left panel**, the number of spontaneous consecutive premature ventricular complexes that followed premature stimulation (Y axis) is plotted against the premature interval (X axis) during pacing at a basic cycle length of 450 msec. Single premature atrial stimulation resulted in H_1-H_2 intervals (*solid circles*) during pacing at a basic cycle length of 450 msec. Single premature atrial stimulation resulted in H_1-H_2 intervals (*solid circles*) and H_2-H_3 intervals (*open circles*) connected by straight lines. The atria were paced at the basic cycle length of 450 msec during premature atrial stimulation. The ventricles were paced at a basic cycle length of 450 msec during premature ventricular stimulation. For the latter, the V_1-V_2 interval is indicated by a cross. The *inset* indicates the results after premature ventricular stimulation during pacing at a basic cycle length of 550 msec. During atrial pacing at a basic cycle length of 550 msec, premature atrial stimulation did not induce any spontaneous premature ventricular complexes (not shown). In the **right panel** are displayed the data obtained during the second study, while the patient was receiving propranolol. Two testing methods were used. In the first, the ventricles were paced without premature stimulation at a fixed cycle length (X axis) for a variable number of cycles (Y axis). Ventricular tachycardia (*open circle*) only followed when the ventricle was paced at a cycle length of 350 msec for 19 cycles. In the second method, the ventricles were prematurely stimulated after a train of eight paced beats. The *inset* indicates the response to premature ventricular stimulation during ventricular pacing at a cycle length of 550 msec. The V_1-V_2 interval is indicated on the X axis and the number of spontaneous consecutive premature ventricular complexes is indicated on the Y axis. (From Zipes *et al.*[13] Reproduced by permission.)

from clinical use due to side effects; alprenolol is not available in the United States; and the results of the sulfinpyrazone study are being questioned. The effects these drugs exerted on ventricular arrhythmias were not assessed. The role of propranolol in preventing sudden death after myocardial infarction is currently being investigated in a large cooperative study supported by the National Institutes of Health. While the results from the practolol and alprenolol studies are encouraging, it is important to remember that left ventricular dysfunction is a significant risk factor for sudden cardiac death after myocardial infarction, making treatment with beta-adrenergic blocking drugs limited in many of those patients at high risk. Most recently, the beta-adrenergic blocking drug timolol [104] has been shown to reduce mortality and reinfarction in patients surviving acute myocardial infarction.

A recent report suggested that in survivors of out-of-hospital cardiac arrest, quinidine and procainamide, in dosages tailored specifically to maintain therapeutic plasma levels, protected against recurrent cardiac arrest without significantly reducing the frequency of complex ventricular arrhythmias, compared with results in a group that did not have therapeutic plasma levels of the drug. The provocative data from this study [105] are inconclusive and need to be confirmed in large numbers of patients.

Sudden cardiac death appears to be a multifactorial event. Most importantly, the extent of left ventricular dysfunction directly and independently correlates with risk of subsequent sudden cardiac death.[103] Appropriate treatment of congestive heart failure, for example, may be a very important antiarrhythmic approach, as may be the use of antiischemic agents. It may be naïve to think that one drug will suppress all episodes of ventricular fibrillation. For example, if the electrophysiologic mechanisms causing occlusion–fibrillation and release–fibrillation are different, and it is likely that they are, different antiarrhythmic agents may be more effective for one event than for the other. Similarly, fibrillation beginning after an episode of rapid ventricular tachycardia may be electrophysiologically different from fibrillation that begins after just several premature ventricular complexes, and it may respond to different drugs.

However, if ischemia is the common denominator of the various electrophysiologic mechanisms responsible for ventricular fibrillation, then prevention of, or reduction in the extent of, myocardial ischemia could be antiarrhythmic. Slow-channel blockers have been shown to improve blood flow to ischemic zones [106, 107] and to reduce the extent of myocardial damage,[108–110] contractile impairment,[111, 112] and prevalence of arrhythmias after coronary arterial occlusion in animals.[84–87] They also prevent catecholamine-induced myocardial damage [113] and ventricular arrhythmias related to hydrocarbon–epinephrine sensitization [84] that could be a cause of arrhythmias in some instances. Slow-channel blockers produce coronary vasodilation [23, 114] and prevent coronary vasospasm,[115] actions that could certainly prevent ischemic-related arrhythmias. Whether slow-channel blockers prevent reperfusion ventricular arrhythmias has not been unequivocally established.[109, 116, 117] Finally, unlike beta-adrenergic blockers that may be contraindicated in patients who have congestive heart failure—the very patients at great risk of dying suddenly—it is possible that the slow-channel blockers can be given safely to this group of patients because of potentially beneficial, or at least not significantly adverse, hemodynamic effects.[118] Other effects on myocardial metabolism, contractility, platelet function, and several other factors could be important.[23]

In conclusion, the existing data suggest numerous reasons why slow-channel blockers might play a critically important role in reducing sudden cardiac death from ischemic heart disease and possibly from other etiologic factors as well. This is a testable hypothesis that should and probably will be explored in the near future. The data suggest that the drug should be given prophylactically since it may not be as effective when given after coronary arterial occlusion.[119] Finally, if verapamil is used, it might be preferable to treat with the (−) isomer. It is possible that verapamil or diltiazem is preferable to nifedipine in order to modulate AV nodal conduction, should a supraventricular tachycardia occur.

REFERENCES

1. HODKGIN, A. L. & B. KATZ. 1949. Ionic current underlying activity in the giant axon of the squid. J. Physiol. (London) **108:** 37.
2. HODKIN, A. L. & A. F. HUXLEY. 1952. A quantitative description of membrane current and its application to conduction and excitation in nerve. J. Physiol. (London) **117:** 500.
3. NOBLE, D. 1962. A modification of the Hodgkin-Huxley equations to Purkinje fibre action and pacemaker potentials. J. Physiol. (London). **160:** 317.
4. CORABOEUF, E. & M. OTSUKA. 1956. L'action des solutions hyposodiques sur les potentials cellulaires de tissu cardiaque de mammiferes. C. R. Acad. Sci. **243:** 441.
5. WEIDMANN, S. 1974. Heart: Electrophysiology. Annu. Rev. Physiol. **36:** 155.
6. TRAUTWEIN, W. 1973. Membrane currents in cardiac muscle fibers. Physiol. Rev. **53:** 793.
7. REUTER, H. 1973. Divalent cations as charge carriers in excitable membranes. Prog. Biophys. Mol. Biol. **26:** 1.
8. CRANEFIELD, P. F. 1975. The Conduction of the Cardiac Impulse. Futura Publishing Company. Mount Kisco, NY.
9. ZIPES, D. P., J. C. BAiLEY & V. ELHARRAR, Eds. 1980. The Slow Inward Current and Cardiac Arrhythmias. Martinus Nijhoff. The Hague.
10. NEIDERGERKE, R. & R. K. ORKAND. 1966. The dependence of the action potential of the frog's heart on the external and intracellular sodium concentration. J. Physiol. (London) **184:** 312.
11. HAGIWARA, S. & S. NAKAJIMA. 1966. Differences in Na and Ca spikes as examined by application of tetrodotoxin, procaine and manganese ions. J. Gen. Physiol. **49:** 793.
12. REUTER, H. 1967. The dependence of slow inward current in Purkinje fibres on the extracellular calcium concentration. J. Physiol. (London) **192:** 479.
13. ENGSTFELD, G., H. ANTONI & A. FLECKENSTEIN. 1961. Die Restitution der Erregungsfortleitung und Kontraktionskraft des K+- gelahmten Frosch und Saugertiermyokards durch Adrenalin. Pfluegers Arch. **273:** 145.
14. CARMELIET, E. & J. VEREECKE. 1969. Adrenaline and the plateau phase of the cardiac action potential. Importance of Ca^{++}, Na^+ and K^+ conductance. Pfluegers Arch. **313:** 300.
15. NARAHASHI, T., J. W. MOORE & W. SCOTT. 1964. Tetrodotoxin blockade of sodium conductance increase in lobster giant axons. J. Gen. Physiol. **47:** 965.
16. PAPPANO, A. J. 1970. Calcium-dependent action potentials produced by catecholamines in guinea pig atrial muscle fibers depolarized by potassium. Circ. Res. **27:** 379.
17. THYRUM, P. 1974. Inotropic stimuli and systolic transmembrane calcium flow in depolarized guinea pig atria. J. Pharmacol. Exp. Ther. **188:** 166.

18. WATANABE, A. M. & H. R. BESCH, JR. 1974. Cyclic adenosine monophosphate modulation of slow calcium influx channels in guinea pig
hearts. Circ. Res. **35:** 316.
19. WATANABE, A. M. & H. R. BESCH, JR. 1974. Subcellular myocardial effects
of verapamil and D600: Comparison with propranolol. J. Pharmacol Exp.
Ther. **191:** 241.
20. CRANEFIELD, P. F. & B. F. HOFFMAN. 1971. Conduction of the cardiac
impulse: II. Summation and inhibition. Circ. Res. **28:** 220.
21. CRANEFIELD, P. F., A. L. WIT & B. F. HOFFMAN. 1972. Conduction of the
cardiac impulse. III. Characteristics of very slow conduction. J. Gen.
Physiol. **59:** 227.
22. FLECKENSTEIN, A. 1971. Specific inhibitors and promoters of calcium action
in the excitation-contraction coupling of heart muscle and their role in
the prevention or production of myocardial lesions. *In* Calcium and the
Heart. Academic Press. NY.
23. ANTMAN, E. M., P. H. STONE, J. E. MUELLER & E. BRAUNWALD. 1980.
Calcium channel blocking agents in the treatment of cardiovascular disorders. Ann. Intern Med. **93:** 875–904.
24. ZIPES, D. P. & C. MENDEZ. 1973. Action of manganese ions and tetrodotoxin
on AV nodal transmembrane potentials in isolated rabbit hearts. Circ. Res.
32: 447–454.
25. GARVEY, H. L. 1969. The mechanism of action of verapamil on the sinus
and AV nodes. Eur. J. Pharmacol. **8:** 159–166.
26. ZIPES, D. P. & J. C. FISCHER. 1974. Effects of agents which inhibit the
slow channel on sinus node automaticity and atrioventricular conduction in
the dog. Circ. Res. **34:** 184–192.
27. WIT, A. L. & P. F. CRANEFIELD. 1974. Effect of verapamil on the sinoatrial
and atrioventricular nodes of the rabbit and the mechanism by which it
arrests reentrant atrioventricular nodal tachycardia. Circ. Res. **35:** 413.
28. BRICHARD, G. & P. E. ZIMMERMAN. 1970. Verapamil and cardiac dysrhythmias during anesthesia. Br. J. Anaesth. **42:** 1005–1012.
29. ZIPES, D. P., H. R. BESCH & A. M. WATANABE. 1975. Role of the slow
current in cardiac electrophysiology. Circulation **51:** 761–766.
30. WELLENS, H. J. J., S. L. TAN, F. W. H. BAR, D. R. DUREN, K. I. LIE & H. M.
DOHMER. 1977. Effect of verapamil studied by programmed electrical
stimulation of the heart in patients with paroxysmal reentrant supraventricular tachycardia. Br. Heart J. **39:** 1058–1066.
31. RINKENBERGER, R. L., D. P. ZIPES, P. J. TROUP, W. M. JACKMAN & E. N.
PRYSTOWSKY. 1980. Clinical and electrophysiologic effects of intravenous
and oral verapamil in patients with supraventricular tachyarrhythmias.
Circulation **62:** 996–1010.
32. SCHAMROTH, L., D. M. KRIKLER & C. GARRETT. 1972. Immediate effects of
intravenous verapamil in cardiac arrhythmias. Br. Med. J. **1:** 660–662.
33. GOTSMAN, M. S., B. S. LOUIS, A. BAKST & A. S. MITHA. 1972. Verapamil
in life-threatening tachyarrhythmias. S. Afr. Med. J. **46:** 2017–2019.
34. GOMES, J. A. C., M. S. DHATT, D. S. RUBENSON & A. N. DAMATO. 1979.
Electrophysiologic evidence for selective retrograde utilization of a specialized conducting system in atrioventricular nodal reentrant tachycardia.
Am. J. Cardiol. **43:** 687–698.
35. SUNG, R. J., B. ELSER & R. G. MCCALLISTER. 1980. Intravenous verapamil
for termination of reentrant supraventricular tachycardias. Ann. Int. Med.
93: 682–689.
36. GALLAGHER, J. J., E. L. C. PRITCHETT, W. C. SEALY, J. CASELL & A. G.
WALLACE. 1978. The pre-excitation syndromes. Prog. Cardiovasc. Dis. **20:**
285–327.
37. PRYSTOWSKY, E. N., E. L. C. PRITCHETT, W. M. SMITH, A. G. WALLACE, W. C.

SEALY & J. J. GALLAGHER. 1979. Electrophysiologic assessment of the atrioventricular conduction system after surgical correction of ventricular preexcitation. Circulation **59:** 789–796.

38. HAN, J., A. M. MALOZZI & G. K. MOE. 1968. Sinoatrial reciprocation in the isolated rabbit heart. Circ. Res. **22:** 355–362.

39. CHILDERS, R. W., M. F. ARNSDORF, D. deLAFUENTE, M. GAMBETA & R. SVENSON. 1973. Sinus node reentry: Clinical case report and canine studies. Am. J. Cardiol. **31:** 220–231.

40. NARULA, O. S. 1974. A mechanism for supraventricular tachycardia. Circulation **50:** 1114–1128.

41. WU, D., F. AMAT-y-LEON, P. DENES, R. C. DHINGRA, R. J. PIETRAS & K. M. ROSEN. 1975. Demonstration of sustained sinus and atrial reentry as a mechanism of paroxysmal supraventricular tachycardia. Circulation **51:** 234–243.

42. WEISFOGEL, G. M., W. P. BATSFORD, K. L. PAULAY, M. E. JOSEPHSON, J. B. OGUNKELU, M. AKHTAR, S. F. SEIBES & A. N. DAMATO. 1975. Sinus node reentrant tachycardia in man. Am. Heart J. **90:** 295–304.

43. CURRY, P. V. L. & D. M. KRIKLER. 1977. Paroxysmal reciprocating sinus tachycardia. In Reentrant Arrhythmias. H. E. Kulbertus, Ed.: 39–62. University Park Press. Baltimore, MD.

44. ALLESSI, M. A. & F. I. M. BONKE. 1979. Direct demonstration of sinus node reentry in the rabbit heart. Circ. Res. **44:** 557–568.

45. MANGIARDIL, M., R. J. HARIMAN, R. G. McALLISTER, V. BHARGAVA, B. SURAWICZ & R. SHABETAI. 1978. Electrophysiologic and hemodynamic effects of verapamil. Correlation with plasma drug concentrations. Circulation **57:** 366–372.

46. CARRASCO, H. A., A. FUENMAYOR, J. S. BARBOZA & G. GONZALEZ. 1978. Effect of verapamil on normal sinoatrial node function and on sick sinus syndrome. Am. Heart J. **96:** 760–771.

47. BREITHARDT, G., L. SEIPEL & E. WIEBRINGHAUS. 1978. Dual effect of verapamil on sinus node function in man. In The Sinus Node. Bonke F.I.M., Ed.: 129–138. Martin Nijhoff. The Hague.

48. ALLESSIE, M. A., F. I. M. BONKE & F. J. G. SCHOPMAN. 1973. Circus movement in rabbit atrial muscle as in mechanism of tachycardia. Circ. Res. **33:** 54–62.

49. ALLESSIE, M. A., F. I. M. BONKE, & F. J. G. SCHOPMAN. 1976. Circus movement in rabbit atrial muscle as a mechanism of tachycardia. The role of nonuniform excitability in the occurrence of unidirectional block, as studied with multiple microelectrodes. Circ. Res. **39:** 168–177.

50. ALLESSIE, M. A., F. I. M. BONKE & F. J. G. SCHOPMAN. 1977. Circus movement in rabbit atrial muscle as a mechanism of tachycardia. III. The 'leading circle' concept: A new model of circus movement in cardiac tissue without the involvement of an anatomical obstacle. Circ. Res. **41:** 9–18.

51. BOINEAU, J. P., C. R. MOONEY, R. D. HUDSON, D. G. HUGHES, R. A. ERDIN, JR. & A. C. WILDS. 1977. Observations on reentrant excitation pathways and the refractory period distributions in spontaneous and experimental atrial flutter in the dog. In Reentrant Arrhythmias. H. E. Kulbertus, Ed.: 72–98. University Park Press. Baltimore, MD.

52. WU, D., P. DENES, R. BAUERNFEIN, R. KEHOE, F. AMAT-y-LEON & K. M. ROSEN. 1978. Effects of procainamide on atrioventricular nodal reentrant paroxysmal tachycardia. Circulation **57:** 1171–1179.

53. COUMEL, P., D. FLAMMANG, P. ATTUEL & J. F. LECKERCQ. 1979. Sustained intra-atrial reentrant tachycardia. Electrophysiologic study of 20 cases. Clin. Cardiol. **2:** 176–178.

54. ALLESSIE, M. A., F. I. M. BONKE & W. J. E. P. LAMMERS. 1977. The effects of carbamylcholine, adrenaline, ouabain, quinidine and verapamil on circus

movement tachycardia in isolated segments of rabbit atrial myocardium. *In* Reentrant Arrhythmias. H. E. Kulbertus, Ed.: 63–71. University Park Press. Baltimore, MD.

55. PAES DECARVALHO, A., W. C. DEMELLO & B. F. HOFFMAN. 1959. Electrophysiologic evidence for specialized fiber types in rabbit atrium. Am. J. Physiol. **196:** 483–488.

56. HOGAN, P. M. & L. D. DAVIS. 1971. Electrophysiological characteristics of canine atrial plateau fibers. Circ. Res. **28:** 62–73.

57. MAKARYCHEU, V. A., I. L. KOSHARSKAYA & L. S. ULYNINSKY. 1976. Automatic activity of the pacemaker cells of the atrioventricular valves in the rabbit heart. Biul. Eksp. Biol. Med. **81:** 646–649.

58. BASSETT, A. L., J. J. FENOGLIO, JR., A. L. WIT, R. J. MYERBURG & H. GELBAND. 1976. Electrophysiological and ultra structural characteristics of the canine tricuspid valve. Am. J. Physiol. **230:** 1366–1373.

59. WIT, A. L. & P. F. CRANEFIELD. 1976. Triggered activity in cardiac muscle fibers of the simian mitral valve. Circ. Res. **38:** 85–98.

60. WIT, A. L., J. J. FENOGLIO, A. J. HORDOFF & K. REEMTSMA. 1979. Ultrastructure and transmembrane potentials of cardiac muscle in the human anterior mitral valve leaflet. Circulation **59:** 1284–1292.

61. WIT, A. L. & P. F. CRANEFIELD. 1977. Triggered and automatic activity in the canine coronary sinus. Circ. Res. **41:** 435–445.

62. CRANEFIELD, P. F. & R. S. ARONSON. 1974. Initiation of sustained rhythmic activity by single propagated action potentials in canine cardiac Purkinje fibers exposed to sodium-free solution or to ouabain. Circ. Res. **34:** 477–481.

63. CRANEFIELD, P. F. 1977. Action potentials and arrhythmias. Circ. Res. **41:** 415–423.

64. SAITO, T., M. OTOGURO & T. MATSUBARA. 1978. Electrophysiological studies on the mechanism of electrically induced sustained rhythmic activity in rabbit right atrium. Circ. Res. **42:** 199–206.

65. VASSALLE, E. M., N. COMMINS, C. CASTRO & J. H. STUCKEY. 1976. The relationship between overdrive suppression and overdrive excitation in ventricular pacemaker in dogs. Circ. Res. **38:** 367–374.

66. ROSEN, M. R. & A. J. HORDOF. 1980. The slow response in human atrium. *In* Zipes *et al.*[9] : 295–308.

67. GOLDREYER, B. N., J. J. GALLAGHER & A. N. DAMATO. 1973. The electrophysiologic demonstration of atrial ectopic tachycardia in man. Am. Heart J. **85:** 205–215.

68. WYNDAM, C. R., M. F. ARNSDORF, S. LEVITSKY, T. C. SMITH, R. C. DHINGRA, P. DENES & K. M. ROSEN. 1980. Successful surgical excision of focal paroxysmal atrial tachycardia. Circulation **62:** 1365–1372.

69. PICK, A. & P. DOMINGUEZ. 1957. Nonparoxysmal AV nodal tachycardia. Circulation **16:** 1022–1032.

70. GARDON, A. & P. C. GILLETTE. 1979. Junctional ectopic tachycardia in children: Electrocardiography, electrophysiology and pharmacologic response. Am. J. Cardiol. **44:** 298–302.

71. ZIPES, D. P., W. E. GAUM, B. C. GENETOS, R. D. GLASSMAN, R. J. NOBLE & C. FISCH. 1977. Atrial tachycardia without P waves masquerading as an AV junctional tachycardia. Circulation **55:** 253–260.

72. ROSEN, M. R., C. FISCH, B. F. HOFFMAN, P. DANILO, D. E. LOVELACE & S. B. KNOEBEL. 1980. Can atrioventricular junctional escape rhythms be explained by delayed after-depolarizations. Am. J. Cardiol. **45:** 1272–1284.

73. MOE, G. & J. A. ABILDSKOV. 1969. Atrial fibrillation as a self-sustaining arrhythmia independent of focal discharge. Am. Heart J. **58:** 59–70.

74. PASTELIN, G., R. MENDEZ & G. K. MOE. 1978. Participation of atrial specialized conduction pathways in atrial flutter. Circ. Res. **42:** 386–393.

75. ZIPES, D. P. & P. J. TROUP. 1978. New antiarrhythmic agents. Amiodarone,

aprindine, disopyramide, ethmozin, mexiletine, tocainide, verapamil. Am. J. Cardiol. **41:** 1005–1024.

76. CARMELIET, E. 1980. Non-voltage-clamp studies. *In* Zipes *et al.*[0]: 97–110.

77. SURAWICZ, B. 1980. Depolarization-induced automaticity in atrial and ventricular myocardial fibers. *In* Zipes *et al.*[0]: 375–396.

78. ELHARRAR, V. & D. P. ZIPES. 1980. Voltage modulation of automaticity in cardiac Purkinje fibers. *In* Zipes *et al.*[0]: 300–416.

79. GILMOUR, R. F., JR. & D. P. ZIPES. 1980. Electrophysiologic characteristics of rodent myocardium damaged by adrenaline. Cardiovasc. Res. **14:** 582–589.

80. ROSEN, M. R. & P. DANILO, JR. 1980. Digitalis-induced delayed afterdepolarizations. *In* Zipes *et al.*[0]: 417–435.

81. KASS, R. S., R. W. TSIEN & R. WEINGART. 1978. Ionic basis of transient inward current induced by strophanthidin in cardiac Purkinje fibers. J. Physiol (London) **281:** 209–226.

82. ELHARRAR, V. & D. P. ZIPES. 1977. Cardiac electrophysiologic alterations during myocardial ischemia. Am. J. Physiol. **233**(3): H239–H345.

83. ELHARRAR, V., W. E. GAUM & D. P. ZIPES. 1977. Effect of drugs on conduction delay and the incidence of ventricular arrhythmias induced by acute coronary occlusion in dogs. Am. J. Cardiol. **39:** 544–549.

84. SCHMID, J. R. & C. HANNA. 1967. A comparison of the antiarrhythmic actions of two new synthetic compounds, iproveratril and MJ1999, with quinidine and pronetholol. J. Pharmacol. Exp. Ther. **156:** 331–338.

85. KAUMANN, A. J. & P. ARAMENDIA. 1968. Prevention of ventricular fibrillation induced coronary ligation. J. Pharmacol. Exp. Ther. **164:** 326–332.

86. KAUMANN, A. J. & J. R. SERUR. 1975. Optical isomers of verapamil on canine heart. Naunyn Schmiedeberg's Arch. Pharmacol. **291:** 347–358.

87. FONDACARO, J. D., J. H. HAN & M. S. JOON. 1978. Effects of verapamil on ventricular rhythm during acute coronary occlusion. Am. Heart J. **96:** 81–86.

88. KUPERSMITH, J., H. SHIANG, R. S. LITWAK & M. V. HERMAN. 1976. Electrophysiologic effects of verapamil in canine myocardial ischemia. Am. J. Cardiol. **37:** 149A.

89. NATTEL, S., D. H. PEDERSEN & D. P ZIPES. 1981. Alterations in regional myocardial distribution and antiarrhythmic effects of aprindine produced by coronary artery occlusion in the dog. Cardiovasc. Res. **15:** 80–85.

90. LAZZARA, R. & B. J. SCHERLAG. 1980. Role of the slow current in the generation of arrhythmias in ischemic myocardium. *In* Zipes *et al.*[0]: 399–416.

91. GILMOUR, R. F., D. G. MORRICAL & D. P. ZIPES. 1979. Response of vascularized hamster cardiac allographs to ischemia (abstract). Circulation. **59 & 60** (Suppl. II): 111.

92. SPEAR, J. F., L. N. HOROWITZ & E. N. MOORE. 1980. The slow response in human ventricle. *In* Zipes *et al.*[0]: 309–326.

93. ZIPES, D. P., P. R. FOSTER, P. J. TROUP & D. H. PEDERSON. 1979. Atrial induction of ventricular tachycardia: Reentry versus triggered automaticity. Am. J. Cardiol. **44:** 1–8.

94. SCHAMROTH, L., D. M. KRICKLER & C. GARRETT. 1972. Immediate effects of intravenous verapamil—cardiac arrhythmias. Br. Med. J. **1:** 660–662.

95. FILIAS, N. 1974. Verapamil—Behandlung bei Herzrhythmusstörungen Schweiz. Rundschau. Med. **3:** 66–74.

96. SINGH, B. N., J. T. COLLETT & C. Y C.. CHEW. 1974. New perspectives in the pharmacologic therapy of cardiac arrhythmias. Prog. Cardiovasc. Dis. **22:** 243.

97. FAZZINI, P. F., F. MARCHI & P. PUCCI. 1978. Effects of verapamil on ventricular premature beats of acute myocardial infarction. Acta. Cardiol. **33:** 25–29.

98. PICKERING, T. G. & L. GOULDING. 1978. Suppression of ventricular extrasystole by perhexiline. Br. Heart J. **40:** 851–855.
99. WELLENS, H. J. J., J. FARRE & F. W. BÄR. 1980. The role of the slow inward current in the genesis of ventricular tachyarrhythmias in man. *In* Zipes *et al.*⁹: 507–514.
100. COBB, L. A., J. A. WERNER & G. B. TROBOUGH. 1980. Sudden cardiac death: I. A decade's experience with out-of-hospital resuscitation. Mod. Concepts Cardiovasc. Dis. **49:** 31–36. II. Outcome of resuscitation management and future directions. **49:** 37–42.
101. ZIPES, D. P. 1975. Electrophysiological mechanisms involved in ventricular fibrillation. Circulation **51** & **52**(Suppl. III): 120–130.
102. ZIPES, D. P., J. J. HEGER & E. N. PRYSTOWSKY. 1981. Sudden cardiac death. Am. J. Med. **70:** 1151–1154.
103. HEGER, J. J., E. N. PRYSTOWSKY & D. P. ZIPES. Clinical choice of antiarrhythmic drugs. *In* Ventricular Tachycardia—Mechanisms and Management. M. E. Josephson, Ed. Futura Publishing Company. Mount Kisco, NY. In press.
104. NORWEGIAN MULTICENTER STUDY GROUP. 1981. Timolol-induced reduction in mortality and reinfarction in patients surviving acute myocardial infarction. N. Engl. J. Med. **304:** 801.
105. MYERBURG, R. J., C. CONTE, D. S. SHEPS, R. A. APPEL, I. DIEM, R. J. SUNG & A. CASTELLANOS. 1979. Antiarrhythmic drug therapy in survivors of prehospital cardiac arrest: Comparison of effects on chronic ventricular arrhythmias and recurrent cardiac arrest. Circulation **59:** 855–863.
106. JOLLY, S. R. & G. J. GROSS. 1980. Improvement in ischemic myocardial blood flow following a new calcium antagonist. Am. J. Physiol. **239:** H163–H171.
107. NAKAMURA, M., Y. KIKUCHI, Y. SENDA, A. YAMADA & Y. KOIWAYA. 1980. Myocardial blood flow following experimental coronary occlusion. Effects of diltiazem. Chest **78:** 205–209.
108. SMITH, H. J., B. N. SINGH, H. D. NISBET & R. M. NORRIS. 1975. Effects of verapamil on infarct size following experimental coronary occlusion. Cardiovasc. Res. **9:** 569–578.
109. REIMER, K. A., J. E. LOWE & R. B. JENNINGS. 1977. Effect of calcium antagonist verapamil on necrosis following temporary coronary artery occlusion in dogs. Circulation **55:** 581–587.
110. NAYLER, W. G., R. FERRARI & A. WILLIAMS. 1980. Protective effect of pretreatment with verapamil, nifedipine and propranolol on mitochondrial function in the ischemic and reperfused myocardium. Am. J. Cardiol. **46:** 242–248.
111. PEREZ, J. E., B. E. SOBEL & P. D. HENRY. 1980. Improved performance of ischemic canine myocardium in response to nifedipine and diltiazem. Am. J. Physiol. **239:** H658–H663.
112. SHERMAN, L. G., C. LIANG, W. E. BODEN & W. B. HOOD. 1981. The effect of verapamil on mechanical performance of acutely ischemic and reperfused myocardium in the conscious dog. Circ. Res. **48:** 224–232.
113. FLECKENSTEIN, A. 1971. Specific inhibitors and promoters of calcium action in the excitation–contraction coupling of heart muscle and their role in the prevention or production of cardiac lesions. *In* Calcium and the Heart. P. Harris and L. H. Opie, Eds.: 135–188. Academic Press. New York, NY.
114. MELVILLE, K. I. & B. G. BENFEY. 1965. Coronary vasodilatory and cardiac adrenergic blocking effects of iproveratril. Can. J. Physiol. Pharmacol. **43:** 339–342.
115. MASERI, A. & S. CHIERCHIA. 1980. Coronary vasopasm in ischemic heart disease. Chest **78:** 210–215.
116. RIBEIRO, L. G., T. L. DEBAUCHE, T. A. BRANDON, L. A. REDUTO, P. R. MAROKO

& R. R. MILLER. 1979. Verapamil and nifedipine during coronary artery reperfusion: Effects on ventricular arrhythmias and regional myocardial blood blow. Clin. Res. **27:** 773A.

117. NAITO, M., J. J. KMETZO & L. S. DREIFUS. 1979. Prevention of reperfusion-induced ventricular fibrillation by antiarrhythmic agents (abstract). Circulation (Suppl. II) **60:** 88.

118. VINCENZI, M., T. MORLINO, P. ALLEGRI, E. BARBIERI, F. CAPPELLETTI, U. DEHIO, R. OMETTO & P. MAIOLINO. 1981. Changes in cardiovascular function induced by verapamil in healthy subjects and in patients with ischemic heart disease. Clin. Cardiol. **4:** 15–21.

119. KARLSBERG, R. P., P. D. HENRY, S. A. AHMED, B. E. SOBEL & R. ROBERTS. Lack of protection of ischemic myocardium by verapamil in conscious dogs. Eur. J. Pharm. **42:** 339–346.

120. ELHARRAR, V., J. C. BAILEY, D. A. LATHROP & D. P. ZIPES. 1978. Effects of aprindine HCl on slow channel action potentials and transient depolarizations in canine Purkinje fibers. J. Pharmacol. Exp. Ther. **205:** 410–417.

121. FOSTER, P. R., R. M. KING, A. B. NICOLL & D. P. ZIPES. 1976. Suppression of ouabain-induced ventricular rhythms with aprindine HCl. A comparison with other antiarrhythmic agents. Circulation **53:** 315–321.

DISCUSSION

DR. BIGGER: There is a great deal of interest in the role of calcium in the cell and in calcium antagonists and differences among the drugs. During your presentation, Dr. Zipes, you have used the word verapamil. Can the words calcium antagonist be substituted? Or have you used it advisedly because you think verapamil is selectively better than the others?

DR. ZIPES: I used it in a generic sense because verapamil has been around for so long and it is the drug that we have had the greatest experience with.

DR. BIGGER: Is the time ripe for reaching a consensus and picking a drug for trial? Or do you think that the field is not advanced to the stage where it would be possible to do that? What kind of further information do we need?

DR. ZIPES: We need more data about the differences between diltiazem, verapamil, nifedipine, and some of the other drugs. Once we have a little bit more data we might be able to pick one of the drugs that would be useful. I firmly believe that this kind of an approach will affect the cardiac mortality. I don't think that the drug that will reduce sudden cardiac death related to ischemia is going to be one of the classical antiarrhythmic agents; and we have heard a lot of data as to why that might not be so.

DR. BIGGER: Do you then regard the diverse actions of calcium antagonists as an advantage rather than a disadvantage?

DR. ZIPES: Yes. I would also like to mention the results of a study we performed in which we administered aprindine to dogs before and after coronary occlusion. As you might predict, there were profoundly different concentrations of the drug in the myocardial ischemic zone determined by whether the drug was given before or after coronary arterial occlusion. When there is such heterogeneity of myocardial drug concentration there is bound to be electrical heterogeneity as well. Consequently, some of the classical antiarrhythmic agents can be harmful by those mechanisms.

Another study showed that verapamil had much less effect or no effect on conduction delay when it was given after the coronary artery was occluded. The drug probably did not reach the ischemic zone in high enough concentrations when given after occlusion. I would predict this on the basis of our data in dogs. Prophylaxis with slow channel blockers needs to be studied, since pretreatment might be better than administering verapamil to a patient after an acute infarction in a coronary care unit.

DR. BIGGER: Drug concentration in the ischemic zone varies unpredictably from drug to drug; procainamide, for example, readily reaches the ischemic zone, whereas verapamil did not in some studies in dogs.

DR. RIBEIRO: Dr. Zipes, do you think it's possible that verapamil prevents ventricular fibrillation after coronary arterial occlusion by blocking the sodium fast channel?

DR. ZIPES: I don't think so. In one study in dogs the investigators compared the preservation of ischemic myocardium with the *dextro* isomer with that of the negative *levo* isomer. The *levo* isomer gave superior results. It is the d-verapamil that affects the slow inward current rather than the l-verapamil. So, if I were to pick verapamil to study cardiac mortality, I would use the *levo* form.

DR. RIBEIRO: Is the afterdepolarization caused by digitalis due to a slow response?

DR. ZIPES: No, not entirely. In afterdepolarization, there is probably a sodium current, but it is linked to calcium. Calcium probably moves into the cell and affects the channel through which this sodium current is moving. The mechanism is very complex and has not entirely been worked out. The afterdepolarizations occur at resting potentials of about -80 mV, which is clearly in the range of the fast response, not the slow response at -40 mV. The afterdepolarizations are probably due to sodium, but they may be linked to transmembrane calcium movements. That is how this slow response may be implicated in some forms of triggered activity that can be suppressed by verapamil.

DR. RIBEIRO: Can you suppress by overdrive pacing the arrhythmias generated by digitalis-induced afterdepolarizations?

DR. ZIPES: Generally, you would make them worse; the only way afterdepolarizations could be suppressed by overdrive is by pacing so rapidly that you actually get entrance block. The more rapidly you pace, the more prominent the afterdepolarizations become; that is how afterdepolarizations are so distinct from normal automaticity.

DR. MOSS: What is the current status of slow channel blockers on digitalis-induced rhythm problems?

DR. ZIPES: Experimentally *in vitro* one can eliminate many of the arrhythmogenic effects that digitalis produces. However, the triggered activity that I showed is a very specific form of digitalis-induced arrhythmia and occurs very early. It may not be related to the chaotic ventricular arrhythmia that digitalis may produce.

We created triggered activity *in vivo* and tested the effects of verapamil. Verapamil had very little effect, whereas *in vitro* it profoundly eliminates the triggered response. I think that the sympathetic nervous system will, by affecting the slow inward current, counteract some of verapamil's effects *in vivo*.

DR. P. J. SCHWARTZ: In my paper I showed that the interaction between acute myocardial ischemia and short-lasting sympathetic stimulation often results in either ventricular tachycardia or fibrillation. In that setting, verapamil is quite effective in eliminating these arrhythmias, as has been already discussed. It is relevant to the problem that we are discussing here today. Would you comment on the possible mechanism?

DR. ZIPES: Verapamil's effect in the models that we have studied is, I think, primarily protection of the ischemic myocardium. This drug affords this protection by a variety of ways, including influences on myocardial metabolism and blood flow. No compelling data exist to indicate that the slow inward current is responsible for the early electrophysiologic changes produced by myocardial ischemia.

There are data that suggest that the slow inward current plays a role in chronic ventricular arrhythmia. Dr. Spear impaled cells of patients who had ventricular aneurysms removed, and he found that there were some cells that had very reduced resting potentials which were eliminated by verapamil. We have similar data.

The chronic situation may be quite different. In that setting there may be some cells that are slow-response-dependent. So the situation becomes very complex if you superimpose an acute event on a chronic event. A variety of mechanisms may be operative.

I also do not want to leave the impression that verapamil is going to be the cure-all. Even if the end result is ventricular fibrillation, the electrophysiologic mechanism by which it is obtained may be complex and not necessarily uniform. I don't think there's one "magic bullet" that will benefit every patient, but I do think that the present data very strongly suggest giving the slow channel blockers a trial in preventing mortality from coronary heart disease.

DR. DWYER: One of the groups that is going to be targeted are patients with relatively poor ventricular function. Will you comment about the use of these agents in that particular group?

DR. ZIPES: Verapamil has been fairly extensively studied in a variety of settings. Its negative hemodynamic effects are very mild. It does have a negative inotropic effect and if one removes sympathetic stimulation then one can clearly worsen heart failure.

Verapamil has mild detrimental effects in patients with diminished myocardial function; I suspect that the minimal effects may be due to its peripheral vasodilating action, which helps to eliminate its direct negative inotropic effect. This is another reason why verapamil may be more beneficial in the postinfarct patient, so many of whom have myocardial dysfunction and would not qualify for propranolol. I think that we could probably safely give verapamil to such patients.

ANTIPLATELET AGENTS: THEIR ROLE IN THE PREVENTION OF SUDDEN DEATH

J. Hirsh

Departments of Pathology and Medicine
McMaster University
Hamilton, Ontario, Canada L8N 3Z5

The rationale for studying antiplatelet drugs in postmyocardial infarction patients is based on the recognized role of platelets in the pathogenesis and complications of coronary artery disease.[1, 2] There is a possibility, however, that some of these drugs may reduce sudden death by mechanisms that are independent of their effects on platelet function.[3-5] These include an effect on coronary blood flow to ischemic areas and a direct antiarrhythmic effect, both of which may be independent of their inhibitory actions on platelet function.

Myocardial infarction and coronary death may be caused by thrombotic occlusion or possibly by sustained coronary spasm,[6] even in the absence of thrombosis. Moschos and associates [7] and Capurro and associates [8] have shown that platelet thromboemboli may also play a role in determining the extent of myocardial necrosis after coronary occlusion. Thromboxane A_2, a powerful coronary vasoconstrictor,[9] is produced by stimulated platelets and could contribute to coronary arterial spasm, which in turn could lead to myocardial necrosis and arrhythmias in the absence of coronary arterial thrombosis. It is possible, therefore, that part of the effectiveness of aspirin (and possibly sulfinpyrazone) in patients with coronary artery disease could be through inhibiting the synthesis of thromboxane A_2 by platelets.

Although preclinical studies (*in vitro* studies and experimental models of thrombosis) have been useful in identifying antiplatelet agents with clinical potential, the final assessment of their effectiveness must be based on results of clinical trials. These studies are tedious, expensive, and difficult to perform so that considerable care should be taken with drug and patient selection and with the design and analysis.

MODE OF ACTION OF ANTIPLATELET AGENTS

Three drugs which inhibit platelet function have been evaluated in well-designed clinical studies. These are acetylsalicylic acid (aspirin), sulfinpyrazone, and dipyridamole.

Aspirin

Aspirin is rapidly absorbed in the stomach and upper intestine and has a half-life of absorption of 4 to 16 minutes.[10] Absorption from enteric-coated tablets may be delayed and is sometimes incomplete.[11] Peak plasma levels are obtained 15 to 20 minutes after aspirin ingestion and the plasma concentration decays in a biexponential manner, with a half-life of 13 to 20 minutes.[12, 13]

289

0077–8923/82/0382–0289 $1.75/0 © 1982, NYAS

Aspirin is rapidly hydrolyzed into salicylic acid by esterase enzymes, which are found in the gastrointestinal tract, various tissues, and in the blood.[14] The most common side effect of aspirin is through its effect on the gastric mucosa. Aspirin produces gastric erosions[15] and most individuals receiving aspirin for prolonged periods have an increase in gastrointestinal blood loss.[16]

Effect of Aspirin on Platelet Function

Aspirin has no effect on platelet adhesion at physiologic rates of shear and at physiologic hematocrit levels.[17-19] Aspirin inhibits platelet function by acetylating platelet cyclooxygenase.[20-22] Doses as low as 160 mg/day inhibit platelet cyclooxygenase activity by more than 80%.[22] As a consequence of this effect, aspirin inhibits the oxidation of arachidonic acid to the endoperoxide PGG_2 and PGH_2 and, therefore, inhibits thromboxane A_2 production.[23]

Platelets exposed to aspirin have impaired aggregation with agonists such as adrenalin, collagen and adenosine diphosphate[24] (second wave), which induce the platelet release reaction mediated by thromboxane A_2. Aspirin does not inhibit the platelet release reaction induced by strong concentrations of collagen or even moderate concentrations of thrombin since these reactions are mediated by mechanisms that are independent of thromboxane A_2 production. Aspirin does not inhibit the primary wave of aggregation with adenosine diphosphate.[24-26]

The acetylation of cyclooxygenase by aspirin is irreversible and the effect of aspirin on platelet function is maintained for the life-span of the platelet.[20-24, 27] There is evidence that aspirin also acetylates platelets before they are released into the circulation and while they are still within megakaryocytes,[22] although there is not general agreement on this point.[28] When used in therapeutic doses, salicylate does not inhibit platelet function.[29]

Effect of Aspirin on Vascular Wall Prostaglandin Synthesis

When the prostaglandin synthetic pathway is activated in vessel wall cells (endothelial cells and smooth muscle cells), prostaglandin I_2 is formed.[30-34] This prostaglandin is a powerful inhibitor of platelet aggregation and a vasodilator and so has an opposing effect to thromboxane A_2.[9, 35] Arachidonic acid in vascular wall cells is oxidized to PGG_2 and PGH_2 by the enzyme cyclooxygenase, and PGH_2 is converted into prostaglandin I_2.[9, 35] The synthesis of PGI_2 by vascular wall cells is inhibited by aspirin but, compared with that of the platelet, this effect is relatively short-lived and may require larger doses of aspirin,[30, 31] although there is disagreement on this point.[36] In vivo studies in rabbits indicate that when complete inhibition of PGI_2 synthesis is achieved by treating the animals with very high doses of aspirin, thrombogenesis is augmented.[37-39] Both the thrombogenic effect and the inhibitory effect on PGI_2 synthesis is short-lived (presumably because de novo synthesis of cyclooxygenase can occur in vascular wall cells) and lasts longer in arteries than veins.[39, 40]

Effect of Aspirin on the Bleeding Time

Aspirin prolongs the bleeding time in normal volunteers over a dosage range that varies between 300 mg and 3.6 grams per day.[41-50] This effect is exaggerated in patients with associated hemostatic abnormalities.

Effect of Aspirin on Shortened Platelet Survival

A number of studies have demonstrated that aspirin does not normalize the reduced platelet survival seen in patients with prosthetic heart valves, but that it has a potentiating effect on dipyridamole in achieving this effect.[51, 52]

Effects of Aspirin on Coagulation and Fibrinolysis

High doses of aspirin have been reported to prolong the prothrombin time.[53, 54] The mechanism of this effect is unclear, but the prolongation is corrected by the administration of vitamin K.[55] Sodium salicylate increases blood fibrinolytic activity, an effect that is thought to be independent of the plasminogen/plasmin system and one that is related to an increase in cellular fibrinolysis.[56]

Effect of Aspirin on Animal Models of Thrombosis

Aspirin prevents thrombosis in a variety of experimental animal models.[57–61] Kelton and associates reported that aspirin reduced the size of thrombi only in male rabbits.[62] These experiments were performed to further explore clinical reports that aspirin was effective in preventing thromboembolism in patients with hip replacement [63] and with transient cerebral ischemia [64] but that this beneficial effect was limited to males.

Aspirin has been reported to have a variable effect on the bleeding time in experimental animal models.[65–70] A number of investigators have demonstrated that, in very high doses, aspirin shortens the bleeding time, presumably by inhibiting vascular wall PGI_2 formation.[69, 70]

Other Effects of Aspirin

Aspirin has been reported to improve collateral coronary blood flow after temporary coronary occlusion in dogs [8] and to have an antiarrhythmic effect.[71] This latter effect is induced by the salicylate moiety of the aspirin molecule and appears to be independent of platelets. Verrier and associates demonstrated that sodium salicylate improved ventricular electrical stability in dogs by raising the ventricular fibrillation threshold in normal hearts after a 10-minute occlusion of the left anterior descending coronary artery.[71]

Sulfinpyrazone

Sulfinpyrazone had been used as a uricose uric agent for a number of years before it was found by chance to lengthen the reduced platelet survival seen in patients with hyperuricemia.[72]

Sulfinpyrazone is derived from phenylbutazone by sulfoxide substitution. Its absorption after oral administration is rapid and complete and peak plasma concentrations are reached at 1 to 2 hours.[73] It is extensively protein-bound and has a plasma half-life of 2 to 3 hours. More than 50% of sulfinpyrazone is excreted unchanged and the remainder is metabolically transformed, mainly by β glucuronidation before excretion.[73] When given in doses of 800 mg/day (200 mg four times daily), plasma concentrations of 30 to 40 mg/ml are obtained.[74] There is experimental evidence that part of the inhibitory effect of sulfinpyrazone on platelet function is mediated by a sulfinpyrazone metabolite.[75]

Side Effects of Sulfinpyrazone

Side effects of sulfinpyrazone are minimal and consist of gastrointestinal intolerance and gastrointestinal bleeding in patients with peptic ulcer disease.[64]

The Effects of Sulfinpyrazone on Platelet Function

Sulfinpyrazone does not inhibit platelet adhesion at pharmacologic concentrations.[76] It is a competitive inhibitor of cyclooxygenase.[77] It is a relatively weak inhibitor of platelet aggregation when tested either *in vitro* or *ex vivo*. *In vitro*, at concentrations of 1 to 20 μmol/liter, sulfinpyrazone inhibits adrenalin- and collagen-induced aggregation, but has little effect on ADP-induced aggregation.[78, 79] Sulfinpyrazone does not inhibit aggregation induced by high concentrations of collagen or even moderate concentrations of thrombin.[78, 80] When administered in high concentrations to experimental animals, sulfinpyrazone inhibits platelet function *ex vivo* in a similar manner to its effects *in vitro*.[81] Sulfinpyrazone has been reported to be synergistic with aspirin on inhibition of collagen-induced aggregation [82] and there is suggestive evidence from the Canadian Stroke Study for synergism between these two drugs in stroke prevention.[64]

A metabolite of sulfinpyrazone inhibits platelet aggregation *in vivo* for as long as 18 hours after drug administration (at which time the drug had been cleared from the plasma).[75] This effect is associated with inhibition of platelet prostaglandin synthesis.[75] An active metabolite has also been reported in other animals treated with sulfinpyrazone [83] and there is suggestive evidence that it exists in man.[84] Its significance is uncertain.

Sulfinpyrazone did not prolong the bleeding time in patients treated with the drug during the Canadian Stroke Study.

In 1970, Weily and Genton [85] reported that the decreased platelet survival in patients with prosthetic mitral valves was not influenced by sulfinpyrazone in a daily dose of 400 mg but that it was lengthened when a dose of 800 mg was used. Since then, a number of reports have appeared indicating that reduced platelet survival time is lengthened by sulfinpyrazone in patients with valvular heart disease, ischemic heart disease, and transient cerebral ischemia.[86-88]

Effect of Sulfinpyrazone on Animal Models of Thrombosis

Sulfinpyrazone reduced thrombus formation and prolonged the reduced platelet survival in a number of animal models.[89-91] Sulfinpyrazone has also been reported to reduce death from disseminated platelet thrombi produced by arachidonic acid infusion.[92, 93]

Sulfinpyrazone has been reported to normalize the reduced platelet survival associated with implantation of arteriovenous cannulas in rabbits [94] and baboons [95] and of Dacron arterial prostheses in dogs and rats.[96]

Other Effects of Sulfinpyrazone

Like aspirin, sulfinpyrazone has effects on coronary blood flow and arrhythmias that appear to be independent of its inhibitory effects on platelet function. Goldstein and associates reported that sulfinpyrazone increases collateral endocardial flow and endocardial flow after temporary myocardial ischemia and that it increases blood flow to the ischemic myocardium.[97, 98] Although these changes were not associated with a reduction in infarct size, these investigators suggested that they may contribute to the decreased incidence of potentially lethal arrhythmias reported after administration of either of these drugs prior to acute myocardial ischemia in dogs. Verrier and associates reported that sulfinpyrazone enhanced ventricular electrical stability by raising the ventricular fibrillation threshold and the excitability threshold and by prolonging the effective refractory period in dogs.[71] Moschos and associates reported that sulfinpyrazone decreased the incidence of ventricular fibrillation after acute nonthrombotic coronary occlusion.[5] These investigators occluded the left anterior coronary artery in thrombocytopenic animals using a balloon and demonstrated that animals treated with sulfinpyrazone had significantly fewer episodes of ventricular fibrillation than did those in the control group. Beamish and associates have reported that sulfinpyrazone reduced the incidence of arrhythmia and death caused by adrenochrome (an oxidation product of catecholamines) in experimental animals.[99]

These observations support the possibility that part of the beneficial effect of sulfinpyrazone in patients with myocardial ischemia could be through non-platelet-mediated mechanisms.

Dipyridamole

Dipyridamole is a pyrimido-pyrimidine compound that was initially used clinically as a vasodilator. Intravenous administration of the drug produces a decrease in blood pressure, but oral administration is associated with only minimal hypotensive effects. The major side effects of dipyridamole are nausea, vomiting, and diarrhea and occasionally headaches and vertigo. After oral administration in therapeutic doses, a blood level of 1 to 3 μmol/liter of dipyridamole is achieved.

Effect of Dipyridamole on Platelet Function

Dipyridamole inhibits platelet adhesion to collagen in a nonflowing system [100] and inhibits platelet adhesion to damaged rabbit aortas both *in vitro* and *in vivo*.[101] Dipyridamole has been reported to inhibit ADP-induced platelet aggregation [102] and adrenalin and collagen-induced serotonin release.[103] It is likely that a major mechanism for its effect on platelet function is through inhibition of platelet phosphodiesterase activity.[104] Inhibition of this enzyme results in an elevation of platelet cyclic AMP levels, which in turn is associated with a decrease in the levels of cytoplasmic calcium, a modulator of platelet aggregation and the platelet release reaction. When tested *ex vivo*, the inhibitory effect of dipyridamole is proportional to its blood concentration.[105] Dipyridamole is bound to an acid glycoprotein, which limits its availability to platelets.[106] Dipyridamole appears to have a greater effect *ex vivo* than *in vitro* on platelet function tested, a difference that may be related to the anticoagulant used for drawing blood in the preparation of platelet-rich plasma for testing *in vitro*.[107] There has been a report that dipyridamole inhibits prostaglandin synthesis,[108] but this has been challenged.[109] It has also been suggested that there is synergism between the effects of PGI_2 and dipyridamole on platelet function since both compounds elevate platelet cyclic AMP levels.[109, 110]

Dipyridamole does not prolong the bleeding time in normal volunteers.[111]

Harker and Slichter reported that dipyridamole normalizes reduced platelet survival in a dose-dependent manner in a variety of thrombovascular disorders.[51, 52, 112] Aspirin, which had no effect on the shortened platelet survival in these patients in a dose of 1 gram/day, augmented the effect of dipyridamole in doses of 100 mg/day on normalizing reduced platelet survival.

The Effect of Dipyridamole on Animal Models of Thrombosis

The reported effects of dipyridamole on inhibiting experimental thrombosis in animals have been variable. In most experimental models of arterial thrombosis, it has been effective,[113-117] but there have been a number of exceptions.[118, 119] A synergistic antithrombotic effect between aspirin and dipyridamole on thrombosis has been reported.[61]

CLINICAL EVALUATION OF ANTIPLATELET DRUGS IN CORONARY ARTERY DISEASE

During the last 5 years, a number of well-designed clinical trials have been performed evaluating the effectiveness of drugs that suppress platelet function in patients who have suffered from myocardial infarction. No studies have been performed in the primary prevention of myocardial infarction.

Although none of the studies performed is beyond criticism, a number do meet many of the methodologic requirements for acceptable clinical trials.

Clinical Results

Elwood and associates[120] reported a randomized double-blind study of aspirin (300 mg/day) in 1,239 men with a recent myocardial infarction. The observed reduction in total mortality was 25% after 1 year, which was not statistically significant. However, in the patients whose qualifying infarction occurred less than 6 weeks prior to entry into the study, there was a statistically significant reduction in mortality from 13.2% in the placebo group to 7.8% in the aspirin-treated group. Since this observation was based on retrospective subgroup analysis, it cannot be regarded as definitive, but should be considered in the design of subsequent trials.

The Coronary Drug Project Group [121] reported on 1,529 males who had myocardial infarction approximately 7 years previously and who were randomly assigned into an aspirin-treated group (975 mg/day) or a placebo group. There was a 30% reduction in mortality from 8.5% in the placeba group to 5.8% in the aspirin-treated group, which was not statistically significant. Twice as many patients on aspirin (12.3%) complained of gastrointestinal upset during the study period.

Breddin [122] randomly allocated 946 patients (80% males) within 6 weeks of myocardial infarction to treatment with aspirin (1.5 g daily), a placebo, or phenprocoumon, and followed them for as long as 2 years. There was little difference in total mortality, but the coronary death rate (sudden death or fetal myocardial infarction) was only 4.1% in the aspirin-treated patients compared with 7.1% in the placebo group (a nonsignificant trend). Nine of the 317 patients on aspirin had their treatment stopped because of hemorrhage compared with none of 309 patients in the placebo group. Twenty patients in the aspirin-treated group and 12 in the placebo group had treatment stopped because of gastrointestinal upset.

In 1979, Elwood and Sweetnam [123] reported on a randomized trial of 1682 patients (85% males). Most of the patients were admitted within 1 week of their qualifying infarction. Total mortality was reduced by 17% in the aspirin-treated (900 mg daily), the mortality being 12.3% in the aspirin group compared with 14.8% in the placebo group. The corresponding reduction for total mortality plus nonfatal myocardial infarction was 28%, and for ischemic heart disease, mortality was 22%. None of these differences was statistically significant. Side effects resulting in withdrawal from the study were only slightly higher in the aspirin-treated group (30.9% versus 28.8%); eight patients in the aspirin-treated group had gastrointestinal bleeding compared with four in the placebo group.

The Aspirin Myocardial Infarction Study Research Group [124] recruited 4524 patients (89% males) who had a documented myocardial infarction 2 to 60 months previously and followed them for 3 years. The total mortality was 10.8% in the aspirin-treated group and 9.7% in the placebo group. There were fewer nonfatal myocardial infarctions in the aspirin-treated group, and the incidence of coronary events (coronary heart disease mortality or definite nonfatal myocardial infarction) was 14.1% in the aspirin-treated group compared with 14.8% in the placebo group.

There were significantly more side effects reported in the aspirin-treated group. These included constipation, heartburn, epigastric discomfort, nausea, vomiting, hematemesis and melena and symptomatic gout.

The Persantine-Aspirin Reinfarction Study Research Group [125] recruited 2026 patients (87% males) with a documented myocardial infarction 2 to 60 months previously and followed them for a mean time of 41 months. Within the groups treated with aspirin (975 mg daily) or treated with aspirin (975 mg daily) plus dipyridamole (225 mg daily), the total mortality, coronary heart disease mortality, cardiovascular mortality, and incidence of coronary events incidence (coronary death or nonfatal myocardial infarction) were each quite similar and consistently less than in the placebo group, but none was statistically significant. For coronary mortality and coronary events, the rates were about 50% lower in the group treated with aspirin plus dipyridamole than the placebo group from 8 to 24 months of follow-up study and were statistically significant by the study criteria; the corresponding reduction for the aspirin-treated group was 30% during this follow-up period.

For the subgroup of 447 patients entered within 6 months of their qualifying infarction, it was found that the mortality was 51% less in the aspirin-treated group and 44% less in the group treated with aspirin plus dipyridamole when compared with the placebo group (comprising only 95 patients). In contrast, for patients enrolled more than 6 months after their myocardial infarction, the mortality differences were very small.

The reported side effects were similar between the two active treatment groups, but permanent or temporary discontinuation of study medication occurred more frequently in the active treatment groups; the reasons for discontinuation included abdominal pain, heartburn, nausea and vomiting, hematemesis, and melena.

There have been other relevant studies of aspirin, both prospective and retrospective. Elwood and Williams [126] carried out a randomized double-blind trial in which 1705 patients (75% males) with myocardial infarction were given a single dose of aspirin (300 mg) or a placebo on their first contact with a general practitioner. They found no effect on the 28-day mortality.

A number of retrospective case control studies have also been performed.[127-129] The possibility of selection bias is always a problem in retrospective studies and the results of these studies have not been consistent.

There has been only one study reported with dipyridamole in postmyocardial infarction patients,[130] but the number of patients studied was too small to allow satisfactory evaluation.

In the Anturane Reinfarction Trial Research Group,[131] 1558 patients were randomly assigned to treatment with sulfinpyrazone (800 mg daily) or placebo 25 to 35 days after a myocardial infarction. The initial communication reported a statistically significant reduction in cardiac mortality from 9.5% per annum to 4.9%. The trial was continued until all 1558 eligible patients (87% males) had completed at least 1 year of follow-up (average follow-up 16 months). The second report was then published [132] in which an overall reduction of 32% in cardiac mortality was reported ($p = 0.06$). This was due almost entirely to a 75% reduction in sudden death during the first 6 months of treatment ($p = 0.003$), after which time there seemed to be no further benefit of treatment.

None of the observed differences in reported side effects between the two treatment groups was statistically significant.

The methods of the Anturane Myocardial Reinfarction Study have been criticized on two grounds: departures from the protocol and the classification of sudden death.[133-135] Patients were excluded from the analysis after randomization on the basis of a number of prospectively defined criteria. These included end-point within the first 7 days of randomization, the discovery that the patient was ineligible after he or she had been randomly assigned to a group, and the reaching of the end-point more than 7 days after the prescribed treatment was stopped. If the analysis had been performed on the basis of an intention to treat, there would have been 60 deaths in the placebo group and 41 in the sulfinpyrazone, a difference that is not statistically significant because in each group there were 16 deaths in patients who were either ineligible, who had had treatment for less than 7 days, or for whom the assigned treatment had stopped more than 7 days before the end-point was reached. When these patients were removed from consideration, the number of deaths in each group was 44 and 25, a much greater difference that almost reaches statistical significance. The second problem in the analysis of the Anturane Myocardial Reinfarction Study relates to the definition of sudden death versus myocardial infarction. It is thought that some of the patients placed in the sudden death category should have been placed instead in the myocardial infarction group. Since the differences found between the sulfinpyrazone and placebo groups was almost exclusively in the sudden death category, taking patients from the sudden death category and placing them in the myocardial infarction group could remove part of the impressive difference found for anturane using sudden death as the end-point. The first problem is a philosophic one, which does not have an easy resolution. The second issue is currently being investigated and, it is hoped, will be resolved to the satisfaction of the study group and the scientific community.

Summary of Current Status

Evidence relating to the efficacy of aspirin comes from the six long-term secondary prevention studies, in five of which there was an observed reduction in mortality with the use of aspirin. None of these six individual studies showed differences in mortality that were statistically significant. However, the observed benefits in each of the six trials are statistically consistent with one another. If the results of the studies are pooled, the risk reduction with aspirin is 16% ($p < 0.01$) for cardiovascular deaths and for the outcome of first infarction, fatal or nonfatal, the pooled estimate of the risk reduction with aspirin is 21% ($p < 0.001$).

Questions remain about the best time to initiate treatment, about aspirin dose, and about possible gender differences in response to aspirin. The evidence that the combination of dipyridamole plus aspirin is better than aspirin alone is not persuasive.

A number of concerns have been raised about the Anturane Reinfarction Trial and it is not possible to make recommendations until the question of classification of sudden deaths is resolved. If an independent group concludes that the study group was not in error in their classification of sudden deaths, then it would be reasonable to conclude that sulfinpyrazone reduces the incidence of sudden deaths in patients after myocardial infarction.

REFERENCES

1. ROBERTS, W. C. 1971. The pathology of acute myocardial infarction. Hosp. Pract. **6**: 89.
2. HAEREM, J. W. 1972. Platelet aggregates in intramyocardial vessels of patients dying suddenly and unexpectedly of coronary artery disease. Atherosclerosis **15**: 199.
3. MOSCHOS, C. B., B. HAIDER, C. DELA CRUZ, M. M. LYONS & T. J. REGAN. 1978. Antiarrhythmic effects of aspirin during nonthrombotic coronary occlusion. Circulation **57**: 681.
4. CUDDY, T. E., N. DONEN, H. KARLINSKY, J. MCMANUS & H. LARSON. 1980. Holter 24 hour recordings in post myocardial infarction patients in double blind treatment with sulfinpyrazone. Am. J. Cardiol. **45**: 455.
5. MOSCHOS, C., A. EXCOBINAS, O. JORGENSEN & T. REGAN. 1979. Effect of

sulfinpyrazone on survival following experimental non-thrombotic coronary occlusion. Am. J. Cardiol. **43:** 372.

6. MASERI, A., A. L'ABBATE, G. BAROLDI, S. CHIERCHIA, M. MARZILI, A. M. BELLESTRA, S. SEVERI, O. PARODI, A. BRAGINI, A. DISTANTE & A. PESOLA. 1978. Coronary vasospasm as a possible cause of myocardial infarction. N. Engl. J. Med. **299:** 1271.

7. MOSCHOS, C. B., K. LAHIRI, M. LYONS, A. B. WEISSE, H. A. OLDEWURTEL & T. J. REGAN. 1973. Relation of microcirculatory thrombosis to thrombus in the proximal coronary artery: Effect of aspirin, dipyridamole and thrombolysis. Am. Heart J. **86:** 61.

8. Capurro, N. L., K. C. Marr, R. Aamodt, R. E. Goldstein & S. E. Epstein. 1979. Aspirin-induced increase in collateral flow after acute coronary occlusion in dogs. Circulation **59:** 744.

9. NEEDLEMAN, P., A. WYCHE & A. RAZ. 1979. Platelet and blood vessel arachidonate metabolism and interactions. J. Clin. Invest. **63:** 345.

10. ROWLAND, M., S. RIEGELMAN, P. A. HARRIS & S. D. SHOLKOFF. 1972. Absorption kinetics of aspirin in man following oral administration of an aqueous solution. J. Pharm. Sci. **61:** 379.

11. LEVY, G. 1978. Clinical pharmacokinetics of aspirin. Pediatrics **62:** 867.

12. ROWLAND, M. & S. RIEGELMAN. 1968. Pharmacokinetics of acetyl-salicyclic acid and salicylic acid after intravenous administration in man. J. Pharm. Sci. **57:** 1313.

13. ORTON, D., R. T. JONES, T. KASPI & R. RICHARDSON. 1979. Plasma salicylate levels after soluble ann effervescent aspirin. Br. J. Clin. Pharm. **7:** 410.

14. BUCHANAN, W. W., P. J. ROONEY & J. A. N. RENNIE. 1979. Aspirin and the salicylates. Clin. Rheum. Dis. **5(2):** 499.

15. FROMM, D. 1978. Salicylate and gastric mucosal damage. Pediatrics **62:** 938.

16. COHEN, A. 1979. Fecal blood loss and plasma salicylate study of salicylic acid and aspirin. J. Clin. Pharm. **19(4):** 242.

17. LEGRAND, Y. J., F. FAUVEL, G. KARTALIS, J. L. WAUTIER & J. P. CAEN. 1979. Specific and quantitative method for estimation of platelet adhesion to fibrillar collagen. J. Lab. Clin. Med. **94:** 438.

18. TSCHOPP, TH. B. 1977. Aspirin inhibits platelet aggregation on, but not adhesion to, collagen fibrils: An assessment of platelet adhesion and deposited platelet mass by morphometry and ^{51}Cr-labelling. Thromb. Res. **11:** 619.

19. BAUMGARTNER, H. R., T. B. TSCHOPP & H. J. WEISS. 1977. Platelet interaction with collagen fibrils in flowing blood. II. Impaired adhesion-aggregation in bleeding disorders. A. comparison with subentothelium. Thromb. Haemostas. (Stuttgart) **37:** 17.

20. ROTH, G. J., N. STANFORD & MAJERUS, P. W. 1975. Acetylation of prostaglandin synthetase by aspirin. Proc. Natl. Acad. Sci. USA **72(8):** 3073.

21. ROTH, G. J. & P. W. MAJERUS. 1975. The mechanism of the effect of aspirin on human platelet. I. Acetylation of a particulate fraction Protein. J. Clin. Invest **56:** 624.

22. BURCH, J. W., N. STANFORD & P. W. MAJERUS. 1978. Inhibition of platelet prostaglandin synthetase by oral aspirin. J. Clin. Invest. **61:** 314.

23. SMITH, J. B. 1980. The prostanoids in hemostasis and thrombosis: a review. Am. J. Pathol. **99:** 743.

24. PACKHAM, M. A. & J. F. MUSTARD. 1977. Clinical pharmacology of platelets. Blood **50:** 555.

25. PACKHAM, M. A., R. L. KINLOUGH-RATHBONE, H.-J. REIMERS, S. SCOTT & J. F. MUSTARD. 1977. *In* Prostaglandins in Hematology. M. J. Silver, J. B. Smith & J. J. Kocsis, Eds. 247–276. Spectrum Publications. New York, NY.

26. PACKHAM, M. A. 1976. Stages in the interaction of platelets with collagen. Thromb. Haemost. **36:** 269.

27. STUART, R. K. 1970. Platelet function studies in human beings receiving 300 mg of aspirin per day. J. Lab. Clin. Med. **75:** 463.
28. ALI, M., J. W. D. McDONALD, J. J. THIESSEN & P. E. COATES. 1980. Plasma acetylsalicylate and salicylate and platelet cyclo-oxygenase activity following plain and enteric-coated aspirin. Stroke **11:** 9.
29. ZUCKER, M. B. & K. G. ROTHWELL. 1978. Differential influences of salicylate compounds on platelet aggregation and serotonin release. Curr. Ther. Res. **23:** 194.
30. CZERVIONKE, R. L., J. B. SMITH, G. L. FRY, J. C. HOAK & D. L. HAYCRAFT. 1979. Inhibition of prostacyclin by treatment of endothelium with aspirin. J. Clin. Invest. **63:** 1089.
31. BAENZIGER, N. L., M. J. DILLENDER & P. W. MAJERUS. 1977. Cultured human skin fibroblasts and arterial cells produce a labile platelet-inhibitory prostaglandin. Biochem. Biophys. Res. Commun. **78**(1): 294.
32. MONCADA, S. & J. R. VANE. 1979. The role of prostacyclin in vascular tissue. Fed. Proc. **38:** 66.
33. MONCADA, S., R. GRYGLEWSKI, S. BUNTING & J. R. VANE. 1976. An enzyme isolated from arteries transforms prostaglandin endoperoxides to an unstable substance that inhibits platelet aggregation. Nature **263:** 663.
34. WEKSLER, B. B., A. J. MARCUS & E. A. JAFFE. 1977. Synthesis of prostaglandin I_2 (prostacyclin) by cultured human and bovine endothelial cells. Cell Biology **74:** 3922.
35. NEEDLEMAN, P. 1979. Prostacyclin in blood vessel-platelet interactions: Perspectives and questions. Nature **279:** 14.
36. JAFFE, E. A. & B. B. WEKSLER. 1979. Recovery of endothelial cell prostacyclin production after inhibition by low doses of aspirin. J. Clin. Invest. **63:** 532.
37. KELTON, J. G., J. HIRSH, C. J. CARTER & M. R. BUCHANAN. 1978. Thrombogenic effect of high-dose aspirin in rabbits. Relationship to inhibition of vessel wall synthesis of prostaglandin I_2-like activity. J. Clin. Invest. **62:** 895.
38. ZIMMERMAN, R., M. THIESSEN, H. MORL & G. WECKESSER. 1979. The paradoxical thrombogenic effect of aspirin in experimental thrombosis. Thromb. Res. **16:** 843.
39. BUCHANAN, M. R., E. DEJANA, M. GENT, J. F. MUSTARD & J. HIRSH. 1981. Enhanced platelet accumulation onto injured carotid arteries in rabbits following aspirin treatment. J. Clin. Invest. **67:** 503.
40. BUCHANAN, M. R., E. DEJANA, J.-P. CAZENAVE, M. RICHARDSON, J. F. MUSTARD & J. HIRSH. 1980. Differences in inhibition of PGI_2 production by aspirin in rabbit artery and vein segments. Thromb. Res. **20:** 447.
41. HIRSH, J., D. STREET, J. F. CADE & H. AMY. 1973. Relation between bleeding time and platelet connective tissue reaction after aspirin. Blood **41** (3): 369.
42. MIELKE, C. H., JR., J. C. RAMOS & A. F. H. BRITTEN. 1973. Aspirin as an antiplatelet agent: template bleeding time as a monitor of therapy. Am. J. Clin. Path. **59:** 236.
43. FRICK, P. G. 1956. Haemorrhagic diathesis with increased capillary fragility caused by salicylate therapy. Am. J. Med. Sci. **231:** 402.
44. WEISS, H. J., L. M. ALEDORT & S. KOCHWA. 1968. The effect of salicylates on the hemostatic properties of platelet in man. J. Clin. Invest. **47:** 2169.
45. KUMAR, R., J. E. ANSELL, R. T. CANOSO & D. DEYKIN. 1978. Clinical trial of a new bleeding-time device. Am. J. Clin. Path. **70**(4): 642.
46. SUTOR, A. H., E. J. W. BOWIE & C. A. OWEN, JR. 1970. Clinical application of a new quantitative bleeding time test. Blood **36:** 92.
47. BICK, R. L., T. ADAMS & W. R. SCHMALHORST. 1976. Bleeding times, platelet adhesion and aspirin. Am. J. Clin. Path. **65:** 69.
48. BUCHANAN, G. R., V. MARTIN, P. H. LEVINE, K. SCOON & R. I. HANDIN.

1977. The effects of 'anti-platelet' drugs on bleeding time and platelet aggregation in normal human subjects. Am. J. Clin. Path. 68(3): 355.
49. HARKER, L. A. & S. J. SLICHTER. 1972. The bleeding time as a screening test for evaluation of platelet function. N. Engl. J. Med. 287(4): 155.
50. MIELKE, C. H. & A. F. H. BRITTEN. 1970. Aspirin as an antithrombotic agent: template bleeding time—test of antithrombotic effect. Blood 36: 855.
51. HARKER, L. A. & S. J. SLICHTER. 1970. Studies of platelet and fibrinogen kinetics in patients with prosthetic heart valves. N. Engl. J. Med. 283: 1302.
52. RITCHIE, J. L. & L. A. HARKER. 1977. Platelet and fibrinogen survival in coronary atherosclerosis. Am. J. Cardiol. 39: 595.
53. COLDWELL, B. B. & Z. ZAWIDZKA. 1968. Effect of acute administration of acetylsalicylic acid on the prothrombin activity of bishydroxycoumarin-treated rats. Blood 32(6): 945.
54. LOEW, D. & H. VINAZZER. 1976. Dose-dependent influence of acetylsalicylic acid on platelet functions and plasmatic coagulation factors. Haemostasis 5: 239.
55. GOLDSWEIG, H. G., M. KAPUSTA & J. SCHWARTZ. 1976. Bleeding, salicylates and prolonged prothrombin time. Three case reports and a review of the literature. J. Rheumat. 3: 37.
56. MOROZ, L. A. 1977. Increased blood fibrinolytic activity after aspirin ingestion. N. Engl. J. Med. 296(10): 525.
57. DANESE, C. A., CH. D. BOLETI & H. J. WEISS. 1971. Protection by aspirin against experimentally induced arterial thrombosis in dogs. Thromb. Diath. Haemorrh. 25: 288.
58. MOSCHOS, C. B., K. LAHIRI, M. LYONS, A. B. WEISSE, H. A. OLDEWURTEL, T. J. REGAN & N. J. NEWARD. 1973. Relationship of microcirculatory thrombosis to thrombus in the proximal coronary artery: effect of aspirin, dipyridamole and thrombolysis. Am. Heart J. 86(1): 61.
59. HONOUR, A. J., R. D. CARTER & J. I. MANN. 1977. The effects of treatment with aspirin and an antithrombotic agent SH1117 upon platelet thrombus formation in living blood vessels. Br. J. Exp. Pathol. 58: 474.
60. GERTZ, S. D., A. KURGAN, R. S. WAJNBERG & E. NELSON. 1979. Endothelial cell damage and thrombus formation following temporary arterial occlusion. J. Neurosurg. 50: 578.
61. HONOUR, A. J., T. D. R. HOCKADAY & J. I. MANN. 1977. The synergistic effect of aspirin and dipyridamole upon platelet thrombi in living blood vessels. Br. J. Exp. Pathol. 58: 268.
62. KELTON, J. G., J. HIRSH, C. J. CARTER & M. R. BUCHANAN. 1978. Sex differences in the antithrombotic effects of aspirin. Blood 52: 1073.
63. HARRIS, W. H., E. W. SALZMAN, C. A. ATHANASOULIS, A. C. WALTMAN & R. W. DeSANCTIS. 1977. Aspirin prophylaxis of venous thromboembolism after total hip replacement. N. Engl. J. Med. 297: 1246.
64. Canadian Cooperative Study Group. 1978. A randomized trial of aspirin and sulphinpyrazone in threatened stroke. N. Engl. J. Med. 299: 53.
65. DAVIS, J. W., P. E. PHILLIPS, J. M. ELLISON & S. R. LUCAS. 1974. Effect of aspirin on bleeding time and survival of rats after head trauma. J. Clin. Exp. Theoret. Med. 5: 229.
66. STELLA, L., M. B. DONATI & G. DE GAETANO. 1975. Bleeding time in laboratory animals. I. Aspirin does not prolong bleeding time in rats. Thromb. Res. 7: 709.
67. MINSKER, D. H. & P. J. KLING. 1977. Bleeding time in rats is prolonged by aspirin. Thromb. Res. 10: 619.
68. DEJANA, E., A. QUINTANA, A. CALLIONI & G. DE GAETANO. 1979. Bleeding time in laboratory animals. III. Do tail bleeding times in rats only measure a platelet defect? (The Aspirin Puzzle). Thromb. Res. 15: 199.
69. BUCHANAN, M. R., M. A. BLAJCHMAN, E. DEJANA, J. F. MUSTARD, A. F. SENYI & J. HIRSH. 1979. Shortening of the bleeding time in thrombocytopenic

rabbits after exposure of jugular vein to high aspirin concentration. Prostagland. Med. **3:** 333.

70. BLAJCHMAN, M. A., A. F. SENYI, J. HIRSH, Y. SURYA, M. BUCHANAN & J. F. MUSTARD. 1979. Shortening of the bleeding time in rabbits by hydrocortisone due to inhibition of prostacyclin (PGI_2) generation by the vessel wall. J. Clin. Invest. **63:** 1026.

71. VERRIER, R. L., E. RADDER & B. LOWN. 1981. Comparative effects of sodium salicylate and sulphinpyrazone on ventricular vulnerability in the normal and ischemic heart. *In* The Effect of Platelet-Active Drugs on the Cardiovascular System. University of Colorado Press. Denver. In press.

72. SMYTHE, H. A., M. A. OGRYZLO, E. A. MURPHY & J. F. MUSTARD. 1965. The effect of sulphinpyrazone (Anturan) on platelet economy and blood coagulation in man. Can. Med. Assoc. J. **92:** 818.

73. DIETERLE, W., J. W. FAIGLE, H. MORY, W. F. TICHTER & W. THEOBALD. 1975. Biotransformation and pharmacokinetics of sulphinpyrazone (Anturan) in man. Eur. J. Clin. Pharm. **9:** 135.

74. ROSENFELD, J., M. BUCHANAN, P. POWERS, J. HIRSH, H. J. M. BARNETT & R. K. STUART. 1978. Determination of sulphinpyrazone by gas chromatography. Thromb. Res. **12:** 247.

75. BUCHANAN, M. R., J. ROSENFELD & J. HIRSH. 1978. The prolonged effect of sulphinpyrazone on collagen-induced platelet aggregation in vivo. Thromb. Res. **13:** 883.

76. DAVIES, J. A., E. ESSIEN, J.-P. CAZENAVE, R. L. KINLOUGH-RATHBONE, M. GENT & J. F. MUSTARD. 1979. The influence of red blood cells on the effects of aspirin or sulphinpyrazone on platelet adherence to damaged rabbit aorta. Br. J. Haematol. **42:** 283.

77. ALI, M. & J. W. D. McDONALD. 1977. Effects of sulphinpyrazone on platelet prostaglandin synthesis and platelet release of serotonin. J. Lab. Clin. Med. **89:** 868.

78. MUSTARD, J. F. & M. A. PACKHAM. 1970. Factors influencing platelet function: adhesion, release and aggregation. Pharm. Rev. **22**(2): 97.

79. WILEY, J. S., C. N. CHESTERMAN, F. J. MORGAN & P. A. CASTALDI. 1979. The effect of sulphinpyrazone on the aggregation and release reactions of human platelets. Thromb. Res. **14:** 23.

80. PACKHAM, M. A., M. A. GUCCIONE, P. L. CHANG & J. F. MUSTARD. 1973. Platelet aggregation and release: effects of low concentrations of thrombin or collagen. Am. J. Physiol. **225:** 38.

81. PACKHAM, M. A., E. S. WARRIOR, M. F. GLYNN, A. SENYI & J. F. MUSTARD. 1967. Alteration of the response of platelets to surface stimuli by pyrazole compounds. J. Exp. Med. **126:** 171.

82. WONG, L. T., Z. ZAWIDZKA & R. B. THOMAS. 1978. Effect of acetylsalicylic acid, sulphinpyrazone and their combination on collagen-induced platelet aggregation in guinea pigs. Pharm. Res. Commun. **10:** 993.

83. PEDERSON, A. K. & P. JAKOBSEN. 1979. Two new metabolites of sulphinpyrazone in the rabbit: a possible cause of the prolonged in vivo effect. Thromb. Res. **16:** 871.

84. BUTLER, K. D., W. DIETERLE, E. MAGUIRE, G. F. PAY, R. B. WALLIS & A. M. WHITE. 1979. *In* Cardiovascular Actions of Sulfinpyrazone: Basic and Clinical Research. M. McGregor, J. F. Mustard, M. F. Oliver & S. Sherry, Eds.: 17–35. Symposia Specialist, Inc. Miami, FL.

85. WEILY, H. S. & E. GENTON. 1970. Altered platelet function in patients with prosthetic mitral valves. Effects of sulphinpyrazone therapy. Circulation **42:** 967.

86. WEILY, H. S., P. P. STEELE, H. DAVIES, G. PAPPAS & E. GENTON. 1974. Platelet survival in patients with substitute heart valves. N. Engl. J. Med. **290:** 534.

87. STEELE, P., D. BATTOCK & E. GENTON. 1975. Effects of clofibrate and

sulphinpyrazone on platelet survival time in coronary artery disease. Circulation **52:** 473.

88. STEELE, P., J. CARROLL, D. OVERFIELD & E. GENTON. 1977. Effect of sulphinpyrazone on platelet survival time in patients with transient cerebral ischaemic attacks. Stroke **8:** 396.

89. PHILP, R. B., I. FRANCY & B. A. WARREN. 1978. Comparison of antithrombotic activity of heparin, ASA, sulphinpyrazone and VK 744 in a rat model of arterial thrombosis. Haemostasis **7:** 282.

90. HLADOVEC, J. 1979. Is the antithrombotic activity of "antiplatelet" drugs based on protection of endothelium? Thromb. Haemostas. (Stuttgart) **41:** 774.

90. BREAM, M. L., R. B. PHILP & G. G. FERGUSON. 1979. Antiplatelet drugs in a rat microsurgical model of arterial thrombosis. Thromb. Res. **16:** 381.

92. KOHLER, C., W. WOODING & L. ELLENBOGEN. 1976. Intravenous arachidonate in the mouse: a model for the evaluation of antithrombotic drugs. Thromb. Res. **9:** 67.

93. CERSKUS, A. L., M. ALI, J. ZAMECNIK & J. W. D. McDONALD. 1981. Effects of indomethacin and sulphinpyrazone on in vivo formation of thromboxane B_2 and prostaglandin D_2 during arachidonate infusion in rabbits. Thromb. Res. **12:** 549.

94. MUSTARD, J. F., H. C. ROWSELL, H. A. SMYTHE, A. SENYI & E. A. MURPHY. 1967. The effect of sulphinpyrazone on platelet economy and thrombus formation in rabbits. Blood **29:** 859.

95. HARKER, L. A., S. R. HANSON & T. R. KIRKMAN. 1979. Experimental arterial thromboembolism in baboons: mechanism, quantitation and pharmacologic prevention. J. Clin. Invest. **64:** 559.

96. WILKINSON, A. R., R. J. HAWKER & L. M. HAWKER. 1979. The influence of antiplatelet drugs on platelet survival after aortic damage or implantation of a dacron arterial prosthesis. Thromb. Res. **15:** 181.

97. GOLDSTEIN, R. E., N. J. DAVENPORT, N. L. CAPURRO, L. C. LIPSON, R. O. BONOW, N. R. SHULMAN & S. E. EPSTEIN. 1980. Relative effects of sulfinpyrazone and ibuprofen on canine platelet function and prostaglandin-mediated coronary vasodilation. J. Cardiovasc. Res. **2:** 399.

98. CAPURRO, N. L., L. C. KIPSON, R. O. BONOW, R. E. GOLDSTEIN, N. R. SHULMAN & S. E. EPSTEIN. 1980. Relative effects of aspirin on platelet aggregation and prostaglandin-mediated coronary vasodilatation in the dog. Circulation **62:** 1221.

99. BEAMISH, R. E., K. S. DHILLON, P. K. SINGAL & N. S. DHALLA. 1981. Protective effect of sulfinpyrazone against catecholamine metabolite adrenochrome-induced arrhythmias. Am. Heart J. **102**(2): 149.

100. CAZENAVE, J.-P., M. A. PACKHAM, M. A. GUCCIONE & J. F. MUSTARD. 1974. Inhibition of platelet adherence to a collagen-coated surface by nonsteroidal anti-inflammatory drugs, pyrimido-pyrimidine and trycyclic compounds and lidocaine. J. Lab. Clin. Med. **83:** 797.

101. GROVES, H. M., R. L. KINLOUGH-RATHBONE, J.-P. CAZENAVE, M. RICHARDSON & J. F. MUSTARD. 1978. Effect of dipyridamole and aspirin on platelet adherence to damaged rabbit aortas in vitro and in vivo. Fed. Proc. **37:** 260.

102. EMMONS, P. R., M. J. G. HARRISON, A. J. HONOUR & J. R. A. MITCHELL. 1965. Effect of dipyridamole on human platelet behavior. Lancet **2:** 603.

103. ZUCKER, M. B. & J. PETERSON. 1970. Effect of acetylsalicyclic acid, other non steroidal anti-inflammatory agents and dipyridamole on human blood platelets. J. Lab. Clin. Med. **76:** 66.

104. MILLS, D. C. B. 1977. *In* Platelets and Thrombosis. 63–70. Academic Press. London.

105. RAJAH, S. M., M. J. CROW, A. F. PENNY, R. AHMAD & D. A. WATSON. 1977. The effect of dipyridamole on platelet function: Correlation with blood levels in man. Br. J. Clin. Pharm. **4:** 129.

106. SUBBARAO, K., B. RUCINSKI, M. A. RAUSCH, K. SCHMID & S. NIEWIAROWSKI. 1977. Binding of dipyridamole to human platelets and to an acid glycoprotein and its significance for the inhibition of adenosine uptake. J. Clin. Invest. **60:** 936.

107. BUCHANAN, M. R. & J. HIRSH. 1978. A comparison of the effects of aspirin and dipyridamole on platelet aggregation in vivo and ex vivo. Thromb. Res. **13:** 517.

108. ALLY, A. I., M. S. MANKU, D. F. HORROBIN, R. O. MORGAN, M. KARMAZIN & R. A. KARMALI. 1977. Dipyridamole: A possible potent inhibitor of thromboxane A_2 synthetase in vascular smooth muscle. Prostaglandins **14:** 607.

109. MONCADA, S. & R. KORBUT. 1978. Dipyridamole and other phosphodiesterase inhibitors act as antithrombotic agents by potentiating endogenous prostacyclin. Lancet **1:** 1286.

110. DiMINNO, G., G. DE GAETANO & S. GARATTINI. 1978. Dipyridamole and platelet function. Lancet **2:** 1258.

111. DALE, J., E. MYHRE & K. ROOTWELT. 1975. Effects of dipyridamole and acetylsalicylic acid on platelet functions in patients with aortic ball-valve prostheses. Am. Heart J. **89:** 613.

112. HARKER, L. A., S. J. SLICHTER & L. R. SAUVAGE. 1977. Platelet consumption by arterial prostheses: The effect of endothelialization and pharmacologic inhibition of platelet function. Ann. Surg. **186:** 594.

113. ARFORS, K.-E., D. BERGQVIST & O. TANGEN. 1975. The effect of platelet function inhibitors on experimental venous thrombosis formation in rabbits. Acta Chir. Scand. **141:** 40.

114. PHILP, R. B. & J. R. V. LEMIEUX. 1968. Comparison of some effects of dipyridamole and adenosine on thrombus formation, platelet adhesiveness and blood pressure in rabbits and rats. Nature **218:** 1072.

115. DIDISHEIM, P. 1968. Inhibition by dipyridamole of arterial thrombosis in rats. Thromb. Diath. Haemorrh. **20:** 257.

116. MAYER, J. E., JR. & G. L. HAMMOND. 1973. Dipyridamole and aspirin tested against an experimental model of thrombosis. Ann. Surg. **178:** 108.

117. MASON, R. G., R. H. WOLF, W. H. ZUCKER, B. A. SHIMODA & S. F. MOHAMMAD. 1976. Effects of antithrombotic agents evaluated in a non-human primate vascular shunt model. Am. J. Path. **83:** 557.

118. DANESE, C. A. & M. HAIMOV. 1971. Inhibition of experimental arterial thrombosis in dogs with platelet-deaggregating agents. Surgery **70:** 927.

119. JUSTICE, C., E. PAPAVENGELOU & W. S. EDWARDS. 1974. Prevention of thrombosis with agents which reduce platelet adhesiveness. Am. Surgeon **40:** 186.

120. ELWOOD, P. C., A. L. COCHRANE, M. L. BURR, P. M. SWEETNAM, G. WILLIAMS, E. WELSBY, S. J. HUGHES & R. RENTON. 1974. A randomized controlled trial of acetyl-salicylic acid in the secondary prevention of mortality from myocardial infarction. Br. Med. J. **1:** 436.

121. Coronary Drug Project Research Group. 1976. Aspirin in coronary heart disease. J. Chron. Dis. **29:** 625.

122. BREDDIN, K. 1977. Multicenter two-year prospective study on the prevention of secondary myocardial infarction by ASA in comparison with phenprocoumon and placebo. *In* Multicenter Controlled Trials: Principles and Problems. J. P. Buissel & C. R. Klimt, Eds.: 79–92. INSERM, Paris.

123. ELWOOD, P. C. & P. M. SWEETNAM. 1979. Aspirin and secondary mortality after myocardial infarction. Lancet **2:** 1313.

124. Aspirin Myocardial Infarction Study Research Group. 1980. A randomized controlled trial of aspirin in persons recovered from myocardial infarction. J. Am. Med. Assoc. **243:** 661.
125. The Persantine-Aspirin Reinfarction Study Research Group. 1980. Persantine and aspirin in coronary heart disease. Circulation **62:** 449.
126. ELWOOD, P. C. & W. O. WILLIAMS. 1979. A randomized controlled trial of aspirin in the prevention of early mortality in myocardial infarction. J. Roy. Coll. Gen. Pract. **29:** 413.
127. HAMMOND, E. C. & L. GARFINKEL. 1975. Aspirin and coronary heart disease: findings of a prospective study. Br. Med. J. **2:** 269.
128. Boston Collaborative Drug Surveillance Group. 1974. Regular aspirin intake and acute myocardial infarction. Br. Med. J. **1:** 440.
129. HENNEKENS, C. H., L. K. KARISON & B. ROSNER. 1978. A case-control study of regular aspirin use and coronary deaths. Circulation **58:** 35.
130. GENT, A. E., C. G. D. BROOK, T. H. FOLEY & T. N. MILLER. 1968. Dipyridamole: A controlled trial of its effect in myocardial infarction. Br. Med. J. **4:** 366.
131. Anturane Reinfarction Trial Research Group. 1978. Sulfinpyrazone in the prevention of cardiac death after myocardial infarction. The Anturane Reinfarction Trial. N. Engl. J. Med. **298:** 289.
132. Anturane Reinfarction Trial Research Group. 1980. Sulfinpyrazone in the prevention of sudden death after myocardial infarction. N. Engl. J. Med. **302:** 250.
133. Editorial. 1978. Sulfinpyrazone and prevention of myocardial infarction. Food and Drug Admin. Drug Bull. **8:** 3.
134. Editorial. 1978. Sulfinpyrazone, cardiac infarction, and the prevention of death: a successful trial or another tribulation? Br. Med. J. **1:** 941.
135. Editorial. 1980. FDA says no to Anturane. Science **208:** 1130.

DISCUSSION

UNIDENTIFIED SPEAKER: Dr. Hirsh, do you think the Paris study would have been more revealing had a lower dose of aspirin been used, and the vascular component not been activated?

DR. HIRSH: Yes, that is reasonable on theoretical grounds. If the study is repeated, a case could be made for using a smaller dose of aspirin on the basis of that pharmacologic principle.

DR. SHAND: My plea is not for another 25-million dollar study to look at low-dose aspirin, but for a few thousand dollars to find out whether the pharmacology in man is really appropriate for that hypothesis in the first place.

DR. HIRSH: Your point is well taken. Nevertheless, the difficulty is that until you actually do the study you cannot extrapolate. We should perform the study using the best information available in terms of dosages.

BETA BLOCKING AGENTS: CURRENT STATUS IN THE PREVENTION OF SUDDEN CORONARY DEATH *

Å. Hjalmarson

Department of Medicine I
Sahlgren's Hospital
University of Göteborg
Göteborg, Sweden

In the West ischemic heart disease is the main cause of death.[1-3] Most of these deaths are sudden and occur within the first few hours of onset of symptoms and before the patient reaches the hospital.[1, 4, 5] It is generally accepted that sudden death is due to ventricular fibrillation in most cases, but the pathogenesis and the factors predisposing to ventricular fibrillation are not well defined.[6-8] In order to prevent deaths occurring outside the hospital risk factors such as tobacco smoking and hypertension must be eliminated and prophylactic medication must be instituted in patients at high risk for cardiac death.

Beta-adrenoceptor blocking agents have been widely used in various conditions for more than 15 years. Today beta blockade is a well-established means of therapy in the treatment of patients with hypertension, angina pectoris, and tachyarrhythmias. During the last few years long-term treatment with beta blocking agents has been suggested as potentially useful therapy for reduction of morbidity and mortality in ischemic heart disease. The aim of this presentation is to review the studies of long-term beta blockade in the prevention of cardiac death.

NONRANDOMIZED STUDIES

In 1965 it was first suggested by Snow[9] that oral administration of propranolol, 10–20 mg three times daily, during the first weeks of acute myocardial infarction could reduce the total number of deaths from 35% in the control group to 16% in the active treatment group. This study was small, however, and included only 91 patients treated in an open fashion for less than 1 month. A few years later, Amsterdam and coworkers[10] suggested that long-term treatment with propranolol of patients with angina pectoris or previous myocardial infarction, or both, could reduce total mortality as compared with results in patients on long-acting nitroglycerin therapy or after implantation of an internal mammary artery. Some years later, Lambert[11] reported that propranolol in patients with angina pectoris or hypertension, or both, reduced the total number of deaths as well as the number of sudden deaths. All these retrospective studies suggested a favorable effect of long-term beta blockade on morbidity and mortality in ischemic heart disease.

* This investigation was supported by grants from the Swedish Medical Research Council (projects No. B80–19X–2529–11A and B81–19X–2529–12B), the Swedish National Association against Heart and Chest Diseases, the Göteborg Medical Society, and AB Hässle, subsidiary of AB Astra, Sweden.

0077–8923/82/0382–0305 $1.75/0 © 1982, NYAS

RANDOMIZED AND PROSPECTIVE STUDIES

After the first report appeared by Snow in 1965 claiming a reduction in mortality with propranolol given early in the progress of acute myocardial infarction, a number of similar studies were performed. The positive effect suggested for propranolol could not be confirmed in prospective trials.[12-16] Besides propranolol the other available beta blocking agent during the 1960s was alprenolol, a beta-adrenergic blocking drug with intrinsic stimulatory activity. Also, this beta blocking agent was given to patients with acute myocardial infarction in comparison with patients given placebo tablets under double-blind conditions.[17, 18] Neither of these early alprenolol studies demonstrated any favorable effect of beta blockade on survival. However, all these early studies were either very short term or included only a small number of patients. Data from two such studies on propranolol and alprenolol, respectively, are given in TABLE 1. These first negative prospective trials with beta blocking agents in patients after myocardial infarction were followed by three studies claiming a reduction in mortality by beta blockade (TABLE 1).[19-22] As can be seen from the Table, the duration of double-blind treatment was now longer (up to 2 years) and/or more patients were included in the trial.[21, 22]

The two studies from Sweden [19, 20] consisted of a rather small number of patients (230 and 162, respectively). However, in these two trials the patients were divided into four prognostically homogeneous subgroups, causing an accumulation of deaths in smaller groups at high risk. The subgroups included patients with no extensive cardiac damage (subgroup I), those with mechanical damage to the myocardium (subgroup II), those with significant arrhythmias (subgroup III), and patients with a combination of mechanical damage and arrhythmias (subgroup IV). All deaths but one in the two studies occurred in the subgroups II and IV, comprising patients with more marked mechanical damage of the heart. Sudden deaths in the two studies were defined as deaths within 24 hours of onset of any symptoms, and this figure was significantly reduced by alprenolol (FIG. 1, TABLE 1). The total mortality was reduced by 50% or more in both studies, but this reduction reached significance in only one of the studies.[20] In the study from Göteborg,[19] all women and men aged 57 to 67 years who had suffered an acute myocardial infarction and were discharged alive from hospital were included in the double-blind study. In the study from Falun,[20] patients aged 35 to 65 years were randomly assigned to an alprenolol group or to a control group. In contrast to the study from Göteborg, this was an open study and the patients were somewhat younger. The treatment was started 3 to 4 weeks after onset of acute infarction and it was well tolerated. In the study from Falun there was also a significant reduction in the number of reinfarctions, which was not the case in Göteborg. This could have resulted from several factors: The Falun study was an open study, with no special standardized follow-up study of the patients in a postinfarction clinic with careful control of possible risk factors, as was the case in Göteborg. Furthermore, patients in Falun were 5 years younger.

The results from the Multicentre International Study on practolol were first reported in 1975, followed by an additional report in 1977. More than 3000 patients from 67 centers were included and the mean duration of follow-up was 14 months, ranging from less than 1 month to 2 years. The trial was originally planned to include 4000 patients all treated for at least 1 year, but had to be terminated earlier because of the serious oculocutaneous and peri-

TABLE 1

PROSPECTIVE STUDIES

Drug (daily dose)	No. of Patients	Start after Acute Myocardial Infarction	Duration of therapy	Mean age (yr)	No. of Sudden Deaths:* Placebo/ Active Therapy (no.)	Total No. of Deaths:* Placebo/ Active Therapy (no.)	Author and Year of Report
Propranolol (20 mg×4)	454	Day 1	3 wk	(<70)	17/20	24/31	Norris et al.[16] (1968)
Alprenolol (100 mg×4)	87	Day 1	1 yr	54 (<70)	2/3	3/3	Reynolds and Whitlock[18] (1972)
Alprenolol (200 mg×2)	230	4 wk	2 yr	62 (57–67)	11/3 †	14/7	Wilhelmsson et al.[19] (1974)
Alprenolol (100 mg×4)	162	3 wk	2 yr	57 (35–65)	9/1 †	11/5 †	Ahlmark et al.[20] (1974)
Practolol (200 mg×2)	3053 (2282)	2 wk	14 mo	55 (<70)	?/? (55/31 ‡)	124/96 (83/54 †)	Multicentre International Study[21,22] (1975, 1977)

* Deaths in all patients randomly (blindly) assigned to treatment or to placebo group.
† p <0.05.
‡ p <0.01.

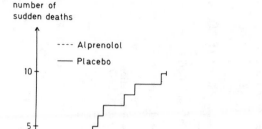

FIGURE 1. Cumulative numbers of sudden deaths in the group treated with alprenolol and in the placebo group during a 2-year follow-up period. (From Wilhelmsson *et al.*[10] Reproduced by permission.)

toneal reactions induced by practolol. The treatment was started 1 to 4 weeks after onset of infarction (mean 2 weeks) and patients younger than 70 years were included. The information provided by the two reports published in 1975 and 1977 makes it possible to calculate the number of total deaths for all patients randomly assigned to treatment or placebo in the trial. However, the causes of death in patients withdrawn from drug treatment are only characterized as cardiac and noncardiac. Furthermore, some conflicting data occur in the two studies The total number of deaths was lower in the group treated with practolol, but the difference did not reach statistical significance (TABLE 2). There was no difference in mortality in the patients withdrawn from the blind oral treatment. In the patients remaining on blind treatment (n = 2282), total deaths, cardiac deaths, and sudden deaths (deaths within 2 hours of onset of any symptoms) were significantly lower in the group treated with practolol. The number of sudden deaths in the treatment group to which the patient belonged first ("intention to treat") cannot be found from the two reports. In this study there was a trend towards a lower number of nonfatal reinfarctions

TABLE 2

MULTICENTRE INTERNATIONAL STUDY ON PRACTOLOL [21, 22]

	Placebo	Practolol	Significance
Total no. of patients	1533	1520	
Total no. of deaths	124	96	NS
No. of patients withdrawn	382	389	
All deaths	41	42	NS
Patients on blind treatment	1151	1131	
All deaths	83	54	$p < 0.02$
Cardiac deaths	78	48	$p < 0.01$
Sudden deaths	55	31	$p < 0.01$
Death from other causes	5	6	NS

Note: NS = not significant.

in the practolol-treated group (4.5 versus 5.8%; p < 0.1). Retrospectively, it was demonstrated that patients with anterior wall infarction and low diastolic blood pressure did particularly well on practolol.[21] TABLE 3 shows that when anterior and inferior wall infarctions are compared, a similar reduction in sudden deaths was found in the practolol-treated group, while contrasting results were seen in those with nonsudden deaths. In anterior wall infarction practolol was associated with a much lower number of nonsudden deaths, whereas in inferior infarction nonsudden deaths were much more frequent in the practolol-treated group than in the placebo-treated group. An analysis of the time of the deaths in the study showed a high incidence of fatal complications during the first 4 weeks in patients with posterior wall infarction in the practolol-treated group.[23] When prophylactic treatment was instituted 4 weeks after infarction there was no difference between patients with different sites of infarction.

In a study from Belfast,[24] patients were given practolol or placebo immediately after arrival at the hospital. This study comprised 298 patients with myocardial infarction and included 2 years of follow-up data (TABLE 4). In the study there was no significant difference in mortality between practolol- and placebo-treated groups at any time. A retrospective analysis of 53 patients with

TABLE 3

MULTICENTRE INTERNATIONAL STUDY [21]: RELATIONSHIP OF INFARCT SITE

Infarct Site	No. of Patients		Cardiac Death		Sudden Death		Nonsudden Death	
	Prac- tolol	Pla- cebo	Prac- tolol	Pla- cebo	Prac- tolol	Pla- cebo	Prac- tolol	Pla- cebo
Anterior	764	768	22 *	48 *	19	33	3	15
Inferior	760	746	25	25	11	19	14	6

initial heart rate higher than 100 beats per minute shows significantly lower mortality in the practolol-treated group compared with that of the placebo-treated group. This was mainly due to beneficial effects during the first 3 months. In this study a fairly high dose of practolol was given (600 mg daily) from the first day of acute myocardial infarction and the tolerance to the treatment was very good, with a low dropout rate despite the fact that patients with clear signs of congestive heart failure were included. The total 3-month mortality for all patients in the study was 16% and the 3-month to 2-year follow-up mortality was 13%, which can be compared with a 12% 3-month mortality in a similar study of metoprolol in Göteborg and a 3-month to 2-year mortality of 8.7% in the alprenolol study in Göteborg. It could be speculated that the inclusion of more severely ill patients in the practolol study in Belfast could have counteracted the beneficial results with practolol in the whole series of patients.

After the practolol study from Belfast was reported in 1975, the next post-infarction study with beta-adrenergic blockade/placebo treatment was reported in 1979 from Sundby Hospital in Copenhagen.[25] Most of the large long-term studies with beta-adrenergic blockade had thus far been performed in post-infarction patients below 70 years of age. Immediately after admission to the

TABLE 4

PROSPECTIVE STUDIES

Drug (daily dose)	No. of Patients	Start after Acute Myocardial Infarction	Duration	Mean age (yr)	No. of Sudden Deaths* Placebo:/Active Therapy (no.)	Total No. of Deaths* Placebo:/Active Therapy (no.)	Author and Year of Report
Practolol (300 mg×2)	298	Day 1	2 yr	63 (32–87)	Not reduced	46/41	Barber et al.[24] (1975)
Alprenolol (200 mg×2)	282	Day 1	1 yr	≤65	—	29/13 †	Andersen et al.[25] (1979)
	198	Day 1	1 yr	>65	—	35/48	
Atenolol (50 mg×2)	388	Day 1	1 yr	All ages	—	19/19	Wilcox et al.[26] (1980)
Propranolol (40 mg×3)					—	19/17	
Oxprenolol (40 mg×3)	315	Day 1	6 wk	All ages	—	10–14	Wilcox et al.[27] (1980)
Propranolol (40 mg×3)	720	1 wk	6 mo (3–9)	54	—	27–28	Baber et al.[28] (1980)
Timolol (10 mg×2)	1884	1–4 wk	17 mo (12–33)	61 (20–75)	95–47 †	152–98 †	The Norwegian Multicenter Study[29] (1981)

* Deaths in all patients randomly (blindly) assigned to a treatment or a placebo group.
† $p < 0.01$.
† $p < 0.001$.

hospital, the patients fulfilling the criteria for the study were divided into risk groups according to age, heart rate, and degree of conciousness. One group consisted of patients 65 years old or younger, and another group of patients was more than 65 years of age. Alprenolol was given, 5 to 10 mg intravenously, followed by 200 mg twice daily as a slow-release preparation. In the first report from this study in 1979 only data on total mortality were given. As can be seen from TABLE 4, alprenolol significantly reduced mortality in the younger group of patients ($\leq$65 years), whereas in the older group of patients ($>$65 years) there was a trend towards higher mortality in the alprenolol-treated group. The cumulative number of deaths in patients $\leq$65 years of age is shown in FIGURE 2. There is a significantly lower mortality in patients treated with alprenolol within 3 months. There are no further deaths in this group from 3 to 12 months. In the patients older than 65 years (FIG. 3), there was a

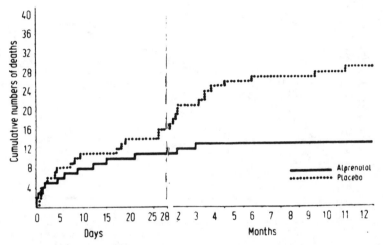

FIGURE 2. Cumulative numbers of deaths in all patients less than 65 years of age treated with alprenolol or placebo during the year of treatment. (From Andersen et al.[25] Reproduced by permission.)

trend towards higher mortality in the alprenolol-treated group that seemed to occur within the first few days of treatment. This difference did not reach statistical significance, but when this trend was detected, the Independent Safety Monitoring Board advised the exclusion from the study of patients older than 65 years. The reason for the negative results with alprenolol in the older group of patients might not be due to the higher age *per se*. The group of patients above 65 years had a higher number of previous infarctions and more often left ventricular heart failure compared with conditions in the younger group, which may be the reason for the early mortality in the alprenolol-treated group and the lack of positive effects on survival.

In 1980 two double-blind studies were reported on propranolol-atenolol and oxprenolol in patients with suspected myocardial infarction.[26, 27] Treatment was started immediately on entry to the coronary care unit and in one study, atenolol, propranolol, or placebo was given for 1 year to 388 patients and in another study oxprenolol or placebo was given for 6 weeks to 315 patients. In neither of the studies was the number of sudden deaths given. Furthermore, there was no significant reduction in total mortality by any of the three beta blocking agents. In the study with intention to treat patients with atenolol, propranolol, or placebo for 1 year, 31 to 40% of the patients in these groups were withdrawn from treatment within 6 weeks.[26] In the second study, which had a duration of only 6 weeks, 29% of the patients in the oxprenolol-treated group and 27% in the placebo-treated group were withdrawn from blind treatment.[27] A serious problem with these two studies is the high withdrawal rate from the trial. It was thought by the authors that this was mainly due to the fact that treatment was started immediately after admission to the coronary care unit. However, in an early intervention trial with metoprolol and placebo in Göteborg, starting with intravenous administration of the drug followed by

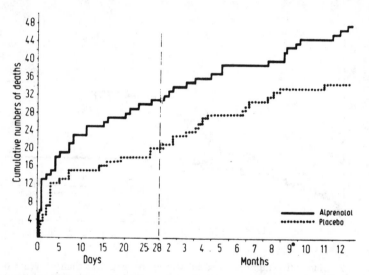

FIGURE 3. Cumulative numbers of deaths in all patients older than 65 years treated with alprenolol or placebo during the years of treatment. (From Andersen et al.[25] Reproduced by permission.)

oral treatment, fewer than 19% of the patients were withdrawn from treatment after 3 months. The reason might just as well be problems of patient selection and physician compliance.

Since the findings of the Multicentre Study with practolol[21] suggested that patients with anterior wall infarction did particularly well on practolol, a new Multicentre Postinfarction Trial was started comprising 720 patients.[28] This was a double-blind placebo controlled study with propranolol, 40 mg three times a day, from a total of 49 hospitals. The mean age of the patients was 54 years, ranging up to 70 years of age. Treatment started 2 to 14 days (mean 8 days) after onset of acute myocardial infarction. Duration of treatment was 3 to 9 months (mean duration, 170 days). As can be seen from TABLE 4, the total number of deaths in the propranolol and the placebo groups was identical. The number of sudden deaths was not given. The number of cardiac deaths in the trial was 18 in the placebo and 19 in the propranolol-treated group. There was no difference in mortality between the two groups at any time during the trial. The trial was designed to detect a 50% reduction in mortality, which was not shown. However, as mentioned by these authors, propranolol may still produce a reduction in mortality of less than 50%, and this is still possible within the confidence limits of the results. It is suggested that the lack of difference between the two groups in the study could be due to an inadequate sample size. Since the patients in the International Multicentre Study with practolol [21] with an anterior wall infarction and a diastolic blood pressure of 78 mm Hg or lower responded especially well to practolol, similar subgroups were analyzed in this propranolol study. However, in none of the subgroups studied was there a significant difference between the propranolol- and the placebo-treated groups.

Early in April 1981, the Norwegian Multicenter Study with timolol in patients surviving acute myocardial infarction was published.[29] As can be seen from TABLES 1 and 4, this Norwegian study, comprising 1884 patients, is the second largest after the Multicenter Study with practolol.[21] Furthermore, patients have been followed for a longer period of time than in the practolol study (mean time, 17 months and 14 months, respectively). In the Norwegian study, timolol was given in doses of 10 mg twice daily starting 1 to 4 weeks

TABLE 5

THE NORWEGIAN MULTICENTER STUDY: SELECTION OF PATIENTS

Number of screenings	11,125
Number with criteria for infarction	4155
Number alive evaluated for entry	3647
Exclusions from entry	1763
(contraindications for beta-adrenergic blockade in 18%)	
Number of randomized patients participating	1884

after onset of acute myocardial infarction. Patients aged 20 to 75 years (mean, 61 years) were included. The number of sudden deaths as well as total number of deaths in all patients "randomized" (intention to treat) was significantly lower in the timolol-treated group. The number of sudden deaths was reduced by about 50%. As can be seen from TABLE 5, 11,125 patients were screened in 20 clinical centers in Norway with a total catchment population of 1.3 million (one-third of the Norwegian population). Of the patients fulfilling criteria for infarction who were alive at the time of evaluation for entry to the trial, 48% were excluded and 52% were randomly assigned to the trial groups (n = 1184). All patients were classified into three different risk groups, as can be seen from TABLE 6. TABLE 7 shows the number of patients randomized and withdrawn and the total number of deaths in the three risk groups. It can be seen that there was a significantly lower total number of deaths in the timolol-treated group compared with that of the placebo group in risk groups II and III. It can also be seen that risk group II, consisting of patients with more marked damage to the left ventricle, has significantly more patients who were withdrawn from blind treatment in the timolol-treated group compared with that of the placebo group. The number of withdrawals in the placebo and the timolol-treated groups are very similar in risk groups I and III. It is reasonable that

TABLE 6

THE NORWEGIAN MULTICENTER STUDY: RISK GROUP STRATIFICATION

I	Recurrent myocardial infarction
II	First infarct with high-risk conditions: (1) heart failure (2) enlarged heart (3) atrial flutter or fibrillation (4) Systolic blood pressure <100 mm Hg (5) ASAT > four times normal limit
III	Remaining patients

patients with more marked damage to the left ventricle should have more adverse reactions to beta-adrenergic blockade compared with patients with better left ventricular function despite this. There is a marked reduction in total number of deaths in timolol-treated patients in risk group II.

FIGURES 4 and 5 show the life-table-cumulated rates of deaths from all causes and sudden deaths (defined as deaths occurring within 24 hours of onset of any symptoms), and both Figures show a significantly lower mortality rate in the timolol-treated patients. As can be seen from TABLE 8, timolol reduced the number of cardiac deaths to the same extent in patients 64 years or less as in patients 65 to 75 years old. This observation is in contrast with the poor results reported in subjects older than 65 years treated with alprenolol in Copenhagen.[25] TABLE 8 also shows that the reduction in number of cardiac deaths was, if anything, more marked in patients with inferior wall infarction and in patients with uncertain localization of infarction compared with those with anterior wall infarction. It was suggested from the Multicentre International Study on practolol[21] that, on the contrary, patients with anterior wall

TABLE 7

THE NORWEGIAN MULTICENTER STUDY: TOTAL NUMBER OF DEATHS AND WITHDRAWAL OF PATIENTS

	Risk Groups						All Groups	
	I		II		III			
	Placebo	Timolol	Placebo	Timolol	Placebo	Timolol	Placebo	Timolol
Number randomized	174	178	543	547	222	220	939	945
Number withdrawn	61	68	120	167 *	38	40	219	275 *
Total deaths (in all randomized patients)	42	34	89	54 *	21	10 †	152	98 ‡

* p <0.01.
† p <0.05.
‡ p <0.001.

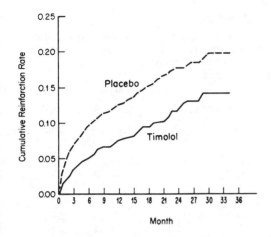

FIGURE 4. Life-table cumulative rates of death from all causes. (These deaths occurred while patients were taking the test medication or within 28 days of administration of last dose). (From the Norwegian Multicenter Study Group.[29] Reproduced by permission.)

infarction should benefit more from treatment with beta-adrenergic blockade than should those with anterior wall infarction. TABLE 8 further shows that the number of reinfarctions in the different groups was significantly reduced by timolol. It can thus be concluded that the reduction in mortality by timolol in the Norwegian Multicenter Study was more marked than that in the International Multicentre Study on practolol.[21] In the practolol study there was a low mortality in the placebo group during the first year (5%) compared with that of the Norwegian study (10%), indicating that there were more high-risk patients in the Norwegian study. It is obvious that a better reduction in mortality can be reached by prophylactic treatment when the mortality in the placebo group is relatively high.

As can be seen from TABLE 9 there are four randomized double-blind studies on beta blocking agents in postinfarction patients in which a prognostic stratification of the patients has been made. All four studies have shown a reduction in sudden deaths and/or total number of deaths by alprenolol or timolol, despite the fact that the numbers of patients in the three alprenolol studies are relatively small. This prognostic stratification may explain why

FIGURE 5. Life-table cumulated rates of sudden cardiac death during administration of medication or within 28 days of the last dose. (From the Norwegian Multicenter Study Group.[29] Reproduced by permission.)

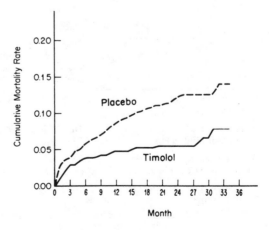

TABLE 8

THE NORWEGIAN MULTICENTER STUDY: CARDIAC DEATHS AND REINFARCTIONS DURING
TREATMENT OR WITHIN 28 DAYS OF WITHDRAWAL, ACCORDING TO AGE AND SITE
OF INFARCTION BEFORE ENTRY INTO THE STUDY

| | No. of Patients: | | | |
| | Cardiac Death | | Initial Reinfarction | |
Category	Placebo	Timolol	Placebo	Timolol
Age				
≤64 yr	54	30 *	72	55 †
65–75 yr	59	28 *	69	33 ‡
Infarction location				
Anterior	44	29	61	38 †
Inferior	36	16 *	52	24 ‡
Other or uncertain	33	13 ‡	28	26

* $p < 0.01$.
† $p < 0.05$.
‡ $p < 0.001$.

these three alprenolol studies reached significance despite the small number of patients.

ONGOING PROSPECTIVE TRIALS

There are at least 11 ongoing prospective trials with beta-adrenergic blocking agents after acute myocardial infarction and these trials include about 17,000 patients (TABLE 10). The beta₁-selective blocker, metoprolol, is being used in five of the studies and in two of these, treatment is started on admission to the hospital, with intravenous administration followed by oral treatment with the drug. In the two Swedish studies on metoprolol patients have been classified

TABLE 9

STUDIES WITH PROGNOSTIC STRATIFICATION

Study	No. of Patients	No. of Sudden Deaths	Total No. of Deaths
Wilhelmsson et al.[19] Alprenolol (Göteborg)	230	Reduced	Reduced (not significant)
Ahlmark et al.[20] Alprenolol (Falun)	162	Reduced	Reduced
Andersen et al.[25] Alprenolol (Copenhagen)	282 (≤65 yrs)	—	Reduced
The Norwegian Multicenter Study Group[29]	1884	Reduced	Reduced

TABLE 10A

ONGOING PROSPECTIVE TRIALS WITH BETA-ADRENERGIC BLOCKING AGENTS AFTER ACUTE MYOCARDIAL INFARCTION

Center	Drug	No. of Patients	Early Intravenous Administration	Prognostic Stratification	Duration
Multicenter, France	Acebutolol	500	—	—	1 yr
Belfast, Northern Ireland	Metoprolol	400	+	—	2 yr
Göteborg, Sweden	Metoprolol	800	+	+	3 mo
Stockholm, Sweden	Metoprolol	250	—	+	2 yr
Amsterdam, The Netherlands	Metoprolol	600	—	—	1 yr
Multicenter, United States	Metoprolol	3000	—	—	1 yr
Total		5600			

by prognosis into various risk groups. Several of these studies will be terminated in 1981 and the results will be available before end of the year. This is true for at least the metoprolol study from Göteborg, the multicenter study with propranolol in the United States (the Beta-blocker Heart Attack Trial [BHAT]), and the multicenter study on sotalol in England. These studies will add important information to our present knowledge of the effects of beta-adrenergic blockade in the early and late phase of myocardial infarction. These studies ought to clarify whether beta-adrenergic blockade can also reduce early mortality (within 3 months) when administered from day of admission. Since various beta blocking agents, $beta_1$-selective and nonselective blockers, with

TABLE 10B

ONGOING PROSPECTIVE TRIALS WITH BETA-ADRENERGIC BLOCKING AGENTS AFTER ACUTE MYOCARDIAL INFARCTION

Center	Drug	No. of Patients	Early Intravenous Administration	Prognostic Stratification	Duration
Multicenter, Europe	Oxprenolol	1400	—	—	1 yr
Multicenter, United States	Propranolol	4200	—	—	1 yr
Multicenter, Norway	Propranolol	800	—	—	1 yr
Multicenter	Pindolol	700	—	—	1 yr
Multicenter, England	Sotalol	1600	—	—	1 yr
Total		11,400			

and without intrinsic stimulatory activity, are used in the various studies, it should be possible to find out whether a certain property of the beta blocker is of importance or if cardioprotection will be obtained by all types of beta blockers.

POSSIBLE MECHANISMS OF THE BENEFICIAL EFFECT OF BETA-ADRENERGIC BLOCKING AGENTS IN ISCHEMIC HEART DISEASE

A large number of studies, both in experimental animals and in patients, have shown that beta-adrenergic blocking agents can reduce the severity of myocardial ischemia. In experimental animals pretreatment with beta blocking agents will limit experimental infarct size [30, 31] and also reduce the incidence of experimental ventricular fibrillation.[8] In our own studies from Göteborg, it has been found that administration of beta blocking agents in the early phase of acute myocardial infarction can reduce heart work, ischemic chest pain, and S-T segment elevation in man.[32, 33] It has also been suggested that early administration of beta blockers to patients with acute myocardial infarction can limit infarct size.[34] It has been reported that beta blocking agents will reduce stress-induced thrombocyte aggregation in patients with ischemic heart disease. At the Symposium on Acute and Long-Term Management of Myocardial Ischemia held recently in Oslo, Thaulow reported that in a subgroup of patients of the Norwegian timolol study timolol had no significant effect on thrombocyte aggregation, either at rest or during exercise.[35] The possible mechanisms involved in the cardioprotective effect of beta-adrenergic blockade are listed in TABLE 11. Further studies will be needed to clarify which mechanisms are of importance.

The properties of various beta blocking agents are given in TABLE 12. As discussed, alprenolol, practolol, and timolol have all been reported to reduce cardiac death during long-term treatment after myocardial infarction. The only property of the beta blocking agents in common for all three drugs is the $beta_1$-selective blockade. It therefore seems reasonable to believe that $beta_1$-selective blockade is the most important and perhaps the only important property for cardioprotection in man. It has also been known for several years that $beta_1$-selective blocking agents can prevent experimental ventricular fibrillation as well as can nonselective drugs.

SELECTION OF PATIENTS FOR CARDIOPROTECTION

A number of studies have been performed in which beta blocking agents are given to patients after acute myocardial infarction. Some of these studies have shown positive results on survival and incidence of reinfarction, while others have shown no beneficial effects at all. There are definite contraindications to both acute and chronic beta-adrenergic blockade, such as severe heart failure, bradycardia, atrioventricular block, and hypotension. The effects of beta-adrenergic blockade in these patients can be harmful. It seems, however, that the majority of patients in a state of either acute myocardial infarction or postmyocardial infarction will tolerate long-term treatment with beta blocking agents. In our experience of the last 10 years, in which more than 1000 patients with acute myocardial infarction in Göteborg have been given intra-

TABLE 11

WHICH MECHANISMS ARE INVOLVED IN CARDIOPROTECTION BY BETA BLOCKADE?

1. Reduced heart work?
2. Reduced thrombocyte aggregation?
3. Reduced myocardial ischemia?
4. Direct antifibrillatory effects?
5. Other mechanisms?

venous and oral practolol or metoprolol, we have found that about 80% of all patients tolerate beta-adrenergic blockade. In the timolol study, one week after onset of infarction 18% of the patients were found to have contraindications to beta-adrenergic blockade, which is comparable to our figures. Even patients with mild to moderate heart failure could be given beta blocking agents together with digitalis and/or diuretics. In patients at high risk for cardiac death, it seems justified to accept some mild side effects, such as fatigue, at least for some period of time. It seems logical to institute a more aggressive prophylactic treatment in younger patients. In our experience, beta blocking agents are also well tolerated in elderly people, although we recommend a slightly lower dose. The presence of angina pectoris, hypertension, or tachyarrhythmias in postinfarction patients will make it easier to convince patients of the value of long-term treatment with beta-adrenergic blockade. There is no clear evidence that the site of infarction is of importance in the selection of patients for long-term prophylactic treatment with beta blockade. If we accept the concept that long-term treatment with beta-adrenergic blocking agents can reduce the total number of all cardiac events, cardiac deaths, and nonfatal reinfarctions, then all patients at some risk of cardiac events should be considered for long-term beta-adrenergic blockade, unless clear-cut contraindications exist.

CONCLUSION

A great number of studies have been performed in which beta-adrenergic blocking agents have been given to patients after myocardial infarction. Only five of these studies—those utilizing alprenolol, practolol, and timolol—have demonstrated a reduction in sudden death and/or total mortality. The studies showing positive results with beta-adrenergic blockade on survival are the two

TABLE 12

PROPERTIES OF BETA BLOCKING AGENTS IMPORTANT FOR CARDIOPROTECTION

1. Beta$_1$ selective blockade *   (alprenolol, practolol, timolol) †
2. Beta$_2$ selective blockade   (alprenolol, timolol)
3. Intrinsic stimulation   (alprenolol, practolol)
4. Membrane stability   (alprenolol, timolol)

* Beta$_1$ selective blockade is the most important property (only?) for cardioprotection (in common for all three beta blockers).
† Beta blockers with positive effects on survival.

with the largest populations (multicenter studies with practolol and timolol) and the studies in which a prognostic stratification of patients into various risk groups was made (three studies with alprenolol). In order to demonstrate a significant reduction in mortality from, for example, 10% in the placebo group to 5% in the active group, more than 1000 patients will be needed, unless sufficient mortality cannot be accumulated in some subgroups. In the patients surviving acute myocardial infarction and in whom there are no contraindications for beta-adrenergic blockade, the 1-year mortality is about 10% and seems at best to be reduced to 5%. It therefore seems reasonable to conclude that beta-adrenergic blockade exerts a positive effect on survival after myocardial infarction in the studies of 2000 to 3000 patients. All the other studies are too small to be able to demonstrate with any certainty a 50% reduction in mortality by beta blockade. The results of the available studies strongly suggest that beta-adrenergic blockade can reduce mortality when given for 2 years after acute myocardial infarction. The results of several ongoing studies will be available in 1981 and we will better be able to know whether all patients surviving an acute myocardial infarction without contraindications for beta-adrenergic blockade should be given this treatment for at least 2 years.

REFERENCES

1. KULLER, L. 1962. Sudden and unexpected nontraumatic deaths in adults: A review of epidemiological and clinical studies. J. Chron. Dis. 19: 1165.
2. STAMLER, J. Cardiovascular diseases in the United States. Am. J. Cardiol. 10: 319.
3. VEDIN, J. A., C. WILHELMSSON, A. M. BOLANDER & L. WERKÖ. 1971. Mortality trends in Sweden 1951–1968 with special reference to cardiovascular cause of death. Acta Med. Scand. Suppl 515: 1.
4. ROMO, M. 1973. Factors related to sudden death in acute ischaemic disease. Acta Med. Scand. Suppl 547: 1.
5. WILHELMSEN, L., S. LUNGBERG, H. WEDEL & L. WERKÖ. 1976. A comparison between participants and non-participants in a primary preventive trial. J. Chron. Dis. 29: 331.
6. HAN, J. & B. G. GOEL. 1972. Electrophysiological precursors of ventricular tachyarrhythmias. Arch. Intern. Med. 129: 749.
7. VISMARA, L. A., E. A. AMSTERDAM & D. T. MASON. 1975. Relation to ventricular arrhythmias in the late hospital phase of acute myocardial infarction to sudden death after hospital discharge. Am. J. Med. 59: 6.
8. HJALMARSON, A. 1978.
9. SNOW, P. J. D. 1965. Effect of propranolol in myocardial infarction. Lancet 2: 551.
10. AMSTERDAM, E. A., S. WOLFSON & R. GORLIN. 1968. Effect of therapy on survival in angina pectoris. Ann. Intern. Med. 63: 115.
11. LAMBERT, D. M. D. 1974. Hypertension and myocardial infarction (abstract). Br. Med. J. 3: 685.
12. BALCON, R., D. E. JEWITT, J. P. H. DAVIES & S. ORAM. 1966. A controlled trial of propranolol in acute myocardial infarction. Lancet 2: 917.
13. CLAUSEN, J., M. FELSBY, F. SCHÖNAU JÖRGENSEN, B. LYAGER NIELSEN, J. ROIN & B. STRANGE. 1966. Absence of prophylactic effect of propranolol in myocardial infarction. Lancet 2: 920.
14. MULTICENTRE TRIAL. 1966. Propranolol in acute myocardial infarction. Lancet 2: 1435.
15. BARBER, J. M., F. M. MURPHY & J. D. MERRETT. 1967. Clinical trial of propranolol in acute myocardial infarction. Ulster Med. J. 36: 127.

16. NORRIS, R. M., D. E. CAUGHEY & P. J. SCOTT. 1968. Trial of propranolol in acute myocardial infarction. Br. Med. J. 2: 398.

17. BRIANT, R. B. & R. M. NORRIS. 1970. Alprenolol in acute myocardial infarction: Double-blind trial. N.Z. Med. J. 71: 135.

18. REYNOLDS, J. L. & WHITLOCK. 1972. Effects of a beta-adrenergic receptor blocker in myocardial infarction treated for one year from onset. Br. Heart J. 34: 242.

19. WILHELMSSON, C., J. A. VEDIN, L. WILHELMSEN, G. TIBBLIN & L. WERKÖ. 1974. Reduction of sudden deaths after myocardial infarction by treatment with alprenolol. Preliminary results. Lancet 2: 1157.

20. AHLMARK, G., H. SAETRE & M. KORSGREN. 1974. Letter: Reduction of sudden deaths after myocardial infarction. Lancet 2: 1563.

21. MULTICENTRE INTERNATIONAL STUDY. 1975. Improvement in prognosis of myocardial infarction by long-term beta-adrenoceptor blockade using practolol. Br. Med. J. 3: 735.

22. Multicentre International Study. 1977. Supplementary report: Reduction in mortality after myocardial infarction with long-term beta-adrenoceptor blockade. Br. Med. J. 2: 419.

23. GREEN, K. G.

24. BARBER, J. M., D. McC. BOYLE, N. C. CHATURVEDI, N. SINGH & M. J. WALSH. 1975. Practolol in acute myocardial infarction. Acta Med. Scand. (Suppl) 587: 213.

25. ANDERSEN, M. P., P. BECHSGAARD, J. FREDERIKSEN, D. A. HANSEN, H. J. JÜRGENSEN, B. NIELSEN, F. PEDERSEN, O. PEDERSEN-BJERGAARD & S. L. RASMUSSEN. 1979. Effect of alprenolol on mortality among patients with definite or suspected acute myocardial infarction. Lancet 2: 865.

26. WILCOX, R. G., J. M. ROLAND, D. C. BANKS, J. R. HAMPTON & J. R. A. MITCHELL. 1980. Randomized trial comparing propranolol with atenolol in immediate treatment of suspected myocardial infarction. Br. Med. J. 280: 885.

27. WILCOX, R. G., J. M. ROWLEY, J. R. HAMPTON & J. R. A. MITCHELL. 1980. Randomized placebo-controlled trial comparing oxprenolol with disopyramide phosphate in immediate treatment of suspected myocardial infarction. Lancet 2: 765.

28. BABER, N. S., D. WAINWRIGHT EVANS, G. HOWITT, M. THOMAS, C. WILSON, J. A. LEWIS, P. M. DAWES, K. HANDLER & R. TUSON. 1980. Multicentre postinfarction trial of propranolol in 49 hospitals in the United Kingdom, Italy, and Yugoslavia. Br. Heart J. 44: 96.

29. NORWEGIAN MULTICENTER STUDY GROUP. 1981. Timolol-induced reduction in mortality and reinfarction in patients surviving acute myocardial infarction. N. Engl. J. Med. 304: 801.

30. BRAUNWALD, E. & P. R. MAROKO. 1974. The reduction of infarct size—an idea whose time (for testing) has come. Circulation 50: 206.

31. WALDENSTRÖM, A. P. & Å. C. HJALMARSON. 1977. Factors modifying ischemic injury in the isolated rat heart. Acta Med. Scand. 201: 533.

32. WAAGSTEIN, F. & Å. C. HJALMARSON. 1975. Effect of cardioselective beta-blockade on heart function and chest pain in acute myocardial infarction. Acta Med. Scand. Suppl 587: 193.

33. WAAGSTEIN, F. & Å. C. HJALMARSON. 1975. Double-blind study of the effect of cardioselective beta-blockade on chest pain in acute myocardial infarction. Acta Med. Scand. Suppl 587: 201.

34. HJALMARSON, Å., R. ARINIEGO, J. HERLITZ, S. HOLMBERG, I. MÁLEK, K. SWEDBERG, F. WAAGSTEIN, A. WALDENSTRÖM, J. WALDENSTRÖM, A. VEDIN, L. WILHELMSEN & C. WILHELMSSON. 1979. Limitation of infarct size in man by the beta$_1$-blocker metoprolol (abstract). Circulation 60 (Suppl II): 164.

35. THAULOW, E. The effect of timolol on platelet aggregation in coronary heart

disease. *In* Symposium on Acute and Long Term Management of Myocardial Ischemia, Oslo, April 3–5, 1981. In press.
36. HJALMARSON, Å. 1980. Myocardial metabolic changes related to ventricular fibrillation. Cardiology **65:** 226.

DISCUSSION

DR. BIGGER: Do you think that it is important to begin therapy with beta blockers early the hospitalization period after acute infarction?

DR. HJALMARSON: The earlier you can start, the better off you will be.

DR. BIGGER: Do you think that it is reasonable to stop beta blockade in a patient who is taking it and is then admitted with acute infarction?

DR. HJALMARSON: No; beta blockade should not be stopped, for this is when the patient needs it most. In the same way, patients also need beta blockade as protection during surgery and it should not be discontinued.

DR. DWYER: Some of the believers in beta blockade have extended its use to the congestive cardiomyopathies; has this given you the additional courage to use beta blockade in patients with significant left ventricular dysfunction after myocardial infarction?

DR. HJALMARSON: We have performed a number of studies in patients with idiopathic primary congestive myopathy. We reported that compared with a matched control group we can reduce mortality by about 50% in the group of patients with myopathy. Pump function will improve dramatically in about 50% of all patients. Some patients go from New York Heart Association class IV to class I and return to work. It's simply unbelievable. We don't know the mechanism for such drastic improvement, but we must remember that this subgroup is special, and therefore it doesn't mean that all patients with heart failure can be given beta blocking agents. All patients with myocardial ischemia should have treatment aimed at reduction of ischemia, which in turn will improve left ventricular pump function and reduce symptoms. But again, I'm a believer that all the patients with coronary artery disease and pump failure might benefit from beta blockade if it is started early enough.

DR. STEWART: Are the mortality and morbidity of the patients who were taking beta blockers but who had recurrent myocardial infarction any different from those of the control group?

DR. HJALMARSON: The only study available so far is our own study and since that has just terminated our results are not available yet.

DR. STEWART: In the timolol study weren't the patients started on timolol several weeks after their infarction?

DR. HJALMARSON: The time varied from about 1 to 4 weeks; I think that the average was a bit more than 2 weeks.

DR. GREENBERG: Could you comment on the development of a rapid, intravenous beta blocker that would deteriorate very rapidly? One of the problems in deciding whether or not to put a patient on a beta blocker after an acute myocardial infarction is the state of the left ventricle, and the clinical state can be misleading. There is a reluctance to initiate therapy with an agent that may stay around a long time.

DR. HJALMARSON: At least two companies in the world are working on this, although it will take some time before it will be available. In the meantime we are working on beta blockade on the one hand and beta stimulation on the other. In myocardial infarction in patients with pulmonary edema, we give 80 mg of furosemide intravenously and 2 hours later we start beta blockade. Most of the patients will tolerate that treatment very well, but we have at the ready the beta stimulating agent that could immediately neutralize the beta blocking agent.

THE ROLE OF ORGANIZED MEDICINE IN PROVIDING EDUCATION ABOUT CARDIOPULMONARY RESUSCITATION *

Richard Crampton

Cardiology Division and Emergency Medical Service
University of Virginia Medical Center
Charlottesville, Virginia 22908

Why should organized medicine attempt to educate the public about cardiopulmonary resuscitation (CPR)? Since the initiation in 1971 of the Medic II community program of CPR in Seattle,[1] this life-saving technique [2] and the subsequently added technique of abdominal thrust (the Heimlich maneuver) for choking [3] have been disseminated widely.[4] The rationale and proof of efficacy of out-of-hospital CPR carried out by lay persons has emerged in reports from Oslo, Birmingham, Seattle, Los Angeles, and Winnepeg (TABLE 1).[5-8, 25]

Acquiring the technique of CPR in a classroom or by poster or television portrayal, the public in Seattle doubled the number of lives saved when citizen-initiated CPR preceded rapid prehospital defibrillation (TABLE 1).[7] A 50% long-term survival rate was achieved when CPR was initiated 4 minutes or less after collapse from ventricular fibrillation and a defibrillating shock was delivered 8 minutes or less from the time of collapse.[9]

Examination of the sequential data emerging from the Seattle reports indicates that the substantial, steadily increasing number of lives saved each year by prehospital CPR and emergency care now approaches 90 to 95 long-term survivors annually.[1, 7, 10-13] In 1971, CPR was initiated by a citizen in 5% of out-of-hospital cardiac arrests, in 1975 by 19%, and in 1976 by 34%.[12, 13] When Acton's value is used of $21,000 per 100,000 population for a saved livelihood in 1969,[14] and adjusted upward for the 137% increase in consumer price index of January 1981, the citizens and fire department in Seattle have generated $4.5 million worth of "lifesaves" per year in 1981 dollars. TABLE 1 shows the favorable impact of CPR performed by the citizens of Seattle. The rates are derived from a large sample of collapsed individuals, all found in a state of ventricular fibrillation upon the arrival of paramedics. In each instance, CPR was begun by a citizen before arrival of either an emergency medical technician (EMT) in an aid car or paramedical personnel in a mobile intensive/coronary care unit. The contribution of CPR by lay persons in the reduction of morbidity (TABLE 2) as well as mortality (TABLE 1) in Seattle is impressive.[7] Similar survival rates (TABLE 1) were obtained by prompt citizen-performed CPR in Oslo,[5] suburban Seattle,[9] Los Angeles, and Winnepeg.[8, 15, 25]

---

* This work was supported in part by the Charles A. Frueauff Foundation, New York, New York, the Robert Wood Johnson Foundation, Emergency Medical Communications Network Project 1420, and the Thomas Jefferson Emergency Medical Services System, Department of Health, Education and Welfare Project 03–M–000, 366–02.

0077-8923/82/0382-0324 $1.75/0 © 1982, NYAS

TABLE 1

RELATION OF PREHOSPITAL CARDIOPULMONARY RESUSCITATION (CPR) BY A CITIZEN
TO DISCHARGE FROM HOSPITAL

Community	No. of Cases	Cardiac Event	Survival	
			Citizen CPR	No Citizen CPR
Oslo [6]	631	Unstated	27/75 (36%)	43/556 (8%)
Suburban Seattle [9]	487	All cardiac arrests	25/108 (23%)	45/379 (12%)
Seattle [7]	316	Ventricular fibrillation	47/109 (43%)	43/207 (21%)
Los Angeles [15]	120	Ventricular fibrillation	12/49 (24%)	4/71 (6%)
	170	Not documented as ventricular fibrillation	9/55 (16%)	3/115 (3%)
Winnepeg [25]	226	Ventricular tachycardia and fibrillation	16/65 (25%)	8/161 (5%)
Total	1950		136/461	146/1489

One-third of Seattle's citizens learned CPR by 1976.[13] Is this the desirable minimum? Should more be trained?

Attempts have been made to evaluate interrelationships among costs, impact and benefits of out-of-hospital emergency cardiac care.[16-20] Prehospital CPR and advanced life support doubled the number of admissions to the hospital cardiac intensive care units in one community.[21, 22] Preliminary theoretical[14] and pragmatically derived[23] models have been constructed to assess cardiac emergency services, and the latter model included costs of citizen-initiated CPR. Another survey yielded a complementary cost-benefit ratio of 1:40 for adding emergency cardiac care to an extant system,[20] but did not include the cost of citizen CPR. Thus, the relationship of the costs and benefits has not yet been clearly determined for citizen-performed CPR.

TABLE 2

BENEFITS OF CARDIOPULMONARY RESUSCITATION INITIATED BY SEATTLE CITIZENS
OUTSIDE THE HOSPITAL [7]

Outcome	Likelihood
Long-term saving of life	Doubled
Hospital mortality	Halved
Patient conscious at entry	Increased 8 times
Patient awake on first day	Increased 7 times
Patient awake eventually	Increased 1.5 times
Brain disaster averted	Increased 14 times

In Seattle, the cost of training 175,000 people was $1.25 per citizen by 1976[12] for a total of $220,000 expended. The consequent annual 47 long-term lives saved (9.4 per 100,000 people) attributed to citizen-performed CPR[7] are worth $2.3 million or $468,327 per 100,000 people. This calculation employed Acton's estimate that a lost livelihood cost the community $21,000 per 100,000 people in 1969.[14] In that year, the consumer price index was 109.8 and adjustment upward to the index of 260.5 for January 1981 yields the contemporary estimated cost to the community of $49,823 per 100,000 people for a lost livelihood. The similarly derived 1981 cost for educating Seattle citizens in CPR using the 1976 consumer price index of 170.5 would be $336,129 or $7,152 per life saved. A complementary crude cost ($336,129)-benefit ($2.3 million) ratio would indicate that 1 dollar of training expenses for CPR yielded 7 dollars in lifesaves to the city of Seattle. This performance of CPR by the citizens contributed $2.3 million, or just over half the annual lifesaves worth $4.5 million. The presumption is that efforts by and costs to the citizens of Seattle justified the derived quantifiable and unquantifiable benefits of saved livelihoods. Despite the favorable impact in a community with more than one-third of the citizens trained in CPR, the minimal necessary number and distribution of citizens trained in CPR remains unknown. The lay person's ability to perform CPR can diminish with time,[13] and the frequency, type, cost and benefits of retraining citizens are unknown.

The standards for CPR in the United States, revised twice in 6 years and now incorporating the abdominal thrust for choking,[2-4] have not always been promptly or enthusiastically adopted by all the representatives of organized medicine and its surrogate institutions. The American Red Cross procrastinated for years before adding CPR to the body of knowledge and elements of psychomotor performance expected of a competent first-aid technician. Now, however, the local, regional, and state chapters of the Red Cross and the American Heart Association (AHA) find themselves competing for pupils to learn CPR. Much needless acrimony and redundant effort by these two surrogates of organized medicine could be eliminated by pragmatic cooperation of the type recently attempted by the local chapters of the Red Cross and the American Heart Association in Charlottesville and Albemarle County, Virginia. The Joint Commission on Accreditation of Hospitals once required all physicians on hospital staffs to learn CPR. Recently this regulatory body exempted certain physician specialists. The public, and perhaps quite importantly, its lawyers, expect *all* health-care professionals to be competent at CPR. No one has yet been sued successfully for a reasonably competent attempt at CPR rendered in good faith.[4]

The proclaimed role of the American Heart Association with respect to CPR is an extensive one.[4] This organization has dedicated itself to the establishment and periodic revision of the standard concepts and techniques of CPR. It has created standards and guidelines for training and for aids and materials used to train and retrain in CPR and promotes their distribution. The American Heart Association collaborates with other national medical and allied health organizations to promote and establish training programs in CPR. It trains and certifies instructor-trainers and trainers for a variety of organizations. Presumably such groups should include workers in Federal agencies, industries, and large transportation carriers and terminals. Schoolteachers and schoolchildren, ushers at concerts, stadia and large gatherings of people, and individuals employed in public services such as policemen, firemen and rescue workers are also important candidates for learning and using CPR. The American Heart Association professes to encourage and expedite the community-wide teaching of the public in CPR. It also disseminates criteria nationally of when not to resuscitate. The American Heart Association promulgates criteria for nationally standardized courses (content and texts) to its affiliates and chapters. It attempts to make clear that no individual who has rendered CPR in good faith with reasonable performance has been legally punished in the United States. The American Heart Association indicates that many victims of prehospital cardiac arrest who have had CPR as the first applied rescue attempt have returned to their jobs and activities. Finally, this organization is ready to assist in legislation of the "Good Samaritan" type for lay and professional individuals performing CPR in good faith in or out of a life-support unit.

On the other hand, the American Heart Association charges the public money for teaching CPR; it also solicits money from that same public. Thus, many volunteer emergency medical technicians and teachers of CPR have been alienated by what they perceive as the American Heart Association's undermining of the Judeo-Christian ethic of the Good Samaritan. The American Heart Association also requires time-consuming demonstration of psychomotor proficiency at CPR for certification and for annual recertification. In Seattle, the triple-tiered response quickly adds an EMT or paramedic to the citizen's effort at CPR, and time-consuming recertification may be irrelevant in this system.[13] The measured loss of skill at CPR [13, 24] by lay persons might be dealt with by briefer episodic reinforcement.

McElroy [8] recently reviewed a number of approaches to CPR that merit study, if not adoption, by organized medicine to promote the learning of CPR by citizens. Enough individuals should be taught CPR to assure the likely presence of several trained persons in every neighborhood. In families with a member whose risk of sudden cardiac death is great, the spouse, offspring and others should learn CPR. Presumably the education in CPR of such a selected population would prove cost-effective. The education of those civil servants who are the first responders among police, firemen, rescue workers and custodians (such as rangers in national forests and parks) is imperative. In the school system, children from the eighth grade upward should learn CPR. Selected persons in industry, offices, factories, and major transport carriers and terminals should be trained in CPR, as should attendants at stadia, theaters and concerts.

Efforts by segments of organized medicine to educate the public in CPR have clearly borne fruit (TABLES 1 and 2), but the full potential has probably not yet been realized. Cardiopulmonary resuscitation performed by the citizen, when coupled with the rapid response of EMTs and paramedics, is patently cost-effective as a component of the emergency medical system on both theoretical [23] and practical [5, 7-9] grounds. Therefore the widespread education of the public in CPR is more than justified—it is required.

SUMMARY

Since the initiation in 1971 of the community program in Seattle, the techniques of CPR have been widely disseminated. Acquiring the CPR technique in the classroom or by poster or television portrayals, citizens doubled the number of lives saved and reduced mortality and neurologic morbidity in those undergoing cardiac arrest. The standards for CPR in the United States, twice revised in 6 years with the abdominal thrust (Heimlich maneuver) added, were incorporated by the Red Cross and the Joint Commission on Accreditation of Hospitals, although the latter exempted certain physician specialists. However, unresolved issues and unanswered questions abound for organized medicine. The public expects all health-care professionals to be competent at CPR. The American Heart Association charges the citizens money for teaching them CPR, yet solicits charitable gift funds annually from these same citizens; it also requires lengthy proof of psychomotor proficiency at CPR and demands frequent retraining. The former posture mocks the idea of the Good Samaritan; the latter, theoretically commendable, proved irrelevant in Seattle where the tiered response quickly added professional basic and advanced cardiac life support. More than 30% of the public in Seattle learned CPR, but retention of CPR techniques declined over time. Is 30% the critical minimal number for community impact? Addition of prehospital mobile intensive care can yield a complementary cost-benefit ratio of 1:40 for an extant emergency service. For citizen-initiated CPR in Seattle, a crude complementary cost-benefit ratio of 1:7 can be estimated. Organized medicine justifiably should continue to promote education of the public in cardiopulmonary resuscitation.

REFERENCES

1. ALVAREZ, H. & L. A. COBB. 1975. Experience with CPR training of the general public. *In* Proceedings of the National Conference on Standards for Cardiopulmonary Resuscitation and Emergency Cardiac Care: 33–37. American Heart Association. Dallas, Texas.
2. AMERICAN HEART ASSOCIATION—NATIONAL ACADEMY OF SCIENCE—NATIONAL RESEARCH COUNCIL. 1974. Standards for cardiopulmonary resuscitation (CPR) and emergency cardiac care (ECC). J. Am. Med. Assoc. 277: 833–868.
3. HEIMLICH, H. J. 1975. A life-saving maneuver to prevent food-choking. J. Am. Med. Assoc. 234: 398–401.
4. AMERICAN HEART ASSOCIATION. 1980. Standards and guidelines for cardiopulmonary resuscitation (CPR) and emergency cardiac care (ECC). J. Am. Med. Assoc. 244: 451–509.
5. LUND, I. & A. SKULBERG. 1976. Cardiopulmonary resuscitation by lay people. Lancet 2: 702–704.
6. COPLEY, D. P., J. A. MANTLE, W. J. ROGERS, R. O. RUSSELL & C. E. RACKLEY. 1977. Improved outcome for prehospital cardiopulmonary collapse with resuscitation by bystanders. Circulation 56: 901–905.
7. THOMPSON, R. G., A. P. HALLSTROM & L. A. COBB. 1979. Bystander-initiated cardiopulmonary resuscitation in the management of ventricular fibrillation. Ann. Intern. Med. 90: 737–740.
8. McELROY, C. R. 1980. Citizen CPR: The role of the lay person in prehospital care. Topics in Emergency Med. 1: 37–46.
9. EISENBERG, M., L. BERGNER & A. HALLSTROM. 1979. Paramedic programs and out-of-hospital cardiac arrest: I. Factors associated with successful resuscitation. Am. J. Public Health 69: 30–38.
10. BAUM, R. S., H. ALVAREZ, III & L. A. COBB. 1974. Survival after resuscitation from out-of-hospital ventricular fibrillation. Circulation 50: 1231–1235.
11. COBB, L. A., R. S. BAUM, H. ALVAREZ, III & W. A. SCHAFFER. 1975. Resuscitation from out-of-hospital ventricular fibrillation: 4 years followup. Circulation 51 & 52 (Suppl III): 223–228.

12. COBB, L. A., H. ALVAREZ & M. K. COPASS. 1976. A rapid response system for out-of-hospital emergencies. Med. Clin. N. Am. **60:** 283–290.
13. COBB, L. A., A. P. HALLSTROM, R. G. THOMPSON, L. P. MANDEL & M. K. COPASS. 1980. Community cardiopulmonary resuscitation. Ann. Rev. Med. **31:** 453–462.
14. SIDEL, V. W., J. ACTON & B. LOWN. 1969. Models for the evaluation of prehospital coronary care. Am. J. Cardiol. **24:** 674–688.
15. GUZY, P. M., M. L. PEARCE, S. GREENFIELD, L. BECK & C. R. MCELROY. 1979. Effectiveness of citizen cardiopulmonary resuscitation during out-of-hospital emergencies in metropolitan Los Angeles. Circulation (Part II) **60:** 46.
16. CRAMPTON, R. S. & L. A. PIZZARELLO. 1976. Prehospital advanced life support: Cost benefit to a rural-urban community. Circulation **54** (Suppl II): 171.
17. CRAMPTON, R. S. 1978. Mobile coronary care: Evaluation of efficiency. *In* Acute Myocardial Infarction. E. Donoso & J. Lipski, Eds.: 27–36. Stratton Intercontinental. New York, NY.
18. CRAMPTON, R. S., J. GASCHO & E. MARTIN. 1978. Taking coronary care to the patient. Lancet **1:** 1145–1146.
19. SHERMAN, M. A. 1979. Mobile intensive care units: An evaluation of effectiveness. J. Am. Med. Assoc. **241:** 1899–1901.
20. CRAMPTON, R. 1980. Prehospital advanced cardiac life support: Evaluation of a decade of experience. Topics in Emergency Medicine **1:** 27–36.
21. CRAMPTON, R. S., S. P. MICHAELSON, R. F. ALDRICH & J. A. GASCHO. 1974. Prehospital care for myocardial infarction. N. Engl. J. Med. **291:** 418.
22. CRAMPTON, R. S., R. F. ALDRICH, J. A. GASCHO, J. R. MILES, JR. & R. STILLERMAN. 1975. Reduction of prehospital, ambulance, and community coronary death rates by the community-wide emergency cardiac care system. Am. J. Med. **58:** 151–165.
23. HALLSTROM, A., M. S. EISENBERG & L. BERGNER. 1981. Modeling the effectiveness and cost-effectiveness of an emergency service system. Soc. Sci. Med. **15C:** 13–17.
24. WEAVER, F. J., A. G. RAMIREZ, S. B. DORFMAN & A. E. RAIZNER. 1979. Trainees' retention of cardiopulmonary resuscitation—how quickly they forget. J. Am. Med. Assoc. **241:** 901–903.
25. TWEED, W. A., G. BRISTON & N. DORREN. 1980. Resuscitation from cardiac arrest: Assessment of a system providing only basic life support outside of hospital. Canad. Med. Assoc. J. **122:** 297–300.

DISCUSSION

DR. RAYMOND BAHR (*Baltimore, Maryland*): I would like to see CPR taught in high schools; furthermore I would also like taught the early warning signs, the association of denial and procrastination, and the need for spouses of high risk patients to learn CPR.

DR. CRAMPTON: Your points about denial and the role of the spouse are well taken.

COMMUNITY-BASED CARDIOPULMONARY RESUSCITATION: WHAT HAVE WE LEARNED? *

Leonard A. Cobb † and Alfred P. Hallstrom

Departments of Medicine and Biostatistics
University of Washington
Seattle, Washington 98104

Harborview Medical Center
Seattle, Washington 98104

Although the number of potentially effective measures for the containment of sudden cardiac death is sizable, few interventions have as yet been shown to be definitely useful. In spite of the widespread application of coronary arterial bypass grafting, as well as the introduction of new pharmacologic agents, the syndrome of sudden cardiac death remains an everyday occurrence, affecting several hundred persons each day in the United States. One established intervention is the provision of emergency medical services to persons with out-of-hospital cardiac arrest. However, even the successful resuscitation of a patient found in cardiac arrest is not an ideal solution to the problem of sudden cardiac death. The desirability of primary prevention of coronary heart disease is obvious, as is the need for development of safe and effective measures to prevent lethal arrhythmias in patients with recognized heart disease. Nevertheless, emergency cardiac care has therapeutic implications affecting thousands of persons each year in the United States.

During the past two decades, major advances have been made in the application of cardiopulmonary resuscitation (CPR). Of particular note were the rediscovery of mouth-to-mouth ventilation,[1] the development of external chest compression,[2] and the application of external defibrillation.[3] Finally, in 1966, Pantridge and colleagues in Belfast devised and utilized a portable defibrillator powered by automobile batteries. The Belfast group showed that even with such an unwieldy, prototype instrument, defibrillation was feasible outside the hospital.[4]

Mobile coronary care, originally proposed by Pantridge and Geddes,[4] has evolved in the United States in two major directions. First the scope of the service has been substantially expanded to provide care for all out-of-hospital medical emergencies. Additionally, the implementation of rapid response systems, particularly by fire departments, has provided the ability to treat patients within a very few minutes after circulatory arrest.[5-8] As predicted from previous epidemiologic reports,[9] out-of-hospital cardiac arrest is commonly encountered in urban emergency care systems. Each year in Seattle, about 300 persons with ventricular fibrillation are treated by the fire department paramedics—an incidence of about six per 10,000 population[10] (FIG. 1). In suburban King

* This work was supported by Grants R18–HS–01943 from the National Center for Health Services Research, Hyattsville, Maryland and HL 18805 from the National Heart, Lung and Blood Institute, Bethesda, Maryland.

† Address for correspondence: Leonard A. Cobb, M.D., Division of Cardiology, Harborview Medical Center, 325 9th Avenue, Seattle, Washington 98104.

0077-8923/82/0382-0330 $1.75/0 © 1982, NYAS

County, that area immediately adjacent to Seattle, the annual incidence of cardiac arrest attributed to heart disease approximated 5.7 per 10,000 population.[11]

DETERMINANTS OF SURVIVAL IN PATIENTS TREATED FOR OUT-OF-HOSPITAL VENTRICULAR FIBRILLATION

Although prompt intervention is important in many medical emergencies, cardiac arrest is a situation in which delays in treatment are of enormous consequence. The time from collapse to initiation of CPR as well as the time to provision of advanced life-support techniques are both major determinants of outcome in patients with cardiac arrest.[11-13] In fact, such clinical factors as age of the patient and history of prior cardiovascular disease appear to have but little significance as predictors of successful resuscitation or ultimate survival compared with the overwhelming importance of delays in treatment. The rela-

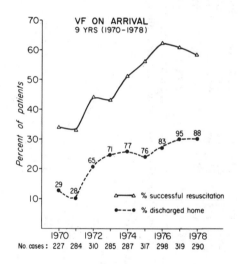

FIGURE 1. Resuscitation and survival rates in patients treated for out-of-hospital ventricular fibrillation (VF) during a 9-year period. The number of cases seen each year is shown in the bottom row. (From Cobb et al.[10] Reproduced by permission.)

tionship of survival to the response times of the secondary (advanced life-support) units and to the rapidity of initiating CPR are shown in TABLE 1.

Strategy to Reduce Delays in Resuscitation

In the Seattle emergency-care system, we have employed several measures to provide care more rapidly to victims of out-of-hospital cardiac arrest.

First, we made efforts to utilize more effectively the resources of the fire department. The Seattle Fire Department has 30 stations with some 200 firefighters on duty. All firefighters were taught when and how to initiate CPR, and fire engines were simultaneously dispatched with medical care units to ensure a more rapid response in instances of suspected cardiac arrest.

Second, the number of advanced life-support (ALS) units was increased over a period of a few years. In 1970, Seattle had only a single such unit. By

TABLE 1

SURVIVAL RELATED TO TIME TO INITIATION OF CPR AND TO RESPONSE TIME OF ADVANCED LIFE SUPPORT UNITS IN 221 WITNESSED EPISODES OF OUT-OF-HOSPITAL VENTRICULAR FIBRILLATION IN SEATTLE *

		Time from Collapse to Initiation of CPR (minutes)					Total
		0, 1	2, 3	4, 5	6, 7	7, 8	
Response Time † of Advanced Life Support Units (minutes)	0–3	56% (9)	14% (8)	36% (14)	50% (2)	0% (2)	34% (35)
	4–7	48% (27)	45% (44)	24% (25)	0% (9)	8% (12)	34% (117)
	8–11	40% (15)	11% (9)	29% (17)	0% (6)	0% (2)	24% (49)
	12 or more	50% (6)	20% (5)	0% (3)	0% (1)	0% (5)	20% (20)
	Total	47% (57)	35% (66)	27% (59)	6% (18)	5% (21)	31% (221)

* Entries are the percent of patients in each time block who were discharged alive. Numbers in parentheses represent the total numbes of cases in each time block.

† Time from dispatch to arrival at the site of collapse.

1973, three units were in operation, and by 1976, there were four. The average response time after dispatch is 3 minutes for the first arriving fire department unit and 5 to 6 minutes for the secondary response, ALS units.

A third action was to establish a program to provide CPR training to a substantial proportion of the general public in Seattle. This project, Medic II, was initiated in 1971 with the goal of providing CPR training to 100,000 persons.[14] By 1980, 175,000 Seattle citizens plus an additional 90,000 suburban King County residents had received instruction. Recently, CPR training has also been provided by other local agencies, including the American Red Cross and several schools. By 1980, 40% of resuscitations had been initiated by bystanders on the scene. The comparable figure in 1970 was but 5%.

COMMUNITY CPR INSTRUCTION

Seattle's community CPR training program (Medic II) is organized and operated by the fire department. Operational costs have been derived mainly from United Way; the cost per student currently averages $2.05. In recent years, approximately 25,000 persons have received training annually.

Assumptions and Rationale

As just indicated, citizen CPR training was proposed as a means of increasing the survival rate in victims of cardiac arrest by early initiation of CPR. In virtually all instances of cardiac arrest in which the emergency-care system is involved, someone is on the scene with the victim. We anticipated that persons who demonstrated competence in CPR skills on a manikin would be able to transfer this capability, or a portion thereof, to a real-life situation under appropriate conditions. We also postulated that the likelihood of a trained rescuer inflicting serious harm was negligible when weighed against the potential for improved survival for a victim of cardiac arrest.

Course Description

The curriculum was developed by the Seattle Fire Department in cooperation with local physicians, medical educators, and the Washington State Heart Association. Classes are typically given in a single 3-hour session consisting of a lecture/demonstration, question and answer period, a training film on CPR, and supervised practice sessions on a life-like manikin. Sessions for high-school students are usually given in three or more shorter periods. The classes are given at any location within the area and at virtually any time convenient for the participants. An important objective of the training is to instill the concept that cardiac arrests do occur and that they are potentially treatable. The importance of responding quickly and the need for obtaining skilled assistance are heavily emphasized. Approximately 25 instructors are active in citizen CPR teaching; the majority are experienced Seattle Fire Department paramedics who have received training in basic elements of instruction. The fire department CPR instructors were subsequently certified by the American Heart Association when that certification process was developed.[15]

The instruction is designed to expose citizens to the indications for—and the technique of—CPR and to afford trainees an opportunity to practice skills and receive critique. Neither routine, formal testing nor certification is carried out in our program.

The Students

A survey of 1,700 randomly selected students showed the following:

- Their average age was 33 years—30 percent were less than 26 years, and only 18 percent were over age 55.
- The male/female ratio was equal.
- The students were predominantly middle or upper-middle class with under-representation of minority populations. Three-fourths of the students had received formal education beyond high school.
- Most students had learned about the availability of CPR classes through communication media, jobs or from acquaintances. Only 10% had been referred by a physician, nurse, or other health worker.
- The most frequently stated reason for taking the course was simply to learn about CPR. For about 20 percent of participants, however, CPR instruction was required for employment or school.
- Eighty-five percent of students indicated a positive attitude toward the CPR training program and the instructors. The manikin practice and the instructor's feedback were regarded as especially useful. Eighty-seven percent indicated a desire to be able to practice their skills periodically and would be willing to take a yearly refresher course.

Testing

Competency testing of randomly selected students showed that citizens trained in a 3-hour class performed satisfactorily on most skills when tested immediately after class. However, 6 months after training, performance on many variables had declined; and by 1 year there was further loss of both knowledge and performance. Students who were evaluated at 6 months and then retested 1 year after training achieved higher scores than those who were only tested at 1 year, presumably because of the reinforcement provided by the interim testing.[16] It is clear that simple, effective reinforcement sessions would be useful, and efforts to develop refresher training are in progress.[17]

INFLUENCE OF BYSTANDER-INITIATED CPR ON RESUSCITATION RATE, SURVIVAL AND NEUROLOGIC RECOVERY

Although it would be desirable to compare outcomes in a community before and after implementation of a community CPR program, an epidemiologically sound evaluation is difficult, if not impossible, to carry out because the development of a citizen CPR training program is commonly associated with other improvements in the delivery of emergency medical services. Furthermore, much of the general public now has an appreciation of CPR, but has not had formal training. Hence the data here will compare the outcome of patients who received bystander-initiated CPR with that of victims treated by the same emergency care system, but without such early CPR.

Association of Bystander-Initiated CPR with Improved Survival

An association of bystander-initiated CPR with improved outcomes has been reported in four communities (TABLE 2). When bystanders initiated CPR in Seattle, 43% of patients with ventricular fibrillation ultimately survived versus 21% of such patients who were not aided by bystanders.[18] In suburban Seattle (the area of King County immediately surrounding the city), the survival rates to hospital discharge were 23% and 12%, respectively, for circulatory arrests attributed to cardiac disease.[11] In Oslo, Norway, the figures were 36% com-

TABLE 2

ASSOCIATION OF SURVIVAL * WITH BYSTANDER-INITIATED CPR
IN FOUR COMMUNITIES

	No. of Cases (Type)	Average Initial Response Time (min)	Site of ALS	Survival With BYS-CPR	Without BYS-CPR
Seattle [18]	316 (VF)	2.9	COLL	43%	21%
Suburban King County, Washington [11]	487 (All cardiac causes)	4.2	COLL/ER	23%	12%
Oslo, Norway [19]	631 (NA)	NA	ER	36%	8%
Winnipeg [20]	226 (VF or VT)	NA	ER	25%	5%

NOTE: ALS=advanced life support; BYS-CPR=bystander-initiated cardiopulmonary resuscitation; COLL=site of collapse; ER=hospital emergency room; NA=information not available; VF=ventricular fibrillation; VT=ventricular tachycardia.
* Survival=alive at time of hospital discharge.

pared with 8 percent.[19] And in Winnipeg [20] the reported survival was 25% when bystanders initiated CPR and 5% otherwise (in patients with ventricular fibrillation or tachycardia). Hence, the available data are in general agreement: survival after cardiac arrest was increased two- to 5-fold when bystanders initiated CPR prior to arrival of emergency-care personnel in urban and suburban communities.

In the Seattle experience (TABLE 3), there was little influence of bystander-initiated CPR on the rate of *immediate* resuscitation, that is, restoration of spontaneous circulation and admission to a hospital. Reversion of ventricular fibrillation with reestablishment of spontaneous perfusion was accomplished in about an equal proportion of the two groups (67% with bystander-CPR and 61% in the others). Presumably, the similar rates for immediate resuscitation reflect the prompt arrival of fire department personnel, whose response time

TABLE 3

INFLUENCE OF BYSTANDER-INITIATED CPR IN SEATTLE: 316 CONSECUTIVE PATIENTS
TREATED FOR OUT-OF-HOSPITAL VENTRICULAR FIBRILLATION *

Outcome	With Bystander-Initiated CPR (n=109) No. (%)	Without Bystander-Initiated CPR (n=207) No. (%)	†
Survived and discharged home	47 (43%)	43 (21%)	< 0.001
Survived, but resided in nursing home at follow-up	0 (0%)	3 (1%)	0.3
Resuscitated, but died in a hospital ‡ or nursing home	26 (24%)	80 (39%)	< 0.02
Unable to be resuscitated	36 (33%)	81 (39%)	0.3

* Adapted from Thompson, Hallstrom and Cobb.[18]
† Significance of group differences by Chi-square test.
‡ Resuscitated patients were transported to any of the city's 14 hospitals.

from dispatch to arrival on the scene averages about 3 minutes. *Importantly, however, hospital mortality in resuscitated patients was halved if bystanders had initiated CPR.* In a separate group of patients admitted consecutively to Harborview Medical Center after resuscitation, we again noted a substantially lower mortality in patients who had received bystander-initiated CPR compared with others (50% versus 25% hospital mortality). Deaths due to shock, congestive heart failure, and anoxic coma were all reduced in the patients who had been assisted by bystanders.[18]

A report by Copley and colleagues in Birmingham was in accord with the aforementioned observations.[21] These investigators studied 12 patients admitted to hospital after resuscitation. In those who had received bystander-initiated CPR, cardiac outputs were greater and left ventricular filling pressures lower compared with those measurements in patients who had delayed onset of CPR but who were nevertheless resuscitated. Although substantiation and extension of these data are necessary, it is reasonable to expect that ventricular function may be preserved when CPR has been initiated promptly after circulatory arrest.

Association of Bystander-Initiated CPR with Neurologic Outcomes

An obvious benefit of bystander-initiated CPR was shown in the neurologic course of the resuscitated patients (TABLE 4). At the time of hospital admission, half of our patients who had received bystander CPR showed at least some form of conscious behavior. In contrast, only 6% of the patients for whom resuscitation had been delayed until the arrival of the fire department showed such responses at the time of admission. Similarly, there was significantly less neurologic impairment at hospital discharge as manifested by disorientation, anoxic coma, or the need for extended-care placement. Although patients with neurologic disability usually showed substantial improvement in the weeks after hospital discharge, the early neurologic course was remarkably better in those who had received bystander-administered CPR.

Relationship Between Outcomes and the Apparent Quality of Bystander CPR

We examined survival in patients stratified according to characteristics of the persons who initiated CPR (Tables 5 and 6). In this analysis, we were unable to detect an obvious difference when the bystanders were grouped according to occupation, training, or retrospectively determined estimates of CPR performance. We found a trend toward a relationship of survival to the estimated performance of CPR, but this was not statistically significant. Although it is possible that the quality of CPR makes little difference in patient outcome, such a position is intuitively difficult to accept, at least without modification. It should be noted that several factors in the setting of out-of-hospital cardiac arrest might obscure a relationship between the apparent quality of CPR and survival. First, it is probable that early application of CPR is not the only benefit of the availability of a trained bystander. A person who initiates CPR is also likely to be familiar with the emergency-care system, and better prepared to summon fire department emergency personnel. Second, it must be remembered that our observations were made in an urban setting where rapid response by the fire department is regularly achieved. The bystander usually performs CPR on his own for only a few minutes. In situations where it would be necessary for a bystander to perform CPR for substantially longer periods, it is possible that the quality of CPR would have a greater impact on survival. Evidence in support of this is shown in Figure 2, which demonstrates that survival was lower in instances where the bystanders were required to carry out CPR more than 2 to 3 minutes. Another explanation for this lack of association is that survival may be only an insensitive reflection of the quality of CPR, and that a detailed assessment of neurologic outcome might be better correlated with indicators of CPR proficiency. Finally, we should consider the possibility that the quality of CPR administered in the field was, in fact, comparable regardless of formal instruction or occupation.

Whatever the correct explanations for these discrepancies, it is evident that bystander-initiated CPR, even when performed in a less than perfect manner,

Table 4

Neurologic Course After Resuscitation:
Relationship to Bystander-Initiated CPR *

	With Bystander-Initiated CPR (n=36)	Without Bystander-Initiated CPR (n=82)	†
Could carry out purposeful activity at time of admission	18/36 (50%)	5/82 (6%)	<.001
Conscious by 24 hours	22/36 (61%)	7/82 (9%)	<.001
Confused at time of discharge	1/27 (4%)	18/38 (47%)	<.001
In a vegetative state at time of discharge	0 (0%)	3/38 (8%)	<.001

* 118 consecutive patients admitted to Harborview Medical Center after resuscitation from out-of-hospital ventricular fibrillation.

† Significance of group differences by Chi-square test.

TABLE 5

RELATIONSHIP OF SURVIVAL TO CHARACTERISTICS OF THE BYSTANDERS
AND TO THE ESTIMATED PERFORMANCE OF CPR PROVIDED BY BYSTANDERS

	Proportion of Patients * Who Survived
CPR training of bystanders	
Medic II training or equivalent	33/65 (51%)
No formal training	8/15 (53%)
Occupation of bystander	
Medical background	11/26 (42%)
All others	29/57 (51%)
Estimated CPR performance score (see TABLE 6)	
< 50	12/28 (43%)
50–99	24/53 (45%)
100	5/9 (56%)

* Consecutive patients treated for ventricular fibrillation by Seattle Fire Department paramedics; witnessed cardiac arrests only.

is associated with an improved outcome. A potentially important consideration in this matter is in the mechanism through which circulation is achieved by external chest compression. Recent studies have pointed out that most blood flow during CPR is accomplished through a "chest pump" mechanism due to generalized increase in intrathoracic pressure, rather than to cardiac compression.[22-24] Although the issue of adequate versus inadequate CPR has not been carefully examined, it is possible that "bad CPR" may not be as useless as heretofore envisioned. While it seems prudent to strive for CPR that is performed as well as possible, it is at the same time unrealistic to expect near-

TABLE 6

ESTIMATED CPR PERFORMANCE SCORE ACCORDING TO INTERVIEWS OF THE
BYSTANDERS

Item	Maximum Number of Points	Scoring
Head tilted (HT)	20	Yes = 20; probably = 15; unknown = 5; other = 0
Ventilation rate (VR)	25	0 = 0; <8 = 15; 8–17 = 25; >17 = 15; unknown = 15
Hand position (HP)	20	Lower ½ or ⅓ of sternum = 20; upper = 5; other = 0
Compression rate (CR)	35	<40 = 15; 40–59 = 30; 60–79 = 35; 80–100 = 30; >100 = 20; unknown = 15
Interrupted CPR (I)	0	Yes = −10; oth = 0

NOTE: Performance score = HT + VR + HP + I + CR(15 + VR)/40. The score is a simple sum of the individual components, except that CR is weighted by VR, the weight going from 15/40 at VR = 0 to 40/40 at VR = 25.

perfect performance by persons who are unlikely to have the opportunity to perform this procedure more than once or twice in a lifetime.

CONCLUSIONS

Although there are unanswered questions concerning community CPR programs, it is evident that early involvement of bystanders in CPR represents a useful adjunct to an emergency-care system. It is important to emphasize, however, that citizen-initiated CPR is a temporizing measure, only one of many links in the emergency medical services chain. It is our position that virtually everyone of high-school age and older should be taught when and how to perform CPR. With continued early application of CPR and more rapid deployment of advanced life-support measures, it seems possible that a survival rate approaching 50% in patients with ventricular fibrillation can be obtained

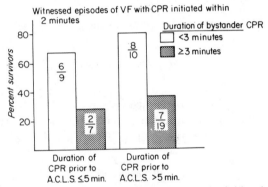

FIGURE 2. Survival related to the duration of bystander-initiated CPR prior to arrival of fire-department personnel. Survival rate was significantly lower in cases where bystanders were required to perform CPR for 3 minutes or more (p <0.03). The slightly greater survival rate in cases with longer delay to onset of advanced cardiac life support (ACLS) can be explained by a shorter time to initiation of CPR (1.5 versus 1.1 minutes).

in some urban communities. Additional improvement will await the development of means for providing more rapid application of defibrillation. If defibrillation is applied to victims of out-of-hospital ventricular fibrillation within 1 or 2 minutes, a high proportion of patients can be expected to survive.[25]

SUMMARY

During the past 9 years, more than 175,000 residents of Seattle have received basic training in cardiopulmonary resuscitation (CPR). On the basis of experience in that city and of observations from three other communities, there is little doubt that early initiation of CPR by a bystander is associated with a substantially improved survival. In one year, 43% of patients (47/109) found in a state of ventricular fibrillation survived to hospital discharge when bystanders initiated CPR. In comparison, only 21% (43/207) lived when CPR was delayed until fire department personnel arrived on the scene (p < 0.001). As expected, there are questions regarding community CPR programs, particularly concerning the level of skills attained and retained. However, in the setting of a rapid-response emergency-care system, we have been unable to relate survival to the apparent quality of CPR as judged by the bystanders' training and occupation or by assessment of what was done on the scene. This discrepancy is likely related to the rapid initial response of the fire department, averaging 3 minutes from dispatch to arrival on the scene.

It is important to emphasize that CPR is almost always a temporizing measure and that most victims who require CPR will also need defibrillation, special airway management, and administration of medications. In patients with out-of-hospital ventricular fibrillation, the factors that determine survival are predominantly related to the rapidity with which care is provided, namely, the time from collapse to initiation of CPR and the time to provision of advanced life-support measures. In many communities a 50% survival rate from ventricular fibrillation is probably attainable. Further improvement might accrue from the extensive deployment of inexpensive defibrillators capable of detecting ventricular fibrillation and suitable for use by the general public.

ACKNOWLEDGMENT

The proposal to develop a community CPR program was first advanced in 1971 by Gordon F. Vickery, then Chief of the Seattle Fire Department. Chief Vickery's concept of public participation in CPR was an important contribution to the delivery of emergency care in this country.

REFERENCES

1. ELAM, J. O. & D. G. GREENE. 1961. Mission accomplished: Successful mouth-to-mouth resuscitation. Anesth. Analg. **40:** 578–580.
2. JUDE, J. R., W. B. KOUWENHOVEN & G. G. KNICKERBOCKER. 1961. Cardiac arrest: Report of application of external cardiac massage on 118 patients. J. Am. Med. Assoc. **178:** 1063–1070.
3. ZOLL, P. M., A. J. LINENTHAL, W. GIBSON, M. H. PAUL & L. R. NORMAN. 1956. Termination of ventricular fibrillation in man by externally applied electric countershock. N. Engl. J. Med. **254:** 727–732.
4. PANTRIDGE, J. F. & J. S. GEDDES. 1967. A mobile intensive care unit in the management of myocardial infarction. Lancet **ii:** 271–273.
5. BAUM, R. S., H. ALVAREZ & L. A. COBB. 1974. Survival after resuscitation from out-of-hospital ventricular fibrillation. Circulation **50:** 1231–1235.
6. LIBERTHSON, R. R., E. L. NAGEL, J. C. HIRSCHMAN & S. R. NUSSENFELD. 1974. Prehospital ventricular defibrillation: Prognosis and followup course. N. Engl. J. Med. **291:** 317–321.
7. LEWIS, A. J. & J. M. CRILEY. 1974. An integrated approach to acute coronary care. Circulation. **50:** 203–204.
8. LEWIS, R. P., J. M. STANG, P. K. FULKERSON, K. L. SAMPSON, A. SCOLES & J. V. WARREN. 1979. Effectiveness of advanced paramedics in a mobile coronary care system. J. Am. Med. Assoc. **241:** 1902–1904.
9. GORDON, T. & W. B. KANNEL. 1971. Premature mortality from coronary heart disease—The Framingham Study. J. Am. Med. Assoc. **215:** 1617–1625.

10. COBB, L. A., J. A. WERNER & G. B. TROBAUGH.   1980.   Sudden cardiac death.
    I. A decade's experience with out-of-hospital resuscitation. Mod. Concepts
    Cardiovasc. Dis. **49:** 31–36.
11. EISENBERG, M. S., L. BERGNER & A. HALLSTROM.   1979.   Paramedic programs
    and out-of-hospital cardiac arrest: 1. Factors associated with successful re-
    suscitation. Am. J. Public Health **69:** 30–38.
12. HALLSTROM, A. P., M. S. EISENBERG & L. BERGNER.   1981.   Modeling the
    effectiveness and cost-effectiveness of an emergency service system. Soc. Sci.
    Med. **15C:** 13–17.
13. MAYER, J. D.   1979.   Paramedic response time and survival from cardiac
    arrest. Soc. Sci. Med. **13D:** 267–271.
14. ALVAREZ, H. & L. A. COBB.   1975.   Experience with CPR training of the
    general public. *In* Proceedings of The National Conference on Standards for
    Cardiopulmonary Resuscitation and Emergency Cardiac Care.: 33–37. Ameri-
    can Heart Association. Dallas, Texas.
15. AMERICAN HEART ASSOCIATION.   1978.   A Manual for Instruction of Basic
    Cardiac Life Support. Dallas, Texas.
16. COBB, L. A., A. P. HALLSTROM, R. G. THOMPSON, L. P. MANDEL & M. K.
    COPASS.   1980.   Community cardiopulmonary resuscitation. Ann. Rev. Med.
    31: 453–462.
17. MANDEL, L. P. & L. A. COBB.   1980.   Three methods of CPR refresher training
    for lay citizens (abstract). Circulation (Suppl. III) **62:** III–123.
18. THOMPSON, R. G., A. P. HALLSTROM & L. A. COBB.   1979.   Bystander-initiated
    cardiopulmonary resuscitation in the management of ventricular fibrillation.
    Ann. Intern. Med. **90:** 737–740.
19. LUND, I. & A. SKULBERG.   1976.   Cardiopulmonary resuscitation by lay people.
    Lancet **ii:** 702–705.
20. TWEED, W. A., G. BRISTOW & N. DONEN.   1980.   Resuscitation from cardiac
    arrest: Assessment of a system providing only basic life support outside of
    hospital. Can. Med. Assoc. J. **122:** 297–300.
21. COPLEY, D. P., J. A. MANTLE, W. J. ROGERS, R. O. RUSSELL, JR. & C. E.
    RACKLEY.   1977.   Improved outcome for prehospital cardiopulmonary col-
    lapse with resuscitation by bystanders. Circulation **56:** 901–905.
22. RUDIKOFF, M. T., W. L. MAUGHAN, M. EFFRON, P. FREUND & M. L. WEISFELDT.
    1980.   Mechanisms of blood flow during cardiopulmonary resuscitation. Cir-
    culation **61:** 345–352.
23. CRILEY, J. M., A. H. BLAUFUSS & E. L. KISSEL.   1976.   Cough-induced cardiac
    compression: Self administered form of cardiac resuscitation. J. Am. Med.
    Assoc. 1246–1249.
24. WERNER, J. A., H. L. GREENE, C. L. JANKO & L. A. COBB.   1981.   Visualization
    of cardiac valve motion in man during external chest compression using two-
    dimensional echocardiography. Circulation **63:** 1417–1421.
25. MEAD, W. F., H. R. PYFER, J. C. TROMBOLD & R. C. FREDERICK.   1976.   Suc-
    cessful resuscitation of two near simultaneous cases of cardiac arrest with a
    review of fifteen cases occurring during supervised exercise. Circulation **53:**
    187–189.

DISCUSSION

DR. P. J. SCHWARTZ: I believe that you mentioned earlier that 25 episodes
of ventricular fibrillation were observed and successfully treated in a cardiac
exercise rehabilitation program in Seattle. Were these 25 patients actively

engaged in exercise at the time? Also do you know whether thump-version resuscitation was successfully attempted before electrical defibrillation was resorted to?

Dr. Cobb: The point at which these patients developed cardiac arrest was looked at very carefully. A few had cardiac arrest during exercise, but in many cardiac arrest developed as long as 4 or 5 minutes after exercise and in most cases at heart rates below what was thought to be reasonably safe. Interestingly, almost all of the patients had been in the exercise program for several months before they experienced cardiac arrest. I do not believe that thump-version resuscitation was tried in these patients.

Dr. Kastor: I'm sure that you've been called to other cities to advise them about developing teams of this sort. What have been some of your observations when you visit other places that might indicate why other cities have such problems in equalling or coming close to the records in Seattle?

Dr. Cobb: There are many differences from one community to another. I believe that not only the geographic and logistic characteristics of the community, but also the general attitude of its public make an enormous difference in the ability to carry out such a program.

Dr. Dwyer: Have you any thoughts about other mechanisms that may be operating in the patients in whom you've not been successful? They may represent an entirely different group.

Dr. Cobb: The patients in whom we've failed, in general, appear to be quite comparable to those in whom successful resuscitation has been effected, at least as judged by the amount of coronary obstruction we've seen at autopsy compared with findings on angiography, history of prior myocardial infarction or congestive heart failure, and age of the patients.

Dr. Bigger: Dr. Pantridge has said, to dramatize the point, that anywhere there's a fire extinguisher there should be a defibrillator. Do you believe that defibrillators should be made more available?

Dr. Cobb: We've made more progress thinking than doing—what we require is a "smart," but simple defibrillator, so that one or two defibrillatory shocks can be made in a patient with ventricular fibrillation. The instrument should be inexpensive, should be able to detect ventricular fibrillation and be relatively fool-proof. I don't think that the amount of energy makes much difference, but it should provide about 100 or 200 joules.

EXERCISE CONDITIONING SOON AFTER MYOCARDIAL INFARCTION: EFFECTS ON MYOCARDIAL PERFUSION AND VENTRICULAR FUNCTION *

Robert F. DeBusk † and Joseph Hung

Division of Cardiology
Department of Medicine
Stanford University School of Medicine
Palo Alto, California 94304

Exercise conditioning improves the physiologic response of the cardiovascular system in patients with coronary heart disease. These effects include a lower heart rate and blood pressure response to submaximal physical effort,[1] a greater submaximal workload at the onset of ischemic S-T segment depression and angina pectoris,[2] a greater peak workload and oxygen uptake,[3] and, in many patients, the abolition of angina pectoris. These favorable changes are mediated largely by peripheral rather than by central mechanisms, that is, the physiologic benefits do not appear to require direct improvement in myocardial perfusion or in the contractile state of the left ventricle. Whether these improved physiologic responses also improve the prognosis in patients with coronary heart disease is not well established despite the performance of several controlled clinical trials.

The conceptual basis for the prevention of sudden cardiac death by exercise conditioning is also not well established. Information is lacking about the precise linkage between the *pathophysiologic substrate* for sudden cardiac death, that is, myocardial ischemia and ventricular dysfunction, and the *electrophysiologic mechanisms* responsible for sudden cardiac death. Newer cardiac imaging techniques, especially myocardial perfusion imaging and radionuclide angiography, will extend our understanding of the pathophysiologic substrate for sudden cardiac death and the role of exercise conditioning in favorably altering this substrate. But even if these advanced techniques demonstrate unequivocally that exercise conditioning directly improves myocardial perfusion and left ventricular function, it is not certain that these benefits are clinically valuable in improving prognosis in coronary heart disease. Further, exercise conditioning is only one of several competing techniques available for improving cardiovascular performance in patients with coronary heart disease. Exercise conditioning requires longer to manifest its cardiovascular effects and is generally more cumbersome than medical or surgical therapy. Its risks, costs, and benefits must be weighed against those of pharmacologic therapy and cardiac surgery.

* This work was supported by Grant HL18907 from the National Heart, Lung and Blood Institute, Bethesda, Maryland. Dr. Hung is an Overseas Fellow supported by the Postgraduate Committee in Medicine, University of Sydney, Australia.

† Address for correspondence: Robert F. DeBusk, M.D., 730 Welch Road, Palo Alto, California 94304.

0077–8923/82/0382–0343 $1.75/0 © 1982, NYAS

Patients who have survived a myocardial infarction constitute the largest identifiable population at risk for sudden cardiac death and we will discuss primarily this population. We will address three major questions concerning the role of exercise conditioning in the prevention of sudden cardiac death: (1) What are the best methods for identifying patients with clinically significant myocardial ischemia and left ventricular dysfunction, which constitute the pathophysiologic substrate for sudden cardiac death? (2) What is the evidence that exercise conditioning diminishes these abnormalities within this susceptible population? (3) Assuming that exercise conditioning bestows physiologic or clinical benefits, what are the most effective strategies for implementing this therapy within the susceptible population?

First, what are the best methods for identifying patients susceptible to sudden cardiac death after myocardial infarction? More to the point, how can patients be identified in whom the balance of risk and benefit is favorable for exercise conditioning? For example, in very ill patients, the risks of exercise conditioning appear to outweigh the benefits and in very well individuals, it is hard to lower the recurrence rate still further by any currently available means.

Our group has emphasized exercise testing for the evaluation of prognosis in part because this technique also provides the basis for exercise conditioning.[4, 5] In a subset of 196 patients undergoing treadmill exercise testing 3 weeks after myocardial infarction we identified a high-risk subset on the basis of the following characteristics: exercise-induced ischemic S-T segment depression ≥ 0.2 mV, a rate–pressure product less than 18,000, and a maximal workload of less than 4 METs (multiples of resting energy expenditure). Patients with one or more of these abnormalities had a 12% rate of subsequent medical events (sudden death, nonfatal cardiac arrest, myocardial infarction) in the 6 months after infarction compared with a rate of 1.4% in patients without significant test abnormalities—a nearly nine-fold difference. Further, 75% of all cardiac events and 88% of all fatal cardiac events occurred in this high-risk subset, which comprised only 25% of the patients. Thus, three-quarters of patients were identified as having a low risk for subsequent cardiac events. It is important to emphasize that within the group as a whole, the incidence of all cardiac events was only 4%. It is not surprising that the incidence of cardiac events was low within this population, for patients with clinically significant left ventricular dysfunction and unstable angina pectoris, who constitute a clinically definable population at high risk, were excluded from exercise testing.[6]

Radionuclide angiography and thallium myocardial perfusion imaging have also been used to evaluate prognosis after myocardial infarction. Whether radionuclide imaging performed in conjunction with exercise significantly increases the yield of prognostic information in postinfarction patients compared with the information obtained by imaging at rest is not well established. For example, Borer et al. followed 45 postinfarction patients for 1 year after the performance of radionuclide angiography at rest and during exercise on the day prior to hospital discharge.[7] While all four patients who died had a resting ejection fraction of less than 35%, the change in ejection fraction with exercise provided no additional prognostic information within the group as a whole. The prognostic significance of thallium defects at rest has been evaluated in postinfarction patients by Silverman et al.[8] In contrast, the prognostic significance of exercise-induced thallium defects in postinfarction patients is largely unknown, although such defects correlate well with the presence of multivessel coronary artery disease and regions of jeopardized myocardium.[9]

Experience with another population of coronary patients provides insight into the prognostic value of exercise radionuclide imaging. Trobaugh *et al.* evaluated survivors of out-of-hospital ventricular fibrillation attributable to coronary artery disease and found a lower resting ejection fraction and more extensive regional wall motion abnormalities in patients who had a subsequent cardiac arrest than in those who did not.[10] However, the magnitude of decrease in left ventricular ejection fraction with exercise, which was small, was not greater in nonsurvivors than in survivors. The same investigators noted a similar phenomenon with thallium myocardial perfusion imaging in survivors of out-of-hospital ventricular fibrillation: while patients with subsequent cardiac arrest had more extensive resting thallium defects than those who did not, the change in defect size with exercise did not further stratify the risk of subsequent cardiac arrest.[11]

The apparent inability of exercise to augment the prognostic power of radionuclide imaging at rest has important implications not only for the identification of coronary patients at high risk for sudden cardiac death, but also for evaluating the effects of exercise conditioning in such patients. For example, if a very sensitive technique such as exercise thallium myocardial perfusion imaging is required to demonstrate improved myocardial perfusion after exercise conditioning, it may be that this *physiologic* change is so subtle as to have no significant effect on *prognosis*. In other words, the demonstration that exercise conditioning favorably influences myocardial perfusion or left ventricular function does not assure that exercise conditioning will also favorably influence prognosis.

EFFECTS OF EXERCISE CONDITIONING ON MYOCARDIAL PERFUSION

Inferential evidence can be found that exercise conditioning improves myocardial oxygen delivery: in studies by Redwood *et al.*[12] and by Sim *et al.*[13] triple product or double product at the onset of angina pectoris increased in most patients after exercise conditioning. However, Nolewajka *et al.* noted no increase in the double product at the onset of angina pectoris in postinfarction patients who had undergone 7 months of vigorous exercise conditioning.[14] Further, although Sim *et al.* noted a training-induced increase in the rate–pressure product at angina during exercise, these investigators failed to demonstrate a similar increase in the rate–pressure product during cardiac pacing. Detry *et al.* found the relationship between exercise-induced ischemic S-T segment depression and heart rate after conditioning was not altered: a higher rate–pressure product after training was accompanied by an increase in the extent of ischemic S-T segment depression.[15]

Studies by Nolewajka[14] and by Ferguson *et al.*[16] of coronary patients undergoing exercise conditioning have demonstrated no changes in the extent of angiographically demonstrable collateralization, the progression of coronary artery disease, the extent of myocardial perfusion assessed by labeled microspheres, or in left ventricular function measured at rest. Although the anginal threshold, that is, the amount of external work performed prior to the onset of angina pectoris, was increased, the double product at the onset of angina pectoris was unchanged in patients undergoing training and in control patients. Similarly, the proportion of patients with angina pectoris or ischemic S-T segment abnormalities and the extent of these abnormalities were not altered by exercise conditioning.

EFFECTS OF EXERCISE CONDITIONING ON VENTRICULAR FUNCTION

It is even more difficult to demonstrate the effects of exercise conditioning on ventricular function than to show a direct effect on myocardial perfusion. Part of this difficulty is due to the fact that exercise conditioning simultaneously alters preload, afterload, and heart rate, each of which affects the measurement of ventricular function. For example, exercise conditioning increases total blood volume unaccompanied by major changes in hematocrit. Left ventricular dimensions increase after conditioning: Rerych et al. found in young normal persons that an increased peak cardiac output and stroke volume after exercise conditioning was produced by an increased end-diastolic volume without a change in ejection fraction.[17] Patients with coronary heart disease demonstrate a similar increase in left ventricular dimensions after exercise conditioning. Further, increases in cardiac output and in myocardial oxygen consumption in patients with coronary heart disease are accompanied by an increase in left ventricular end-diastolic pressure and volume during peak exercise.[18]

Afterload reduction at rest and during submaximal exercise appears to be an especially important mechanism for improving cardiac performance in patients with coronary heart disease.[19] A decrease in resting heart rate is also commonly noted after exercise conditioning in patients with coronary heart disease.[20] Because of the complex interactions between these factors, it is technically difficult to demonstrate a direct training-induced improvement in the intrinsic contractile properties of the left ventricle.

Although exercise conditioning improves functional capacity in patients with coronary heart disease, it does not substantially improve *resting* left ventricular function. For example, Lee et al. trained 18 postinfarction patients with depressed ejection fraction (mean 35%, range 27–40%) for an average of 18.5 months. Although the duration of exercise increased 17%, to a level approximating completion of the second stage of the Bruce protocol, indices of resting left ventricular function, including those of left ventricular end-diastolic pressure, volume and ejection fraction, were not significantly altered.[21] This underscores the importance of peripheral adaptations—in this case a decrease in submaximal heart rate—in effecting improvement in functional capacity.

Most evidence suggests that exercise conditioning in coronary patients improves functional capacity primarily by peripheral mechanisms, such as an increase in peak heart rate and in peak arteriovenous oxygen difference, rather than by central mechanisms, such as an increase in peak stroke volume. Further, an increase in stroke volume can result from an increased end-diastolic volume as well as from an increased ejection fraction. Further studies on the effect of exercise conditioning will therefore require measurement of left ventricular volume as well as ejection fraction.

We have recently evaluated the cardiovascular response to exercise soon after myocardial infarction in 21 men of a mean age of 55 years. These patients had not experienced recurrent ischemic pain after 24 hours or major ventricular arrhythmias after 48 hours, and they had not had atrial tachyarrhythmias or heart block greater than first degree or clinical or radiologic evidence of congestive heart failure within the first 6 days after infarction. They were therefore classified as clinically uncomplicated. Such patients are representative of nearly half of all males aged 70 or less who are admitted to the Stanford Medical Center for the treatment of acute myocardial infarction.

On the seventh day after infarction these patients underwent thallium myocardial perfusion imaging immediately and 4 hours after treadmill exercise. On the next day they underwent radionuclide angiography (that is, equilibrium gated cardiac blood pool scanning) during upright multistage bicycle ergometry. One week later they underwent cardiac imaging after the injection of thallium at rest. End-points for these exercise tests were limiting symptoms of angina pectoris, fatigue or dyspnea, a decrease in systolic pressure of 10 mm Hg or more from the peak value attained during an earlier stage of exercise, the appearance of ventricular tachycardia, or attainment of a heart rate of 130 in the absence of any of these prior end-points. These radionuclide exercise evaluations were repeated at 3 weeks and at 11 weeks after infarction, using a protocol that was limited by symptoms rather than by attainment of an arbitrary heart rate maximum.

End-points for testing during each of the three treadmill tests are listed in TABLE 1. Neither angina pectoris nor ventricular ectopic activity was an end-point on any of the tests. Most tests were limited by shortness of breath and by fatigue even at 1 week. Cardiovascular variables measured at peak effort during treadmill exercise are shown in TABLE 2 and during bicycle ergometry in TABLE 3.

TABLE 1
ENDPOINTS FOR EXERCISE TESTING (n = 21)

	Angina	Other Symptoms	↓BP	VEA	HR ≥ 130
1 week	0	14	2	0	5
3 weeks	0	18	3	0	0
11 weeks	0	21	0	0	0

NOTE: ↓BP = systolic hypotension; HR = heart rate; VEA = ventricular ectopic activity.

Peak treadmill workload, heart rate and rate–pressure product increased significantly ($p < 0.05$) among the three tests, especially between 7 and 21 days. A similar increase was noted during the three bicycle exercise tests. Ischemic S-T segment depression was noted at 1 week in two patients, one of whom also demonstrated ischemic S-T segment depression on both of the two later tests and one of whom did not demonstrate ischemic abnormalities subsequently. One additional patient exhibited ischemic S-T segment depression only at 11 weeks. Angina pectoris was not noted during any of the six treadmill or bicycle exercise tests.

Ischemic thallium responses were defined as a qualitative difference in the images obtained immediately after each of the three exercise tests compared with findings on the resting examination performed 2 weeks after infarction. Eleven of the 21 patients or 52% demonstrated reversible thallium defects on one or more of the three visits: these defects were present in 2 patients on all three visits, in 4 patients on two visits, and in 5 patients on only one visit. Both of the patients with exercise-induced thallium defects on all three visits also had exercise-induced ischemic S-T segment depression on at least one visit. The prevalence of reversible thallium defects on the three visits was 19%, 33% and 38%, respectively—a statistically insignificant difference.

TABLE 2
PEAK CARDIOVASCULAR VARIABLES: TREADMILL EXERCISE TESTING (n = 21)

	Workload (METs)	Heart Rate	HR × SBP / 100
1 week	4.9 ± 1.2	125 ± 3	206 ± 10
3 weeks	6.5 ± 1.4	142 ± 3	247 ± 14
11 weeks	7.3 ± 2.0	145 ± 2	265 ± 22

NOTE: HR = heart rate; METs = multiples of resting energy expenditure; SBP = systolic blood pressure.

Ejection fraction at rest and during exercise is depicted in FIGURE 1. Resting ejection fraction was similar on all three visits. In order to facilitate comparison of the three visits, ejection fraction was plotted at the point of exercise at which values of heart rate and rate–pressure product on the two latter tests were similar to those measured on the first test. On tests performed at 3 and 11 weeks, ejection fraction increased initially and decreased during the later stages of exercise. The peak ejection fraction measured at 1 week was similar to the highest values measured at 3 and 11 weeks. The major difference among the three visits was the higher heart rate, rate–pressure product, and workload attained on the latter two tests.

The cardiovascular response to exercise conditioning between 3 and 11 weeks after infarction was evaluated in these 21 patients: 11 underwent individually prescribed training at home and 10 were given no formal instructions regarding training. Exercise conditioning was divided into five 30-minute sessions per week. Two exercise regimens were used: (1) the 9 patients without exercise-induced S-T segment depression on the 3-week test exercised on stationary bicycles at a heart rate between 70% and 85% of the peak treadmill heart rate at 3 weeks. (2) The 2 patients who exhibited exercise-induced ischemic S-T segment depression during the 3-week test walked briskly or jogged slowly in order to achieve a heart rate approximately 10 beats below the heart rate at which ischemic S-T segment depression had appeared during the 3-week test.

All 11 patients used the ExerSentry®, a heart-rate monitor connected to the chest by adhesive electrodes, to regulate their intensity of exercise within pre-set heart rate limits. The ExerSentry emits an audible tone when the heart rate falls outside the pre-set limits. Another device, the CardioBeeper®, was used to transmit the electrocardiographic signal over the telephone to our laboratory twice weekly during the exercise conditioning sessions. The electro-

TABLE 3
PEAK CARDIOVASCULAR VARIABLES: BICYCLE ERGOMETRY (n = 21)

	Workload (kgm)	Heart Rate	HR × SBP / 100
1 week	450 ± 32	126 ± 2	217 ± 10
3 weeks	692 ± 35	143 ± 3	259 ± 16
11 weeks	715 ± 37	141 ± 4	286 ± 24

NOTE: kgm=kilogram meter; HR=heart rate; SBP=systolic blood pressure.

cardiogram was transmitted for 1 minute during a level of exercise that elicited a near-peak training heart rate and during the first 30 seconds of recovery after exercise. Transmission occurred during bicycle exercise in nonischemic patients. Ischemic patients used a 9-inch step in order to increase heart rate prior to transmission. There were no complications of exercise conditioning.

At 11 weeks after infarction we found no significant difference between the groups in their cardiovascular or radionuclide responses to exercise.[22] Short-term home exercise training thus appears safe in clinically low-risk patients, but this conditioning does not dramatically enhance the cardiovascular response to exercise, decrease the prevalence of exercise-induced thallium perfusion defects, or improve the ventricular response to submaximal effort. Further study is required to establish the effects of exercise conditioning on myocardial perfusion and left ventricular function in patients with coronary artery disease.

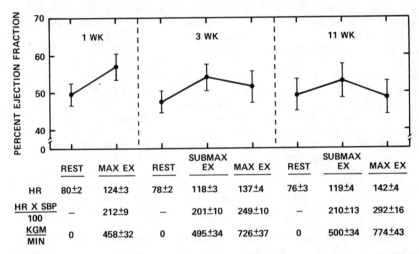

	REST	MAX EX	REST	SUBMAX EX	MAX EX	REST	SUBMAX EX	MAX EX
HR	80±2	124±3	78±2	118±3	137±4	76±3	119±4	142±4
HR X SBP / 100	–	212±9	–	201±10	249±10	–	210±13	292±16
KGM / MIN	0	458±32	0	495±34	726±37	0	500±34	774±43

FIGURE 1. Ejection fraction at rest and during exercise. HR = heart rate; KGM/MIN = kilogram meter per minute; MAX EX = maximal exercise; SBP = systolic blood pressure; and SUBMAX EX = submaximal exercise.

Our findings are generally similar to those of Verani et al.,[23] who carried out exercise conditioning in 16 patients with ischemic heart disease, 10 with prior myocardial infarction. Peak oxygen consumption increased 15% during a 12-week period. Myocardial perfusion imaging with thallium 201 demonstrated no change in perfusion during exercise at comparable rate–pressure products pre- and post-training. Left ventricular functional reserve, assessed by ejection fraction and by regional wall motion responses to exercise at a fixed rate–pressure product, was not altered by training.

CLINICAL EFFICACY OF EXERCISE CONDITIONING IN THE PREVENTION OF SUDDEN CARDIAC DEATH

Even though exercise conditioning favorably affects myocardial ischemia and left ventricular function during submaximal exercise, the efficacy of this therapeutic intervention in preventing sudden cardiac death is difficult to demonstrate. Exercise conditioning studies are invariably confounded by the effects of dropouts, crossovers to coronary arterial bypass graft surgery, and by the effects of cardiac drugs and modification of risk factors. Finally, for the methodologic reasons mentioned previously it is difficult to establish a direct benefit of exercise conditioning on cardiac function.

A recent randomized trial of rehabilitation and secondary prevention underscores several of these difficulties.[24] Compared with control subjects, patients participating in the multifactorial intervention program had a lower rate of sudden death in the 3 years after infarction (5.8% versus 14.4%, p < 0.01). A physical exercise conditioning program was carried out in most patients participating in the intervention group. Physical working capacity was similar in both groups at 1, 2 and 3 years after infarction, but systolic and diastolic blood pressure was significantly lower in the intervention group than in the control group. Risk factors including cholesterol and triglyceride levels and body weight were also slightly, but significantly, lower in the intervention group. Patients in the intervention group received higher doses of beta blocking agents and these patients' contact with their physicians was much more frequent than in the control group. Because of these confounding effects, this study provides little evidence that exercise conditioning contributed significantly to the differential in the rate of sudden cardiac death in these postinfarction patients.

The highest risk for sudden cardiac death occurs in the 3 months after infarction—an interval during which important *spontaneous* changes in cardiovascular performance occur. We have previously documented a 25% spontaneous improvement in functional capacity 3 to 11 weeks after infarction.[25] This resulted in part from an increase in peak heart rate during this interval and probably from an increase in arteriovenous oxygen difference. From the studies of Wohl et al. it appears that improvement in stroke volume does not occur prior to the sixth month after infarction.[26] Thus, the improvement in oxygen transport capacity noted in our patients appears to reflect primarily peripheral mechanisms.

Restoration of left ventricular volume after bedrest contributes to the spontaneous increase in functional capacity after infarction. In a group of 12 normal middle-aged men subjected to 10 days of bedrest, we recently noted a 15% decline in peak VO_2 during upright bicycle exercise but only a statistically nonsignificant 6% decline in peak VO_2 during supine bicycle exercise.[27] After bedrest left ventricular volume measured echographically decreased 17% at rest in the supine position, and there was evidence of an even greater decline in resting left ventricular volume in the upright position. These largely orthostatic influences on functional capacity were reversed within 4 weeks of resumption of usual physical activity or exercise conditioning.

Exercise conditioning is usually equated with an increase in maximal oxygen transport capacity (VO_2 max) and with a decrease in the heart rate and systolic pressure response to a fixed submaximal workload. Recent evidence indicates that the threshold of physical effort required to diminish the cardiovascular response to submaximal effort may be lower than that required to increase maximal oxygen transport capacity. For example, Dressendorfer et al. noted a significant decrease in the heart rate and systolic pressure response to submaximal effort in patients with ischemic heart disease after a 14 to 20 week walking program even in the *absence* of an increase in VO_2 max.[28] In other words, physiologic benefits may accrue to even relatively low-level physical effort. The threshold of physical effort required to increase VO_2 max is 50%

of the VO_2 max.[29] This level of effort elicits a heart rate equivalent to approximately 60% of the maximal heart rate reserve. For example, in a 55-year-old man with a peak heart rate of 155 and a resting heart rate of 70, the threshold training heart rate required to produce an increase in VO_2 max is 127 beats/minute. Once this threshold of physical effort is reached, the duration of physical effort becomes a major determinant of the cardiovascular effects of training: prolonged low-intensity effort appears to bestow the same benefit on functional capacity as brief high-intensity effort if the total energy cost of the activities is equal.

The traditional rationale for exercise conditioning programs is that physical effort must be near maximal in order to be effective and that such activity is inherently dangerous. This in turn necessitates a supervised exercise conditioning environment in order to guard against untoward cardiovascular events during exercise conditioning. This entails a relatively complex organizational structure, which in turn increases the cost and decreases the availability of exercise conditioning to patients with ischemic heart disease: many patients live in communities too small to support group training programs and many patients in large communities cannot afford them. Supervised exercise conditioning programs offer valuable psychological as well as physical benefits, but their availability is limited for the foregoing reasons.

The precise mechanism by which exercise conditioning may protect against sudden cardiac death and other recurrent cardiac events is unknown. Does the protective effect require an increase in VO_2 max or a decrease in the heart rate and systolic pressure during submaximal effort or both of these, or is it mediated by other mechanisms entirely? Until this point is established, it is important to explore the feasibility of alternatives to high-level supervised exercise conditioning. One such alternative is individualized low-level physical effort carried out in an unsupervised environment.

On the basis of our experience,[25] it seems likely that five or six 30-minute sessions per week at home of low-level physical effort, for example, a workload of 4 METs or 5 calories per minute, may achieve substantially the same cardiovascular benefits as three 1-hour sessions per week in a gymnasium at a workload of 6 METs or 7.5 calories per minute. In our patients the cardiovascular effects of home exercise conditioning are comparable to those of supervised exercise conditioning. It is important to emphasize, however, that this experience concerns relatively low-risk postinfarction patients. The safety and efficacy of exercise conditioning in patients at high risk for sudden cardiac death remains to be established.

In summary, exercise conditioning has favorable effects on myocardial ischemia and on left ventricular dysfunction in patients with coronary heart disease, including those recovering from myocardial infarction. Although these effects are associated with physiologic and symptomatic improvement, their role in altering prognosis and especially the risk of sudden cardiac death is largely unknown. Given the hazards and logistic difficulties of exercise conditioning in high-risk patients and the availability of alternate medical and surgical therapies, it is unlikely that exercise conditioning will contribute substantially to a reduction in the risk of sudden cardiac death in postinfarction patients.

ACKNOWLEDGMENT

We wish to thank Dorothy Potter for preparation of the manuscript.

REFERENCES

1. ROWELL, L. B. 1974. Human cardiovascular adjustments to exercise and thermal stress. Physiol. Rev. **54:** 75–159.
2. DETRY, J. R., M. ROUSSEAU, G. VANDENBROOCKE, F. JUSUMI, L. A. BRASSEUR & R. A. BRUCE. 1971. Increased arterio-venous oxygen difference after physical training in coronary artery disease and angina pectoris. Circulation **44:** 109.
3. CLAUSEN, J. P. 1975. Circulatory adjustments to dynamic exercise and effect of physical training in normal subjects and in patients with coronary artery disease. Prog. Cardiovasc. Dis. **18:** 459–495.
4. DAVIDSON, D. M. & R. F. DeBUSK. 1980. The prognostic significance of a single exercise test 3 weeks after uncomplicated myocardial infarction. Circulation **61:** 236–242.
5. DEBUSK, R. F. & W. HASKELL. 1980. Symptom-limited vs. heart rate-limited exercise testing soon after myocardial infarction. Circulation **61:** 738–743.
6. DEBUSK, R. F. & D. M. DAVIDSON. 1980. The work evaluation of the cardiac patient. J. Occup. Med. **22:** 715–722.
7. BORER, J. S., D. R. ROSING, R. H. MILLER, R. M. STARK, K. M. KENT, S. L. BACHRACH, M. V. GREEN, C. R. LAKE, H. COHEN, D. HOLMES, D. DONOHUE, W. BAKER & S. E. EPSTEIN. 1980. Natural history of left ventricular function during 1 year after acute myocardial infarction: Comparison with clinical, electrocardiographic and biochemical determinations. Am. J. Cardiol. **46:** 1–12.
8. SILVERMAN, K. J., L. C. BECKER, B. H. BULKLEY, R. D. BUROW, E. D. MELLITS, C. H. KALLMAN & M. L. WEISFELDT. 1980. Value of early thallium-201 scintigraphy for predicting mortality in patients with acute myocardial infarction. Circulation **61:** 996–1003.
9. TURNER, J. D., K. M. SCHWARTZ, J. R. LOGIC, L. T. SHEFFIELD, S. KANSAL, D. I. ROITMAN, J. A. MANTLE, R. O. RUSSELL, C. E. RACKLEY & W. J. ROGERS. 1980. Detection of residual jeopardized myocardium 3 weeks after myocardial infarction by exercise testing with thallium-201 myocardial scintigraphy. Circulation **61:** 729–737.
10. RICHIE, J. L., G. B. TROBAUGH, A. P. HALLSTROM, G. W. HAMILTON & L. A. COBB. 1980. Radionuclide ventriculography in 121 survivors of out-of-hospital ventricular fibrillation. Am. J. Cardiol. **45:** 433.
11. TROBAUGH, G. B., J. L. RICHIE, A. P. HALLSTROM, G. W. HAMILTON, J. A. WERNER & L. A. COBB. 1979. Thallium-201 myocardial imaging in survivors of out-of-hospital ventricular fibrillation. Circulation (Suppl II) **60:** II–231.
12. REDWOOD, D. R., D. R. ROSING & S. E. EPSTEIN. 1972. Circulatory and symptomatic effects of physical training in patients with coronary artery disease and angina pectoris. N. Engl. J. Med. **286:** 959.
13. SIM, D. N. & W. A. NEILL. 1974. Investigation of the physiological basis for increased exercise threshold for angina pectoris after physical conditioning. J. Clin. Invest. **54:** 763.
14. NOLEWAJKA, A. J., W. J. JOSTUK, P. A. RECHNITZER & D. A. CUNNINGHAM. 1979. Exercise and human collateralization: An angiographic and scintigraphic assessment. Circulation **60:** 114–121.
15. DETRY, J. & R. BRUCE. 1971. Effects of physical training on exertional S-T-segment depression in coronary heart disease. Circulation **44:** 390–396.
16. FERGUSON, R. J., R. PETITCLERC, G. CLOQUETTE, L. CHANIOTIS, P. GAUTHIER, R. HUOT, C. ALLARD, L. JANKOWSKI & L. CAMPEAU. 1974. Effect of physical training on treadmill exercise capacity, collateral circulation and progression of coronary disease. Am. J. Cardiol. **34:** 764.

17. RERYCH, S. K., P. M. SCHOLZ, D. C. SABISTON & R. H. JONES. 1980. Effects of exercise training on left ventricular function in normal subjects: A longitudinal study by radionuclide angiography. Am. J. Cardiol. **45:** 244–252.
18. WALLACE, A. G., S. K. RERYCH, R. H. JONES & J. K. GOODRICH. 1978. Effects of exercise training on ventricular function in coronary disease. Circulation (Suppl II) **57, 58:** II–97.
19. SCHEUER, J. & C. M. TIPTON. 1977. Cardiovascular adaptations to physical training. Annu. Rev. Physiol. **39:** 221–251.
20. SALTIN, B. 1971. Central circulation after physical conditioning in young and middle-aged men. *In* Coronary Heart Disease and Physical Fitness. O. A. Larsen & E. O. Malmborg, Eds.: 26. Munksgaard. Copenhagen.
21. LEE, A. P., R. ICE, R. BLESSEY & M. E. SANMARCO. 1979. Long-term effects of physical training on coronary patients with impaired ventricular function. Circulation **50:** 1519–1526.
22. HUNG, J., J. McKILLOP, M. GORIS, R. DEBUSK. 1981. The effects of exercise training on myocardial ischemia and left ventricular function soon after myocardial infarction: A randomized study. Circulation (Suppl IV): IV–198.
23. VERANI, M. S., G. H. HARTUNG, J. HOEPFEL-HARRIS, D. E. WELTON, C. M. PRATT & R. R. MILLER. 1981. Effects of exercise training on left ventricular performance and myocardial perfusion in patients with coronary artery disease. Am. J. Cardiol. **47:** 797–803.
24. KALLIO, V., H. HAMALAINEN, J. HAKKILA & O. J. LUURILA. 1979. Reduction in sudden deaths by a multifactorial intervention programme after acute myocardial infarction. Lancet **2:** 1091–1094.
25. DEBUSK, R. F., N. HOUSTON, W. HASKELL, M. PARKER & G. FRY. 1979. Exercise training soon after myocardial infarction. Am. J. Cardiol. **44:** 1223–1229.
26. WOHL, A. J., H. R. LEWIS, W. CAMPBELL, E. KARLSSON, J. T. WILLERSON, C. B. MULLINS & C. G. BLOMQVIST. 1977. Cardiovascular function during early recovery from acute myocardial infarction. Circulation **56:** 931–937.
27. CONVERTINO, V., J. HUNG, D. GOLDWATER, R. F. DEBUSK. 1982. Cardiovascular responses to exercise in middle-aged men following ten days of bedrest. Circulation. In press.
28. DRESSENDORFER, R. H., J. L. SMITH & E. A. AMSTERDAM. 1981. Decreased myocardial demand from exercise training secondary to improved work efficiency: Effect of habituation versus aerobic conditioning. Am. J. Cardiol. **47:** 467.
29. KARVONEN, M., K. KENTALA & O. MUSTALA. 1957. The effects of training heart rate: A longitudinal study. Ann. Med. Exper. Biol. Fenn. **35:** 307–315.

DISCUSSION

DR. VERNON: About 12 years ago in Boston, I heard two Czechoslovakian doctors describe how they had their patients with myocardial infarction exercise a few seconds at a time on the day after infarction. Now, an exercise prescription should have quantitation, including how much and how often. With all the sophisticated gadgetry that we have for research and all the fine nuances to our follow-up studies, sometimes we forget that just simple bedside trial and observation lends itself to accurate prescriptions for patients. Please comment on that.

DR. DEBUSK: No one would disparage the value of clinical evaluation, including bedside evaluation. We feel that the clinical evaluation is extended by the exercise test and that the exercise provides the basis for individualized prescription of activity. We need to find out what minimal level of surveillance might be necessary in order to establish efficacy and to determine the risks involved. I suspect that in the future we will evolve something far simpler in which it will be clinically apparent which patients really have a low risk and therefore can walk. It is something of a conceptual problem right now in postinfarction patients. We are a little reluctant to tell these patients that they can be very physically active because we lack these kinds of quantitative measures of efficacy.

DR. HERLING: How do you deal with the person who has significant S-T segment depression without symptoms? What do you recommend for his level of activity since he has no warning system?

DR. DEBUSK: The level at which the S-T segment depression appears is very important, as has been determined by us and by others. If a patient has ischemic S-T segment depression, for example, at a heart rate of 140 beats per minute 3 weeks after myocardial infarction, it appears that he or she has a much different prognosis than if that S-T segment depression appears at a heart rate of 100.

In general, however, we handle asymptomatic S-T segment depression by having the patients exercise at a heart rate below the onset of the S-T segment depression.

PREVENTION OF VENTRICULAR FIBRILLATION BY USE OF LOW-INTENSITY ELECTRICAL STIMULI *

Richard L. Verrier† and Bernard Lown

Cardiovascular Division
Department of Medicine
Brigham and Women's Hospital
Harvard Medical School Department of Nutrition
Harvard School of Public Health
Boston, Massachusetts 02115

INTRODUCTION

The pioneering studies of Wiggers and Wegria [1] demonstrated more than 40 years ago that ventricular fibrillation (VF) could be induced by delivering a relatively low-energy electrical discharge during the vulnerable phase of the cardiac cycle. Indeed, in the normal heart a transthoracic stimulus of less than 1 joule is sufficient to precipitate ventricular fibrillation.[2] However, once this arrhythmia ensues, energies several hundred times as great are required for its termination.[2] Even when defibrillation is carried out by internal means, considerable energy, ranging between 20 and 30 joules, is required.[3]

Studies conducted by Wolf *et al.*[4] in our laboratory about 9 years ago led to the discovery of a period in the cardiac cycle during which ventricular fibrillation can be prevented by low-intensity electrical stimuli. This interval, designated the protective zone (PZ), was found to closely adjoin the vulnerable period. When a stimulus is delivered during the protective zone, fibrillation can be prevented with less than 1 joule of energy.

The objectives of this paper are to review what is currently known about the protective zone and to suggest directions for future research.

MATERIALS AND METHODS

General

The investigations reported herein were conducted in mongrel dogs of either sex and weighing between 8 and 22 kg. The animals were anesthetized intravenously using either sodium pentobarbital (30 mg/kg) or alpha-chloralose (100 mg/kg, Sigma Chemical) 10% wt/vol in isotonic sodium chloride solution. Ventilation was maintained with room air or 40% oxygen through a cuffed endotracheal tube using a Harvard respirator. The respiratory rate was

* This work was supported by Grant HL–07776 from the National Heart, Lung and Blood Institute of the National Institutes of Health, United States Public Health Service, Bethesda, Maryland.

† Address for correspondence: Richard L. Verrier, Ph.D., F.A.C.C., Assistant Professor of Physiology in Medicine, Harvard University School of Public Health, Department of Nutrition, 665 Huntington Avenue, Boston, Massachusetts 02115.

0077–8923/82/0382–0355 $1.75/0 © 1982, NYAS

adjusted to maintain arterial oxygen tension between 100 and 125 mm Hg and pH between 7.35 and 7.45. A polyethylene catheter was inserted into a femoral artery for sampling arterial blood and for monitoring blood pressure. A Statham P23ID transducer was employed to record systemic arterial pressure. Recordings of blood pressure and electrocardiograms were obtained using a Gould/Brush 220 recorder.

Heart rate was maintained constant at 220 beats/min by ventricular pacing during cardiac testing. This rate was selected since many experimental procedures such as the administration of pentobarbital anesthesia, vagotomy, sympathetic stimulation, and acute coronary arterial occlusion result in high heart rates which require pacing rates of 200 to 220 beats/min to overdrive the spontaneous rhythm.

Defibrillation was accomplished, usually within 5 sec, by a direct current pulse (100–200 joule capacitor discharge from a Lown cardioverter) delivered through a pair of copper plates (150 cm^2), which were previously fastened on either side of the thorax. A rest period of 10 to 15 min was generally allowed before cardiac testing was resumed.

Cardiac Electrical Testing

After our initial study, which involved transthoracic electrical stimulation of the heart, we decided to employ transvenous cardiac catheters and intramyocardial electrodes to investigate the PZ phenomenon. This method enables more precise activation of the ventricular myocardium. In most experiments electrical stimulation was accomplished using an intracavitary lead system consisting of a transvenous bipolar pacing catheter (Medtronic, Inc., Minneapolis, Minnesota) with 3-mm platinum electrodes and an interelectrode distance of 1.5 cm and an electrocardiographic recording catheter (4F semifloating bipolar temporary pacing catheter; USCI, Billerica, Massachusetts). The recording catheter was bound to the pacing catheter with silk ligatures, approximately 3 cm proximal to the tip of the latter. This catheter system was introduced via an external jugular vein and positioned in the apex of the right ventricle under direct fluoroscopic visualization. Heart rate was controlled using a variable-rate pacemaker that delivered constant-current rectangular pulse stimuli of 2 msec duration. The current of the pacemaker was set at twice the value of the diastolic threshold. The distal pole of the pacemaker catheter was made cathodal with reference to the proximal pole. Testing stimuli of variable duration were generated using Grass S88 and S44 stimulators (Grass Instrument Company, Quincy, Massachusetts) in conjunction with an optically isolated constant-current source of our own manufacture. The optically isolated constant-current source uses voltage-controlled voltage-source circuitry to generate constant current pulses directly proportional to the voltage input pulses. The output of the device has a voltage compliance of 300 volts direct current. Current output of the optically isolated constant-current source can be verified by taking the voltage across a variety of dummy load resistors (10 ohms to 10 kilohms) and employing Ohm's law. Current output under actual operating conditions can be verified by taking the voltage across a small resistor (~10 ohms) with an oscilloscope with a differential input amplifier and once again using Ohm's law. Timing of stimuli was controlled by a digital timer with a crystal-controlled time base having an accuracy of ±0.01% or better. Timing synchronization was from the pacemaker stimulus for dogs that were paced ventricularly, and from the R wave for supraventricularly paced animals. The stimulation system is equipped with appropriate circuitry to inhibit the output of the pacemaker from 1 to 5 seconds after delivery of the test stimuli. The test impulses were delivered after every 10th to 15th paced beat and were synchronized from the pacer impulse.

Determination of the Vulnerable Period Threshold

Ventricular Fibrillation Threshold

The single-stimulus technique was generally employed to determine the vulnerable period threshold for ventricular fibrillation. This was carried out in the following manner: The duration of the test stimulus was set at 5 msec, and the initial current of the stimulus was set at 8 milliamperes (mA). Electrical diastole was then scanned in 5-msec decrements beginning at the apex of the T wave and ending at the border of the refractory period. If VF was not induced with an 8-mA stimulus, current was increased in 2-mA steps and scanning was continued until VF resulted. The lowest stimulus intensity that elicited VF defined the VF threshold.

Repetitive Extrasystole (RE) Threshold

The repetitive extrasystole (RE) rather than the ventricular fibrillation threshold was selected as an end-point of cardiac testing in many experiments since RE and ventricular fibrillation share a common protective zone.[5] Repetitive extrasystole threshold testing precludes the disruptive effects of defibrillation. The RE threshold has been shown to be a reliable and constant index of vulnerability to ventricular fibrillation. Specifically, it has been shown that when a single RE occurs, approximately two-thirds of the fibrillatory current has been delivered. Furthermore, the nadir of the ventricular vulnerability threshold coincides precisely with the locus in the cardiac cycle where RE can be elicited. The relationship between RE and VF is maintained under diverse experimental conditions.[6, 7]

To determine the RE threshold, the initial current of the stimulus was set at 8 mA and increased in 2-mA steps while scanning was continued until an RE was evoked. The lowest stimulus intensity that consistently elicited RE defined its threshold. The timing in the cardiac cycle at which the RE threshold was determined defined the RE nadir.

Determination of the Protective Zone

Once the RE threshold was determined, the temporal boundaries of the PZ were defined. To accomplish this, the intensity of a second stimulus was set at the RE threshold value and the delay between this stimulus and the RE stimulus was increased in 5-msec steps until the elicitation of RE was prevented. The earliest time in the cardiac cycle for suppression of RE defined the inner boundary of the PZ. This interval usually occurred 10 to 15 msec after the

RE nadir. To determine the outer boundary of PZ, the delay between the RE stimulus and the protective stimulus was further increased until RE was not prevented. The outer boundary of the PZ was usually located 20 to 50 msec beyond the inner boundary.[8]

The PZ threshold was defined as the minimal current required to consistently prevent RE by a stimulus in the midportion of the PZ.

Effects of Varying Stimulation Site and Electrode Arrangement

The influence of stimulating differing anatomic sites by means of various electrode configurations was studied with plunge electrodes[5] which consisted of Teflon®-coated stainless steel wires (diameter 0.007 inch). The wires were passed through a hypodermic needle and bent at the tip to form a small hook. The needle was then inserted into the myocardium and subsequently withdrawn, leaving the wires hooked into the myocardium. Unless specified otherwise, the electrode pairs, consisting of an anode and cathode, were separated by a distance of 7 to 10 mm.

Experimental Interventions

Parasympathetic and Sympathetic Nerve Stimulation

Isolation of the vagus nerves and stellate ganglia for electrical stimulation was carried out as previously described.[8] Briefly, cervical vagosympathetic trunks were sectioned bilaterally 2 cm below the level of the carotid bifurcation. The left ganglion was exposed by left thoracotomy in the second interspace. An insulated, Teflon-coated stainless steel bipolar stimulator was positioned over the isolated nerves. Stellate nerve stimulation was accomplished by means of a Tektronic square-wave pulse generator, using a pulse train of 5 V and having a duration of 5 msec at 40 Hz. Vagus nerves were stimulated bilaterally using a pulse train of 5 msec duration at 10 Hz. Voltages were adjusted (5 to 15 V) during vagus nerve stimulation to produce asystole at the time of pacemaker inhibition. Left stellate ganglion stimulation was considered adequate if the mean systemic pressure increased by at least 40 mm Hg above control level. Effectiveness of nerve stimulation could be demonstrated for at least 10 min, a period adequate for obtaining RE and PZ thresholds.

Myocardial Ischemia and Reperfusion

The main device used in the animals in these experiments included a balloon occluder positioned around the left anterior descending (LAD) coronary artery.[9] The coronary vessel was obstructed for 10 minutes, after which time the balloon was abruptly deflated. This model was selected because it results in a reproducible time course of vulnerability changes that closely parallels spontaneous susceptibility to ventricular fibrillation.[10] The VF rather than the RE threshold was used as an end-point of electrical testing in these experiments because total coronary occlusion of a major vessel disrupts the RE/VF threshold relationship.[11] Thus, the PZ threshold was determined by delivering the fibrillatory stimulus in the midpoint of the zone using stimuli of 20 mA above the VF threshold. The time of the protective stimulus was varied and the PZ boundaries mapped. The LAD was occluded and the PZ was determined at 0–3 min, 3–6 min, 6–10 min, and upon release.[9]

All results were analyzed for statistical significance by either analysis of variance or Student's t test. Values are expressed as mean ± standard error of the mean.

RESULTS

Basic Characteristics of the Protective Zone (PZ)

Detailed study of the PZ confirmed the initial observation regarding the general characteristics of this phenomenon. Specifically, the PZ was found to be a relatively broad interval, which occurs shortly after the vulnerable period and persists for nearly the entire remainder of the repolarization phase (FIGS. 1 and 2). A striking feature of the PZ phenomenon is that only a fraction of the fibrillatory current is required for its activation and the consequent prevention of ventricular fibrillation.

It was also found that the PZ could be effectively engaged by administering a train of stimuli.[12] The effect of varying the timing and duration of a 100-Hz train of 5-msec stimuli was studied. When the train traversed the PZ, the elicitation of repetitive extrasystoles by a prior stimulus delivered during the vulnerable period was prevented (FIG. 3). However, when the train of stimuli extended beyond the boundaries of the PZ, no suppression of the RE response was observed. Administration of a train of stimuli during the PZ also increased the current required to induce ventricular fibrillation (FIG. 4).

Influence of Heart Rate Change, Autonomic Nervous System Stimulation, and Myocardial Ischemia on the Protective Zone

The effects of these diverse physiologic interventions on the characteristics of the PZ have been studied in some detail. The main findings can be summarized as follows:

Effect of heart rate change: The boundaries of the PZ change considerably as a function of heart rate (FIG. 5). With increasing heart rate, the vulnerable period occurs progressively earlier in the cardiac cycle and the width of the PZ narrows. There is also a shortening of the interval between the vulnerable period and the inner boundary of the PZ.

Vagal influence: In bilaterally vagotomized animals, stimulation of the distal nerve stump raised the RE threshold by 20% ($p < 0.05$). At the same time, both the PZ was shifted later into diastole and the duration of the zone was increased (FIG. 6).

Sympathetic neural influence: Left stellate ganglion stimulation in previously vagotomized animals markedly lowered the RE threshold by 38% ($p < 0.05$). There was a concomitant shift earlier into diastole of both the RE nadir and the midpoint of the protective zone. Left stellate ganglion stimulation also moved PZ boundaries earlier into diastole without significantly altering its duration (FIG. 7). The inner and outer boundaries of the PZ were changed

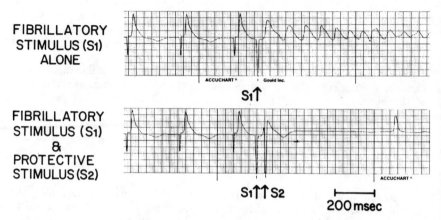

FIGURE 1. Protective zone for ventricular fibrillation (VF). Fibrillation is induced by delivering a 30-mA stimulus, S_1 (*upper tracing*), during the vulnerable period. The protective stimulus, S_2, which is half this intensity, is delivered 40 msec after the fibrillatory impulse (*lower tracing*). In the latter situation, VF is averted and sinus rhythm prevails. Heart rate is maintained constant by ventricular pacing.

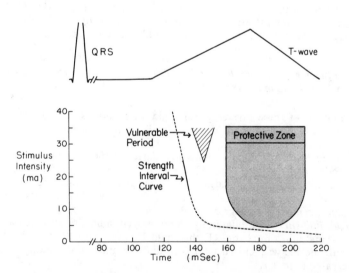

FIGURE 2. Location of the protective zone (PZ). Temporal relationships between T wave, vulnerable period, strength–interval curve, and protective zone. The vulnerable-period curve has a characteristic V shape, the nadir of which coincides temporally with that for provoking ventricular fibrillation. The PZ is a relatively broad zone which occurs 10 to 20 msec after the VP nadir and is approximately 50 msec in duration.

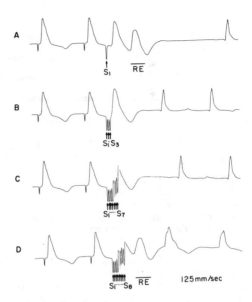

FIGURE 3. Activation of the protective zone (PZ) by a 100-Hz train of stimuli. (A) Single 5-msec stimulus, S_1, of 20 mA delivered 125 msec after last pacer stimulus elicits a repetitive extrasystole (RE) and defines the RE threshold. (B) When S_1 is followed by two stimuli, S_2 and S_3, of equal intensity, no RE is evoked. (C) Suppression of RE continues up to a maximum of 7 stimuli. (D) When train consists of 8 stimuli, RE reemerges.[12]

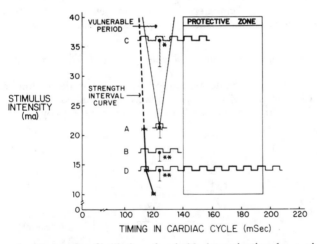

FIGURE 4. Ventricular fibrillation threshold determination by a single stimulus and by trains of stimuli of varying duration. (A) Timing in the cardiac cycle of the VP for VF was first determined using a single 5–msec stimulus. Thereafter, VF thresholds were redetermined using a train of 5–msec stimuli of varying duration. Trains were initiated at identical times in the cardiac cycle just after the ventricular refractory period. (B) When a train consisting of three stimuli was delivered, the VF threshold was significantly lower than that observed using a single stimulus (**$p < 0.01$). (C) When the train was extended to five stimuli, the PZ was activated and VF threshold was elevated (*$p < 0.05$). (D) When the train was increased to ten stimuli and the PZ boundary was exceeded, elevation in VF threshold failed to occur.[12]

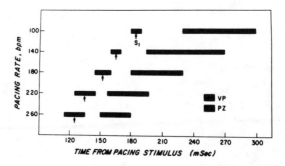

FIGURE 5. Relationship between the vulnerable period (VP) and protective zone (PZ) as a function of heart rate. As heart rate is increased from 100 to 280 beats per minute, the VP occurs progressively earlier in the cardiac cycle. With increasing heart rate, the PZ narrows and the interval between the VP and PZ shortens. Values are means obtained from ten dogs.[2]

from 141 ± 3 to 122 ± 3 msec ($p < 0.001$) and 172 ± 4 to 151 ± 4 msec ($p < 0.01$), respectively.

Sympathetic–parasympathetic interactions: Stimulation of the peripheral cut end of the vagus nerve during concurrent left stellate ganglion activation prevented both the decrease in the RE threshold and the earlier occurrence of the PZ observed during left stellate ganglion stimulation alone. Thus, parasympathetic stimulation completely annulled the effects of the sympathetic nervous system on the characteristics of the protective zone.

Influence of Myocardial Ischemia on the Protective Zone

The effects of a 10-minute period of left anterior descending coronary arterial occlusion on the PZ phenomenon were also studied.[9] Epicardial electrodes or right ventricular endocardial electrodes were employed. Significant

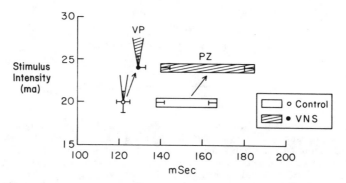

FIGURE 6. Influence of vagus nerve stimulation (VNS) on the protective zone (PZ) and vulnerable period (VP) in bilaterally vagotomized dogs. Vagus stimulation raised the RE threshold coincident with a parallel shift of the RE nadir and PZ later into electrical diastole. A concomitant prolongation of the PZ duration is also in evidence.[8]

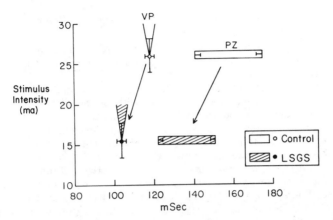

FIGURE 7. Effect of left stellate ganglion stimulation (LSGS) on the protective zone and vulnerable period threshold in vagotomized and stellate decentralized dogs. LSGS decreased the RE threshold coincident with a parallel shift of the RE nadir and PZ earlier into electrical diastole.[8]

narrowing of the PZ occurred during occlusion of the coronary vessel (FIG. 8); this was independent of the test site. Upon release of the obstruction, the PZ returned to control values. Five additional dogs were studied using a two-stage LAD occlusion. The vulnerable period (VP) and PZ were determined at 30–60 min and 120–150 min. A significant constriction of the PZ ($p < 0.01$) and lengthening of the VP ($p < 0.05$) occurred at 30–60 min. At 120–150 min both the VP and PZ had returned to control values.

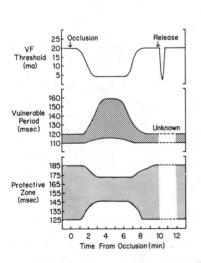

FIGURE 8. Effect of a 10-minute period of left anterior descending coronary arterial occlusion on ventricular fibrillation (VF) threshold and the characteristics of the vulnerable period and the protective zone. Upon occlusion of the coronary vessel there is a fall in the VF threshold to extremely low levels within 2 minutes. This period of enhanced vulnerability to VF persists for about 4 minutes, after which time spontaneous recovery of the fibrillation threshold occurs. A second period of extreme susceptibility to VF is observed upon release of the occlusion. This effect is observed within 10 to 15 seconds of release and is transient, lasting less than 1 minute. Coronary occlusion also results in a significant broadening of the vulnerable period and constriction of the protective zone. The transient nature of the release-reperfusion phenomenon does not permit reliable delineation of these zones.

Electrophysiologic Basis for the Protective Zone

To gain further insight into the mechanisms responsible for the PZ, we studied the effects of varying stimulation site and electrode configuration on the characteristics of the protective zone.[5]

Effect of varying stimulation site: In these experiments, RE rather than VF was induced to permit repeated testing without the disruptive effects of defibrillation. Plunge electrodes were positioned epicardially and transmurally midway between the apex and base of the right and left ventricles, and across the interventricular septum. Effective activation of the PZ was achieved by stimulation of each of these sites with a current of 8 mA or less (TABLE 1).

Effect of electrode configuration on the PZ: Two types of bipolar epicardial electrode configurations were employed (FIGS. 9 and 10). In both cases the provocative stimulus for inducing RE was delivered from the reference point designated 0 cm. In one situation (type A electrode configuration), the protective stimulus was delivered at increasing distances from the provocative stimulus (FIG. 9). When this electrode configuration was used, the stimulus intensity required to suppress repetitive extrasystoles increased as a function of distance.

TABLE 1

PROTECTIVE ZONE THRESHOLD AT DIFFERENT SITES

Electrode Location	No. of Animals	Protective Zone Threshold * (mA)
Right ventricle, epicardium	3	2 ± 1
Left ventricle, epicardium	5	3 ± 1
Interventricular septum	2	4 ± 1
Right ventricle, transmural	4	5 ± 1
Left ventricle, transmural	2	4 ± 2

* Values are means ± the standard error of the mean.

When the provocative and protective stimuli were separated by more than 0.5 cm, repetitive extrasystoles could no longer be prevented by the PZ impulse (TABLE 2).

The second electrode arrangement (type B electrode configuration, FIG. 10) was such that the protective pulse shared a common anode with the provocative stimulus. While the position of the anode remained fixed, the location of the cathode of the PZ stimulus was varied. Using this electrode arrangement, suppression of RE could be achieved at the maximal distance tested, which was 3 cm, practically the long axis of the heart (FIG. 10; TABLE 3).

DISCUSSION

These observations indicate that the PZ is a highly reproducible phenomenon that can be demonstrated under a variety of experimental conditions. The existence of the PZ has also been confirmed by other investigators.[13, 14] When the electrical stimuli are delivered during a discrete interval that adjoins the

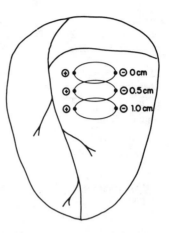

FIGURE 9. Type A electrode configuration. Several pairs of bipolar plunge electrodes were implanted in the left ventricular myocardium. The provocative stimulus, S_1, was always delivered from the reference point, designated 0 cm. The protective stimulus, S_2, was delivered at increasing distances from the site of the provocative stimulus. Using this electrode configuration, suppression of repetitive extrasystoles could not be achieved beyond a distance of 0.5 cm.

vulnerable period, ventricular fibrillation is prevented. The temporal boundaries of the PZ are not fixed, but are dynamically altered by physiologic interventions such as changes in heart rate, autonomic nervous system stimulation, and myocardial ischemia. Activation of the PZ does not require selective excitation of the specialized conducting system.

Electrophysiologic Basis for the Protective Zone

Activation of the PZ is a critically time-dependent phenomenon. To prevent ventricular fibrillation, the protective stimulus must be delivered between 10 to 50 msec after the fibrillatory pulse. The PZ stimulus must also be administered within a certain distance from the site where VF is initiated. As the physical separation between the fibrillatory and protective impulse increases, the duration of the PZ progressively decreases and the current required for protection increases. These findings suggest that the protective stimulus may block the occurrence of VF by a local phenomenon rather than a more diffuse myocardial effect. Tamargo et al.[13] have provided evidence that the PZ stimulus may

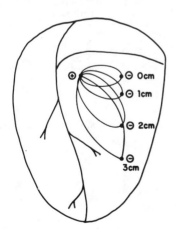

FIGURE 10. Type B electrode configuration. As indicated in Figure 9, S_1 and S_2 refer to the provocative and protective stimulus, respectively. As with the type A electrode configuration, provocative stimulus was delivered from the pair of electrodes, designated 0 cm. However, in this case the position of the cathode was varied while the anode was shared with that of the provocative stimulus. Using this electrode arrangement, suppression of RE could be achieved at the maximal distance tested, which was 3 cm, essentially the long axis of the heart.[5]

TABLE 2

PROTECTIVE ZONE THRESHOLD USING TYPE A ELECTRODE CONFIGURATION *

Electrode Location	Distance (cm) Between S_1 and S_2 †	Protective Zone Threshold (mA) ‡
Right ventricle, epicardium	0.0	3 ± 1
	0.5	9 ± 3
	1.0	No protection §
	2.0	No protection
	3.0	No protection
Left ventricle, epicardium	0.0	2 ± 1
	0.5	7 ± 1
	1.0	No protection
	2.0	No protection
	3.0	No protection

* See FIGURE 9.
† S_1 and S_2 = Provocative and protective stimulus, respectively.
‡ Values are means ± standard error of the mean.
§ Maximal current of 40 mA was tested.

TABLE 3

PROTECTIVE ZONE THRESHOLD USING TYPE B ELECTRODE CONFIGURATION *

Electrode Location	Distance (cm) Between S_1 and S_2 †	Protective Zone Threshold (mA) ‡
Right ventricle, epicardium	0.0	2 ± 1
	1.0	5 ± 1
	2.0	5 ± 1
	3.0	3 ± 2
Left ventricle, epicardium	0.0	3 ± 1
	1.0	6 ± 2
	2.0	4 ± 1
	3.0	12 ± 5

* See Figure 10.
† S_1 and S_2 = Provocative and protective stimulus, respectively.
‡ Values are means ± standard error of the mean.
§ Maximal current of 40 mA was tested.

prevent the induction of VF by "occluding" a major reentrant pathway. This hypothesis is consistent with our observations that delivery of the protective stimulus must be both temporally and spatially located to block the propagating wave front which otherwise degenerates into ventricular fibrillation. The studies of Euler and Moore [14] provide additional support for this hypothesis. They found that electrograms recorded from muscle adjacent to the site of the fibrillatory stimulus exhibited fragmented activation complexes which heralded the onset of ventricular fibrillation. Activation of the PZ consistently abolished the fractionated electrical activity and aborted the induction of ventricular fibrillation. Moreover, it was noted that the PZ occurs at a time when reentrant activity should be relatively localized and that delivery of a strong stimulus during this period could effect blockade of a propagating wavefront by depolarizing unexcited fibers in the circuit.

Mechanisms Responsible for the Effects of Heart Rate Changes, Autonomic Nervous System Stimulation, and Myocardial Ischemia on the Protective Zone

A number of well-established effects of adrenergic stimulation on ventricular excitability properties are likely to be involved in the observed changes in PZ characteristics. In particular, stellate ganglion stimulation has been shown to accelerate repolarization of both ventricular and specialized conducting tissue.[15-17] The shift of the inner boundary of the PZ earlier into the cardiac cycle during sympathetic stimulation may be the result of hastened recovery of excitability. It is of interest in this regard that stellate ganglion excitation resulted in nearly identical shifts in vulnerable period threshold and inner boundary of the protective zone. This would indicate that a related electrophysiologic process accounts for the temporal changes in these electrical properties during adrenergic stimulation.

Effects of sympathetic nerve stimulation: How does sympathetic nerve activation abbreviate the duration of the protective zone? Our supposition is that the protective stimulus aborts the induction of ventricular fibrillation by blocking conduction in major reentrant pathways. Accordingly, adrenergic stimulation, by augmenting the number of potential reentrant circuits, would decrease the effectiveness of a given protective stimulus. This could result in an increase in PZ threshold current or a decrease in the interval during which the PZ stimulus is capable of preventing ventricular fibrillation. While stellate ganglion stimulation did not significantly alter the threshold of the PZ, a substantial abbreviation of its duration was observed.

Effects of vagus nerve stimulation: Considerable evidence indicates that parasympathetic neural influences affect ventricular excitability properties.[6, 18, 19] Kent and coworkers [19] have shown that vagus nerve stimulation increases the VF threshold in the normal and ischemic canine heart. They demonstrated a rich cholinergic innervation of the specialized conducting system through which the antifibrillatory action of the vagus nerve is thought to occur.[20] Our view has been that the effect of the vagus nerve on ventricular vulnerability is contingent on the level of preexisting cardiac sympathetic tone.[7, 21-23] Sympathetic–parasympathetic interactions also appear to play a role in altering the protective zone. The present study demonstrated that vagus nerve excitation during concurrent stellate ganglion stimulation restored PZ properties to control values, but did not alter them beyond this. Thus, further proof is provided that vagal effects on diverse electrical properties of the heart result from opposition of adrenergic influences.

Influence of myocardial ischemia: The constriction of the PZ boundaries during acute coronary arterial occlusion is likely to be due to both direct effects of myocardial ischemia and indirect influences related to reflex activation of potent cardiocardiac sympathetic reflexes.[24, 25] Myocardial ischemia would be expected to increase the PZ threshold and narrow its temporal boundaries by enhancing the number of potential reentrant circuits. These effects should be further augmented by the presumed elevation in sympathetic drive in response to coronary arterial occlusion. We would therefore anticipate that reduction of adrenergic tone by surgical or pharmacologic interventions should markedly blunt the changes in PZ associated with myocardial ischemia. Indeed, this has been shown to be the case with respect to ischemia-induced changes in the vulnerable period properties.[10] Whether substantial changes in the characteristics of the PZ also occur during adrenergic blockade remains to be determined.

FINAL COMMENTS

These observations indicate that the repolarization phase of the cardiac cycle contains not only a vulnerable period, as originally suggested by Wiggers and Wegria,[1] but also a closely adjoining protective zone. This finding has important theoretical as well as practical implications. An intriguing possibility is that the protective zone may serve to prevent spontaneous ventricular arrhythmias. Exploitation of this potential therapeutic modality will require further study.

REFERENCES

1. WIGGERS, C. J. & R. WEGRIA. 1940. Ventricular fibrillation due to single localized induction and condenser shocks applied during the vulnerable phase of ventricular systole. Am. J. Physiol. **128:** 500–505.
2. WOLFF, G. A., F. VEITH & B. LOWN. 1968. A vulnerable period for ventricular tachycardia following myocardial infarction. Cardiovasc. Res. **2:** 111–121.
3. MIROWSKI, M., P. R. REID, M. M. MOWER, L. WATKINS, V. L. GOTT, J. F. SCHAUBLE, A. LANGER, M. S. HEILMAN, S. A. KOLENIK, R. E. FISCHELL & M. L. WEISFELDT. 1980. Termination of malignant ventricular arrhythmias with an implanted automatic defibrillator in human beings. N. Engl. J. Med. **303:** 322–324.
4. WOLF, M., E. SEROPPIAN, B. LOWN, J. TEMTE, A. GARFEIN & R. L. VERRIER. 1972. Protective zone for ventricular fibrillation (abstract). Am. J. Cardiol. **29:** 298.
5. KINNARD, M. S., R. L. VERRIER & B. LOWN. 1978. Prevention of ventricular fibrillation by low intensity stimuli delivered during the protective zone (abstract). Fed. Proc. **37:** 656.
6. MATTA, R. J., R. L. VERRIER & B. LOWN. 1976. Repetitive extrasystole as an index of vulnerability to ventricular fibrillation. Am. J. Physiol. **230:** 1469–1473.
7. LOWN, B. & R. L. VERRIER. 1976. Neural activity and ventricular fibrillation. N. Engl. J. Med. **294:** 1165–1170.

8. BROOKS, W. W., R. L. VERRIER & B. LOWN. 1981. Influence of autonomic nervous system stimulation on the protective zone. Cardiovasc. Res. **15:** 92–97.

9. LANIGAN, J., G. A. COOK, J. V. TEMTE & B. LOWN. 1974. The protective zone following acute coronary occlusion (abstract). Am. J. Cardiol. **33:** 150.

10. AXELROD, P. J., R. L. VERRIER & B. LOWN. 1975. Vulnerability to ventricular fibrillation (VF) during acute coronary occlusion and release. Am. J. Cardiol. **36:** 776–782.

11. KOWEY, P. R., R. L. VERRIER & B. LOWN. 1981. The repetitive extrasystole as an index of vulnerability to ventricular fibrillation during myocardial ischemia (abstract). Am. J. Cardiol. **47:** 391A.

12. VERRIER, R. L., W. W. BROOKS & B. LOWN. 1978. Protective zone and the determination of vulnerability to ventricular fibrillation. Am. J. Physiol.: Heart Circ. Physiol. **3:** H592–H596.

13. TAMARGO, J., B. MOE & G. K. MOE. 1975. Interaction of sequential stimuli applied during the relative refractory period in relation to determination of fibrillation threshold in the canine ventricle. Circ. Res. **37:** 534–541.

14. EULER, D. E. & E. N. MOORE. 1980. Continuous fractionated electrical activity after stimulation of the ventricles during the vulnerable period: Evidence for local reentry. Am. J. Cardiol. **46:** 783–791.

15. WIT, A. L., B. F. HOFFMAN & M. R. ROSEN. 1975. Electrophysiology and pharmacology of cardiac arrhythmias. IX. Cardiac electrophysiologic effects of beta adrenergic receptor stimulation and blockade. Part A. Am. Heart. J. **90:** 521–533.

16. WIT, A. L., B. F. HOFFMAN & M. R. ROSEN. 1975. Electrophysiology and pharmacology of cardiac arrhythmias. IX. Cardiac electrophysiologic effects of beta adrenergic receptor stimulation and blockade. Part C. Am. Heart. J. **90:** 795–803.

17. SCHWARTZ, P. J., R. L. VERRIER & B. LOWN. 1977. Effect of stellectomy and vagotomy on ventricular refractoriness. Circ. Res. **40:** 536–540.

18. KOLMAN, B. S., R. L. VERRIER & B. LOWN. 1975. The effect of vagus nerve stimulation upon vulnerability of the canine ventricle: Role of sympathetic-parasympathetic interactions. Circulation **52:** 578–585.

19. KENT, K. M., E. R. SMITH, D. R. REDWOOD & S. E. EPSTEIN. 1973. Electrical stability of acutely ischemic myocardium: Influence of heart rate and vagal stimulation. Circulation **47:** 291–298.

20. KENT, K. M., S. E. EPSTEIN, T. COOPER & D. M. JACOBOWITZ. 1974. Cholinergic innervation of the canine and human ventricular conduction system: Anatomic and electrophysiologic correlation. Circulation **50:** 948–955.

21. RABINOWITZ, S. H., R. L. VERRIER & B. LOWN. 1976. Muscarinic effects of vagosympathetic trunk stimulation on the repetitive extrasystole threshold. Circulation **53:** 622–627.

22. LEVY, M. N. & B. BLATTBERG. 1976. Effect of vagal stimulation on the overflow of norepinephrine into the coronary sinus during cardiac sympathetic nerve stimulation in the dog. Circ. Res. **38:** 81–85.

23. WATANABE, A. M. & H. R. BESCH. 1975. Interaction between cyclic adenosine monophosphate and cyclic guanosine monophosphate in guinea pig ventricular myocardium. Circ. Res. **37:** 309–317.

24. MALLIANI, A., P. J. SCHWARTZ & A. ZANCHETTI. 1969. A sympathetic reflex elicited by experimental coronary occlusion. Am. J. Physiol. **217:** 703–709.

25. MALLIANI, A. & F. LOMBARDI. 1978. Neural reflexes associated with myocardial ischemia. *In* Neural Mechanisms in Cardiac Arrhythmias. P. J. Schwartz, A. M. Brown, A. Malliani & A. Zanchetti, Eds.: 209–219. Raven Press. New York, NY.

DISCUSSION

Dr. Cobb: I noticed, Dr. Verrier, that you have used the strength of the intensity stimulus as an index of the ease of producing a repetitive ventricular response (RVR), implying a VF threshold. This is generally overlooked in most electrophysiologic studies. Should more attention be paid to this?

Dr. Verrier: Yes, this is an important difference between experimental studies on repetitive response testing and the procedures used clinically. In the clinical setting the intensity of stimuli is not varied substantially, and the repolarization phase is explored with one, two, or three stimuli. The end-point of testing is RVR or ventricular tachycardia. In the animal laboratory, we vary the current, increasing it until a response is elicited, and the current required to provoke a repetitive response is taken as an index of susceptibility to fibrillation.

There are important differences between the repetitive extrasystole threshold, which is a vulnerable period phenomenon and is located within the first half of the T wave. The RVR end-point is frequently elicited on the downslope of the T wave and thus may not necessarily be a vulnerable-period phenomenon.

Unidentified Speaker: Can you speculate on the underlying mechanism for this phenomenon in terms of altered membrane potentials, altered membrane currents, or altered time constants?

Dr. Verrier: That would be difficult. We have no data with respect to action potentials. We believe that by delivering a relatively strong stimulus, unexcited fibers are activated, providing a refractory field which interrupts the propagating wavefront.

Unidentified Speaker: Then for this to become an effective therapeutic mode it would seem that one would have to know the site of the ectopic extrasystole. Is that your impression?

Dr. Verrier: Actually not. If the two poles are to encompass the long axis of the heart, the assumption is that any fibrillating wavefront that originated between the two could be extinguished. This is what the data suggest. What we do need to study is the effectiveness of the protective zone in suppressing the spontaneous arrhythmias such as those generated during recovery from myocardial infarction in the experimental model. We are planning to focus on this question in the near future.

Dr. Cobb: What, if any, therapeutic implication does this observation have?

Dr. Verrier: The problem with the protective zone phenomenon is that it necessitates anticipation of the development of an arrhythmia and this requires the continuous delivery of pulses. If there are any shifts in temporal relationships, a protective stimulus might become a trigger for ventricular fibrillation.

IMPLANTABLE AUTOMATIC DEFIBRILLATORS: THEIR POTENTIAL IN PREVENTION OF SUDDEN CORONARY DEATH

M. Mirowski, Morton M. Mower, Philip R. Reid, and
Levi Watkins, Jr.

Department of Medicine
Sinai Hospital of Baltimore
Baltimore, Maryland 21215

Departments of Medicine and Surgery
The Johns Hopkins Medical Institutions
Baltimore, Maryland 21205

BACKGROUND

The multifaceted strategy necessary to decrease the current prohibitive toll of sudden cardiac death has recently been complemented by the development of a clinically applicable automatic implantable defibrillator.[1-3] This electronic device is designed to continuously monitor cardiac rhythm, to recognize ventricular fibrillation and sinusoidal ventricular tachycardias, and then to deliver corrective defibrillatory discharges. Conceptually, the implantable defibrillator can be viewed as analogous to an implantable demand pacemaker, except that malignant ventricular arrhythmias instead of asystole are sensed and that the output pulse has appropriate defibrillating characteristics.

The main impetus behind the development of such a device was the realization that sudden cardiac death usually reflects electrical instability of the heart culminating in ventricular fibrillation, an arrhythmia for which the only treatment is the delivery to the fibrillating heart of a sufficiently strong electrical countershock. The effectiveness of this maneuver, however, is totally dependent upon the prompt availability of specialized personnel and equipment. Because this essential prerequisite to successful defibrillation is difficult to satisfy outside the hospital, we[4] as well as others[5] have been convinced that an urgent need exists for a diagnostic-therapeutic system capable of detecting and treating malignant arrhythmias automatically, without medical assistance or additional equipment.

Since the development of the first working model of such a device in the late 1960s,[4] various aspects of the automatic implantable defibrillator concept have been investigated.[1-3, 6-15] Recently, this effort has culminated in the development of a device the structural and functional characteristics of which made it suitable for implantation in human beings.

DESCRIPTION OF THE DEVICE

The automatic implantable defibrillator currently used in patients is shown on FIGURE 1. This device,* similar in size and configuration to early pace-

---

* Developed and manufactured under the name of AID™ defibrillator by Medrad, Inc./Intec Systems, Inc., Pittsburgh, Pennsylvania.

0077-8923/82/0382-0371 $1.75/0 © 1982, NYAS

makers, is encased in titanium and is hermetically sealed with a laser weld; it weighs 250 grams and occupies a volume of 145 ml. All materials in contact with body tissue are biocompatible. The defibrillating electrodes are made from titanium and silicone rubber; one, designed for placement in the superior vena cava, is located on an intravascular catheter. The second electrode, in the form of a flexible rectangular patch, is placed over the apex of the heart. The outer surface of the apical electrode is insulated to achieve optimal current distribution.

The device establishes the diagnosis of ventricular fibrillation by continuously analyzing the probability density function of cardiac electrical activity.[12] This function reflects the time spent by the slope of the input electrogram between two amplitude limits, located in our system near zero potential. In essence, ventricular fibrillation is identified by the striking absence of isoelectric segments. Ventricular tachycardias which satisfy the probability density criteria and which are faster than a preset cut-off rate are also recognized by the device.

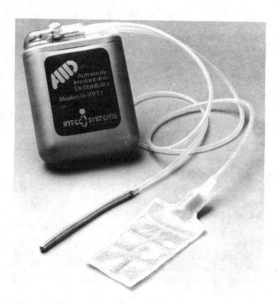

FIGURE 1. The automatic implantable defibrillator with its superior vena caval catheter electrode and the apical patch electrode.

When a suitable ventricular arrhythmia is detected, the device delivers Schuder's truncated exponential pulse [16] of 25 joules some 20 seconds after onset of the arrhythmia; the pulse duration is 3 to 8 msec, depending on the interelectrode resistance. The device can recycle as many as three times if the previous discharge is ineffective; the strength of the third and fourth pulses being increased to 30 joules. After the fourth discharge, about 35 seconds of nonfibrillating rhythm is required to reset the counter, allowing a full series of pulses to be delivered again at the next episode.

EXTERNAL ANALYZER

The operational readiness of the automatic defibrillator can be tested prior to and periodically after implantation by an external analyzer.† This simple and noninvasive method is based on triggering the capacitor charging cycle of the defibrillator with a magnet briefly placed over the skin in the area of the implanted device. After becoming fully charged, the capacitors are automatically discharged into a built-in test-load resistor rather than through the leads to the patient. The capacitor charging time is measured with an electromagnetic transducer. Progressive increases in this time, normally 10 seconds or less, reflect battery depletion, whereas failure to initiate the cycle indicates an abnormal condition resulting in self-deactivation of the device. Continuous application of the magnet over the pulse generator can be used to disable the device completely and to deplete the batteries if needed.

PRECLINICAL TESTING PROGRAM

The first clinical version of the automatic implantable defibrillator was subjected to extensive preclinical testing.[2] In addition to acute and chronic animal electrophysiologic and pathologic studies, an experimental model was designed [1] in which the clinical syndrome of sudden death from ventricular fibrillation was reproduced in active, conscious dogs. In these animals, ventricular fibrillation could be induced by magnetically triggering an implanted alternating-current generator connected to the dog's heart through a right ventricular catheter. The resulting arrhythmia led to circulatory arrest and syncope within seconds. However, in contrast to patients stricken by ventricular fibrillation, the animals are automatically defibrillated and resuscitated by the chronically implanted defibrillator (FIG. 2).

The preclinical testing [2] also included the analysis of the long-term bench performance of the implantable defibrillator and of the effects of its exposure to various physical stresses such as vacuum, pressure, temperature cycling, mechanical vibration, mechanical shock, and to electromagnetic interference signals. Despite the fact that many of the test conditions exceeded the standards required of implantable pacemakers, the results were generally satisfactory and the few detected failure modes were analyzed and corrected. In addition, the automatic implantable defibrillator underwent an independent evaluation by the Applied Physics Laboratory of The Johns Hopkins University, which included basic device design, provocative challenges to the sensing system, and analysis of components, manufacturing, quality control procedures, and preclinical test results. On the basis of this information the device was found suitable for use in a clinical setting.

PATIENT POPULATION

A clinical evaluation study of the automatic defibrillator began in February 1980 at The Johns Hopkins Hospital.[3, 14, 15] The criteria for entry into the

---

† Developed and manufactured under the name of AIDCHECK™ by Medrad, Inc./Intec Systems, Inc., Pittsburgh, Pennsylvania.

pilot study were stringent. The prospective candidates for implantation must have survived at least two episodes of cardiac arrest outside the setting of acute myocardial infarction, with ventricular fibrillation or sinusoidal ventricular tachycardia documented electrocardiographically at least once. One such epi-

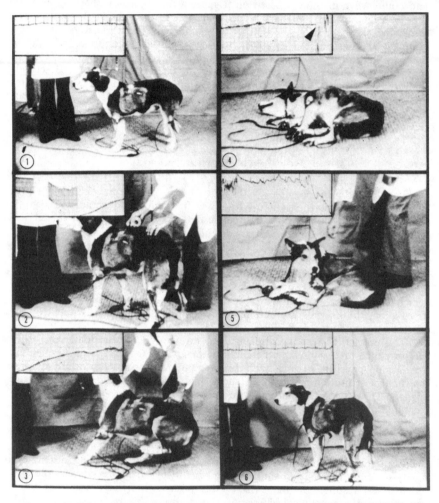

FIGURE 2. Selected movie frames of a typical automatic fibrillation–defibrillation episode. Simultaneous electrocardiographic monitoring is displayed in the left upper corner. *Panel 1:* The animal prior to the procedure. *Panel 2:* Induction of ventricular fibrillation. *Panel 3:* Syncope secondary to the arrhythmia. *Panel 4:* The delivery of the countershock 15 seconds after the onset of the arrhythmia (*arrowhead*). *Panels 5 and 6:* The animal at 3 and 5 seconds, respectively, after automatic defibrillation.

sode must have occurred despite treatment with a medication suppressing all complex ventricular arrhythmias present or, failing that, despite treatment with two antiarrhythmic agents given simultaneously and resulting in satisfactory levels of the drugs in the blood. Patients were excluded if they had other chronic or acute illness, were on drugs (other than antiarrhythmic agents) known to influence electrical activity of the heart, or had psychological disabilities. The extremely poor prognosis of patients fulfilling these criteria is exemplified by the fact that eight patients identified as potential candidates for implantation of the automatic defibrillator died before they could be transferred to The Johns Hopkins Hospital.

Up to March 1981, 12 men and 4 women have undergone AID defibrillator implantation; their ages at the time of surgery ranged from 16 to 74 (mean: 51 years). Coronary artery disease was the underlying heart lesion in 11 patients and nonischemic cardiomyopathy in 5 (congestive in 2, hypertrophic in 2, and sarcoid in 1 patient). Three patients had previous coronary bypass surgery, one an aneurysmectomy, one placement of a mitral valve prosthesis, one a septal myectomy, and three had pacemakers implanted. The average follow-up period was 6 months, the longest being 14 months.

The left lateral thoracotomy approach was used in seven patients and median sternotomy in nine. Associated surgical procedures were frequently performed along with the implantation, including coronary bypass grafting (three patients), endocardial resection (one), aneurysmectomy and endocardial resection (two), and coronary bypass grafting with mitral valve replacement (one); a total of seven patients (44%) underwent these additional procedures. Also, three patients received permanent demand pacemakers. The initially implanted pulse generators were replaced with units incorporating improved circuitry in six patients. There was no surgical or hospital mortality and the postoperative morbidity was unremarkable; in general, the device has been well tolerated by the implantees. Three additional patients not included in this analysis have undergone implantation of the defibrillating electrodes alone during a thoracotomy for unrelated conditions. In these patients the pulse generators may be implanted at a later stage if indicated.

RESULTS

Twenty-five episodes of malignant arrhythmias were documented in the hospital after implantation; eight episodes occurred spontaneously, while seventeen were induced during electrophysiologic studies. All spontaneous arrhythmias and fourteen of the seventeen induced arrhythmias were correctly identified and reverted to sinus rhythm with a single 25-joule pulse (FIGS. 3 and 4).

In three instances the induced arrhythmias were properly identified, but the first shock was ineffective and the device did not recycle promptly as expected; in one of these episodes a ventricular tachycardia accelerated into flutter–fibrillation. These three arrhythmias were terminated with an external countershock. The delay in recycling was due to transient polarization of the electrodes caused by the discharge and which led to attenuation of the input signal. Appropriate design modifications have been implemented and in one subsequent case, when the initial discharge and an ensuing external countershock were both ineffective, the device did recycle as programmed, delivering a second pulse, which restored normal rhythm. Arrhythmias that were not expected to be corrected by the device because they were slower than the preset cut-off rate or had a nonsinusoidal waveform were not included in the present analysis.

With only the one just-described exception, the automatic discharges were not associated with ventricular irritability, bradyarrhythmias, or asystole. Cor-

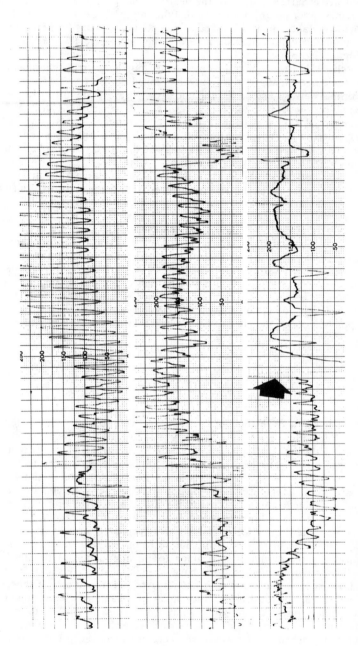

FIGURE 3. Electrocardiogram of a patient in whom atrial flutter developed with rapid and irregular ventricular response of 28 minutes' duration, during which the implanted automatic defibrillator remained quiescent. The last few beats of this supraventricular rhythm are seen in the left part of the *upper strip*. Two spontaneous premature ventricular beats then induced ventricular flutter–fibrillation, which was automatically terminated (*arrow*) 23 seconds later. The strips are continuous.

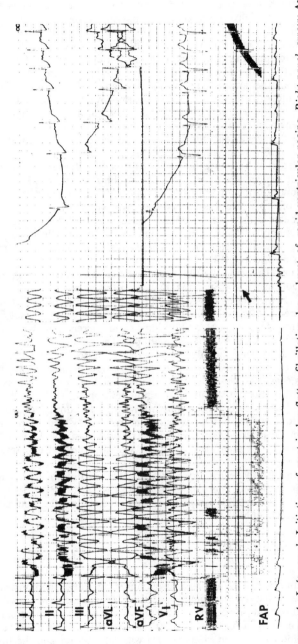

FIGURE 4. *Left panel*: Initiation of ventricular flutter–fibrillation by a burst of rapid ventricular pacing. *Right panel, arrow*: Automatic reversion of the arrhythmia to normal sinus rhythm by the implanted defibrillator. I, II, III, aVF, and V₁ are standard electrocardiographic leads.   RV = right ventricular electrogram; FAP = femoral arterial pressure.

rection of the malignant rhythm with restoration of normal circulation was usually uneventful and virtually instantaneous. On many occasions the defibrillatory pulses were delivered to conscious patients without producing undue discomfort or pain.

In three patients a number of spurious discharges occurred during sinus rhythm but did not produce untoward effects or induce arrhythmias. In two of these patients the cause for the unwarranted discharges was found to be a poor connection in the apical lead producing signals that fulfilled the probability density function criteria. Appropriate improvements in lead construction were implemented and the original pulse generators were replaced with units made insensitive to the interfering signals; subsequently, no further spurious discharges have been observed in these patients. In a third patient, the false-positive pulses were related to the presence of prominent P waves in the bipolar electrogram resulting in signals that satisfied the sensing criteria. These huge atrial deflections were due to a combination of right atrial overloading with a low position of the catheter electrode in the right atrium.

Miscounting of heart rate was observed in two patients with relatively slow (130 and 171 beats/min), well-tolerated, ventricular rhythms, one induced during pacemaker implantation. The problem was corrected by incorporating into the design a special circuit more responsive to the actual heart rate and less subject to errors due to QRS aberrancy.

No interference between the AID defibrillator and functioning demand pacemakers (Medtronic 5984 Spectrax™) was noted in patients with both devices implanted. The effect of the AID defibrillator on external defibrillation is less clearly defined. Although supportive clinical evidence did not become apparent, laboratory tests suggested shunting of the current flow when a transthoracic countershock is delivered through paddles having an inappropriate polarity, possibly decreasing the effectiveness of the pulse. Practically, such an effect can easily be eliminated by the reversal of the paddles if an external discharge is unsuccessful. Design modifications aimed at completely excluding the possibility of such current-shunting are being developed.

After nearly 100 pulse generator implant-months accumulated to date, no evidence of random component failure, premature battery depletion, malfunctioning capacitors, hermeticity loss, or case fracture was noted. One patient was found to have a permanent lead fracture, which prompted explantation of the pulse generator.

There were three late deaths: two patients died in pulmonary edema and one was found in asystole. The explanted devices were found to be operating properly and the autopsy did not disclose myocardial damage that could be attributed to the AID defibrillator.

CONCLUSIONS

These preliminary results are clearly encouraging. They demonstrate that the automatic defibrillator can reliably monitor cardiac electrical activity for a prolonged period of time, recognize ventricular fibrillation as well as sinusoidal ventricular tachycardias faster than a preset heart rate, and then deliver effective treatment when indicated. The safety record was satisfactory and the problems that became apparent were identified and corrected.

Although its ultimate value has yet to be determined, this new therapeutic modality represents a new and promising approach to prevention of sudden death in patients who are at a particularly high risk of developing malignant ventricular arrhythmias.

REFERENCES

1. MIROWSKI, M., M. M. MOWER, A. LANGER, M. S. HEILMAN & J. SCHREIBMAN. 1978. A chronically implanted system for automatic defibrillation in active conscious dogs: Experimental model for treatment of sudden death from ventricular fibrillation. Circulation **58:** 90–94.
2. MIROWSKI, M., M. M. MOWER, B. S. BHAGAVAN, A. LANGER, S. A. KOLENIK, R. E. FISCHELL & M. S. HEILMAN. 1980. *In* Proceedings of the VIth World Symposium on Cardiac Pacing. C. Meere, Ed.: chapt. 27–2. PACE-SYMP. Montreal, Canada.
3. MIROWSKI, M., P. R. REID, M. M. MOWER, L. WATKINS, V. L. GOTT, J. F. SCHAUBLE, A. LANGER, M. S. HEILMAN, S. A. KOLENIK, R. E. FISCHELL & M. L. WEISFELDT. 1980. Termination of malignant ventricular arrhythmias with an implanted automatic defibrillator in human beings. N. Engl. J. Med. **303:** 322–324.
4. MIROWSKI, M., M. M. MOWER, W. S. STAEWEN, B. TABATZNIK & A. I. MENDELOFF. 1970. An approach to prevention of sudden coronary death. Arch. Intern. Med. **126:** 158–161.
5. SCHUDER, J. C., H. STOECKLE, J. H. GOLD, J. A. WEST & P. Y. KESKAR. 1970. Experimental ventricular defibrillation with an automatic and completely implanted system. Trans. Am. Soc. Artif. Intern. Organs **16:** 207–212.
6. MIROWSKI, M., M. M. MOWER, W. S. STAEWEN, R. H. DENNISTON, B. TABATZNIK & A. I. MENDELOFF. 1971. Ventricular defibrillation through a single intravascular catheter electrode system. Clin. Res. **19:** 328.
7. MIROWSKI, M., M. M. MOWER, W. S. STAEWEN, R. H. DENNISTON & A. I. MENDELOFF. 1972. The development of the transvenous automatic defibrillator. Arch. Intern. Med. **129:** 773–779.
8. MIROWSKI, M., M. M. MOWER, V. L. GOTT & R. K. BRAWLEY. 1973. Feasibility and effectiveness of low-energy catheter defibrillation in man. Circulation **47:** 79–85.
9. MOWER, M. M., M. MIROWSKI, J. F. SPEAR & E. N. MOORE. 1974. Patterns of ventricular activity during catheter defibrillation. Circulation **49:** 858–861.
10. HEILMAN, M. S., A. LANGER, M. M. MOWER & M. MIROWSKI. 1975. Analysis of four implantable electrode systems for automatic defibrillator. Circulation **52**(Suppl. II):II–194.
11. MIROWSKI, M., M. M. MOWER, A. LANGER & M. S. HEILMAN. 1976. Miniaturized implantable automatic defibrillator for prevention of sudden death from ventricular fibrillation. *In* Proceedings of the Vth International Symposium on Cardiac Pacing, Tokyo, Japan. 103. Excerpta Medica. Amsterdam.
12. LANGER, A., M. S. HEILMAN, M. M. MOWER & M. MIROWSKI. 1976. Considerations in the development of the automatic implantable defibrillator. Med. Instrum. **10:** 163–166.
13. MIROWSKI, M., M. M. MOWER, B. S. BHAGAVAN, A. LANGER, M. S. HEILMAN & J. SCHREIBMAN. 1978. The automatic implantable defibrillator: Toward the development of the first clinical model. *In* Proceedings of the Symposium on Management of Ventricular Tachycardia: Role of Mexiletine, Copenhagen, Denmark. E. Sandøe, D. G. Julien, and J. W. Bell, Eds.: 655. Excerpta Medica. Amsterdam.
14. MIROWSKI, M., M. M. MOWER & P. R. REID. 1980. The automatic implantable defibrillator. Am. Heart J. **100:** 1089–1092.

15. MIROWSKI, M., P. R. REID, L. WATKINS, M. L. WEISFELDT & M. M. MOWER. 1981. Clinical treatment of life-threatening ventricular tachyarrhythmias with the automatic implantable defibrillator. Am. Heart J. **102:** 265–270.
16. SCHUDER, J. C., G. A. RAHMOELLER & H. STOECKLE. 1966. Transthoracic ventricular defibrillation with triangular and trapezoidal waveforms. Circ. Res. **19:** 689–694.

DISCUSSION

DR. COBB: It is quite fair to say that 10 years ago many of us here would not have anticipated this presentation. You are indeed to be congratulated.

Do you anticipate that fibrosis increasing the energy requirements will appear in coming years? How often should you check for these?

DR. MIROWSKI: There is no evidence as of today that such a situation will develop or has developed. But obviously we have to be very careful and be aware that this is a possibility.

SURGERY FOR RECURRENT SUSTAINED VENTRICULAR TACHYCARDIA ASSOCIATED WITH CORONARY ARTERY DISEASE: THE ROLE OF SUBENDOCARDIAL RESECTION *

Mark E. Josephson,†‡ Leonard N. Horowitz,§ and
Alden H. Harken

Clinical Electrophysiology Laboratory
Cardiovascular Section, and
Cardiothoracic Surgery Section
Departments of Medicine and Surgery
University of Pennsylvania School of Medicine
Philadelphia, Pennsylvania 19104

Recurrent sustained ventricular tachycardia is a well-known complication of ischemic heart disease. It is a major cause of postinfarction morbidity and is frequently the initiating arrhythmia in "sudden cardiac death" among patients with ischemic heart disease.[1] The most common anatomic substrate for recurrent sustained ventricular tachycardia is prior myocardial infarction associated with left ventricular wall motion abnormalities, in particular, left ventricular aneurysms.[1, 2] In view of the fact that an anatomic substrate potentially responsible for generating these arrhythmias could be identified, it was logical to attempt to remove the substrate by surgical intervention as a treatment for such refractory arrhythmias.

The first surgical approach to the treatment of ventricular arrhythmias was simple aneurysmectomy.[3] Since the appearance of the initial report some 22 years ago, a variety of surgical procedures have been employed in an attempt to deal with life-threatening arrhythmias, but with rather limited success.[4-17] With the advent of invasive electrophysiologic investigations, a greater understanding of the mechanisms of ventricular tachycardia was obtained. These data suggested that ventricular tachycardia was due to reentry and that the reentrant circuit was located near the endocardium.[18-24] The ability to potentially locate the site of tachycardia with catheter and intraoperative mapping suggested the possibility of more directed surgical interventions to ablate the site of the arrhythmia.[14, 16, 23-26] The present study reviews our experience with

* This work was supported in part by Grants No. RO1 HL24278 and 1 RO1 HL22315 from the National Heart, Lung, and Blood Institute, Bethesda, Maryland, and by grants from the American Heart Association, Southeastern Pennsylvania Chapter, Philadelphia, Pennsylvania, and the Fannie Rippel Foundation, Morristown, New Jersey.

† Address for correspondence: Mark E. Josephson, M.D., Director, Clinical Electrophysiology Laboratory, Box 683, Hospital of the University of Pennsylvania, 3400 Spruce Street, Philadelphia, Pennsylvania 19104.

‡ Recipient of Research Career Development Award No. 1 KO4 HL00361 from the National Heart, Lung, and Blood Institute, Bethesda, Maryland.

§ Recipient of Young Investigator Award No. 1 R23 HL21292 from the National Heart, Lung, and Blood Institute, Bethesda, Maryland.

0077–8923/82/0382–0381 $1.75/0 © 1982, NYAS

subendocardial resection guided by activation mapping for the management of recurrent sustained ventricular tachycardia.

METHODS

Patient Population

Sixty consecutive patients with recurrent sustained ventricular tachycardia underwent subendocardial resection to eliminate tachycardia. There were 52 men and 8 women, ranging in age from 39 to 74 years (TABLE 1). The primary indication for surgery in each patient was medically refractory arrhythmia. All patients had coronary artery disease and had had a prior myocardial infarction 1 week to 11 years prior to surgery. Three patients required surgery within 10 days of a myocardial infarction; in the remaining patients surgery was performed at least 4 weeks after an acute myocardial infarction. The resting electrocardiogram revealed a transmural myocardial infarction in 55 patients, nontransmural myocardial infarction in 2 patients, and no identifiable infarction in the remaining 3 patients (two due to preexisting left bundle branch

TABLE 1

ENDOCARDIAL RESECTION FOR VENTRICULAR TACHYCARDIA WITH CORONARY ARTERY DISEASE *

Cardiac index	2.7 liters/min per m²
Ejection fraction	27%
Left ventricular end-diastolic pressure	17.5 mm Hg
Aneurysms (no.)	52

* This procedure was performed in 60 patients (52 men and 8 women) from 39 to 74 years of age.

block and one due to a permanent right ventricular pacemaker). In 35% of our patients, ventricular tachycardia had produced a cardiac arrest. Empirical therapy had failed in all patients, as had at least two standard antiarrhythmic agents (range, two to six drugs) during serial electrophysiologic studies. In 10 patients experimental antiarrhythmic agents also failed to prevent initiation of the tachycardia by programmed ventricular stimulation.

Fifty-eight of the 60 patients underwent catheter endocardial mapping, as previously described.[23, 25] Two patients were unable to undergo this procedure: one due to lack of access sites because of prior cardiac catheterization and cardiac surgery (that is, aneurysmectomy and coronary bypass grafts), and extensive peripheral vascular disease; and one who was too sick to undergo mapping. In our remaining patients, 8 to 20 endocardial sites in both ventricles were mapped, including 6 to 15 left ventricular sites (FIG. 1). In all patients operated upon, electrical activity preceding the onset of the QRS complex could be recorded from the area of infarction and/or border of left ventricular aneurysm. In six patients, continuous activity was recorded at these sites. In each of these six patients the initiation and maintenance of the tachycardia was critically dependent upon the presence of this continuous electrical activity.

The area in which the earliest activity or continuous activity was recorded was considered to be the segment where the ventricular tachycardia originated. If multiple morphologic patterns of ventricular tachycardia were present, mapping of each distinct configuration was attempted.

All patients underwent complete angiographic and hemodynamic catheterization. All patients had coronary artery disease, most with multivessel disease (mean, 2.0 vessels with $\geq 50\%$ obstruction). The mean cardiac index was

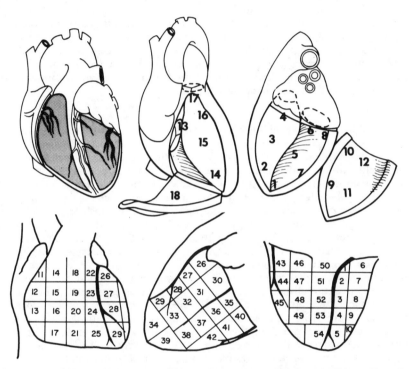

FIGURE 1. Schema of catheter and epicardial mapping sites. (*Top*) schematic diagram of the heart opened and the standard left ventricular (sites 1–12) and right ventricular (sites 13–18) catheter mapping sites. (*Bottom*) the schema for intra-operative epicardial mapping. From *left to right* the heart is displayed in the anterior, left lateral, and inferior views. There are 54 standard mapping sites.

2.7 liters/min per m², mean ejection fraction was 27%, and mean left ventricular end-diastolic pressure was 17.5 mm Hg. Fifty-two patients had left ventricular aneurysms, including two who had had prior aneurysmectomy for recurrent ventricular tachycardia. Eight patients had infarctions without aneurysms; in each of these the infarction was inferior in location. Thirty-nine aneurysms were anteroapical, involving the septum, five were anterolateral without septal involvement, and eight were inferoposterior.

Intraoperative Studies

Intraoperative mapping was performed after the cannulation of cardiopulmonary bypass, as previously described.[14, 16, 25, 26] A bipolar plunge electrode (0.005-inch diameter, Teflon®-coated stainless steel wire) was inserted into the left ventricle by means of a 23-gauge needle to record a left ventricular reference electrogram. An additional plunge electrode, or more commonly a quadrapolar electrode catheter, was inserted into the right ventricle and used for a second reference. The catheter was also utilized for pacing. Three electrocardiographic leads, usually I, aVF, and either V_5 or V_6 or V_5R, V_6R, were recorded simultaneously with both the right and left ventricular reference electrograms. Bipolar (1–1.5 mm interelectrode distance) electrograms were recorded using a ring electrode from at least 54 preselected epicardial sites on both ventricles during both sinus rhythm and ventricular tachycardia (FIG. 1). Particular attention was directed toward the margin of the aneurysm or infarction, where more detailed mapping was performed.

Method of Surgical Resection

Once the area of earliest activity was identified, cold potassium cardioplegia was instituted and undermining of the endocardium was performed in the area from which the earliest activity was recorded. In the 52 patients with discrete aneurysms, the edge of the aneurysm was grasped in clamps and the endocardium was undermined with scissors (FIG. 2). In this fashion, an 8–25 cm² piece of endocardium extending 2 to 3 cm beyond the edge of the aneurysm was removed. In each case, this involved 25 to 40% of the circumference of the aneurysmectomy. In the eight patients with no aneurysm, an inferior infarction was present. Then, after ventriculotomy through the center of the infarction, endocardial resection of local areas of the infarction or the posterior septum was accomplished in each patient. In these eight cases, the area of tissue removed was usually less than 10 cm². The majority of the endocardial resections were from the septum, either anterior (34 patients) or posterior (3 patients). The remaining patients had endocardial resections from the inferoposterior free wall (14 patients) or the left ventricular free wall border of either an anteroapical or anterolateral aneurysm (16 patients). Six patients had two areas of origin; hence, endocardial resection was performed at 66 regions. After endocardial resection, the ventriculotomy or aneurysmectomy was closed. Forty patients also had concomitant coronary artery bypass grafts to vessels with greater than 70% stenosis. This was performed after endocardial resection in all instances.

Postoperative Evaluation and Follow-Up

All but one surviving patient underwent postoperative electrophysiologic testing 9 to 27 days after surgery. The one patient who refused study had no spontaneous arrhythmias and was discharged without medication. Forty-nine patients underwent complete angiographic and hemodynamic catheterization the same day or within 2 days of the electrophysiologic study. A minimum of 7 days of continuous electrocardiographic monitoring on telemetry and at least one 24-hour Holter monitoring were obtained prior to discharge. In patients in whom the tachycardia could be reinduced after surgery, serial electrophysiologic studies were undertaken to ascertain which drug or drug combination could either prevent initiation of the tachycardia or make it more difficult to initiate.

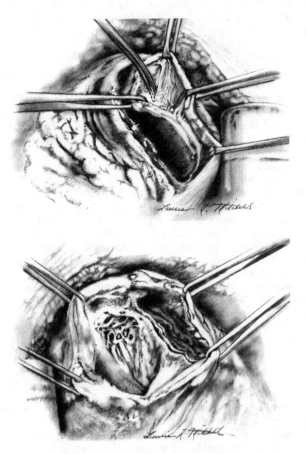

FIGURE 2. Method of endocardial resection. The orientation of both figures is with the patient's head at the bottom so that the anterior septum is the site of endocardial resection. After standard aneurysmectomy the septal endocardium is undermined with a scissors (*top*). The endocardial resection is 1–3 mm thick and approximately 10 cm² in area (*bottom*). (Adapted from Josephson *et al.*[14] Reproduced by permission.)

RESULTS

Activation Mapping Studies

Ninety-five morphologically distinct ventricular tachycardias were induced and mapped either epicardially, endocardially, or both. Thirty-one patients had more than one morphologically distinct ventricular tachycardia mapped (27 had two ventricular tachycardias and 4 had three ventricular tachycardias). Complete epicardial and endocardial activation maps could not be obtained during all morphologically distinct ventricular tachycardias. The reasons for failure to perform endocardial mapping included: the presence of a large mural thrombus, rapid degeneration of the tachycardia to ventricular fibrillation, or failure to induce the arrhythmia. In one patient a surgical complication prohibited induction and mapping of the arrhythmia. In this latter patient as well as in those in whom endocardial mapping could not be accomplished, the results of the preoperative catheter map were used to guide surgical ablation of the site of arrhythmia.

Epicardial activation typically followed the onset of the QRS complex during ventricular tachycardia. In one patient, epicardial breakthrough was coincident with the onset of the QRS complex during the tachycardia and in the remaining patients epicardial breakthrough appeared 10 to 76 msec after the onset of the QRS complex. In all tachycardias with right bundle branch block patterns, epicardial breakthrough appeared on the left ventricle. In ventricular tachycardias with left bundle branch block configuration, epicardial breakthrough was on the right ventricle adjacent to the anterior or inferior interventricular groove in all but three cases, in which early epicardial breakthrough was on the left ventricle adjacent to the anterior (two patients) or inferior (one) interventricular groove. In two-thirds of those patients with ventricular aneurysms, low amplitude, fractionated or no activity was seen over the aneurysm. Exit block of varying degrees was not infrequently seen, but it was usually found at the border of an aneurysm. Endocardial activation always preceded epicardial activation (14–85 msec) and activity could always be recorded prior to the onset of the QRS complex during the tachycardia (FIG. 3). During three ventricular tachycardia morphologic patterns, continuous activation spanning the cardiac cycle in a sequential fashion (so that activation at any site would depend upon activation at a prior site) was recorded around the border of the aneurysm (FIG. 4). In the remaining patients, activation could be recorded 2 to 80 msec prior to the onset of the QRS complex. In one-third of the patients, discrete potentials in systole and diastole could be recorded at sites within a small area of 4 to 6 cm². Within this region, electrical activity could be seen as presystolic to systolic activity. These findings were compatible with recordings near the completion of the reentrant circuit. In all instances, the catheter endocardial map actually predicted the earliest area found intraoperatively, and in those tachycardias that were not mapped it was the only method of guiding endocardial resection.

The earliest recorded activity was most commonly on the septum (36 patients): it was on the anterior half of the septum in 33 and on the posterior half in 3 patients. The area of origin was on the inferoposterior free wall in 14 patients and was on either the superior-lateral or inferior border of an anteroapical or anterolateral aneurysm in 16 patients. There were six patients in whom there appeared to be two widely separate areas of origin of two tachycardias (hence the total of 66 areas of origin). In 25 other patients with multiple patterns of ventricular tachycardia, the earliest recorded activity during each configuration of ventricular tachycardia was at the same or closely adjacent (within 3 cm) area. Of the six patients with ventricular tachycardia arising from multiple areas, in only three patients was the second ventricular tachycardia observed preoperatively.

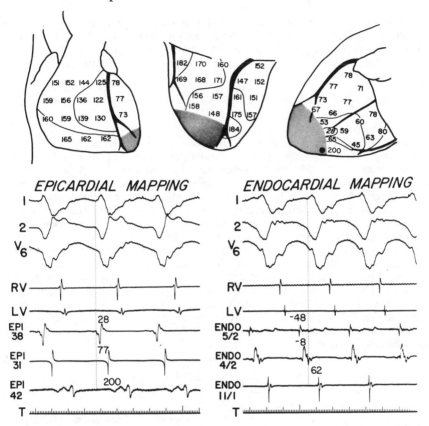

FIGURE 3. Epicardial and endocardial mapping of ventricular tachycardia. Epicardial activation is shown on **top** with the heart in the anterior, inferior, and left lateral position (from *left to right*). The shaded area represents an apical aneurysm. The earliest epicardial breakthrough occurs 28 msec after the onset of the QRS complex. The solid circle in the aneurysm is the site of early endocardial activation, which is 3 cm away from the site of epicardial breakthrough. On the **bottom** are data during epicardial (*left*) and endocardial (*right*) mapping of the tachycardia. Leads 1, 2 and V₆ are shown with right (RV) and left ventricular (LV) reference electrograms. Epicardial (EPI) site 38, the site of epicardial breakthrough, is shown with activation from sites 31 and 42 (see FIGURE 1). Endocardial (ENDO) activation is shown at the lower right. The earliest endocardial activity is recorded 2 cm from the cut edge of the aneurysm at 5 o'clock (ENDO 5/2) and precedes the QRS complex by 42 msec. Other sites of endocardial activity occur later. See text for further explanation.

Comparison of epicardial breakthrough with endocardial area of origin revealed that there was no correlation of epicardial breakthrough when the origin was on the septum. In such cases, epicardial breakthrough was always along the anterior inferior interventricular groove, either on the left or right ventricle. When the origin of tachycardia arose on the free wall, there was a reasonable correlation of epicardial breakthrough and area of origin (that is, within 2 cm) in half the patients. In the remaining half of these patients, the endocardial origin was greater than or equal to 3 cm away from the point of epicardial breakthrough. Therefore, the earliest epicardial breakthrough only gave adequate localization to the area of origin in 25% of the cases.

Surgical Results

Endocardial resection was accomplished in 60 patients, 52 of whom had concomitant aneurysmectomies. Forty patients also received coronary artery bypass grafts, with an average of 1.6 grafts per patient. There were five operative deaths (within 30 days). Three patients died from pump failure in the first week, two of whom had prior myocardial infarction within a week prior to surgery. One patient had an acute infarction on the eighth postoperative day and died in electrical-mechanical dissociation. Both bypass grafts were widely patent and infarction was assumed to be secondary to spasm. The remaining death occurred in a patient in whom ventricular tachycardia arose in the posterior papillary muscle; thus, only partial subendocardial resection could be accomplished. Ventricular tachycardia was inducible by programmed stimulation 2 weeks postoperatively (see later) in this patient, and he was placed on disopyramide therapy to control the inducible arrhythmia. Two days after therapy was initiated, acute cardiogenic shock developed and he died. At the time of death he was in sinus rhythm. There was no evidence of myocardial infarction; therefore we attributed his death to disopyramide-induced cardiac dysfunction.

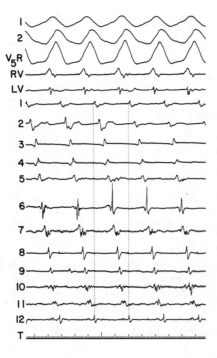

FIGURE 4. Endocardial electrograms recorded around the perimeter of an aneurysm during ventricular tachycardia (VT) in patient 2. Electrocardiographic leads 1, 2 and V_5R were recorded with right (RV) and left (LV) ventricular reference electrograms and electrograms from 12 consecutive sites equally spaced around the edge of a ventricular aneurysm and 10-msec time marks. Sites 1 and 12 were adjacent. The endocardial electrograms were recorded individaully and are time-aligned in this Figure. The dotted lines are placed arbitrarily to allow temporal comparison. Note that discrete electrograms occur throughout the cardiac cycle. The VT terminated after digital pressure at sites 4, 9 and 12, which were anterior, posterior and septal, respectively. (From Horowitz et al.[26] Reproduced by permission.)

The remaining 55 patients underwent programmed ventricular stimulation 10 to 28 days postoperatively. The study included single and double, and on occasion, triple ventricular extrastimuli from the right and, when necessary, from the left ventricle. In 42 patients no ventricular tachycardia was inducible (group 1) and they were discharged without medication. Ventricular tachycardia was inducible in the remaining 13 patients (group 2), in three of whom ventricular tachycardia occurred spontaneously prior to electrophysiologic study. Each underwent serial electrophysiologic studies to assist pharmacologic therapy. In five patients ventricular tachycardia was no longer inducible on antiarrhythmic agents, while in eight patients ventricular tachycardia was still inducible, although in most patients it was both more difficult and slower to induce tachycardia than it was prior to administration of antiarrhythmic therapy. All patients in group 2 were discharged on a regimen of those drugs that made the tachycardias either noninducible or more difficult to induce.

Forty-nine patients underwent cardiac catheterization prior to discharge, the preliminary results of which have been reported.[27] As noted earlier, 52 patients had aneurysmectomies and the remaining patients had ventriculotomy and endocardial resection alone. Sixty-three coronary bypass grafts were placed in 40 patients. In the patients studied, all but two grafts were patent (96%). Both included grafts to vessels with poor distal runoff, one of which required endarterectomy prior to placement into the graft. In the patients with aneurysmectomy, the mean ejection fraction rose from 27 to 39% (p < 0.0005), and the mean left ventricular end-diastolic pressure decreased from 17 to 12 mm Hg (p < 0.001), while cardiac index was unchanged. No thrombus was observed, nor was there any evidence of ventricular septal defect at the time of left ventricular angiography.

Follow-Up Data

Of the 55 surviving patients, 42 were discharged with no antiarrhythmic agent for prevention of ventricular tachycardia. One of these patients was discharged on quinidine therapy for atrial fibrillation, and this drug has subsequently been discontinued. All of the 13 patients with inducible tachycardia (group 2) were discharged on therapy with antiarrhythmic agents. On follow-up of 2 to 41 months, there have been nine late deaths: six in group 1 and three in group 2. Four have been due to progressive heart failure, two have been due to myocardial infarction, one due to pneumonia, one due to aneurysm of the pulmonary artery, and one due to cardiac rupture. The site of rupture was at an area of recent ischemia adjacent to the ventricular suture line. The area of endocardial resection, which was on the septum, was intact and coated with an endothelial fibroplastic layer without evidence of thrombosis. There have been two recurrences of tachycardia in group 1, both of which have been controlled with antiarrhythmic agents. There have been two recurrences in group 2, which were controlled by increasing the medication. No other patient has required hospitalization for arrhythmias. Half of the surviving patients have complex ventricular ectopic activity, which has remained asymptomatic and untreated. The actuarial predicted survival curve is 62% at 40 months (FIG. 5).

DISCUSSION

The most commonly used procedure for the management of recurrent sustained ventricular tachycardia and associated coronary artery disease has been left ventricular aneurysmectomy with or without coronary arterial bypass grafting. The rationale for such surgery was the fact that aneurysms and multivessel coronary disease were frequently present in such patients. The success of such surgical therapy, however, is not uniform and is difficult to assess for many reasons. A variety of arrhythmias, most of which were not well-classified or evaluated, are included; the methods of follow-up have been inadequate, the use of antiarrhythmic therapy after operation is not assessed, objective assessment of therapy has not been attempted, and, importantly, the tendency to report successes rather than failures are several limitations that prohibit adequate analysis of the effects of this type of surgery for ventricular tachycardia. In our experience, successful ablation of the site of tachycardia by this method occurs in less than 30% of the patients.[17]

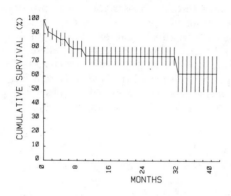

FIGURE 5. Actuarial survival curve of the 60 patients undergoing endocardial resection for ventricular tachycardia. (From Josephson et al.[31] Reproduced by permission.)

On the basis of experimental data by Wittig and Boineau,[28] we believed the major cause of failure to eliminate tachycardia by these procedures was the fact that the tachycardia arose from the region of the border of the infarction and normal tissue and that these areas were not removed by the surgeon. Invariably, at least a 1-cm cuff of aneurysmal scar tissue is left to sew the ventriculotomy together. Moreover, since many ventricular tachycardias arise from the septal border of the aneurysm, these tachycardias would not be altered by simple aneurysmectomy. We therefore decided to explore this hypothesis by developing a technique for catheter endocardial mapping as well as by performing more detailed intraoperative epicardial and endocardial mapping during ventricular tachycardia at the time of surgery.[23, 25, 26] The results of both the catheterization and intraoperative mapping data, as well as prior data demonstrating the ability to reproducibly initiate and terminate the tachycardia, suggested that ventricular tachycardias associated with coronary artery disease were due to reentry at or near the subendocardium at the border of infarctions and/or aneurysms.[18-21, 23-26] These areas are typically not altered by standard aneurysmectomy, and this fact led to the development of subendocardial resection as a means for removing and/or altering these reentrant circuits.

Values and Limitations of Subendocardial Resection

The advantages of subendocardial resection are related to the fact that surgery is directed to the area or areas responsible for the arrhythmia. As a result, the resection is limited and only involves subendocardial border of the aneurysm or infarct. This allows the surgeon to utilize the cuff of fibrous rim of aneurysm to close the aneurysmectomy. This technique also allows the surgeon to abolish tachycardias arising on the septum without either disarticulating or removing large parts of the septum. The hemodynamic results of limited resection are gratifying in that the ejection fraction is improved and left ventricular end-diastolic pressure reduced in the majority of cases.[27] No residual ventricular septal defects have been observed on repeat catheterization. The one death from cardiac rupture 6 months postoperatively was unrelated to the septal subendocardial resection. Autopsy revealed that the rupture was associated with a recent area of necrosis on the free wall adjacent to the ventricular suture line. The septal subendocardial resection was healed and completely endothelialized.

The major limitations of the technique are related to the requirement that the tachycardia be inducible so that it can be mapped intraoperatively or at the very least preoperatively. Intraoperative inducibility is affected by cardiac temperature, anesthetic agents, and other miscellaneous pharmacologic and metabolic factors. Moreover, all the morphologic patterns of tachycardia may not be able to be completely mapped due to other factors, such as: (1) failure to induce the arrhythmia after aneurysmectomy; (2) failure to induce all clinical morphologic patterns during both epicardial and endocardial mapping; (3) rapid degeneration of the tachycardia to ventricular fibrillation; (4) inability to distinguish early from late areas because the rate of tachycardia is too rapid; (5) inability to map the endocardium because of large mural thrombi; and (6) unexpected surgical complications that prohibit detailed mapping. We have been able to prevent the majority of these problems by maintaining normothermia, by using multiple stimulation techniques from both ventricles, by using antiarrhythmic agents (such as procainamide) to slow very rapid tachycardias and/or to prevent their degeneration to ventricular fibrillation, and by relying on the preoperative catheterization map to show morphologic forms that can neither be induced nor completely mapped intraoperatively.

Another limitation of this procedure is the inability to resect the base of papillary muscle should the tachycardia arise there. Although limited resection can be accomplished, other techniques (such as cryosurgery) will probably be required to uniformly ablate the site of such arrhythmias. Activation mapping usually takes 30 to 60 minutes of normothermic cardiopulmonary bypass. Although this might potentially influence surgical mortality and morbidity, we have not found this to be the case. Our data demonstrate a comparable mortality with that occurring after aneurysmectomy and bypass grafting without mapping.

Another factor to be considered is the large investment in personnel and equipment required for this approach which limits its applicability to large university centers. Despite these limitations, most of which we have been able to deal with, subendocardial resection appears to be a very promising surgical approach for the treatment of ventricular tachycardia.

Relationship to Other Surgical Approaches for Ventricular Tachycardia

Two other surgical approaches have recently been developed which offer promise either as isolated procedures or in combination with endocardial resection. The first, encircling endocardial ventriculotomy, was developed by Guiraudon *et al.*[10, 11] as a means of electrophysiologically excluding the area responsible for ventricular tachycardia from the rest of the heart. Since experimental animal and human data suggested that the areas responsible for the arrhythmia were located along the border of an aneurysm, these workers believe that a circular ventriculotomy performed outside the limits of the border zone would isolate the tachycardia from the normal working myocardium.

The procedure is carried out after entrance to the ventricular cavity by standard ventriculotomy through the aneurysm or infarction. A transmural ventriculotomy is then performed around the border of endocardial fibrosis, sparing the epicardium and coronary arteries. Septal infarction required virtual disarticulation of the septum. The ventriculotomy is then repaired with running sutures-buttressed with Teflon® strips or pledgets.

To date, 23 patients have been reported. There were two operative deaths, two patients had recurrent ventricular tachycardia in the perioperative period, but this was controlled by drugs, and there have been two late recurrences. The hemodynamic results of the procedure have not been assessed prospectively, although the French group suggests that the operation should not be performed in patients with very low output. Low output failure from this procedure has been reported by Waldo *et al.*[29] Ungerleider *et al.*[30] from Duke University have demonstrated a potential mechanism for the cardiac dysfunction associated with this procedure. They have demonstrated that the procedure causes an ischemic insult which is comparable to that occurring after ligation of a coronary artery. In man a finite amount of viable tissue exists between the subendocardial fibrosis and epicardial extension of the infarction that is placed in jeopardy by this procedure.

The advantages of the procedure are chiefly that neither induction of the arrhythmia nor mapping is required. Furthermore, it can be more widely applied since sophisticated equipment is unnecessary. Its major limitations are requirement of septal disarticulation to deal with arrhythmias arising in the septum (a common finding) and the impairment of ventricular function in patients with low cardiac output, which unfortunately is also a common finding in this group of patients. The potential effect of endocardial sutures or thrombus formation and/or endocarditis is uncertain.

A second potentially useful procedure is cryosurgical ablation, which has been employed in a few patients.[12, 13] The procedure requires some form of mapping and has theoretical advantages in that reversible arrhythmia can be used to evaluate an area from which the tachycardia appears to originate. Since the regions involved usually have some fibrous stroma, and cryothermia does not influence fibrous tissue, the major structural substrate remains intact. The extent of cryosurgery is limited because of the size of the probe and tissue interface. The use of endocardial mapping should help to improve the efficacy of this procedure. Since transmural cryosurgery is uncommon (usual depth is approximately 6 mm), it seems ideally suited to be combined with subendocardial resection. Further work is necessary to establish the exact role of cryosurgery in the management of ventricular tachycardia.

Conclusion

Recent advances in our understanding of the mechanisms and anatomic substrate of ventricular tachycardia associated with ischemic heart disease have led to the development of new surgical approaches to treat this arrhythmia. We have utilized the technique of subendocardial resection guided by catheter and/or intraoperative mapping in this endeavor and have demonstrated a good success rate with excellent hemodynamic results and an acceptable mortality. An electrophysiologically-based approach to arrhythmia surgery offers great promise for the treatment of ventricular tachycardia.

References

1. JOSEPHSON, M. E., L. N. HOROWITZ, S. R. SPIELMAN & A. M. GREENSPAN. 1980. Electrophysiologic and hemodynamic studies in patients resuscitated from cardiac arrest. Am. J. Cardiol. **46:** 948–955.
2. SPIELMAN, S. R., A. M. GREENSPAN, L. N. HOROWITZ, J. A. KASTOR & M. E. JOSEPHSON. 1979. Anatomic substrates of recurrent sustained ventricular tachycardia (abstract). Clin. Res. **27:** 569.
3. COUCH, O. A., JR. 1959. Cardiac aneurysm with ventricular tachycardia and subsequent excision of aneurysm. Circulation **20:** 251–253.
4. MAGDISON, O. 1969. Resection of post-myocardial infarction ventricular aneurysm for cardiac arrhythmia. Dis. Chest **56:** 211–218.
5. THIND, G. S., W. S. BLAKEMORE & H. P. ZINSSER. 1971. Ventricular aneurysmectomy for the treatment of recurrent ventricular tachycardia. Am. J. Cardiol. **27:** 690–694.
6. BRYSON, A. L., A. F. PARISI, E. SCHECHTER & S. WOLFSON. 1973. Life-threatening ventricular arrhythmias induced by exercise. Cessation after coronary bypass surgery. Am. J. Cardiol. **32:** 995–999.
7. ECKER, R. R., C. B. MULLINS, J. C. GRAMMER, W. J. REA & J. M. ATKINS. 1971. Control of intractable ventricular tachycardia by coronary revascularization. Circulation **44:** 666–670.
8. TILKIAN, A. G., J. F. PFEIFER, W. H. BARRY, M. J. LIPTON & H. N. HULTGREN. 1976. The effect of coronary bypass surgery on exercise-induced ventricular arrhythmias. Am. Heart J. **92:** 707–714.
9. SPURRELL, R. A. J., A. K. YATES, C. W. THORBURN, A. E. SOWTON & D. L. DEUCHAR. 1975. Surgical treatments of ventricular tachycardia after epicardial mapping studies. Br. Heart J. **37:** 115–126.
10. GUIRAUDON, G., G. FONTAINE, R. FRANK, G. ESCANDE, P. ETIEVENT & C. CABROL. 1978. Encircling endocardial ventriculotomy: A new surgical treatment for life-threatening ventricular tachycardias resistant to medical treatment following myocardial infarction. Ann. Thorac. Surg. **26:** 438–444.
11. FONTAINE, G., G. GUIRAUDON, R. FRANK, C. CABROL & Y. GROSGOGEAT. 1979. The surgical management of ventricular tachycardia. Herz **4:** 276–284.
12. GALLAGHER, J. J., R. W. ANDERSON, J. KASELL, J. R. RICE, E. L. C. PRITCHETT, J. H. GAULT, L. HARRISON & A. G. WALLACE. 1978. Cryoablation of drug-resistant ventricular tachycardia in a patient with a variant of scleroderma. Circulation **57:** 190–197.
13. CAMM, J., D. E. WARD, R. CORY-PEARCE, G. M. REES & R. A. J. SPURRELL. 1979. A successful cryosurgical treatment of paroxysmal ventricular tachycardia. Chest **75:** 621–624.
14. JOSEPHSON, M. E., L. N. HOROWITZ & A. H. HARKEN. 1979. Endocardial excision—a new surgical technique for the treatment of ventricular tachycardia. Circulation **60:** 1430–1439.

15. HARKEN, A. H., M. E. JOSEPHSON & L. N. HOROWITZ. 1979. Surgical endocardial resection for the treatment of malignant ventricular tachycardia. Ann. Surg. **190:** 456–460.
16. HOROWITZ, L. N., M. E. JOSEPHSON, J. A. KASTOR & A. H. HARKEN. 1980. Ventricular resection guided by epicardial and endocardial mapping for treatment of recurrent ventricular tachycardia. N. Engl. J. Med. **302:** 589–593.
17. HARKEN, A. H., L. N. HOROWTIZ & M. E. JOSEPHSON. 1980. Comparison of standard aneurysmectomy and aneurysmectomy with directed endocardial resection for the treatment of recurrent sustained ventricular tachycardia. J. Thorac. Cardiovasc. Surg. **80:** 527–534.
18. WELLENS, H. J. J., R. M. SCHUILENBURG & D. DURRER. 1972. Electrical stimulation of the heart in patients with ventricular tachycardia. Circulation **46:** 216–226.
19. WELLENS, H. J. J., K. I. LIE & D. DURRER. 1974. Further observations on ventricular tachycardia as studied by electrical stimulation of the heart. Chronic recurrent ventricular tachycardia and ventricular tachycardia during acute myocardial infarction. Circulation **49:** 647–653.
20. WELLENS, H. J. J., D. R. DUREN & K. I. LIE. 1976. Observations on mechanisms of ventricular tachycardia in man. Circulation **54:** 237–244.
21. JOSEPHSON, M. E., L. N. HOROWITZ, A. FARSHIDI & J. A. KASTOR. 1978. Recurrent sustained ventricular tachycardia. 1. Mechanisms. Circulation **57:** 431–440.
22. FISHER, J. D., H. L. COHEN, R. MEHRA & S. FURMAN. 1977. Cardiac pacing and pacemakers. II. Serial electrophysiologic-pharmacologic testing for control of recurrent tachyarrhythmias. Am. Heart J. **93:** 658–668.
23. JOSEPHSON, M. E., L. N. HOROWITZ, A. FARSHIDI, J. F. SPEAR, J. A. KASTOR & E. N. MOORE. 1978. Recurrent sustained ventricular tachycardia. 2. Endocardial mapping. Circulation **57:** 440–447.
24. JOSEPHSON, M. E., L. N. HOROWITZ & A. FARSHIDI. 1978. Continuous local electrical activity: A mechanism of recurrent ventricular tachycardia. Circulation **57:** 659–665.
25. JOSEPHSON, M. E., L. N. HOROWTIZ, S. R. SPIELMAN, A. M. GREENSPAN, C. VANDEPOL & A. H. HARKEN. 1980. Comparison of endocardial catheter mapping with intraoperative mapping of ventricular tachycardia. Circulation **61:** 395–404.
26. HOROWITZ, L. N., M. E. JOSEPHSON & A. H. HARKEN. 1980. Epicardial and endocardial activation during sustained ventricular tachycardia in man. Circulation **61:** 1227–1238.
27. JOSEPHSON, M. E., L. N. HOROWITZ, A. H. HARKEN & J. A. KASTOR. 1980. Hemodynamic and electrocardiographic changes produced by endocardial resection and aneurysmectomy for ventricular tachycardia (abstract). Circulation **62** (Suppl. III): 320.
28. WITTIG, J. H. & J. P. BOINEAU. 1975. Surgical treatment of ventricular arrhythmias using epicardial, transmural, and endocardial mapping. Ann. Thorac. Surg. **20:** 117–126.
29. WALDO, A. L., J. G. ARCINIEGAS & H. KLEIN. 1981. Surgical treatment of life-threatening ventricular arrhythmias: The role of intraoperative mapping and consideration of presently available surgical techniques. Prog. Cardiovasc. Dis. **23:** 247–264.
30. UNGERLEIDER, R. M., T. E. STANLEY, J. M. WILLIAMS, G. K. LOFLAND & J. L. COX. 1980. Physiologic effects of encircling endocardial ventriculotomy (EEV) for refractory ischemic ventricular tachycardia. Circulation **62** (Suppl. III): 61.
31. JOSEPHSON, M. E., et al. 1982. Long term results of endocardial resection for sustained ventricular tachycardia. Circulation. In press.

DISCUSSION

DR. MORTON GOLDMANN (*Skokie, Illinois*): What evidence is there that either success or failure of programmed stimulation in this type of patient predicts the clinical course?

DR. JOSEPHSON: There are some variabilities among the different laboratories concerning the specificity of the technique. Many of the differences are related to the different techniques of stimulation. There is no assurance of 100% prediction. If you are talking about a lethal arrhythmia, you can be right 80 to 90% of the time; that's the best shot you have.

UNIDENTIFIED SPEAKER: How do you account for the failures? Are these caused by the depth or location of the excision or by some other factor yet unrecognized?

DR. JOSEPHSON: The hardest cases that we have had to date have been the inferior infarcts without aneurysms. In part that is because a papillary muscle usually sits right in the middle of that area and the base of the papillary muscle cannot be resected. We have performed slightly deeper excisions and we have contemplated using an encircling endocardial ventriculotomy. Unfortunately most papillary muscles aren't neat structures; they are matted down and technically it is not feasible to do that surgery.

The other explanation is that we don't make a deep enough excision in some patients. We're building a new surgical cart so that we can record more simultaneous electrograms from intramural as well as endocardial sites. How that will alter the surgery is unclear. One of the "new frontiers" might be to employ cryothermia in these patients. A cryothermal injury does not affect fibrous tissue and will kill whatever living tissue we've not gotten.

DR. ROSSI: What are the histologic results of endocardial resection? Is there a viable subendocardial muscle or scar?

DR. JOSEPHSON: It is mostly scar tissue but there are several layers of muscle. Both muscle and Purkinje fibers are seen and this muscle appears to be in contact with living muscle. We make our resection to the border of living muscle.

DR. ROSSI: I wonder whether recurrences of high-risk ventricular tachyarrhythmias could result from the surgical procedures. I would hope that the operations would be as trauma-free as possible.

DR. JOSEPHSON: I agree that the less you cut, the better. I don't believe that we are doing what is theoretically possible—shifting one scar for another and creating another circuit. The recurrences that we have seen have been remapped and have the identical morphologic pattern and are from the same site as the earlier one.

However, we have also operated on two patients who had a right ventriculotomy for tetralogy of Fallot and both of the tachycardias had reentrant loops around the scar that was created by ventriculotomy. We resected this scar and so far the patients are arrhythmia-free. I don't know whether another circuit will form around our scar, for only time will tell. So far we have followed these patients for 40 months and this has not happened.

INTRAOPERATIVE MAPPING AND SURGERY FOR THE PREVENTION OF LETHAL ARRHYTHMIAS AFTER MYOCARDIAL INFARCTION *

G. Fontaine,† G. Guiraudon, R. Frank, R. Coutte,
C. Cabrol, and Y. Grosgogeat

Service de Rythmologie du Pr. Y. Grosgogeat
Hôpital Jean Rostand
94200 Ivry, France

Service de Chirurgie Cardiovasculaire du Pr. C. Cabrol
Hôpital de la Pitie
75013 Paris, France

About 75% of patients presenting with ventricular tachycardia (VT) have coronary arterial disease.[1, 2] This arrhythmia can occur during acute myocardial infarction or in the chronic stage. Ventricular tachycardia may be observed many years after the initial event [3] in the absence of recurrent acute ischemia.

In the setting of myocardial infarction, ventricular tachycardia may be life-threatening. Rapid rhythms may cause acute myocardial ischemia, which favors degradation to ventricular fibrillation. When the rate is slower and the attack lasts longer, cardiac failure will tend to develop.

The treatment of ventricular tachycardia has two objectives: termination of the arrhythmia and prevention of recurrence. Although the achievement of the first goal is relatively easy, long-term control of recurrent ventricular tachycardia is often difficult. The course of the arrhythmia is unpredictable and it may be difficult to predict definitely the effectiveness of therapy even after several weeks of hospitalization. The introduction of Holter monitoring, provocative exercise electrocardiograms, and stimulation studies have been of particular value in this field.[4-7]

Antiarrhythmic drugs are still the first line of defense in prophylaxis of ventricular tachycardia. Much progress has been made in the last few years and many more effective antiarrhythmic drugs are now available.[8] None are free of side effects or toxicity, but the variety permits a greater choice should one particular drug cause intolerable or troublesome side effects. Some have long half-lives and this property has two advantages: Patient compliance should be enhanced since the medicine need not be taken frequently, and there is less possibility of wide swings of body concentration using a drug with a long half-life. This should reduce the possibility of alternating between high drug concentrations causing side effects or toxicity and low drug concentrations resulting in ineffective therapy.[8] Consequently, a greater number of patients can be stabilized after their first attack of ventricular tachycardia using presently available medication. Should drug therapy fail, other modalities need to be considered.

* This work was supported in part by grants from L'Association de Recherche et d'Entraide Cardiologique et Angéiologique, La Caisse Régionale d'Assurances Maladie de Paris, and La Délégation Générale à la Recherche Scientifique et Technique (Grants No. 76–7–1409 and 79–7–1008).

† Address for correspondence: Dr. G. Fontaine, Service de Rythmologie, Hôpital Jean-Rostand, 93 rue Jean Le Galleu, 94200 Ivry-sur-Seine, France.

0077–8923/82/0382–0396 $1.75/0 © 1982, NYAS

Pacemakers may be used alone or in association with drugs to prevent or terminate ventricular tachycardia.[9] However, this method has some limitations in the context of ventricular tachycardia and, in practice, it is only helpful in a small number of very selected cases.[10, 11]

Surgical treatment of ventricular tachycardia is currently reserved for cases of drug failure.[12] The first successful case was observed after a ventriculoplasty[13] performed by Charles Bailey of Philadelphia in 1955, which was reported by Couch in 1959.[14] The prime objective of ventriculoplasty was to restore a more normal ventricular shape. The effectiveness of the procedure on the arrhythmia was attributed to ablation of the abnormal zone containing the arrhythmogenic areas. Since then, aneurysmectomy undertaken to prevent arrhythmias has been reported to be effective.[15-21] This operation may act by improving the cardiac output and coronary perfusion. Other surgical techniques have been suggested, including plication of dilated zones (without excision of the aneurysm),[22] sympathectomy,[23, 24] and, more recently, myocardial revascularization by aortocoronary saphenous vein bypass grafting.[25-29]

Advances in clinical electrophysiology have led to the development of new techniques to localize and obliterate the origin of the arrhythmia. These include ventriculotomy,[30] cryosurgery,[31-33] subendocardial excision,[34-37] and encircling endocardial ventriculotomy.[38-40]

A surgical procedure for the treatment of ventricular tachycardio guided by data obtained during preoperative electrophysiologic investigation was carried out by our group in 1971.[41] Since that time, 41 patients with chronic ventricular tachycardia complicating myocardial infarction have been managed surgically. The results of this series will be reported in this paper.

CLINICAL MATERIAL

This series comprises 39 male and 2 female patients whose ages ranged from 26 to 76 years (average, 55 years ± 9 months). These patients were considered to be resistant to antiarrhythmic drug therapy. Myocardial infarction dated from 3 weeks to 20 years prior to admission to our department (average, 5 years), 10% being referred during the first year after infarction. The first attack of ventricular tachycardia occurred an average of 3 years after infarction, although 20% of the cases were observed during the first year after necrosis. Three patients had recurrent infarction, 9 years, 5 years, and 1 month, respectively, after the initial event. The principal clinical and follow-up data are shown in TABLE 1.

METHODS

Epicardial Mapping in Supraventricular Rhythm

The epicardial map is a representation of the spread of the activation front over the surface of the heart. It is constructed by determining the time at which electrical activity is recorded at a number of fixed sites on the epicardium. Our technique employs a grid to define 40 recording sites over the right ventricle and 45 recording sites over the left ventricle. These sites are fixed at the intersection of hypothetical lines drawn between obvious anatomic landmarks, such as the line from the origin of left anterior descending artery to

TABLE 1

Patient No.	Age (yr.) & Sex	Site of Infarction *	Time Elapsed †	Date of Operation	Date of Death	Cause of Death	Date of Last Information	Survival Time ‡	Operation
1	48, M	Posterior	4 mo.	12/16/71	11/72	VT		11 mo.	EX
2	62, M	Anterior + Septal	10 yr.	12/07/72			3/81	99 mo.	EX
3	69, F	Anterior + Posterior	10 yr. + 1 yr.	11/21/73	12/73	CHF		23 days	EX
4	53, M	Lateral	3 wk.	10/09/73	1/74	NCC		3 mo.	EX + BJK
5	56, M	Anterior + Septal	2 mo.	12/05/73	12/75	SUD		24 mo.	EX
6	76, F	Anterior + Septal	6 yr.	2/15/74			3/81	85 mo.	EX
7	68, M	Anterior + Septal	7 yr. + 2 yr.	3/17/74	3/74	LOF		0 days	EX
8	64, M	Posterior	3 yr.	5/08/74	5/74	CHF		15 days	EX + BJK
9	56, M	Anterior + Septal	14 yr.	5/29/74	2/77	CHF		33 mo.	EX
10	53, M	Anterior + Septal	10 yr.	9/30/74			4/81	78 mo.	V.
11	66, M	Anterior + Septal	1 mo.	4/10/75			3/81	71 mo.	V.
12	49, M	Anterior + Septal	2 mo.	7/16/75	7/75	VT		12 days	EEV + 1V
13	48, M	Exterior + Anterior	3 yr.	7/04/76			3/81	64 mo.	EEV
14	60, M	Posterior	8 yr.	11/10/75			3/81	56 mo.	EEV
15	55, M	Anterior	3 yr.	2/17/77	11/80	VT		45 mo.	EEV
16	59, M	Anterior	1 yr.	2/21/77	4/77	CHF		2 mo.	EEV
17	40, M	Posterior + Lateral	2 yr.	5/16/77	7/79	MI		26 mo.	EEV + EX
18	39, M	Anterior + Septal + Posterior	36 + 35 mo.	12/19/77				25 mo.	EEV
19	60, M	Posterior + Septal	15 yr.	12/21/77	12/77	LOF	1/80	0 days	EEV
20	50, M	Septal	5 mo.	3/01/78	6/80	MI		27 mo.	EEV
21	66, M	Posterior	11 yr.	11/21/78			1/81	26 mo.	EEV + EX
22	61, M	Anterior	10 yr.	12/06/78	11/80	CHF		13 mo.	EEV
23	61, M	Posterior	15 mo.	12/11/78	12/78	NCC		10 days	EEV
24	55, M	Anterior	3 yr.	1/29/79			4/81	20 mo.	EEV
25	54, M	Posterior	8 yr.	5/14/79			3/81	22 mo.	EEV
26	58, M	Anterior	10 mo.	5/21/79			3/81	22 mo.	EEV
27	48, M	Posterior + Septal	20 yr.	8/06/79			2/81	19 mo.	EEV + EX + 1V
28	60, M	Anterior + Septal	7 mo.	10/15/79			4/81	16 mo.	EEV + EX
29	42, M	Anterior + Septal	8 mo.	12/10/79			4/81	16 mo.	EEV + EX
30	59, M	Posterior	5 yr.	2/04/80				14 mo.	EEV + EX + 1V
31	58, M	Anterior	3 yr.	2/06/80			11/80	9 mo.	EEV + 1V
32	61, M	Posterior	11 yr.	2/13/80			4/81	14 mo.	EEV + EX
33	52, M	Posterior	11 yr.	4/01/80			4/81	7 mo.	EEV + EX
34	59, M	Anterior + Septal	20 mo.	4/21/80	9/80	CHF		5 mo.	V
35	56, M	Anterior + Septal	2 mo.	4/30/80	5/80	NCC		26 days	EEV + EX
36	41, M	Anterior	18 yr.	5/19/80	5/80	LOF		0 days	EEV + EX
37	62, M	Posterior	4 mo.	7/11/80	7/80	LOF		0 days	V
38	52, M	Anterior + Septal	10 yr.	7/16/80			4/81	9 mo.	EEV + EX
39	52, M	Anterior + Septal	1 yr.	9/15/80			4/81	7 mo.	EEV + EX
40	26, M	Exterior + Anterior	10 yr.	10/15/80				6 mo.	EEV + EX
41	49, M	Posterior	2 yr.	11/24/80			4/81	5 mo.	EEV + EX

NOTE: BJK = Björk prosthesis; CHF = congestive heart failure; EEV = encircling endocardial ventriculotomy; EX = excision of necrotic tissue or aneurysmectomy; LOF = low output failure at the end of cardiopulmonary bypass; MI = recurrence of myocardial infarction; NCC = noncardiac cause; SUD = sudden death; V = simple ventriculotomy (endocardial in case 34); 1V = one-vessel bypass grafting; VT = ventricular tachycardia.

* Determined by electrocardiographic pattern.
† Between myocardial infarction and date of operation.
‡ Calculated by the difference between date of operation and last information, in surviving patients.

the apex of the heart or the line from the crux of the heart following the diaphragmatic part of the right atrioventricular groove to the right border of the heart. Test points are defined by the extremities and middle point of each line. Subsequently, the middle point and each extremity defines a segment the middle of which determines a new test point and so on. Finally, the recording sites are all represented in the same plane on a drawing of the heart shown spread out after section along the posterior interventricular groove.

The timing reference in sinus rhythm is obtained by atrial pacing at a rate 20 to 30% faster than the basal rhythm. This completely inhibits the sinoatrial node. Manipulation of the heart or other external conditions may change the atrioventricular conduction time during the investigation. It is therefore important that this be checked by continuous monitoring of the time interval between the atrial stimulus and a fixed ventricular reference electrode. This allows compensation for any change in atrioventricular conduction in the calculation of the activation times.

The exploratory probe used for mapping consists of three electrodes 1 mm apart arranged in a triangular array. This arrangement permits recording from three separate bipolar leads. The tip of the probe is curved to avoid excessive tilting of the heart on its vascular pedicle and to facilitate exploration of the diaphragmatic wall. The potentials recorded by the three exploratory leads and the fixed reference electrode are led into an appropriately filtered (10 Hz– 1 kHz) differential amplifier ($G = 500$).

The sites on the grid are investigated after identification of the anatomic recording sites, while the timing of the occurrence of electrical activity at each site is measured on an oscilloscope. The activation times are then recorded on the grid. The investigation of all 85 test sites takes about 15 minutes.

At surgery, the map is generally drawn manually by interpolation and extrapolation of the values measured so as to obtain isochronic lines. However, this is usually carried out automatically off-line by feeding the activation times into a minicomputer. This saves time and is more objective. When epicardial potentials are not of satisfactory quality to be properly measured, the computer program extrapolates the isochrones from the surrounding available data.

EPICARDIAL MAPPING DURING VENTRICULAR TACHYCARDIA

It has been shown in the Electrophysiological Laboratory that most chronic ventricular tachycardia can be triggered by premature or short bursts of ventricular stimuli.[7, 42, 43] The same technique is used at surgery to initiate the arrhythmia.

When the spontaneous rhythm of the tachycardia is fast enough to produce hemodynamic distress, short-acting antiarrhythmic drugs such as chloracetylajmaline are given intravenously to slow the rate. When there is severe hemodynamic distress, electrical cardioversion is required.

During sustained ventricular tachycardia, electrical activity must be timed with respect to the deflection recorded by a fixed ventricular reference electrode. As a rule, the earliest point of ventricular activation is unknown, so the ventricular reference is simply fixed in an area where large signals are obtained. To measure the activation times with respect to the reference electrode, the signal recorded by the exploratory electrode is delayed so that it is always displayed on the oscilloscope *after* the reference potential.[44]

When mapping during tachycardia is poorly tolerated, the investigation may be hastened by recording the activation times on tape and carrying out the measurements at a later stage. In this way, the procedure may be completed in about 5 minutes.

Peroperative endocardial mapping has been recently carried out in a few cases to try to localize the origin of abnormal activation during sustained ventricular tachycardia.

The earliest point of epicardial breakthrough during ventricular tachycardia can be determined by mapping, but is not necessarily the point of *origin* of the arrhythmia. For example, in cases where ventricular tachycardia originates in the ventricular septum, the earliest epicardial breakthrough may be found in the paraseptal area.

SURGICAL TECHNIQUES

Three surgical techniques have been used:

1. Aneurysmectomy and/or excision of transmural scar. This classical approach involves excising the fibrotic area, leaving a fibrous rim to support the closing sutures.

2. Simple ventriculotomy. This technique has been derived from methods developed in the surgical approach to nonischemic ventricular tachycardia.[45] It is guided by the data obtained by mapping. The abnormal zone is characterized in supraventricular rhythm by slowing of epicardial activation; this approximates the epicardial limits of ischemic damage. In some cases, the earliest point of epicardial breakthrough during ventricular tachycardia was identified on epicardial mapping after induction of ventricular tachycardia by electrical stimulation.

A transmyocardial incision is made at the earliest activated area. Its length is usually 4 to 10 cm and its direction is determined by anatomic considerations.

However, from the outset it was evident that the earliest point of epicardial breakthrough in ventricular tachycardia did not always coincide with the site of myocardial infarction, and this observation was confirmed in one other case in this series.[30]

3. Encircling endocardial ventriculotomy (EEV). Results obtained with the preceding technique led one of us (GG) to develop a new method, the endocardial encircling ventriculotomy mainly on the basis of the anatomic aspect of left ventricular myocardium.[38] The encircling endocardial ventriculotomy is made through the border zone between myocardial scar and normal tissue to isolate the arrhythmogenic area from normal myocardium.

The surgical approach to chronic ventricular tachycardia has been developed over a period of 10 years, during which the pre- and peroperative techniques have changed dramatically. For the sake of clarity, the results of this study have been divided into two parts—those obtained with encircling endocardial ventriculotomy and results with other procedures, almost all of which were done preceding encircling endocardial ventriculotomy, which was still in a developmental state.

The group in which procedures other than encircling endocardial ventriculotomy were performed consists of 14 cases and is considered as a control group (TABLE 2). Information regarding zones of delayed activation in sinus rhythm and the point of earliest epicardial breakthrough in ventricular tachycardia were immediately communicated to the surgeon. The operative technique in 10 cases consisted of excision of the ischemic tissue or aneurysm, whose limits were mainly determined by the epicardial macroscopic appearance rather than by the data obtained by mapping. In two cases simple ventriculotomy was carried out along the left paraseptal area, where the first activation during ventricular tachycardia was observed. These cases have been reported in more detail elsewhere.[46] As regards the two remaining cases, a simple ventriculotomy was performed in one patient with ischemic cardiomyopathy in whom no endocardial fibrosis was observed, and in the other, fibrosis in three distinct endocardial areas led to several endocardial ventriculotomies. All the remaining patients underwent encircling endocardial ventriculotomy.

TABLE 2

MORTALITY IN PATIENTS UNDERGOING ENCIRCLING ENDOCARDIAL VENTRICULOTOMY (EEV)

| | | Patients Undergoing EEV | | |
Mortality *	Control Group	First Period	Second Period	Total EEV Group
Early Mortality				
No. of cases	14	11	16	27
No. of deaths	5 (36%)	2 (18%)	2 (13%)	4 (15%)
Late Mortality				
No. of cases	9	9	14	23
No. of deaths	5 (56%)	5 (56%)	0	5 (22%)
Overall mortality	71%	64%	13%	33%

* Early mortality is defined as that occurring within 1 month of surgery; late mortality is that occurring during the follow-up period.

DEFINITIONS

Mortality

We classify mortality in three groups:

1. Peroperative deaths.

2. Early deaths. These are defined as occurring in the first 30 postoperative days, whatever the cause and whether or not the patients have been discharged from the hospital.

These first two groups taken together constitute the immediate hospital mortality.

3. Late deaths. These are deaths that occurred after the 30th postoperative day.

Relapse

Relapse is defined as the recurrence of ventricular tachycardia considered clinically as a therapeutic failure. As for mortality, these cases are classified as follows: *early relapse* (occurring in the first 30 postoperative days) and *late relapse* (occurring after the 30th postoperative day).

In this study, peroperative deaths were not taken into consideration since it was impossible to know what the surgical result on the arrhythmia would have been.

Survival

All cases in this study were regularly reviewed and none have been lost to follow-up. The results have been updated periodically and the calculated survival rates are based on the latest information (TABLE 1).

RESULTS

Mortality

Before encircling endocardial ventriculotomy

The results in this group of 14 patients studied for an average of 7 years are summarized in TABLE 2. The immediate hospital mortality (peroperative plus early deaths) was 5 of 14 patients (36%). Two patients died of low output failure at the end of cardiopulmonary bypass and two of congestive heart failure. One had recurrent fatal ventricular arrhythmias.

During the follow-up period of this first group five more patients died. One death was caused by documented ventricular tachycardia. One patient died suddenly. Two had congestive heart failure, and the last patient died of an unrelated cause 3 months after operation.

Six patients had a survival period of 2 years or more and four patients survived more than 5 years. The longest survivor has now been followed for more than 8 years.

After encircling endocardial ventriculotomy

The second group comprises a series of 27 patients studied for an average of 2 years. In order to demonstrate improvement of results, we have arbitrarily divided the time into two periods:

The *first* period includes 11 patients operated upon between November 1975 and December 1978. The immediate operative mortality was two (one patient died of low output failure at the end of cardiopulmonary bypass and the other of a noncardiac cause). Five other patients died during the follow-up study: Two deaths were related to progression of coronary arterial disease with probable reinfarction in one case and definite reinfarction confirmed at autopsy in the second, 26 and 27 months after operation, respectively. Two patients died of congestive heart failure during the second and third postoperative months. Cardiac catheterization of one of these patients performed in the immediate postoperative period showed a minor but definite ventricular septal defect associated with mitral regurgitation. The remaining patient died suddenly, probably due to recurrent ventricular tachycardia 45 months after ·operation.

The *second* period includes 16 patients undergoing encircling endocardial ventriculotomy between December 1978 and April 1981. The immediate operative mortality was two (13%), one patient dying of low output failure at the end of cardiopulmonary bypass and the other of noncardiac causes. The remaining patients are still alive.

Postoperative Arrhythmias

This series, excluding the 4 patients (of 41) who died of low output at the end of cardiopulmonary bypass, is summarized in TABLE 3.

TABLE 3

RECURRENCE OF VENTRICULAR TACHYCARDIA AFTER ENCIRCLING ENDOCARDIAL VENTRICULOTOMY (EEV)*

	Control Group	Patients Undergoing EEV		Total EEV Group
		First Period	Second Period	
Early Recurrences				
No. of cases	12	10	15	25
No. of recurrences	1 (1)†	2 (0)	0	2 (8%)
Late Recurrences				
No. of cases	9	7	14	21
No. of recurrences	2 (2)	3 (1)	1	4 (1) (16%)
Total % of Recurrences	25%	50%	7%	24%
Mortality	8%	10%	0%	4%

* After exclusion of the four patients who died from low output failure at the end of cardiopulmonary bypass.
† Numbers in parentheses indicate the number of deaths due to arrhythmias.

Before encircling endocardial ventriculotomy

The control group comprises 12 patients. One had a fatal early relapse of ventricular tachycardia. Of the nine survivors, one had a fatal recurrence of ventricular tachycardia and one patient died suddenly. If we consider that sudden death was related to the recurrence of arrhythmia, this figure gives an overall relapse rate of 25%.

After encircling endocardial ventriculotomy

During the *first* period, early recurrence of ventricular tachycardia was observed in two of ten patients, giving a relapse rate of 20%. These two patients responded to antiarrhythmic treatment. During follow-up, three patients had a late relapse, one 2 months after surgery, but this was well controlled by treatment with amiodarone. After 6 months of therapy without further recurrence of ventricular tachycardia, the drug was completely withdrawn. The second patient had a relapse at 34 months and was successfully treated by antiarrhythmic drugs. The last patient died suddenly 45 months after relapses of ventricular tachycardia that had been seemingly controlled by antiarrhythmic treatment.

In the *second* period after encircling endocardial ventriculotomy, no recurrences of ventricular tachycardia were observed during the early postoperative period, but one patient had a relapse after 3 months, although this was controlled by drug therapy.

The total number of patients treated by encircling endocardial ventriculotomy forms a series of 25 cases in which early recurrent ventricular tachycardia occurred in 2 patients, a relapse rate of 8%, but when the follow-up period alone is taken into consideration, late recurrence of arrhythmia occurred in 3 of 21 cases, a rate of 16%.

Ventricular tachycardia was successfully prevented for a period of 2 years or more in 7 patients and for a period of 1 year or more in 16 patients.

Discussion

Our group started to perform surgical procedures based on epicardial mapping in 1971.[41] The information obtained from this procedure evolved during the developmental period. Consequently, our patients operated upon before encircling endocardial ventriculotomy was developed may be considered as controls for those patients who later underwent this procedure. In particular, we observed at the beginning of our experience[30] that the earliest point of epicardial breakthrough during ventricular tachycardia could occur in healthy myocardium at a distance from the infarcted zone, a fact subsequently demonstrated experimentally[48] and the mechanism of which was extensively documented by endocavitary and epicardial mapping.[49] Although a good correlation may be shown between the point of origin and the earliest point of epicardial breakthrough during ventricular tachycardia when the arrhythmia arises from the free wall of the ventricle, the earliest point of epicardial breakthrough may occur at a distance when the origin of ventricular tachycardia is situated in the septal area.[50] This led us to introduce the technique of encircling endocardial ventriculotomy.[39, 40] Using this approach, our surgical results improved: Although the immediate operative mortality decreased from 36 to 18%, this was not statistically significant because of the small number of cases. The same holds for the long-term mortality, which was identical in both series, and for the short-term recurrence of lethal ventricular tachycardia (although there was an improvement in the long-term results). Therefore, we should focus on the latest results with encircling endocardial ventriculotomy as it is now performed.

In the second of this procedure (EEV) period, the immediate operative mortality was unchanged, but there was a spectacular decrease in long-term morbidity, with total absence of recurrent ventricular tachycardia, both in the immediate postoperative period and, except for one case, during the follow-up period. Even when both operative (EEV) subgroups are considered together and compared with patients in whom other methods were used, both early and late mortality due to recurrent ventricular arrhythmias were reduced and there was, above all, a very significant decrease in the recurrence of ventricular tachycardia, both in the immediate postoperative period and at long term. This demonstrates that encircling endocardial ventriculotomy in our experience gives better results than do previous techniques.

Similar results have been reported by other investigators: In two papers [47, 53] the Stanford group reported the largest experience in this field with a study that was started 7 years ago and was at the beginning mainly based on aneurysmectomy in more than half of their 56 cases and on coronary arterial bypass alone in 7 patients. This series provides useful data, but most publications on this subject are isolated case reports with favorable outcomes or limited series studied for an insufficient length of time.[47]

Relatively poor results have been observed with coronary bypass surgery alone, a fact confirmed by other groups, suggesting that its role in the prevention of chronic ventricular arrhythmias is questionable.[28, 51, 52]

One poor prognostic factor has been emphasized. Mortality is always high when surgery is undertaken in the days or weeks immediately after myocardial infarction.[35, 53] In our series, the earliest operation was performed 3 weeks after myocardial infarction and the fatal outcome was due to an extracardiac cause.

Another poor prognostic factor seems to be related to impaired myocardial contractility, especially in patients with left ventricular end-diastolic pressures greater than 15 mm Hg.[53] Our patients did not have systematic left ventricular pressure measurements at angiography, but we have observed poor results in patients with signs of cardiac failure before operation. Two of our patients (No. 36 and 37) were nevertheless operated on despite their clinical condition, and the results were poor. We would add to these poor prognostic factors the presence of multiple infarctions, present in three of our patients (No. 3, 7 and 19), giving rise to low output states, with death at the end of cardiopulmonary bypass in two patients and progressive cardiac failure leading to death within a few weeks of operation in the other patient.

The differences between these series make the comparison of results difficult. As a rule, our group has not performed surgery in high-risk patients, operated on in the days or weeks immediately after myocardial infarction. Also, it has not been our policy to perform coronary arterial bypass surgery alone for the prevention of chronic ventricular arrhythmias. Coronary bypass surgery associated with encircling endocardial ventriculotomy was only performed in 4 of 29 patients in our series, and in none of our patients did we attempt to prevent ventricular tachycardia by coronary revascularization alone.

Since we have observed an identical overall mortality to that reported by the Stanford group with a similar follow-up period, it may be that the benefits won in the prevention of the arrhythmia and the reduction in mortality due to relapse may have been offset by a greater impairment in myocardial contractility.

In one of our patients, postoperative cardiac catheterization showed the presence of a minor ventricular septal defect associated with mitral regurgitation. A recent experimental study [54] has shown that encircling endocardial ventriculotomy acts by interrupting blood flow to the border zone between the ischemic area and healthy tissue, the zone where intraventricular reentry is thought to arise. This led to a change in our surgical technique, ventriculotomy now being performed in an oblique fashion so as to spare as much contractile muscle as possible.

The Philadelphia team has based its approach to ventricular arrhythmias and their surgical management on the localization of the point of origin of the arrhythmia in order to limit the surgical procedure to a well-defined zone. This involves endocavitary mapping in the catheterization laboratory and perioperative endocardial mapping.[34, 36, 37]

This group [35] recently reported the results of a series of patients undergoing peroperative endocavitary left ventricular electrophysiologic investigation. Diffuse intraventricular conduction defects in the form of fragmented potentials were demonstrated and the endocardial origin of the arrhythmia could be located to within 2 cm, thus increasing the precision of the surgical procedure. At surgery, the arrhythmogenic zone where subendocardial resection was to be performed was even more precisely located by peroperative endocardial mapping. There are, however, notable differences between our series and the American ones. The average age of the patients in the American series was lower than that in our series and the population differed in that the majority had ventricular aneurysms (compared with only about 50% in our series). Aortocoronary bypass was carried out in two-thirds of the patients in the American series compared with only 4 times in our series, in which the indications had no relation to the arrhythmia.

The overall mortality was lower in the Philadelphia series. Given the limited number of published series, it is difficult to compare the relapse and late mortality rates.

The follow-up period is as yet only 13.5 months on the average, the longest follow-up period being 28 months.

We agree with the opinion of the Stanford team that at present it is difficult to know whether one approach is better than the other.[47] Only longer follow-up of larger series of patients will show whether extensive pre- and peroperative electrophysiologic mapping is necessary for surgical treatment of ventricular tachycardia. Peroperative electrophysiologic investigations have the disadvantage of prolonging the operative time and particularly of cardiopulmonary bypass. It also requires specially trained teams and large amounts of equipment. Therefore, these investigations can only be carried out in specialized centers.

CONCLUSIONS

In conclusion, with respect to the present state of the art, we offer the following suggestions in the surgical management of ventricular arrhythmias after myocardial infarction:

1. Risks of surgery are high in the acute phase of myocardial infarction, in cases of multiple myocardial infarctions, and in the presence of a poor reserve of contractility of the myocardium.

2. Coronary arterial bypass and ventricular aneurysmectomy alone are not regularly effective in the prevention of chronic sustained ventricular tachycardia.

3. Surgery based on electrophysiologic concepts seems to increase the prevention of arrhythmias.[55]

REFERENCES

1. ARMBRUST, C. A. & S. A. LEVINE. 1950. Paroxysmal ventricular tachycardia. A study of one hundred and seven cases. Circulation 1: 28.

2. FEDERMAN, J., J. A. WHITFORD, S. T. ANDERSON & A. PITT. 1978. Incidence of ventricular arrhythmias in first year after myocardial infarction. Br. Heart J. **40:** 1243.
3. BOUVRAIN, Y., A. SLAMA, G. MOTTE, M. WAYNBERGER & A. CREVELIER. 1968. Les tachycardies ventriculaires: Etiologie et evolution à propos de 161 malades. Arch. Mal. Coeur **61:** 909.
4. BENDITT, D. G., E. L. C. PRITCHETT, A. G. WALLACE & J. J. GALLAGHER. 1979. Recurrent ventricular tachycardia in man: Evaluation of disopyramide therapy by intracardiac electrical stimulation. Eur. J. Cardiol. **9:** 255.
5. MASON, J. W. & R. A. WINKLE. 1978. Electrode-catheter arrhythmia induction in the selection and assessment of anti-arrhythmic drug therapy in recurrent ventricular tachycardia. Circulation **58:** 971.
6. WINKLE, R. A. 1980. Ambulatory electrocardiography and the diagnosis, evaluation and treatment of chronic ventricular arrhythmias. Prog. Cardiovasc. Dis. **23:** 99.
7. WELLENS, H. J. J. 1978. Value and limitations of programmed electrical stimulation of the heart in the study and treatment of tachycardias. Circulation **57:** 845.
8. ZIPES, D. P. & P. J. TROUP. 1978. New antiarrhythmic agents: Amiodarone, aprindine, disopyramide, ethmozine, mexiletine, tocainide, verapamil. Am. J. Cardiol. **41:** 1005.
9. FONTAINE, G. & F. I. MARCUS. 1980. Current status of pacemaker therapy of arrhythmias. *In* Current Problems in Cardiology, Vol. V. Year Book Medical Publishers. Chicago, IL.
10. MOSS, A. J. & R. J. RIVERS. 1974. Termination and inhibition of recurrent tachycardias by implanted pervenous pacemakers. Circulation **50:** 942.
11. RUSKIN, J. N., H. GARAN, F. POULIN & J. W. HARTHORNE. 1980. Permanent radiofrequency ventricular pacing for management of drug-resistant ventricular tachycardia. Am. J. Cardiol. **46:** 317.
12. GALLAGHER, J. J. & J. L. COX. 1979. Status of surgery for ventricular arrhythmias. Circulation **60:** 1440.
13. BAILEY, C. P., H. E. BOLTON, H. NICHOLS & R. A. GILMAN. 1958. Ventriculoplasty for cardiac aneurysm. J. Thorac. Cardiovasc. Surg. **35:** 37.
14. COUCH, O. A. 1959. Cardiac aneurysm with ventricular tachycardia and subsequent excision of aneurysm. Circulation **20:** 251.
15. FAVALORO, R. G. & L. K. EFFLER. 1968. Ventricular aneurysm. Clinical experience. Ann. Thorac. Surg. **6:** 227.
16. HUNT, D., G. SLOMAN & G. WESTLAKE. 1969. Ventricular aneurysmectomy for recurrent tachycardia. Br. Heart J. **31:** 264.
17. KENAAN, G., A. M. MENDEZ & P. ZUBIATE. 1973. Surgery for ventricular tachycardia unresponsive to medical treatment. Chest **64:** 574.
18. KLUGE, T. H., S. R. ULLAL & J. D. HILL. 1971. Dyskinesia and aneurysm of the left ventricle. Surgical experience in 36 patients. J. Cardiovasc. Surg. **12:** 273.
19. MAGIDSON, O. 1969. Resection of post-myocardial infarction. Ventricular aneurysm for cardiac arrhythmias. Dis. Chest **56:** 211.
20. THIND, G. S., W. S. BLAKEMORE & H. F. ZINSSER. 1971. Ventricular aneurysmectomy for the treatment of recurrent ventricular tachyarrhythmia. Am. J. Cardiol. **27:** 690.
21. GALLAGHER, J. J., H. N. OLDHAM, A. G. WALLACE, R. H. PETER & J. H. KASELL. 1975. Ventricular aneurysm with ventricular tachycardia. Report of a case with epicardial mapping and successful resection. Am. J. Cardiol. **35:** 696.
22. KAY, J. H., E. DUNN & B. G. KROHN. 1970. Left ventricular excision, exclusion or plication for akinetic areas of the heart. J. Cardiovasc. Surg. **59:** 139.
23. SEALY, W. C. & H. N. OLDHAM. 1978. Surgical treatment of malignant ventricular arrhythmias by sympathectomy, coronary artery grafts and heart

wall resection. *In* Advances in the Management of Arrhythmias. D. T. Kelly, Ed. Telectronics Pty. Lane Cove, NSW Australia.

24. LLOYD, R., R. OKADA, J. STAGG, R. ANDERSON, B. HATTLER & F. MARCUS. 1979. The treatment of recurrent ventricular tachycardia with bilateral cervico-thoracic sympathetic-ganglionectomy. A report of 2 cases. Circulation **50:** 382.

25. ECKER, R., C. B. MULLINS & J. C. GRAMMER. 1971. Control of intractable ventricular tachycardia by coronary revascularization. Circulation **44:** 666.

26. CLINE, R. E., R. G. ARMSTRONG & W. STANFORD. 1973. Successful myocardial revasculation after ventricular fibrillation induced by treadmill exercise. J. Thorac. Cardiovasc. Surg. **65:** 802.

27. GRABOYS, T. B., B. LOWN, J. J. COLLINS & L. H. COHN. 1978. Does coronary revascularization reduce the prevalence of ventricular ectopic activity? Am. J. Cardiol. **41:** 401.

28. LEUTENEGGER, F., G. GIGER, P. FUHR, E. A. RAEDER, F. BURKART, H. SCHMITT, E. GRADEL & D. BURCKHARDT. 1979. Evaluation of artocoronary venous bypass grafting for prevention of cardiac arrhythmias. Am. Heart J. **98:** 15.

29. NORDSTROM, L. A., J. P. LILLEHEI, A. ADICOFF, Y. SAKO & F. L. GOBEL. 1975. Coronary artery surgery for recurrent ventricular arrhythmias in patients with variant angina. Am. Heart J. **89:** 236.

30. FONTAINE, G., G. GUIRAUDON, R. FRANK, J. VEDEL, R. COUTTE, C. DRAGODANNE, H. PHAN-THUC & Y. GROSGOGEAT. 1976. Cartographies epicardiques dans 4 cas de tachycardie ventriculaire par reentrée après infarctus du myocarde. I. origine de la tachycardie et attitude chirurgicale. Arch. Mal. Coeur **11:** 1099.

31. GALLAGHER, J. J., R. W. ANDERSON, J. KASELL, J. R. RICE, E. L. C. PRITCHETT, J. H. GAULT, L. HARRISON & A. G. WALLACE. 1978. Cryoablation of drug-resistant ventricular tachycardia in a patient with a variant of scleroderma. Circulation **57:** 190–197.

32. CAMM, J., D. E. WARD, R. CORY-PEARCE, G. M. REES & R. A. J. SPURRELL. 1979. A successful cryosurgical treatment of paroxysmal ventricular tachycardia. Chest **75:** 621.

33. CAMM, J., D. E. WARD, R. A. J. SPURRELL & G. M. REES. 1980. Cryothermal mapping and cryoablation in the treatment of refractory cardiac arrhythmias. Circulation **62:** 67.

34. JOSEPHSON, M. E., A. H. HARKEN & L. N. HOROWITZ. 1979. Endocardial excision: A new surgical technique for the treatment of recurrent ventricular tachycardia. Circulation **60:** 1430.

35. HOROWITZ, L. N., A. H. HARKEN, J. A. KASTOR & M. E. JOSEPHSON. 1980. Ventricular resection guided by epicardial and endocardial mapping for treatment of recurrent ventricular tachycardia. N. Engl. J. Med. **302:** 589.

36. HOROWITZ, L. N., M. E. JOSEPHSON, J. A. KASTOR & A. H. HARKEN. 1979. Intraoperative epicardial and endocardial mapping of ventricular tachycardia in man. Am. J. Cardiol. **43:** 401.

37. JOSEPHSON, M. E., A. H. HARKEN & L. N. HOROWITZ. 1981. This volume.

38. GUIRAUDON, G., G. FONTAINE, R. FRANK, G. ESCANDE, P. ETIEVENT & C. CABROL. 1978. Encircling endocardial ventriculotomy. A new surgical treatment for life-threatening ventricular tachycardias resistant to medical treatment following myocardial infarction. Ann. Thoras. Surg. **26:** 438.

39. GUIRAUDON, G., G. FONTAINE, R. FRANK, B. BAEHREL, V. BORS, P. ETIEVENT & C. CABROL. 1978. Encircling endocardial ventriculotomy: A new surgical management of ventricular tachycardia related to myocardial infarction. *In* Management of Ventricular Tachycardia. Role of Mexiletine E. Sandoe, D. G. Julian & J. M. Bell, Eds.: 630. Excerpta Medica. Amsterdam.

40. GUIRAUDON, G., G. FONTAINE, R. FRANK, Y. GROSGOGEAT & C. CABROL. 1980. Encircling endocardial ventriculotomy. Late follow-up results. Circulation **62:** Suppl. III: 1233.

41. FONTAINE, G., R. FRANK, M. BONNET, C. CABROL & G. GUIRAUDON. 1973. Methode d'étude experimentale et clinique des syndromes de Wolff-Parkinson-White et d'ischemie myocardique par cartographie de la depolarisation ventriculaire epicardique. Coeur Med. Int. **12:** 105.
42. WELLENS, H. J. J., D. R. DURRER & K. I. LIE. 1976. Observations on mechanisms of ventricular tachycardia in man. Circulation **54:** 237.
43. WELLENS, H. J. J., R. M. SCHUILENBURG & D. DURRER. 1972. Electrical stimulation of the heart in patients with ventricular tachycardia. Circulation **46:** 216.
44. FONTAINE, G., G. GUIRAUDON, R. FRANK, R. COUTTE, C. DRAGODANNE, Y. GROSGOGEAT & C. CABROL. 1975. Nouvelles techniques de realisation des cartographies epicardiques. Coeur **6:** 115.
45. FONTAINE, G., G. GUIRAUDON, R. FRANK, A. GERBAUX, J. P. COUSTEAU, A. BARILLON, J. GAY, C. CABROL & J. FACQUET. 1975. La cartographie epicardique et le traitement chirurgical par simple ventriculotomie de certaines tachycardies ventriculaires rebells par réentrée. Arch. Mal. Coeur **68:** 113.
46. FONTAINE, G., G. GUIRAUDON, R. FRANK, J. VEDEL, Y. GROSGOGEAT & C. CABROL. 1978. The concept of reentry and the surgical treatment of ventricular tachycardia. *In* Management of Ventricular Tachycardia. Role of Mexiletine. E. Sandoe, D. G. Julian & J. W. Bell, Eds.: 622. Excerpta Medica. Amsterdam.
47. MASON, J. W., A. J. BUDA, E .B. STINSON & D. C. HARRISON. 1980. Surgical therapy of ventricular tachyarrhythmias in ischemic heart disease using conventional techniques. *In* Medical and Surgical Management of Tachyarrhythmias. Springer-Verlag. Berlin.
48. WITTIG, J. H. & J. P. BOINEAU. 1975. Surgical treatment of ventricular arrhythmias using epicardial transmural and epicardial mapping. Ann. Thoras. Surg. **20:** 117.
49. JOSEPHSON, M. E., L. N. HOROWITZ, S. R. SPIELMAN, A. M. GREENSPAN, C. VANDEPOL & A. H. HARKEN. 1980. Comparison of endocardial catheter mapping with intraoperative mapping of ventricular tachycardia. Circulation **61:** 395.
50. MOORE, E. N., J. F. SPEAR, S. SPIELMAN, E. MICHELSON, A. MODESS, M. JOSEPHSON & L. N. HORWITZ. 1978. Electrophysiological studies on the mechanism of ventricular tachycardia. *In* Advances in the Management of Arrhythmias. D. T. Kelly, Ed.: 175. Telectronics Pty. Lane Cove, NSW Australia.
51. GUINN, G. A. & V. S. MATHUR. 1977. Ambulatory nocturnal and exercise arrhythmias in coronary artery disease: A prospective randomized study to assess the influence of aortocoronary bypass surgery. Am. J. Cardiol. **39:** 270.
52. TILKIAN, A. G., J. F. PFEIFER, W. H. BARRY, M. J. LIPTON & H. N. HULTGREN. 1976. The effect of coronary bypass surgery on exercise-induced ventricular arrhythmias. Am. Heart J. **92:** 707.
53. HARRISON, D. C., A. BUDA & E. B. STINSON. 1978. Surgery for ventricular arrhythmias. *In* Management of Ventricular Tachycardia. Role of Mexiletine. E. Sandoe, D. G. Julian & J. W. Bell, Ed.: 643. Excerpta Medica. Amsterdam.
54. UNGERLEIDER, R. M., T. E. STANLEY, J. M. WILLIAMS, G. K. LUFLAND & J. L. COX. 1980. Physiologic effects of the encircling endocardial ventriculotomy (EEV) for refractory ischemic ventricular tachycardia. Circulation **62**(4) 215.
55. MASON, J. W. & E. B. STINSON. 1980. Comparison of efficacy of map-guided to blind myocardial resection for recurrent ventricular tachycardia. Circulation **62:** Suppl. III: 1007.

DISCUSSION

DR. KASTOR: Is it possible that some of the patients could have been controlled on what are now considered reasonable doses of drugs or do you think they all represent drug failures?

DR. FONTAINE: I don't think that they represent definite drug failures because in the referring centers these patients have been relatively thoroughly studied. In the population of patients referred to our medical department for evaluation we were able to treat roughly 50% with drugs.

DR. WINKLE: I'd like to make a few comments about the Stanford series because although it has often been used as a standard for comparison for the various mapping procedures and surgical operations that are now being done, it is a very difficult series to use to evaluate surgical results. Recently, Dr. Jay Mason has tried to compare our current results using mapping procedures with the older retrospective data in that series, but it is clear that the patients in the older series are not at all comparable with the types of patients now being treated. A large number of the earlier patients were referred directly to the surgeons. Furthermore, by current definitions, a number of them didn't really have a drug-resistant tachycardia. In fact, some of these patients didn't even have sustained ventricular tachycardia of the type that we would now consider treatable by surgery.

In summary in retrospective review, there were roughly 32 patients who seemed somewhat comparable to the kind of patients we are now operating on with prior mapping. Two findings are relevant: The operative mortality really didn't change that much; it was a little bit better in the map-guided group, but still about 15%. What seemed to be dramatically different between the two groups was the recurrence rate of ventricular tachycardia. Far fewer recurrences occurred in the map-guided group compared with the so-called blind resection group.

We feel that the map-directed procedure is clearly superior for ablating the site of tachycardia, at least for a 2-year follow-up period. Beyond that point the outcome is unclear. I wanted to make this point because the Stanford series has been widely used as a standard for comparison, but it has a lot of problems that should be recognized.

LARGE-SCALE CLINICAL TRIALS:
ARE THEY WORTH THE COST?

Robert I. Levy and Edward J. Sondik

National Heart, Lung, and Blood Institute
National Institutes of Health
Bethesda, Maryland 20205

INTRODUCTION

Despite a decline which began in the mid 1960s, cardiovascular disease remains the nation's number one health problem. It accounts for slightly more than 50% of all mortality and costs the nation some $70 billion annually. The biomedical research efforts directed against cardiovascular disease are carried on along a number of fronts, including basic research into etiology and pathophysiology, clinical trials for testing preventive and therapeutic regimens, and demonstration and education programs for translating the results of this research into practice. The National Heart, Lung, and Blood Institute has the responsibility for leading this biomedical research effort, which has been congressionally mandated in a series of legislative acts dating mainly from the National Heart, Blood Vessel, Lung, and Blood Act of 1972.

Clinical trials and clinical research have been components of the biomedical research fight against cardiovascular disease since the formation of the National Heart, Lung, and Blood Institute (NHLBI) as the National Heart Institute in 1948. During the last 15 years, however, large-scale prospective randomized clinical trials have played an increasingly important role in the program.

Prospective randomized experiments are a relatively new tool in the biomedical researchers' armamentarium. The notion of randomization was put forth by R. A. Fisher in 1935 [1] and only during the 1940s was this idea incorporated into human trials. Major large-scale clinical trials (which we define as prospective clinical experiments involving three or more centers and generally involving at least hundreds of patients) began for the National Heart, Lung, and Blood Institute with the Coronary Drug Project (CDP) in 1965. Since that time a number of trials have followed, including the ongoing Coronary Primary Prevention Trial (CPPT/4000 patients), a part of Lipid Research Clinics program, the Beta Blocker Heart Attack Trial (BHAT/4000 patients), the ongoing Multiple Risk Factor Intervention Trial (MRFIT/12,000 patients), the recently completed Hypertension Detection and Follow-up Program (HDFP/ 10,000 patients), and a number of additional ongoing studies. The Institute's large-scale preventive and therapeutic studies now account for about 15% of its extramural program budget, or about $80 million annually. Because of fiscal constraints, these clinical trials necessarily replace or compete with the funding of some fraction of other meritorious biomedical research aimed at the aquisition of new information on the etiology and/or pathophysiology of disease. Our purpose in this paper is to discuss whether this investment in clinical trials is indeed worth the cost. In discussing this issue we will consider first the framework that the Institute uses to plan, evaluate, and manage its program

411

0077-8923/82/0382-0411 $1.75/0 © 1982, NYAS

of clinical trials. We then discuss several examples of the Institute's clinical trial portfolio and consider the potential benefits to be realized from these trials and the justification of the resources devoted to them. We close with a discussion of a possible trial on the prevention of sudden coronary death.

THE CLINICAL TRIAL DECISION FRAMEWORK

Cost is a critical issue in the decision to undertake a clinical trial, but it is only one of several factors that the Institute considers in deciding to initiate a clinical trial. As discussed in an earlier paper [2] first presented at a symposium held by the New York Academy of Sciences entitled "Hypertension: To Treat or Not to Treat," the National Heart, Lung, and Blood Institute uses a structured decision process to address the need for and resources required to launch a clinical trial.[3] The process (FIG. 1) consists of four phases, with a critical decision point separating each phase. The earliest stage, initiation (Phase 0) includes the evolutionary stages of the trial, such as the proposal of the trial concept, preliminary studies of feasibility, and other activities related to an

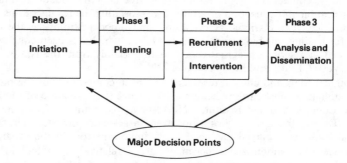

FIGURE 1. Clinical trial decision process.

analysis of the need for the clinical trial. In addition, the state of science must not be in flux; it must be sufficiently stable to assure that the technique or concept under test in a trial will not be outmoded before the trial is concluded.

During Phase 0 the trial design is analyzed along four major lines that form the framework for the decision to undertake the trial. First, the state of the science is addressed. Our scientific knowledge must be sufficient to serve as the foundation for the trial. Sufficient information must be known to show that the therapy proposed for testing has a reasonable chance to succeed. In view of the tremendous resources required—for example, for the Coronary Primary Prevention Trial, the total cost will exceed $80 million—the clinical trial cannot be a "fishing expedition." Sufficient preliminary and pilot studies must have been done to warrant at least the detailed planning of the clinical trial.

Secondly, the trial must be ethically sound. The consensus of opinion of biomedical researchers and practitioners must be that the therapy under evaluation competes with and has a good chance of being an improvement over existing therapies. In addition, the therapy under test cannot be already widely used since in that case the "window" for changing practice may have already passed. Moreover, if the therapy under test is already in widespread practice, it may be difficult, if not impossible, to find suitable control patients.

The third factor concerns the feasibility of the trial and includes an assessment of the number of patients required, the cost, the availability of suitable clinical facilities, end-points and their assessability, and issues relating to randomization and whether physician and patient participants will be aware as to which therapy patients are assigned.

The fourth factor relates to the potential impact of the trial. The trial must be important to health care. With the results appropriately disseminated, it must have the potential to reduce morbidity and mortality in terms sufficiently significant to warrant the cost of the trial. The benefits to be derived from the trial must be more than commensurate with the cost of the trial. For the NHLBI to support the trial, the results must also be of real or potential importance to health research and they must also validate or extend a hypothesis emanating out of basic research.

Before the trial can be undertaken and the detailed planning phase entered, all of these factors are reviewed by Institute Advisory Committees, the Institute staff, the director of the Institute, and the National Heart, Lung, and Blood Advisory Council. Only when approved does a trial enter into the detailed planning phase (Phase 1 in FIGURE 1).

During the planning phase the trial protocol is developed in detail and further studies are undertaken to assess the need for, and feasibility of, the proposed trial. After the planning phase, the four factors discussed earlier are again reviewed, and, if warranted, in light of the information available at that time, the trial will be undertaken.

Phase 2 represents the actual conduct of the trial, which includes the recruitment of subjects and the intervention itself. Throughout the trial, issues of safety, efficacy, advances in our state of knowledge, and other factors are continually reviewed and, if need be, the trial will be halted before its designed concluding point. The final phase of the trial occurs after formal termination of patient follow-up study and consists of the analysis of the data and the dissemination of this information to biomedical researchers, physicians, and the public at large.

The opportunity for the clinical testing of a regimen emerges naturally during the progression of biomedical research from bench to practice. Medical advances progress from basic and clinical research through validation, either formal or informal, to practice (FIG. 2). As regimens emerge from basic and clinical research some are proposed for clinical testing. The factors limiting clinical testing and validation are formidable and include not only limitations on research manpower and Institute staff, but especially, as we will discuss, the Institute's financial limitations.

In addressing its options with respect to a given advance, the Institute has three major decisions: to continue basic research on the topic; to consider and launch an educational and information dissemination program; or to undertake a clinical trial. These decisions are illustrated schematically in FIGURE 3. The strategies are not mutually exclusive; indeed, the Institute's program in high blood pressure, for example, has employed a multiple strategy with basic studies, clinical studies, clinical trials, and a major education program underway simultaneously.[4] The timing, initiation, and coordination of the various aspects of the program reflect the program decisions illustrated in FIGURE 3.

We cannot overemphasize that the key factor in the Institute's programmatic

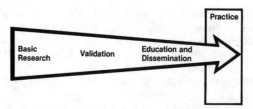

FIGURE 2. The progression of health advances from basic research to practice.

decisions related to investigator-initiated research and clinical trials is the fiscal constraints under which the Institute operates. Investigator-initiated grant research has become increasingly costly over the past 15 years. FIGURE 4 illustrates the rise in the cost of an average research project grant. Even in terms of constant dollars with increasing research opportunities, the cost of maintaining a strong investigator-initiated research program continues to escalate. Clinical trial costs for the major cardiovascular trials are between $1,000 and $2,000 per year per patient and major education efforts, even when their costs are lessened by voluntary support, can cost millions of dollars. The dilemma in decisions posed by the options in FIGURE 3 is difficult to resolve. Basic research gives rise to advances that lead to clinical trials; clinical trials in turn have an impact on health care and they lead to changes in basic research strategy. In turn, basic research advances can prevent the need for future trials. To make the decision to invest in a clinical trial numerous factors must be considered. In addition to fiscal cost we must assess the myriad changes that may occur from its results, the extent of patient benefits from the advances, as well as the length of time that these advances might be employed before still newer advances cause further changes in practice.

ASSESSING CLINICAL TRIAL COSTS AND BENEFITS

How do we assess the costs and benefits of a clinical trial? Costs are relatively easy to determine. The overall cost is estimated from the component resources required for the trial, including such expenditures as patient costs, drug costs, facilities, analysis, data collection, personnel, and laboratory costs. Benefits are more difficult to assess since their assessment involves several steps, including speculation on possible trial outcomes, consideration of the effect of these outcomes, and the quantitative valuation of the effects on health care. The first step in assessing benefits is to analyze the potential trial outcomes

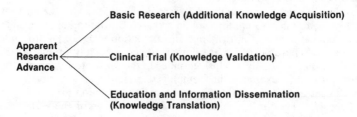

FIGURE 3. A decision tree representing the major Institute program options.

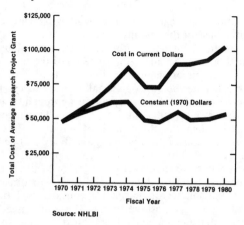

Source: NHLBI

FIGURE 4. Trends in investigator-initiated research costs.

(FIG. 5). First, we might find that the experimental therapy (E) is a significant improvement over the control therapy (C); second, we might find that there is no significant difference between E and C; and third we might find that the experimental therapy is significantly worse than the current therapy. FIGURE 5 shows that in the first and last cases we might undertake an education and dissemination program on the basis of the results. The education program is designed to influence physicians who use the inferior therapy to adopt the alternate therapy. The results of the program would be a change in the event rate associated with the problem under consideration from an average rate near that of the control therapy P_C to either a rate closer to that of the experimental therapy P_E if the first outcome had occurred, or closer to the control therapy if the third outcome had occurred. If there were no differences in outcome, we still might undertake an education and dissemination program toward cost-effective use of the therapies if they differ in cost or resources required. FIGURE 6 shows the estimated impact of a hypothetical education program and corresponding changes in the average event rate assuming that E is an improvement over C. We assume that the nature of the events is such that P_E is lower than P_C. Thus, under a successful education program the percentage of physicians employing the more effective therapy E would increase to some maximal

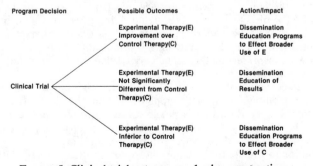

FIGURE 5. Clinical trial outcomes and subsequent actions.

level while the population's average event rate would decrease concomitantly with the more widespread use of the therapy.

The potential or realized impact of the trial can be calculated using a standard economic methodology by analyzing for each of the three outcomes the changes in event rates in terms of changes in direct costs of care, in morbidity, and in mortality. We calculate the cost of mortality in terms of an individual's lost economic productivity, which, for the standard approach, is essentially his projected lifetime earnings, given that he did not die. This income stream is generally discounted to reflect the time value of money. Thus, the cost of mortality becomes a single figure reflective of age and sex and economic status at the time of death. Direct health-care costs include physician, hospital, drug costs, and other factors related to the direct provision of health care. Morbidity costs account for time lost from productive activity due to disease.

To assess the potential impact of a trial we consider first the likelihoods that the trial will find significant positive or negative differences between the therapies or find them statistically equivalent. Next we derive the societal

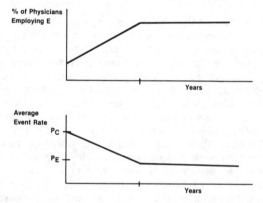

FIGURE 6. Hypothetical education program and impacts on physicians' practice and average event rate.

benefits for each of the outcomes. For example, if differences are found between the experimental and control therapies, society will benefit by adopting the new, effective therapy, and savings are accrued from a reduction in morbidity, mortality and the direct costs of care. If no differences are found between the therapies, then society benefits by choosing the least costly therapy. The information gained from each of the outcomes is important. While specific outcomes are not known *a priori*, estimates can be derived that are indicative of the impact of the potential findings.

The expected value of the trial is found by weighting the three outcomes with their probabilities. It must be emphasized that any of the three outcomes in the examples to be discussed is possible. As we discuss in detail in a later section, the Hypertension Detection and Follow-up Program, a major test of the effectiveness of blood pressure control, found the experimental therapy clearly superior to the control therapy; however, in the Coronary Drug Project (a test of the secondary prevention of coronary heart disease) none of the lipid-lowering drugs under test proved to be effective, and moreover, several proved to be ineffective and associated with severe side-effects.

In considering the decision to undertake a trial, the expected costs of the trial must be compared with the expected benefits to be derived from the trial. Of course, the benefits related to health care are not the full story. Information is gained from the trial that can lead to other research advances or even to other clinical trials. For example, information gained during the Coronary Drug Project on aspirin led to a further trial on aspirin (the Aspirin Myocardial Infarction Study [AMIS]) as a means of preventing subsequent cardiovascular events in patients who have recently suffered a myocardial infarction. Information currently being gained from our Multiple Risk Factor Intervention Trial and our Coronary Primary Prevention Trial has led to an Institute program in behavioral medicine aimed at a better understanding of the factors that influence patients to choose and comply with therapies.

A trial is a complex undertaking and because of its many facets it is difficult to derive a single figure that represents the potential benefits to accrue from the study. Yet for public-policy purposes such figures are essential if we are to justify our allocation of resources and make that allocation maximally effective.

Some Examples

With this framework in mind, let us consider some examples drawn from the clinical trials supported by the National Heart, Lung, and Blood Institute to determine the extent to which potential or realized benefits are commensurate with potential costs.

The Coronary Drug Project

The purpose of the Coronary Drug Project, which was initiated in 1965 and ended in 1973, was to determine whether any of four supposed lipid-lowering drugs were effective in reducing mortality in postmyocardial infarction patients. This was the first major trial undertaken by the Institute and included some 5,000 patients across the United States. The trial found that these drugs led to no significant difference in event rates and, moreover, that most were associated with serious side-effects. The effect of the trial on just one drug is shown in Figure 7. The use of this drug, clofibrate, had been steadily rising until publication of the trial results. It then began to fall and is now approximately at a level of one-half the use before the trial began. Of course it is not possible to conclude that the clinical trial was the only factor related to this decline (clofibrate has other uses besides the treatment of postmyocardial infarction patients), but the correlation with the timing of the publication of the trial results is compelling evidence to conclude that the clinical trial was a major factor in the decline.

The value of this decline in terms of the cost of the drug alone—not including morbidity and mortality associated with the drug—is approximately $50 million annually, which is about the cost of the entire clinical trial. If we estimate conservatively that this drug would continue to have been used for the next 10 years had the clinical trial not been conducted, the value of the reduction in direct health-care costs associated with the drug (discounted at 10% over the next 10 years) is approximately 300 million dollars, or about a six to one ratio between the benefits derived from the trial and its cost. This ratio becomes all the more impressive when we consider that it is based on the savings in drug costs from only one of four drugs tested by the trial and that the benefit as calculated does not include the dollars saved by the future avoidance of the side-effects associated with these drugs and the invaluable information the trial has provided *vis-à-vis* the natural history of postmyocardial infarction patients and the long-term effects of certain lipid-lowering drugs.

The Hypertension Detection and Follow-up Program

This recently concluded clinical trial was designed to test a number of issues about hypertension control. The first and foremost issue was whether a structured program of hypertension control would result in reduced blood pressures,

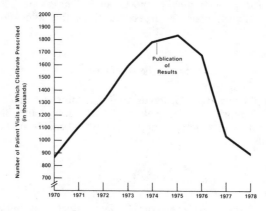

FIGURE 7. Clofibrate usage. Patient visits to physicians during which clofibrate was prescribed from 1970 to 1978. (Source: NDTI.)

which in turn would lead to decreased morbidity and mortality. Second, the trial was designed to assess whether community-based control was possible and whether therapy was effective in blacks, in the relatively young patient, and in women. The dramatic results show that in patients with mild hypertension (90 to 104 mm Hg diastolic blood pressure) the reduction in mortality in the group under the HDFP's structured "stepped-care" approach to hypertension control compared with the patients referred to their physician for (usual) care was about 20%. Overall reductions in mortality comparing the stepped-care group with the usual-care group was approximately 17%. Additional analysis has also shown a significant reduction in left ventricular hypertrophy and in stroke. The study showed that both the young and old as well as blacks benefit from therapy, which dispels the old wives' tale that high blood pressure in blacks is different and less responsive to therapy. In effect, the trial has shown for the first time that systematic blood pressure control in a community setting using a wide spectrum of patients can lead to significant reductions in morbidity and mortality. The trial involved some 10,000 patients and was conducted from 1974 through 1979. The cost of this trial was approximately $60 million.

What Are the Benefits from the Hypertension Detection and Follow-up Program?

Approximately 40 million Americans have mild hypertension. Mortality in the experimental group for this blood pressure range was approximately 5.9 per hundred for 5 years. Cardiovascular-related mortality in the referred-care group was approximately 7.4 per hundred, and we estimate that mortality in an uncontrolled group would be approximately 8.0 per hundred. Therefore, we estimate that if this full group were under effective hypertension control the reduction in mortality could be as many as 100,000 deaths per year (or 10% of cardiovascular deaths or 5% of all deaths occurring in the United States). When conservative figures are used to determine the value of these reduced costs in mortality alone, not including associated health-care costs and morbidity costs, the value of this new information, if acted on, is approximately $10 billion annually; and this does not include the savings in morbidity from fewer cases of stroke, heart failure, and myocardial infarction. Again, the total cost of the trial was approximately $60 million.

This trial clearly more than justifies itself in terms of the enormous magnitude of lives and health-care costs saved, but with every advance new questions and new issues arise. To treat all hypertensive patients with drugs could cost more than 1 billion dollars annually. The Institute does not recommend such universal drug therapy for all patients, but instead endorses aggressive treatment, which in many cases could be simply low-cost diet therapy. The importance of the trial's results argues for urgent, vigorous evaluation of nondrug therapy and the intensive search, through the allocation of additional dollars to basic and clinical research, for the causes of hypertension so that an even more cost-effective outcome can be achieved for the prevention of hypertension.

A Possible Trial of Antiarrhythmic Agents in the Prevention of Sudden Death

This entire symposium has dealt with the state of the science and issues involved in sudden death. In deciding on whether the time is right to undertake a multicenter drug trial in sudden death it is clear that an argument can be made for such a trial in terms of its potential impact on health-care and health research. Each year some 400,000 lives are lost through sudden cardiac death. Approximately 50% of these deaths occur in persons below age 75, with a concomitant value in lives of more than $15 billion dollars, a figure that only indirectly hints at the loss to families and to the Nation of these human resources.

Cardiac rhythm control is a promising possibility to reduce this toll and most certainly is a worthy subject for consideration for a clinical trial. It is clear that one can argue that in high-risk subjects events such as ventricular fibrillation, ventricular tachycardia, and sudden death and the great prevalence of the problem as well as the certainty of the dreadful end-points would make such a study feasible. In addition, in consideration of the current state of our knowledge, the lack of consensus about treatment benefit, and the potential for tragic outcome for the patient, one can make a strongly ethical argument for such a trial. However, the problem with considering support for such a trial today lies in the current state of science in the field. There appears to be little agreement as to which of the more than 16 available drugs should be used, how high-risk subjects should be defined, and on the value of programmed electrical stimulation and Holter monitors. Moreover, there is a need for careful acute-phase metabolic studies to define the nature of the problem and the precise effects and side-effects of appropriate drug regimen(s). Furthermore, the population at risk for sudden death and the response to different drug regimens as well as the nature of the arrhythmic focus still appear to be inhomogeneous. All this argues that any trial begun today would be in danger of being outmoded even before patient recruitment is finished. Thus, the current unsettled state of the field argues strongly against the conduct of a multicenter trial today. The possibility that such a trial would have major impact if and when it can be done, however, strongly calls for support of more basic and clinical research with attention and detail given to the rigor and detail of study design. Rigor is necessary if researchers in this very difficult field will ever be able to compare one another's studies and move us forward to the day when we can seek to prevent sudden cardiac death effectively.

Conclusion

Cost/benefit calculations similar to those in the previous section have been made for a number of other clinical trials in the Institute's portfolio. All show similar results. What are we led to conclude? First we note that the benefit to cost ratio for these undertakings can be impressive. When these trials are well designed and carefully considered, their impact on morbidity and mortality can be enormous. But we must also consider their cost in terms of reduced opportunities for the Institute in other areas. The cost of the Hypertension Detection and Follow-up Program in terms of foregone investigator-initiated research is approximately equivalent to that of 200 3-year investigator-initiated research grants. We are convinced that we need a strong investigator-initiated research program; but we also need a balance between basic research, validation effects, and education and demonstration programs. Decisions on program balance are made on the basis of a careful assessment of competing research opportunities and health-care needs. The Institute's resource allocations attempt to reflect all these needs. Despite the fact that clinical trials can have a major impact on the nation's health in human as well as economic terms, we always must be concerned that too heavy an investment in any one area will reduce the opportunities for further advances for years to come.

Large-scale clinical trials are most certainly worth the cost, but only after careful deliberation and consideration of their potential impact and feasibility and an assessment of the lost opportunities that might derive from shifting funds from basic research into validation.

References

1. FISHER, R. A. 1966. The Design of Experiments, 8th ed. Hafner. New York, NY.

2. LEVY, R. I. & E. J. SONDIK. 1978. Decision making in planning large-scale comparative studies. Ann. NY Acad. Sci. **304:** 441–457.
3. LEVY, R. I., & E. J. SONDIK. 1980. Initiating large-scale clinical trials. *In* Issues in Research with Human Subjects. U.S. Department of Health Education and Welfare, National Institutes of Health. NIH Publication No. 80–1858.
4. LEVY, R. I. 1982. The National Heart, Lung, and Blood Institute Overview–1980. The Director's Report to the National Heart, Lung, and Blood Advisory Council. Circulation. In press.

DISCUSSION

DR. HERLING: Dr. Levy, what would the impact be if the National Heart and Lung Institute and the medical community in general used its resources to make cigarette-smoking illegal? In 30 years from now where would we be in the sudden death issue?

DR. LEVY: If we attempted to use the resources that are for biomedical research to make smoking illegal, the next year Congress would not allocate any money for heart, lung or blood research. We do research on the etiology and pathophysiology of smoking. We have education and demonstration trials; trials that examine the effects of stopping smoking and that attempt to find ways to get people to stop smoking. Our investment in this is about 10 million dollars. The investments of the National Cancer Institute and others are equally high. We get our budget from Congress, and we're delighted that they consider biomedical research important enough to allocate resources there. Unfortunately those same men consider cigarette-smoking important enough to the economy so that they continue to support the growing of tobacco. These are the kinds of contradictions that we live with and we have to accept what we have. My answer is very pragmatic but these are the facts.

DR. HERLING: It seems as if we're addressing the issues "after the barn door has been locked" when we are dealing with the patient with established coronary disease. If our efforts were directed at prevention and with identification of youngsters with a family history of coronary diseases, a lot of money would be saved in the long run.

DR. LEVY: You asked me a different question when you asked me about cigarette-smoking. The major investment of the Institute is in prevention, not in therapy of the high-risk patient who already has coronary disease and is at risk for sudden coronary death. Of those eight trials more than half of them, and in terms of cost more than 75%, are involved with multi-risk-factor intervention. These trials attempt to show that intervention on some of the risk factors can indeed make an impact in terms of lowering mortality. The majority of the resources at our Institute are spent in prevention, but it would not be appropriate to forget the four million Americans who already have coronary artery disease.

DR. DE BUSK: Dr. Levy, in a time of restricted resources, the universities are increasingly turning to arrangements of various kinds with private industries. There are certain issues, such as rehabilitation of patients who have already had a heart attack, which have some very direct applications to industry. So there is a meaningful forum for that kind of interaction between the university and industry. Should government help to increase those interphases and inter-actions with private industry?

DR. LEVY: As you can imagine, especially with the current administration, there is a tremendous emphasis on self-sufficiency. It is suggested by many that we do not need to support biomedical research, industry will. The problem is that I don't think industry will. The area that you cited and others such as drug trials can perhaps interest industry sufficiently so that it will pick up some of the bill. But when we are talking about the area that most of our dollars are invested in, such as knowledge acquisition, finding new facts, and understanding basic etiology and pathophysiology, then we see that this is too early in the developmental process for most industries. It's unlikely that industry will ever foot the bill for basic research activities.

DR. DE BUSK: While I realize that in the past those relationships haven't been very fruitful, I'm asking whether there might be a reevaluation on the part of government so that they will look in a new way at these relationships. I'm not talking about an industry that benefits directly from the manufacture of a device or drug, but industry that is already paying costs that are well hidden from them and for which they have no motivation to make a change in their way of doing things.

DR. LEVY: We have approached both labor and industry in our program of risk reduction, pointing out that while both have large financial programs in accident prevention, cardiovascular disease costs labor and industry more each year than do the accidents. Some of them have been responsive. Obviously we have to try to tap all the resources that we can if we're going to get the job done.

DR. BAHR: Now that the consensus report on coronary bypass surgery has appeared, do you see a trial in the near future for bypass surgery as an anti-ischemic means of reducing sudden death?

DR. LEVY: No. Until we have the results from the European study and from the Coronary Artery Surgery Study (CASS) I would hate to think of enlarging the indications for bypass surgery.

PRIMARY PREVENTION
OF SUDDEN CORONARY DEATH:
A COMMUNITY-BASED PROGRAM IN
NORTH KARELIA, FINLAND

Jukka T. Salonen

North Karelia Project
Research Institute of Public Health
University of Kuopio
70101 Kuopio 10, Finland

OCCURRENCE OF SUDDEN CORONARY DEATH IN NORTH KARELIA

The county of North Karelia is a geographically large and mainly rural area in Eastern Finland with about 180,000 inhabitants. The highest recorded mortality rates for cardiovascular disease have been found among North Karelian men.[1,2] The exceptional occurrence of coronary heart disease (CHD) in men in the area has been confirmed in cross-sectional surveys,[3] follow-up studies of middle-aged male population samples,[3,4] and in community-based myocardial infarction registers.[5,6]

The age-standardized annual incidence of acute myocardial infarction (AMI) was 8.6 per thousand men aged 20–64 in North Karelia in 1973. According to the same diagnostic criteria, it was 5.9 in Helsinki (Southern Finland) in 1973.[6] The methods used in the registration of AMIs in North Karelia are identical with those in the international AMI register study. In 1975 and 1976, the crude annual incidence of sudden coronary death (within 1 hour from the onset of symptoms) was 1.9 per thousand men aged 20–64 years. The respective sudden death rate in Helsinki in 1971 was 1.6 per thousand, and in the rest of Europe it was between 0.2 and 0.9 per thousand.[5]

In the pooled data of the international AMI register study,[5] 40% of all deaths in the first 28 days occurred within the first hour from the onset of symptoms. In North Karelia in 1975–76 this proportion was 57% in men and 45% in women aged 30–64 years.

From these rough figures it is clear that in addition to the high incidence of AMI, its early case-fatality was remarkable in North Karelian men in the early 1970s. The situation among North Karelian women has not been as pathologic as in men. Both the incidence and case-fatality rates of AMI have been of the same magnitude as in Helsinki[6] and in some Central European countries.[5]

RISK FACTORS OF SUDDEN CORONARY DEATH

The high levels of the conventional CHD risk factors in North Karelian men had been observed already in the 1950s.[7] The 1972 baseline survey data confirmed these findings. About 52% of North Karelian men aged 25–59 were current smokers; their mean serum cholesterol was 269 mg/dL and mean casual blood pressure 147/91 mm Hg; 23% of them had systolic blood pressure

423

0077-8923/82/0382-0423 $1.75/0 © 1982, NYAS

of at least 160 mm Hg, 34% had diastolic blood pressure of at least 95 mm Hg, and 19% had both pressures above these values.[8, 9]

Although some epidemiologic knowledge of the factors associated with the risk of sudden coronary death has accumulated,[10] it was not evident whether these risk factors had the same impact in a high-incidence area like North Karelia. Major differences in CHD risk factors were observed in the "seven countries" study between areas with varying occurrence of CHD.[4] Smoking and obesity were found to be important risk factors of sudden death in middle-aged men in the Framingham Study.[11] Serum cholesterol and blood pressure were apparently less powerful predictors of sudden death.

The factors related to the risk of sudden death and to the suddenness of CHD death in North Karelian men were explored in a longitudinal study of a random population sample. A 6.6% sample of the population aged 25–59 in North Karelia was surveyed between February and April of 1972. Eighty-six percent of the men in the sample participated in the field examination. Smoking was recorded by a questionnaire; height, weight and blood pressure were measured; and serum cholesterol was determined for 2455 men. Of these 2455, 173 had a history of AMI or angina in the preceding 12 months. The details of the survey methods are published elsewhere.[8, 9, 12]

Sudden coronary deaths in the cohort examined in 1972 were derived from the community-based AMI register functioning in North Karelia since May 1, 1972.[13, 14] According to the register, 57 fatal AMIs occurred among men in this cohort between May 1, 1972 and December 31, 1978. Of these, 27 were sudden deaths. Of the men suffering a sudden death, 18 had no AMI or angina in the preceding 12 months.

Separate multiple logistic models were constructed in which the following factors were entered: smoking (1, if a smoker), body-mass index (BMI) (1, if 29 kg/m² or more), systolic blood pressure (1, if 190 mm Hg or higher), serum cholesterol (1, if 310 mg/dL or more), physical activity at work and in leisure time (separately) (1, if nonactive), coffee consumption (1, if seven cups a day or more), alcohol consumption (1, if spirits were taken at least twice a week), perception of psychosocial stress (1, if continuously stressed for at least 1 year), history of AMI or angina in parents under the age of 50 years (1, if present in either parent), education (1, if 7 or fewer years in school), and income (1, if 2,000 (United States) dollars or less a year). Age was included as a second predictor for the purpose of adjustment. When analyzed separately, serum cholesterol, smoking, systolic blood pressure, physical activity in leisure time, and education were significantly associated with the risk of sudden death (TABLE 1).

CHD-free men with serum cholesterol of 310 mg/100 ml or more had an age-adjusted sudden death risk of 9.3 (90% confidence interval [CI], 3.9–22.0) relative to those with a lower cholesterol level. Smokers had an age-adjusted relative risk of sudden death of 2.3 (90% CI, 1.0–5.2). The respective relative risk of sudden death associated with the systolic blood pressure of 190 mm Hg or more was 2.2 (90% CI, 0.6–7.7). Low physical activity in leisure time was associated with a relative risk of 2.8 (90% CI, 1.3–12.6).

Among those who died of AMI within 28 days of the event, the only factor that was associated with the suddenness of death was serum cholesterol. Those with a serum cholesterol of 310 mg/100 ml or more had a 3.8 times greater (90% CI, 1.3–10.6) age-adjusted probability of dying within 1 hour than those with serum cholesterol 310 mg/100 ml or less. Cigarette smoking as classified

TABLE 1

AGE-ADJUSTED RELATIVE RISKS * OF SUDDEN CORONARY DEATH ASSOCIATED WITH SELECTED FACTORS IN 2455 MEN AND 2282 MEN AGED 25–59 WITH NO CHD IN THE PRECEDING 12 MONTHS

	All men		CHD-free men	
	Relative Risk	90% CI	Relative Risk	90% CI
Serum cholesterol (≥ 310 mg/dl)	4.8 †	2.5–9.2	9.3 †	3.9–22.0
Smoking (≥ 1 cigarette/day)	1.9 §	1.0–3.7	2.3 §	1.0–5.2
Systolic blood pressure (≥ 190 mm Hg)	2.7 §	1.1–6.7	2.2	0.6–7.7
Low physical activity in leisure time	1.8	1.0–3.3	2.8 §	1.4–6.0
Low education (≤ 7 years in school)	5.0 §	1.7–14.8	4.1 ‡	1.3–12.6
Number of events	27		18	

* Based on multiple logistic models, including age as the second independent variable. Relative risk estimates are computed as antilogarithms of the original coefficients of dichotomized predictors. The high-risk category is defined in parenthesis, one-tailed significance levels are indicated as † if p < 0.001, ‡ if p < 0.01 and § if p < 0.05.

here had no relationship and body-mass index had a weak inverse association with the suddenness of death in this material.

These results differ somewhat from the findings of the Framingham Study.[11] The discordance might be attributable to differences in the means and distributions of the risk factors in the populations at risk.

MODIFICATION OF RISK FACTORS IN AN ENTIRE COMMUNITY

General Principles of the North Karelia Project

When the magnitude and nature of the problem were considered, the fact that cardiovascular diseases (CVDs) were so common and that the risk factors and preceding stages involved a major proportion of the population, it was quite evident that we were dealing with a community problem. Accordingly, our aim was to control these diseases for the whole community.

Because CVDs are related to each other in their natural course and control measures, it appeared sensible to integrate their control activities. It was decided to base the control program on the existing community service structure, and to direct and develop the existing services to meet the program needs.

The North Karelia project was started in North Karelia in 1972 as a comprehensive community-based program to control CVDs. The main program objective was to reduce the population's CVD mortality and morbidity. Although middle-aged men were emphasized, the intermediate objectives were a reduction of smoking, serum cholesterol levels and elevated blood pressure levels among the whole population. Early detection, systematic treatment, and rehabilitation of CVD patients was also a goal. The project protocol called for the first program evaluation to take place over the 5-year period from the spring of 1972 to the spring of 1977.

The program's activities were integrated into the area's service structure and social organization. Comprehensive community action used the mass media and other general health education measures to teach risk-factor-lowering skills. Delivery of practical services, training of local personnel, introduction of environmental changes, and creation of information systems were also part of the program. Official administrative support was combined with motivation and training of personnel. Community involvement and participation were particularly stressed.[8, 15, 16]

Program Implementation

Subprograms were established to work toward alleviating each of three coronary disease risk factors on a community-wide basis. A county-wide campaign to reduce or eliminate cigarette smoking in the population was launched in 1972. Smoking was banned in all public vehicles and public buildings. This action was supplemented by antismoking posters in public places, lectures in schools, and antismoking advertisements in newspapers and on radio and television. Special efforts were made to reduce smoking among health personnel, teachers and among those individuals identified by screening programs as having CVD or being at high risk of developing CVD. Group therapy sessions for confirmed smokers were also established.[8, 16]

The dietary program sought to reduce the total fat consumption in dairy products, sausages and other high-fat meat. With the cooperation of the dairy industry, low-fat and nonfat milk were recommended and became the staple dietary product. Margarine was recommended as a butter substitute and sausage was modified by including 25% mushrooms to lower the fat content. Use of vegetable oil in food and cooking was encouraged. Fresh vegetables, seldom seen in the North Karelian diet, were encouraged, as were family vegetable plots. In addition, drug therapy was recommended for high-risk individuals with hypercholesterolemia not normalized by dietary change.[8]

A county-wide screening program to detect individuals with elevated arterial blood pressure was undertaken. Hypertensive persons were listed in a special register and usually placed on antihypertensive therapy. They were followed up by public health nurses in special dispensaries.[8, 17]

Special efforts were made to identify individuals with clinical coronary heart disease. If such persons were not already under a physician's care, treatment was initiated. Community programs taught cardiopulmonary resuscitation. A rehabilitation program was started for the medical follow-up of patients who had suffered acute myocardial infarction. This included organized group activities for secondary prevention and rehabilitation.[18] A separate, intensified service was established primarily for the middle-aged male population found to be at high risk for CVD.[19] Although most of the intervention was directed towards the general population as environmental changes, general information and regional campaigns, health service activities were individually oriented and directed largely towards patients and population groups at high risk of CVD.

RESULTS OF THE COMMUNITY-BASED PREVENTION PROGRAM

Risk Factor Changes in 1972–77

The evaluation of the program-related changes in the major CHD risk factors was based on comparison of independent population samples from the program area and the matched reference area. The neighboring county of Kuopio was chosen as the reference area because it was the most comparable with regard to demographic, socioeconomic, and epidemiologic characteristics of the population. In each survey separate samples were drawn before (in 1972) and after (in 1977) the first 5 years of the program. A pretest–post-test separate sample design was chosen because of the tendency of the cohort design to overestimate the net changes connected with the program being tested.[20]

About 11,000 persons were examined in each survey, with participation rates of about 90%. The risk factor changes were analyzed both in the birth cohort examined in 1972 (then aged 25–59) and in the same age range (30–59 years) in 1972 and 1977. The results essentially did not differ. Only a brief summary of the risk factor changes that were observed in the birth cohort analysis will be presented here.

Smoking

The proportion of smokers in the population was the same in the two areas before the program. Smoking among men decreased considerably in both areas; a smaller reduction was present among women. After adjustment for changes in the reference area, there was a net reduction of 3% in the prevalence of smoking for men and 6% for women, both within sampling variation. The reported tobacco consumption among men in North Karelia declined 10% more than in the reference area (p < 0.05). This was partly due to North Karelian men's smoking more than men in the reference area in 1972, a difference that disappeared during the program. Otherwise, the findings on tobacco consumption were similar to those on smoking prevalence.

Serum Cholesterol

In 1972 the average serum cholesterol level in North Karelia in all sex and age groups was higher than in the reference area. During the program this difference declined among women and was reversed among men. There was a net reduction in North Karelia of 4% (11 mg/dL) among men and a non-significant net reduction of 1% among women (3 mg/dL). The net reduction in the proportion of elevated serum cholesterol values (≥270 mg/dL or 7.0 mmol/L) was greater than for the means. This net reduction was 16% among men and 9% among women.

Blood Pressure

The average casual systolic blood pressure at the outset in North Karelia was somewhat higher than in the reference area. This difference was reversed during the follow-up period, so that there was a net reduction in North Karelia both for men (4% or 5 mm Hg) and women (5% or 7 mm Hg). In 1972, the average casual diastolic blood pressure for men was lower in North Karelia than in the reference area. No marked difference was found among women. During the follow-up period a net reduction in North Karelia was observed both among men (3% or 3 mm Hg) and among women (4% or 3 mm Hg). Because the aim of the hypertension program was to systematically control elevated blood pressure values, it is relevant to look at the prevalence rates of elevated values according to given criteria: ≥175 mm Hg systolic or ≥100 mm Hg diastolic or both on the resting blood pressure measurements. At the outset these prevalence rates were similar among men in the two areas, but among women the prevalence was higher in North Karelia. The net reduction in the prevalence of elevated values in North Karelia was substantial, both among men (34%) and among women (32%).

The mean of the CHD risk estimate, based on a multiple logistic model derived from a 5-year follow-up of the baseline survey sample,[14] was higher in North Karelia than in the reference area in 1972. During the follow-up period there was a considerable net reduction of estimated CHD risk in North Karelia, both among men (17%) and among women (12%).[8]

There was a clear net reduction—although not great in absolute terms—in the mean levels of all three risk factors among men in the whole intervention community. Among women, similar net changes were found only for systolic and diastolic blood pressure.

The results presented here suggest that the population risk factor levels in North Karelia changed during the intervention period. Five years are a long enough period to say that changes on the individual level are not short-term fluctuations; however, whether there will be further changes in the community after this period is still open to question.[8, 20]

CHANGES IN MORBIDITY AND MORTALITY DUE TO CORONARY HEART DISEASE

The system of CHD surveillance in North Karelia consists of an AMI register and systematic collection of death records in the county medical office. These monitoring methods have been used continuously since the start of the program and cover the whole county. All men and women living in North Karelia in whom AMI is suspected are included in the register as soon as possible, regardless of whether they are alive or dead at the time of registration. Almost all AMI patients are treated as inpatients in the central hospital or the wards of the health centers. This helps the registration considerably. In accordance with the study criteria of the World Health Organization,[5] the registered heart attack cases are classified by a doctor into the following diagnostic categories: "definite AMI," "possible AMI," "no AMI," and "insufficient data." The last category consists of those dead patients in whom AMI as the cause of death can be neither confirmed nor ruled out on the basis of the available information.

To investigate the reliability over time of the diagnostic classification of the cases of heart attack registered, a random sample of 30 cases per year was blindly reclassified by the doctor who made the initial classification. There was no significant disagreement between the two classifications whether by year or when all cases were considered together.[13]

According to the AMI register, the age-adjusted annual incidence of all AMIs decreased by 25% from 1973 (16.7 per 1000; 99% CI, 14.8–18.6) to 1979 (12.6 per 1000; 99% CI, 10.9–14.3) among men aged 35–64 (FIG. 1, TABLE 2). The age-adjusted annual mortality due to ischemic heart disease (IHD) (ICD 410–414, 8th revision) based on national statistics did not change notably between 1973 and 1977 (FIG. 1). Among women there was no consistent trend in AMI incidence or IHD mortality (FIG. 2). When only the diagnostic category of "definite AMI" was considered, the reduction in the incidence among men was even greater. The age-adjusted annual incidence of "definite AMI" in men aged 35–64 fell by 36% from 10.4 (99% CI, 8.9–12.0) per thousand in 1973 to 6.6 (99% CI, 5.4–7.9) in 1979 (FIG. 3). Among women there was no change (FIG. 4).

According to the AMI register there was no change in short-term AMI case-fatality rates from 1973 to 1979. However, there was a nonsignificant trend towards a decreasing age-adjusted prehospital fatality of all AMIs. In both sexes combined, it declined by 22% from 23% in 1973 to 18% in 1979 in the age group of 35–64. The ratio of prehospital deaths to all deaths due to AMI within 28 days in men aged 35–64 was 75% in 1973 and 46% in 1978. The proportion of sudden deaths (death within 1 hour of onset of symptoms) of all deaths within 28 days did not change significantly over time among men or among women. The proportion of sudden deaths in the pooled data of the years 1975–78 was 58% (349 out of 603) of all early deaths (within 28 days) among men and 46% (54 out of 117) among women aged 35–64 years.

The age-adjusted annual incidence of AMI with death in the first 28 days declined nonsignificantly by 21% from 5.6 (99% CI, 4.5–6.7) in 1973 to

4.4 per thousand persons (99% CI, 3.4–5.4) in 1978 among men and did not change among women aged 35–64 (FIG. 5). The age-adjusted annual incidence of prehospital deaths from AMI fell by 51% from 4.2 per thousand persons (99% CI, 3.2–5.2) in 1973 to 2.1 (99% CI, 1.3–2.8) in 1978 among men aged 35–64 (FIG. 6). The respective decrease among women was 55% (nonsignificant) from 0.6 (99% CI, 0.2–0.9) in 1973 to 0.2 (99% CI, 0.0–10.05) in 1978.

Starting in 1975, the time-lag between the onset of symptoms and death was recorded as precoded categorical data. This improved the completeness of information from 20 to 30% of the data missing for those dying within 28 days before 1975 to practically no missing data in the classification of sudden deaths after 1975. For this reason, data on the occurrence of sudden death are presented only for the years 1975–78.

The age-adjusted annual incidence of sudden death among men aged 35–64 was 3.2 per thousand persons (99% CI, 2.3–4.1) in 1975 and 2.8 per thousand

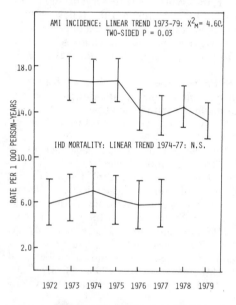

FIGURE 1. Age-adjusted annual incidence of AMI (register data) and mortality from IHD (national statistics) among men aged 35–64 during 1972–79 in North Karelia. Bars indicate 99% confidence limits.

persons (99% CI, 2.0–3.6) in 1978 (FIG. 7). The respective incidence of sudden death among women was 0.4 9(9% CI, 0.1–0.7) in 1975 and 0.3 (99% CI, 0.1–0.6) in 1978.

The evaluation of the effects of the intervention program on mortality and morbidity in North Karelia will be based on the comparison of the changes in the program area and the matched reference area. The data on mortality from AMI, CHD and all CVDs are derived from the national death certificate register. Those on the incidence of AMI and other CVDs are derived from the national hospital discharge data register. The preliminary data for the years 1972–1977 show no significant differences in these indicators between the program and reference area either among men or women aged 35–64. Due to the long latency from data collection to the closure of the national data files, the final results for the period of 1972–79 can only be presented later.

TABLE 2

NUMBER OF AMIs AND DEATHS FROM IHD AND STANDARDIZED RATE RATIOS AMONG
MEN AGED 35–64 IN NORTH KARELIA DURING 1973–79

	Year							Chi-Square for Linear Trend *
	1973	1974	1975	1976	1977	1978	1979	
No. of AMIs	482	465	465	397	397	404	352	4.60, p < 0.05
SRR † for AMI	1.00	0.96	0.96	0.83	0.79	0.85	0.75	
No. of IHD deaths	185	199	178	161	162			1.86, NS
SRR for IHD		1.00	0.90	0.83	0.83			

* Mantel-extension test.
† Standardized rate ratio.

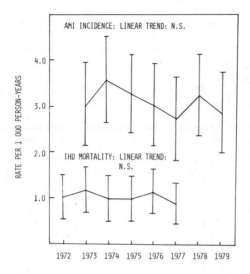

FIGURE 2. Age-adjusted annual incidence of AMI (register data) and mortality from IHD (national statistics) among women aged 35–64 during 1972–79 in North Karelia. Bars indicate 99% confidence limits.

A continuous and prospective community-based disease register is, as a tool of disease surveillance, the only system that can systematically detect sudden deaths in the population. A retrospective investigation of death certificates or hospital records cannot achieve the same result unless strict and rigid standards are effective in recording the diagnostic data and the time-lag between the onset of symptoms and death.

According to the register data, the incidence of AMI declined among middle-aged North Karelian men during and after the program. The decline in AMI mortality was smaller than the decline in incidence. These findings have not yet been confirmed by the national death certificate statistics.

The intervention program in North Karelia was only gradually built into the community and the changes in the risk factor levels occurred gradually over the 5-year period. Since an exposure period of decades is probably needed for an individual to develop CVD, effects of a community program might be expected only after several years of intervention. For this reason, we are continuing to monitor morbidity and mortality in these areas.

FIGURE 3. Age-adjusted annual incidence of "definite" and other AMI (register data) among men aged 35–64 during 1973–79 in North Karelia. Bars indicate 99% confidence intervals.

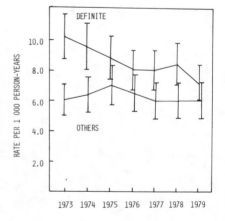

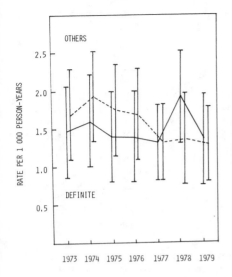

FIGURE 4. Age-adjusted annual incidence of "definite" and other AMI (register data) among women aged 35–64 during 1973–79 in North Karelia. Bars indicate 99% confidence intervals.

CONCLUSION

A comprehensive community-based prevention program for the control of CHD and other CVDs was carried out from 1972 to 1977 in the county of North Karelia, Eastern Finland. This is an area with exceptionally high rates of cardiovascular disease.

The existing studies [21-24] have shown that prevention programs are acceptable and that risk factor levels can be modified to a considerable degree. The greatest reduction in risk factor levels in multifactorial preventive trials is achieved in persons who are at very high risk and who are subjected to intensive counseling. A significant decrease in the incidence of CHD followed the reduc-

FIGURE 5. Age-adjusted annual incidence of fatal (in 28 days) AMI (register data) among men and women aged 35–64 during 1973–78 in North Karelia. Bars indicate 99% confidence intervals.

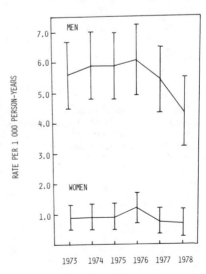

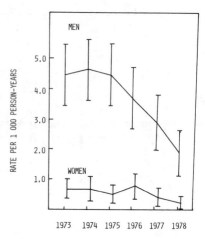

FIGURE 6. Age-adjusted annual prehospital mortality due to AMI (register data) among men and women aged 35–64 during 1973–78 in North Karelia. Bars indicate 99% confidence intervals.

tions in risk factor levels in the Oslo study.[22] However, in our studies in North Karelia [12] we found that those at high risk from one risk factor do not necessarily change their behaviors regarding other risk factors more than do those with low levels of the first risk factor. People seem to pick and choose how they are going to change; they may not choose the factor that puts them at highest risk. The intervention team has to be prepared to deal with this.

The levels of major risk factors declined in North Karelia during the project period. The decline was most marked among men. Although the final effects on CHD incidence are still to be shown, there was also a clear decline in AMI incidence and some reduction in the incidence of sudden death.

In high-occurence areas, more than half of the incidence of CHD is determined by only a few factors. These are to a great extent behavioral in origin and the data from recent intervention studies [22] and the decline in CVD mor-

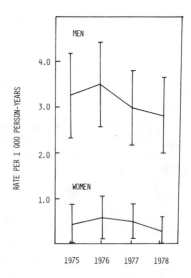

FIGURE 7. Age-adjusted annual incidence of sudden coronary deaths (register data) among men and women aged 35–64 during 1975–78 in North Karelia. Bars indicate 99% confidence intervals.

tality in the United States during the 1970s [25] confirm that it is possible to prevent and control CHD.

About half of the deaths due to acute CHD occur outside of hospitals and more than a third occur in the first half-hour after the onset of symptoms.[5] These deaths are currently beyond the reach of curative activities, but even if more effective emergency services could be developed, nonfatal infarction results in permanent damage to the myocardium. Clinic-based preventive intervention carries with it the costs of identifying high-risk individuals and the problems of missing the bulk of potential disease when only those at high risk in the population are targeted. With community-based programs, the problem of high cost is avoided, while all individuals who are susceptible and amendable to behavior change receive the message. This appears to make community-based programs the method of choice in populations where the mean risk of cardiovascular diseases is high.

REFERENCES

1. BOLANDER, A-M. 1971. A comparative study of mortality by cause in four Nordic countries, 1966–68, with special reference to male excess mortality. Statistic Rep. **9:**

2. LEPPO, K., J. LINDGREN & M. RITAMIES. 1972. Mortality trends in the 1960's. *In* Yearbook of Population Research in Finland XII, 1971. Vammala.

3. KEYS, A. 1970. Coronary heart disease in seven countries. American Heart Association Monograph No. 29. New York, NY.

4. KEYS, A., C. ARAVANIS, H. BLACKBURN, R. BUZINA, B. S. DJORDJEVIC, A. S. DONTAS, F. FIDANZA, M. J. KARVONEN, N. KIMURA, A. MENOTTI, I. MOHACEK, S. NEDELKOVIC, V. PUDDU, S. PUNSAR, H. L. TAYLOR & F. S. P. VAN BUCHEM. 1980. Seven Countries. A Multivariate Analysis of Death and Coronary heart disease. Harvard University Press. Cambridge, MA.

5. WORLD HEALTH ORGANIZATION. 1976. Myocardial infarction community registers. Public Health in Europe 5. WHO/EURO. Copenhagen, Denmark.

6. POHJOLA, S., P. SILTANEN, M. ROMO, J. HAAPAKOSKI, J. SALONEN, P. PUSKA, H. MUSTANIEMI, R. RUOSTEENOJA, M. ARSTILA & V. KALLIO. 1980. Sydäninfarktin esiintyvyys ja ennuste Suomessa vuonna 1973. Helsingin, Turun, Tampereen ja Pohjois-Karjalan rekistereiden vertailua. Duodecim **96:** 18–31.

7. KARVONEN, M., E. ORMA, A. KEYS, F. FIDANZA & J. BROZEK. 1959. Cigarette smoking, serum cholesterol, blood pressure and body fatness. Observations in Finland. Lancet **1:** 492.

8. PUSKA, P., J. TUOMILEHTO, J. SALONEN, A. NISSINEN, J. VIRTAMO, S. BJÖRKQVIST, K. KOSKELA, L. NEITTAANMÄKI, T. TAKALO, T. E. KOTTKE, J. MÄKI, P. SIPILÄ & P. VARVIKKO. 1981. The North Karelia Project: Evaluation of a comprehensive community programme for control of cardiovascular diseases in 1972–77 in North Karelia, Finland. WHO/EURO Monograph series. Copenhagen, Denmark.

9. TUOMILEHTO, J., P. PUSKA, J. VIRTAMO, J. MÄKI, J. SALONEN & K. KOSKELA. 1979. The levels of the major risk indicators of cardiovascular diseases in Eastern Finland prior to a community-based intervention programme (The North Karelia Project). Acta Cardiol. **6:** 359–374.

10. KANNEL, W. B., J. T. DOYLE, P. M. McNAMARA, P. QUICKENTON & T. GORDON. 1975. Precursors of sudden coronary death: Factors related to incidence of sudden death. Circulation **51:** 606–613.

11. THOMAS, H. E., C. B. CLARK, W. B. KANNEL, P. M. McNAMARA & R. J. HAVLIK. 1981. Sudden death from coronary heart disease. The Framingham Study. CVD Epidemiol. Newsletter **30:** 54.

12. SALONEN, J. T. 1980. Smoking and dietary fats in relation to estimated risk of myocardial infarction before and during a preventive community programme. Publications of the University of Kuopio, Community Health, Series Original Reports 1/80.
13. SALONEN, J. T., P. PUSKA & H. MUSTANIEMI. 1979. Cardiovascular morbidity and mortality changes during the comprehensive community programme for the control of cardiovascular diseases during 1972–7 in North Karelia, Finland. Br. Med. J. 2: 1178–1183.
14. SALONEN, J. T., P. PUSKA & T. E. KOTTKE. 1981. Smoking, blood pressure and serum cholesterol as risk factors of acute myocardial infarction and death among men in Eastern Finland. Eur. Heart J. 2: 365–373.
15. PUSKA, P. 1980. The North Karelia Project: Health promotion in action. In Strategies for Public Health, Promoting Health and Preventing Disease. K. Y. Lorenz & L. D. Devra, Eds.: 317–335. Van Nostrand-Reinhold. New York, N.Y.
16. TUOMILEHTO, J., K. KOSKELA, P. PUSKA, S. BJÖRKQVIST & J. SALONEN. 1978. A community anti-smoking programme: Interim evaluation of the North Karelia Project. Int. J. Health Educ. 21: Suppl.
17. TUOMILEHTO, J., A. NISSINEN, J. T. SALONEN, T. E. KOTTKE & P. PUSKA. 1980. Community programme for control of hypertension in North Karelia, Finland. Lancet 2: 900–903.
18. SALONEN, J. & P. PUSKA. 1980. A community programme for rehabilitation and secondary prevention for patients with acute myocardial infarction as part of a comprehensive community programme for control of cardiovascular diseases (North Karelia Project). Scand. J. Rehab. Med. 12: 33–42.
19. VIRTAMO, J. 1978. Effects of mass health examination of a rural population with particular reference to cardiovascular risk factors. Publications of the University of Kuopio, Community Health, Series Original Reports 1/78.
20. SALONEN, J. T., P. PUSKA, T. E. KOTTKE & J. TUOMILEHTO. 1981. Changes in smoking, serum cholesterol and blood pressure levels during a community-based cardiovascular disease prevention program—the North Karelia project. Am. J. Epidemiol. 114: 81–94.
21. FARQUHAR, J. W., N. MACCOBY, P. D. WOOD, J. K. ALEXANDER, H. BREITROSE, B. W. BROWN, JR., W. L. HASKELL, A. L. MCALISTER, A. J. MEYER, J. D. NASH & M. P. STERN. 1977. Community education for cardiovascular health. Lancet 1: 1192–1195.
22. HJERMANN, I., K. VELVE BYRE, I. HOLME & P. LEREN. 1981. Effect of diet and smoking intervention on the incidence of coronary heart disease. Lancet 2: 1303–1310.
23. ROSE, G., R. F. HELLER, H. TUNSTALL-PEDOE & D. G. S. CHRISTIE. 1980. Heart disease prevention project: A randomized controlled trial in industry. Br. Med. J. 1: 747.
24. KORNITZER, M., G. DE BACKER, M. DRAMAIX & C. THILLY. 1980. The Belgian heart disease prevention project. Modification of the coronary risk profile in an industrial population. Circulation 61: 18.
25. HAVLIK, R. J. & M. FEINLIEB. 1979. Proceedings of the Conference on the Decline in Coronary Heart Disease Mortality. National Heart, Lung, and Blood Institute, October 24–25, 1978. Bethesda, MD.

DISCUSSION

DR. MOSS: I would like to congratulate the speaker and his group, for this is clearly a landmark presentation. This study has profound implications and I will ask Dr. Doyle to comment upon it because, to my knowledge, this is the first primary intervention prevention trial that has shown such dramatic findings.

DR. DOYLE: I too would like to congratulate Dr. Salonen on his meticulously conducted trial, which indeed, as Dr. Moss points out, is the first with truly substantive results. This is a matter of considerable interest to the recently dormant Intersociety Commission on Heart Disease Resources. We have been in the process for several years of rewriting the position paper and have been hard pressed to find reliable information that confirms what we all regard as a reasonable hypothesis, that risk factor interventions of the type described are indeed effective.

DR. MOSS: The percentage of the risk factor reduction was remarkably small, yet the effect was unequivocal. Was this a surprise to you?

DR. SALONEN: The magnitude of risk factors changes wasn't exactly a surprise for us because what was shown to you was a change in mean population levels. For individuals the change can be substantial.

DR. DWYER: What percent of the population stopped smoking entirely?

DR. SALONEN: About 10% of current smokers stopped smoking.

DR. TUCKMAN (New York, New York): With respect to your antihypertensive program, was there any sort of cooperation among the treating physicians as to the type of treatment they would deliver?

DR. SALONEN: There was a training program for treatment of hypertension, but no recommendation about drugs was given by the project group. But there was a national hypertension committee that made some recommendations, but that was not part of the North Korelia Project. In Finland, as in all Nordic countries, beta blocking agents are most often used for hypertension.

DR. MOSS: There was a reduction not only in total cardiac death, but also in sudden cardiac death. Did the proportion change? Did the ratio of sudden cardiac death to total cardiac death change or was the effect distributed equally?

DR. SALONEN: The ratio of sudden deaths to all coronary deaths changed only slightly.

THE PATIENT WITH CORONARY ARTERY
DISEASE WITHOUT INFARCTION:
CAN A HIGH-RISK GROUP BE IDENTIFIED?

Jan Erikssen

Cardiological Section, Medical Department B
Rikshospitalet, Oslo 1, Norway

Reidar Mundal

Institute of Work Physiology
Norwegian College of Physical Education
Oslo 3, Norway

Although the ability to predict coronary heart disease in surveys of part of the population is fairly accurate,[1,2] it could be improved by adding diagnostic tests within an acceptable ethical and cost/benefit framework. This implies, however, that methods such as isotopic and angiographic studies cannot be used for the screening of large, apparently healthy populations. However, such methods ought to be used to validate results of the less expensive and cumbersome survey methods commonly used.

The present report deals with baseline and follow-up data from a survey population of apparently healthy, middle-aged men first studied approximately 7 years ago.[3] (The examination program is shown in TABLE 1). The follow-up data gave us the opportunity (1) to assess the misclassification regarding the presence or absence of coronary heart disease (CHD) at the baseline examination in relation to the development of CHD events during follow-up; (2) to study the course of latent, angiographically verified CHD; and (3) to assess the value of risk-factor screening for CHD prediction, with particular reference to the information gained by adding exercise electrocardiographic testing to conventional CHD-screening techniques. Scrutiny of these data may facilitate the identification of subjects at particularly high risk of developing complications of a clinically silent or oligosymptomatic coronary artery disease (CAD).

MATERIAL AND METHODS

Two thousand fourteen apparently healthy working men aged 40–59 years underwent a comprehensive baseline examination during the years 1972–75, and all men still alive have currently been summoned for a reexamination (TABLE 1).

The selection procedures and reasons for exclusion have been presented elsewhere.[3] In particular, men with known or suspected CHD and other heart disease were excluded, as were men with hypertension being treated with drugs, diabetes mellitus, defined disorders of the locomotor system, and miscellaneous other diseases.[3] The participation rate in the baseline study was 86%. Of the 785 men so far summoned for reexamination, 724 (92%) have participated.

438

0077-8923/82/0382-0438 $1.75/0 © 1982, NYAS

The prospective angiographic study during the baseline study was conducted in men who fulfilled one or more of the following criteria, suggesting latent CHD:

1. A positive exercise test during and/or post exercise.[3]
2. A positive World Health Organization (WHO) angina questionnaire on personal interview.[4]
3. Typical angina pectoris developing during near maximal stress on bicycle exercise test.
4. A Minnesota Code (MC) of the 1.1-type on a resting 12-lead electro-cardiogram.[4]

One hundred fifteen men fulfilled one or more of these criteria, and angiography was performed in the 109 who gave their informed consent (four of these were excluded later for various reasons).[3] Sixty-nine had pathologic angiograms (angiopositive men) and 36 had normal coronary angiograms. The details of this angiographic study have been presented elsewhere.[3] All angiographied men have been followed closely.

Thirty-two men had mild angina pectoris according to the clinically oriented New York Health Insurance Plan Survey Questionnaire (NY-Q) (TABLE 1)[5] without fulfilling the criteria for a suspect, latent CHD presented above. These individuals were not studied further during the initial survey. The remaining 1867 were labeled "normals" for practical purposes.

Deaths have been classified as being *cardiac* or *noncardiac*. The Norwegian Central Bureau of Statistics has provided complete data on causes of death as well as additional information (such as autopsy reports, available in 60% of the present series). The 73 deaths (40 noncardiac and 33 cardiac) had been reported by January 31, 1981. Our primary selection procedures[3] probably explain why no case of cardiac death due to chronic congestive heart failure, valvular heart disease, cor pumonale or other specified, chronic heart disease

TABLE 1

BASELINE AND FOLLOW-UP EXAMINATION PROGRAMS *

1. A comprehensive *case history* (including WHO angina questionnaire and New York Health Insurance Plan Survey Questionnaire on Angina).[4, 5]
2. Full clinical examination and spirographic studies.
3. A panel of blood tests (an intravenous glucose tolerance test [IVGT] only in †, and insulin response to the IVGT in ‡)
4. Phonocardiography,† resting electrocardiogram and near maximal bicycle exercise electrocardiographic test.
5. X-ray film of heart and lungs.
6. Platelet studies † and study of coagulation factors †
7. Selective coronary angiography in men with strong suspicion of latent CHD (that is, fulfilling particular survey criteria, informed consent was obtained).[3]‡
8. Isotope studies of myocardial perfusion and left ventricular function at rest and during exercise.§
9. Echocardiography.§
10. Electrokymography at rest and during exercise.§

* Tests not labelled †, ‡, or § were performed in all individuals during both surveys.
† Studied in all, but only during the baseline survey.
‡ Studied in subgroups during baseline study.
§ Studied in subgroups only during follow-up examination.

(apart from CHD) was encountered. Of the 33 cardiac deaths, 26 occurred within 24 hours of the presenting symptoms (mainly instantaneously and witnessed) and 7 during the course of an acute myocardial infarction ≧24 hours after the onset of symptoms.[6]

CHD events among the "normals" disclosed at reexamination were classified as: (A) coronary death; (B) myocardial infarction (MI); (C) angina pectoris de novo; and (D) positive exercise electrocardiographic test de novo.

(A) In view of the available information on modes of death, autopsy findings, and in the absence of information on other chronic heart disease (see above), all cardiac deaths have been attributed to coronary disease. (This approach may cause a slight misclassification.[6]) Thus, all cardiac deaths among the "normals" summoned so far have been labeled CHD deaths.

(B) A diagnosis of myocardial infarction was given to men who became acutely ill during follow-up, and who fulfilled at least two of the following three criteria: (1) typical chest pain of ≧30 minutes' duration; (2) typical enzyme pattern during the acute phase, with a peak value of ASAT, creatine phosphokinase (CPK) or lactic dehydrogenase (LDH) (including isoenzyme) exceeding the upper normal limit of the respective laboratory by a factor of 2; (3) development of a Minnesota Code of the 1.1-type during the acute phase.

If enzymes could not be studied, a myocardial infarction was only diagnosed in the presence of criteria 1 and 3. Since all clinically diagnosed myocardial infarctions were treated in hospitals within a limited geographic area, complete information on all myocardial infarctions was easily obtained.

(C) Angina pectoris de novo was defined as a NY-Q score ≧10.[5] By definition, none of the "normals" had a NY-Q ≧10 on the baseline examination.

(D) A positive exercise electrocardiographic test de novo was said to be present in men who, in the absence of the use of confounding drugs and conditions as specified earlier,[3] had: a horizontal or downward or upsloping S-T segment during and/or post exercise of ≧1.5 mm in either of the chest-head leads 2–7, or ≧1.0 mm in standard leads I, II, aVF, aVL or V leads 2–7 ≧0.08 sec from the J point.[3] In the presence of some S-T segment depression at rest, an additional 1.5-mm S-T depression was necessary for labeling a test positive.

In the presence of more than one CHD event as defined above, only the highest classification has been counted (that is, cardiac death highest and a positive stress test lowest).

CHD progression was said to have occurred in an angiopositive man if he either (a) died from CHD or (b) had a myocardial infarction during follow-up; or (c) developed angina pectoris de novo (that is, had a NY-Q-score ≧10)[5]; or (d) if a mild angina pectoris diagnosed at the baseline examination[3] progressed to a degree that another angiographic study was thought necessary for assessing the possibility of performing a coronary bypass operation. However, if the second angiographic study failed to show more pronounced arterial lesions than on the first angiograms, CHD progression was not said to be present.

Neither did we classify as CHD progression a decline in exercise capacity or the development of a more pathologic exercise electrocardiogram during follow-up.

In order to study the feasibility of pinpointing the men whom follow-up proved to have been at highest risk at the baseline examination, two group comparisons have been performed:

1. The 33 men who died from a cardiac cause have been compared with the 1807 "normals" still alive.

2. Angiopositive men who showed CHD progression have been compared with their counterparts without CHD progression.

A number of baseline data have been compared by means of multiple t tests, as reported previously.[3]

RESULTS

As mentioned earlier, 33 of the 73 men reported dead by January 31, 1981 had died from a cardiac cause. Coronary artery disease was confirmed in the 60% who had an autopsy and was suspected according to the case history/death certificates in the remaining men. FIGURE 1 shows the mortality from CHD in the study group compared with the mean Norwegian CHD mortality during

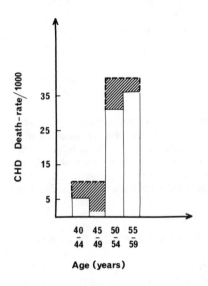

FIGURE 1. Seven-year mortality among 2014 "apparently healthy" men aged 40–59 years at survey examination. *White areas* show CHD mortality rate versus age in survey material. *Crosshatched* areas indicate excess mortality from CHD among the total Norwegian male population.

the same period. In contrast to men below 50 years, men above 50 have a CHD mortality only slightly below the Norwegian mean.[7]

The data on CHD events among the 724 men examined so far are summarized in TABLE 2. There have been 15 deaths and 27 myocardial infarctions, that is, an incidence of "hard CHD events" of 42/739 or 5.7%. Thirty men have developed angina pectoris de novo. Thus, the total incidence of clinical CHD was 72/739 or 9.7%. Sixty-three men have a positive exercise test de novo. Mean values for maximal heart rate (MHR), maximal load (ML) reached, and total work (TW) performed were almost identical with age-corrected exercise test baseline data (not shown).

Coded Q waves without a history suggesting acute myocardial infarction were found in nine men (two had MC 1.2-type and seven MC 1.3-type). These cases are not counted as CHD events.

TABLE 2

SEVEN-YEAR INCIDENCE OF VARIOUS CHD EVENTS AMONG "NORMAL" MEN HAVING
COMPLETED FOLLOW-UP EXAMINATIONS

	Number
(a) Reexamined "normals"	724 ⎫
(b) Died from CHD (among men summoned so far)	15 ⎬ "At risk" ⎭
(c) Acute myocardial infarction	27
(d) Angina pectoris de novo (NY-Q-positive)	30 (16) *
(e) Positive exercise electrocardiogram de novo	63
"Hard" CHD incidence (b + c/a + b)	42/739 (5.7%)
Total clinical CHD incidence (b + c + d/a + b)	72/739 (9.7%)
Clinical CHD events plus de novo positive exercise electrocardiographic tests (= b + c + d + e/a + b)	135/739 (18.3%)

* Number in brackets represents men with angina de novo and a concomitant positive exercise electrocardiographic test.

Comparison Between Men Who Died From Cardiac Disease and "Normals" Still Alive

A number of the variables reported in TABLE 3 differ significantly between the two groups, such as serum lipid levels and blood pressure, as expected from a number of previous CHD surveys (for example, those of Wilhelmsen et al.[1] and Kannel[2]). In addition, men who died were slightly older, had lower age-corrected spirographic values and poorer physical performance, and very low MHR during exercise, as well as unexplained higher erythrocyte sedimentation rates (ESRs).

Comparison of Angiopositive Men with and without CHD Progression

For most of the variables studied (TABLE 4) there are only minor, insignificant differences. However, the CHD progression group had poorer physical performance and higher ESR, and in addition (TABLE 5) men with CHD progression had mainly triple-vessel disease in the baseline angiograms.

FIGURE 2 shows the close positive association between poor physical fitness and (1) the risk of dying from a cardiac cause (among "normals") and (2) the risk for an angiopositive man of developing CHD progression.

As reported earlier,[8] we have divided the "normals" into 16 fitness groups, that is, quartiles for each 5-year age group. Total work (kpm)/body weight (kg) was used as the measure for physical fitness (a variable which to some extent is equivalent with treadmill time as used by others.[9, 10]). It is seen that the majority of those who died belonged to the lowest quartiles of physical fitness, and that clinical CHD progression only rarely occurred in men with high fitness in the angiopositive group.

TABLE 5 shows that clinical CHD progression was mainly found among subjects with triple-vessel disease. The progression events have mainly developed after a quiescent clinical period of 4 to 5 years after the baseline examination. It is noteworthy that of the five men with left main stem disease (LMD), two have died during follow-up, two have had bypass operations performed after the development of serious CHD symptoms, and one has had CHD progression, but his condition is technically inoperable.

Although men with triple-vessel disease had somewhat higher serum lipid levels, were older, and had marginally lower exercise capacity, the differences in TABLE 4 can only in part be explained by the skewed distribution of men with single-, double-, and triple-vessel disease (data not shown).

When data from TABLES 3 and 4 are compared, it is apparent that the men who died and the angiopositive men resemble each other closely, and in particu-

TABLE 3

VARIOUS CLINICAL, PHYSIOLOGIC AND BIOCHEMICAL VARIABLES IN MEN WHO DIED FROM ACUTE CHD DURING 7-YEAR FOLLOW-UP AND MEN INITIALLY CLASSIFIED AS "NORMALS" STILL ALIVE. A STUDY OF POSSIBLE CONTRASTS

Variable	"Normal" Men (n = 1807)		Men who Died (n = 33)		p-value for a Possible Difference *
	X	SE	X	SE	
Age (yr)	49.6	(0.13)	52.6	(0.84)	0.002
Systolic blood pressure (mm Hg)	129.6	(0.41)	140.8	(4.14)	<0.001
Diastolic blood pressure (mm Hg)	87.0	(0.24)	89.7	(2.36)	>0.10
Resting heart rate (beats/min)	61.3	(0.23)	62.4	(1.57)	>0.10
Heart volume (ml/m^2)	402	(1.37)	434	(14.7)	0.003
Hemoglobin (g/100 ml)	15.34	(0.023)	15.25	(0.174)	>0.10
ESR (Westergren) (mm/hr)	7.22	(0.15)	13.30	(1.72)	<0.001
K value (from IVGT)	1.93	(0.002)	1.76	(0.14)	>0.10
Cholesterol (mg/100 ml)	256	(1.08)	287	(7.86)	<0.001
Triglycerides (mg/100 ml)	116	(1.47)	140	(8.87)	0.028
Peak expiratory flow (L/min)	525	(2.05)	490	(14.4)	0.026
Forced expiratory volume (1 sec) (ml)	3468	(17.6)	3218	(112)	0.056
Forced vital capacity (ml)	4480	(19.1)	4163	(119)	0.026
Maximal exercise heart rate (MHR) (beats/min)	163.5	(0.31)	151.4	(2.76)	<0.001
Maximal blood pressure (mm Hg)	215.7	(0.52)	220.3	(5.22)	>0.10
Maximal load reached (ML) (kpm/min)	1094	(84.8)	936	(38.6)	<0.001
Total work performed (TW) (kpm)	11,447	(110)	8145	(668)	<0.001
Maximal heart rate–blood pressure product ($\times 10^{-3}$)	35.15	(0.11)	33.51	(1.12)	0.048

* Corrected for differences in age.

lar angiopositive men with CHD progression and men who died were almost identical for all the variables tested.

No differences in smoking habits, the prevalence of arrhythmias at rest or during exercise, or R wave response to exercise testing [11] were found among the groups (data not shown).

TABLE 4

VARIOUS CLINICAL, PHYSIOLOGIC AND BIOCHEMICAL VARIABLES IN MEN WITH POSITIVE CORONARY ANGIOGRAPHY DURING INITIAL CHD SURVEY EXAMINATION. A STUDY OF POSSIBLE CONTRASTS BETWEEN MEN WITH AND WITHOUT CLINICAL PROGRESSION OF CHD DURING 7-YEAR FOLLOW-UP *

Variable	Men with CHD Progression (n = 29)		Men Without CHD Progression (n = 40)		p Value for a Possible Difference †
Age (yr)	54.2	(0.88)	52.9	(0.84)	>0.10
Systolic blood pressure (mm Hg)	136.7	(3.40)	136.5	(3.18)	>0.10
Diastolic blood pressure (mm Hg)	87.2	(1.55)	87.9	(1.61)	>0.10
Resting heart rate (beats/min)	63.9	(1.47)	62.1	(1.77)	>0.10
Heart volume (ml/m²)	428	(15.4)	415.2	(9.9)	>0.10
Hemoglobin (g/100 ml)	15.18	(0.21)	15.25	(0.16)	>0.10
ESR (Westergren) (mm/hr)	12.46	(1.65)	7.41	(0.90)	0.005
K value (from IVGT)	1.88	(0.17)	1.67	(0.11)	>0.10
Cholesterol (mg/100 ml)	281	(6.49)	268	(7.45)	>0.10
Triglycerides (mg/100 ml)	129	(12.9)	129	(13.4)	>0.10
Peak expiratory flow (L/min)	499	(17.7)	502	(14.5)	>0.10
Forced expiratory volume (1 sec) (ml)	3044	(160)	3068	(106)	>0.10
Forced vital capacity (ml)	3980	(132)	4034	(116)	>0.10
Maximal exercise heart (MHR) rate (beats/min)	151.2	(3.52)	156.1	(2.34)	>0.10
Maximal blood pressure (mm Hg)	209	(4.90)	220	(4.39)	=0.10
Maximal loadreached (ML) (kpm/min)	879	(30.6)	995	(28.6)	0.008
Total work performed (TW) (kpm)	6812	(554)	8914	(491)	0.01
Maximal heart rate–blood pressure product ($\times 10^{-3}$)	31.66	(1.22)	34.33	(1.01)	=0.10

* For definition of CHD progression see the MATERIAL AND METHODS section.
† Corrected for differences in age.

Baseline data from men who have developed myocardial infarction or angina pectoris de novo among the 724 restudied men show that they also closely resemble the angiopositive men and the men who died (data not shown).

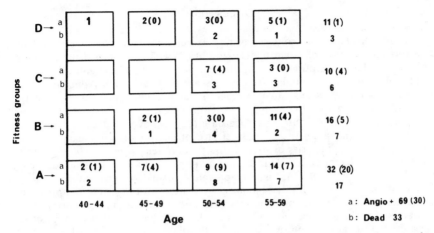

FIGURE 2. Physical fitness classification of angiopositive men (a) and men who died from CHD during 7-year follow-up (b). Comparison with quartiles for physical fitness in 1867 "normals". Lines A and B represent low-fitness groups; lines C and D represent high-fitness groups. (Figures in brackets represent cases with CHD progression.)

TABLE 5

CLINICAL COURSE OF LATENT CHD DURING 7-YEAR FOLLOW-UP. A STUDY OF 69 MEN WITH ANGIOGRAPHICALLY VERIFIED CORONARY ARTERY DISEASE DETECTED DURING A PROSPECTIVE SURVEY STUDY IN APPARENTLY HEALTHY MIDDLE-AGED MEN

No. of Diseased Coronary Vessels	CHD Progres- sion * Present	CHD Progres- sion Absent	Second Coronary Angiogram Taken	Bypass Operation Performed
Single-vessel disease (n = 18)	6(1)†	12	5(1)‡	4
Double-vessel disease (n = 25)	6(1)	19	8(2)	4
Triple-vessel disease (n = 26)	17(5)	9	11(1)	6
Totals (n = 69)	29(7)	40	24(4)	14

NOTE. χ^2 value for CHD progression versus nonprogression in men with single- and double-vessel disease versus men with triple-vessel disease is 9.33 (1 DF), that is, $p < 0.005$.

* For definitions see MATERIAL AND METHODS section.

† Numbers in parentheses represent men in the respective groups who died during follow-up.

‡ Numbers in parentheses represent reangiographed men in whom the second angiogram failed to show progression of atherosclerosis.

Discussion

During the baseline study, a positive exercise test was the most sensitive tool for the detection of latent CHD,[3] and also—with due caution for the lack of angiographic verification—during the second survey. The slightly divergent results obtained in two similar studies[12, 13] are probably mainly due to differences in study populations. In view of (1) our previous angiographic experience, (2) the fact that the men are 7 years older at follow-up, and (3) the fact that a positive exercise electrocardiogram de novo is probably a more serious finding than a positive exercise electrocardiogram on a first examination, we assume that the majority of men with a positive second electrocardiographic stress test have latent CHD. This is even more plausible since previous autopsy studies have shown that CAD is very prevalent in middle-aged men in Oslo.[14] Provided this is true, a considerable misclassification with regard to the presence or absence of CAD was made at the baseline examination, as shown by a combined CHD incidence rate of 18%. The very high incidence of positive exercise electrocardiograms is caused by the inclusion of the upsloping S-T segment response.[3] The inclusion of this electrocardiographic criterion as a sign of latent CHD is justified from our previous angiographic findings,[3] and is in concert with the experiences of many[15, 16] authors but not all.[17, 18] The mortality data (Fig. 1) also indicate that our group of "normals" probably had almost population average of advanced CHD at the baseline examination despite our selection procedures. The combined data from the approximately half-completed follow-up study indicate that one should be extremely cautious in drawing conclusions on the presence or absence of CHD in a population even after comprehensive screening procedures to exclude the presence of CHD.

The clinical course of medically or surgically treated CHD is fairly well known from hospital studies as surveyed recently,[19] whereas there is less information on the prognosis in minimal and moderate CAD.[20] On the other hand the clinical course of latent, angiographically proven CHD is largely unknown, because only a few studies in apparently healthy subjects have used angiography as a diagnostic procedure.[3, 12, 13]

Our follow-up data show that the presence of detectable, largely asymptomatic CHD is not to be considered an innocuous condition. Thus, whereas only seven men died (10% or 1.4% per year), more than 40% (6% per year) fulfilled one or more of the criteria for CHD progression. The mortality in the present, small group of angiopositive men is less than 50% of the mortality found in recent studies[21, 22] in persons with angina pectoris. However, since our 69 angiopositive men have been followed closely and have undergone a variety of treatments (for example, bypass was performed in 14 of the 69), the clinical course cannot be labeled the "natural course." However, the 6% annual progression rate supports and amplifies the notion that latent CHD is a serious clinical condition.

That subjects with triple-vessel disease were more likely to show CHD progression than were men with single- or double-vessel disease only supports previous experience in hospitalized patients.[19] It should be noted, however, that the five men with left main disease showed a poor clinical course. This suggests that a very active approach probably ought to be chosen when such cases are encountered, regardless of symptoms. Thus, only one of the five had symptoms (very mild angina) when the diagnosis was first made. The poor prognosis in patients with left main disease not operated on has been reflected for a long time in clinical studies.[19, 23, 24]

In addition to the well-known unfavorable prognosis related to high serum lipids,[1, 2] low spirographic values proved to be associated with risk of dying from CHD. A low vital capacity has proved to be of predictive value for the development of congestive heart failure.[25] The reason for this finding among our men who died is obscure, although the fact that on the average they have somewhat larger hearts may suggest that incipient heart failure was present in some.

In addition to the study of the S-T segment during exercise, increasing attention has been paid to physiologic responses to exercise in recent years.[14, 15, 26, 27] The study of variables like MHR, ML, TW and blood pressure response to exercise has, for instance, been shown to be of considerable value in predicting the outcome in CHD patients[28] as well as in healthy populations.[14, 15, 26, 27] Our present data corroborate and amplify these aspects of exercise testing. Authors who exclude from further scrutiny[18] those individuals who do not attain 90% of predicted MHR for age inevitably lose significant information from their exercise testing. Although a poor response to exercise of the aforementioned variables may well be caused by poor cooperation and/or considerable lack of training, it seems reasonable to assume that this sort of response may often represent a poorly appreciated sign of advanced, latent CHD when encountered in otherwise asymptomatic middle-aged males.

An additional, simple way of expressing the negative impact of a poor physical performance on the risk of dying from CHD and on the risk of CHD progression is shown in FIGURE 2. It is noteworthy that the majority of those who died belonged to the lowest fitness quartile for their age. It is also noteworthy that 20 of the 32 angiopositive men in the lowest fitness quartile (62.5%) showed CHD progression during follow-up in contrast to only 1 of the 11 within the highest fitness quartiles (9.1%). This difference is highly significant, and should be taken into consideration in risk predictions.

At follow-up we have defined two high-risk, noninfarct CAD groups: (1) men who died and (2) men who showed CHD progression. Such individuals should have been identified earlier for the purpose of prevention, and it is hardly a coincidence that the two groups resemble each other closely. Blood pressure and lipid values classify most of these men to conventional CHD high-risk groups.[1, 2] However, these men show additional stigmata, such as lower spirographic values and a poorer exercise test response, as mentioned earlier. From a cost/benefit view, the implications of these findings may be that the most practical approach for identifying subjects at very high risk for future CHD is (1) to make a simple, conventional, initial screening of serum lipids, blood pressure, and case history, for example; and (2) to add a more comprehensive screening for those classified conventionally as belonging to the high CHD risk groups.[1, 2] Individuals within such high-risk groups should be particular candidates for further scrutiny and prevention if, in addition, they show exercise electrocardiographic changes or have lower spirographic values or the aforementioned particular physiologic stress test response.

REFERENCES

1. WILHELMSEN, L., H. WEDEL & G. TIBBLIN. 1973. Multivariate analysis of risk factors for coronary heart disease. Circulation 48: 950–958.
2. KANNEL, W. B. 1976. Some lessons in cardiovascular epidemiology from Framingham. Am. J. Cardiol. 37: 269–282.
3. ERIKSSEN, J., I. ENGE, K. FORFANG & O. STORSTEIN. 1976. False positive

diagnostic tests and coronary angiographic findings in 105 presumably healthy males. Circulation **54**: 371–376.

4. ROSE, G. & H. BLACKBURN, Eds. 1968. Cardiovascular Survey Methods. World Health Organization Monograph Series No. 56. Geneva.

5. FRANK, C. W., E. WEINBLATT & S. SHAPIRO. 1973. Angina pectoris in men. Prognostic significance of selected medical factors. Circulation **47**: 509–517.

6. KULLER, L., M. COOPER & J. PERPER. 1972. Epidemiology of sudden death. Arch. Intern. Med. **129**: 714–719.

7. CENTRAL BUREAU OF STATISTICS OF NORWAY. Statistical Yearbook of Norway, 1980.

8. ERIKSSEN, J., K. FORFANG & J. JERVELL. 1981. Coronary risk factors and physical fitness in healthy middle aged men. Acta Med. Scand. Suppl. **645**: 57–64.

9. BRUCE, H., F. KUSUMI & D. HOSMER. 1973. Maximal oxygen intake and nomographic assessment of functional aerobic impairment in cardiovascular disease. Am. Heart J. **85**: 546–562.

10. FROELICHER, V. F., YANOWITZ, F., A. THOMPSON & M. C. LANCASTER. 1976. Treadmill exercise testing at the USAF School of Aerospace Medicine. Physiological Responses in Aircrewmen and the Detection of Latent Coronary Artery Disease. Agardograph No. **210**: 1–60.

11. BONOUS, P. E., P. S. GREENBERG, G. W. CRISTISON *et al.* 1978. Evaluation of R wave amplitude changes versus ST-segment depression in stress testing. Circulation **57**: 904–910.

12. FROELICHER, V. F., A. J. THOMPSON, M. R. LONGO, *et al.* 1976. Value of exercise testing for screening asymptomatic men for latent coronary heart disease. Progr. Cardiovasc. Dis. **18**(4): 265–276.

13. BORER, J. S., J. F. BRENSIKE, D. R. REDWOOD, *et al.* 1975. Limitations of the electrocardiographic response to exercise in predicting coronary artery disease. N. Engl. J. Med. **293**: 367–371.

14. STRONG, J. P., L. A. SOLBERG & C. RESTREPO. 1968. Atherosclerosis in persons with coronary heart disease. Lab. Invest. **18**(5): 527–537.

15. McHENRY, P. L. & C. FISCH. 1977. Clinical application of the treadmill exercise test. Mod. Conc. Cardiovasc. Dis. **46**(5): 21–25.

16. ELLESTAD, M. H. & M. K. C. Wan. 1975. Predictive implications of stress testing. Follow-up of 7200 subjects after maximum treadmill testing. Circulation **51**: 363–369.

17. ALLEN, W. H., W. S. ARONOWN, P. GOODMAN & P. STINSON. 1980. Five-year follow-up of maximal treadmill stress test in asymptomatic men and women. Circulation **62**: 522–527.

18. COHN, K., B. KAMM, F. NIZAR, R. BRAND & N. GOLDSCHLAGER. 1979. Use of treadmill score to quantify ischemic response and predict extent of coronary disease. Circulation **59**: 286–296.

19. McINTOSH, H. D. & J. A. GARCIA. 1978. The first decade of coronary bypass grafting 1967–1977. A review. Circulation **57**: 405–431.

20. MARCHANDISE, B., BOURASSA, M. G., B. R. CHAITMAN & J. LESPERANCE. 1978. Angiographic evaluation of the natural history of normal coronary arteries and mild coronary atherosclerosis. Am. J. Cardiol. **41**: 216–220.

21. EUROPEAN CORONARY STUDY GROUP. 1979. Coronary artery bypass surgery in stable angina pectoris. Lancet **i**: 889–893.

22. MURPHY, M. L., H. N. HULTGREN, K. DETRE, J. THOMSEN & T. TAKARO. 1977. Treatment of chronic stable angina. A preliminary report of survival data of the randomized Veterans Administration Cooperative Study. N. Engl. J. Med. **297**: 621–627.

23. COHEN, M. V. & R. GORLIN. 1975. Main left coronary occlusive disease. Clinical experience from 1964–1974. Circulation **52**: 275–285.

24. OBERMAN, A., R. R. HARRELL, R. O. RUSELL, JR., *et al.* 1976. Surgical versus medical treatment of the left main coronary artery. Lancet **ii:** 591–594.
25. KANNEL, W. B., J. M. SEIDMAN, W. FERCHO & W. P. CASTELLI. 1974. Vital capacity and congestive heart failure. Circulation **49:** 1160–1166.
26. BRUCE, R. A., T. A. DEROUEN, & K. F. HOSSACK. 1980. Value of maximal exercise tests in risk assessment of coronary heart disease events in healthy men. Am. J. Cardiol. **46:** 371–378.
27. ERIKSSEN, J., K. RASMUSSEN, K. FORFANG & O. STORSTEIN. 1977. Exercise ECG and case history in the diagnosis of latent coronary heart disease among presumably healthy middle-aged men. Eur. J. Cardiol. **5/6:** 463–476.
28. BRUCE, R. A., T. DEROUEN, D. R. PETERSON, *et al.* 1977. Noninvasive predictors of sudden cardiac death in men with coronary heart disease. Am. J. Cardiol. **39:** 833–840.

DISCUSSION

DR. DE BUSK: Did you do multivariate correlations in order to find which of the clinical and exercise test variables was the most predictive of subsequent cardiac events or coronary anatomy at the time of angiography?

DR. ERIKSSEN: We did perform them, but I find no reason to present them with the variant analysis because of the misclassification that I reported. I shall have to await complete classification of the data on the population until I can finish the multivariate study.

DR. DE BUSK: My question has to do with whether the exercise test variables, for example, were significant even in persons who did not have major risk factors.

DR. ERIKSSEN: It is of poor predictive value in people that have no additional risk factors.

DR. S. KENNETH JACOBSON (*Maplewood, New Jersey*): Do you have any ideas about how the sedimentation rate is involved in predicting coronary events?

DR. ERIKSSEN: I have no idea whatsoever.

VALUE OF EARLY THALLIUM-201 SCINTIGRAPHY AND GATED BLOOD POOL IMAGING FOR PREDICTING MORTALITY IN PATIENTS WITH ACUTE MYOCARDIAL INFARCTION *

Lewis C. Becker,† Kenneth J. Silverman, Bernadine H. Bulkley,
E. David Mellits, Clayton Kallman, and Myron L. Weisfeldt

*Departments of Medicine (Cardiology Division) and
Pediatrics (Division of Biostatistics)
The Johns Hopkins Medical Institutions
Baltimore, Maryland 21205*

Although most cases of sudden coronary death occur in individuals without any prior manifestation of ischemic heart disease, a significant minority of cases occur in patients who have suffered an acute myocardial infarction. Once an infarction occurs, subsequent mortality is related to the extent of left ventricular dysfunction,[1] which in turn is related in largest measure to the combined effects of old and new myocardial ischemic damage. If one could intervene early enough in patients with acute infarction, it might be possible to limit ischemic damage, preserve left ventricular function, and reduce mortality and subsequent sudden coronary death.

Our research has focused on methods for identifying infarct patients at higher risk of death as early as possible after hospital admission in order to select this subgroup for therapeutic interventions. Early identification of those at highest risk should allow optimal application of aggressive therapeutic interventions with the minimal exposure of low-risk patients to possible adverse effects.

A number of approaches have been utilized for early identification of high-risk patients, including clinical classifications based on the degree of heart failure,[2] invasive hemodynamic characterization,[3] and multivariate equations using combinations of clinical variables.[4-6] Patients admitted in pulmonary edema or cardiogenic shock are well known to be at high risk, but comprise only a small proportion of the acute infarct population. Because of larger numbers, most deaths actually occur in patients demonstrating lesser degrees of hemodynamic compromise, in Killip Class I or II, who as a group have a much better prognosis. Myocardial scintigraphy might be anticipated to be useful for identifying a high-risk subset within this lower risk group.

In previous studies thallium-201 perfusion scintigraphy has been useful for detecting and localizing areas of infarction and ischemia.[7-10] Since the extent of perfusion deficit early after infarction represents the sum total of old damage, new necrosis, and surrounding ischemic myocardium—which in turn should be an important determinant of short term prognosis—thallium imaging might be expected to be helpful for selecting the high-risk group.

* This work was supported by United States Public Health Service Grant P 50–HL–17655–04 from the National Heart, Lung and Blood Institute, National Institutes of Health, Bethesda, Maryland.

† Address for correspondence: Lewis C. Becker, M.D., The Johns Hopkins Hospital, 600 N. Wolfe Street, Baltimore, Maryland 21205.

Another approach of potential value is early measurement of global and regional left ventricular function by noninvasive scintigraphic ventriculography. The degree of functional impairment early in the course of infarction would ·also be expected to reflect the combination of old and new damage to the left ventricle plus the amount of jeopardized ischemic myocardium that may be present. Recent reports suggest that early measurements of left ventricular function are helpful in assessing short-term prognosis.[11]

The purpose of our recent studies has been to determine the predictive value of early thallium-201 imaging in hemodynamically stable patients with suspected acute myocardial infarction. We first examined a group of 42 infarction patients identified retrospectively.[12] We then sought to validate the predictive value of thallium scintigraphy in 92 patients gathered prospectively and consecutively, and in this second population we also examined the predictive value of scintigraphic ventriculography.[13, 14] The results from the gated blood pool study were used to further characterize patients with large and small thallium-201 defects. Finally, we performed an autopsy study to determine the pathologic significance of large and small thallium defects in patients with acute myocardial infarction.[15]

RETROSPECTIVE STUDY [12]

Patients

The study population consisted of 42 consecutive patients with acute myocardial infarction presenting within 12 hours of the onset of symptoms and judged to be Killip Class I or II on admission. The diagnosis of acute myocardial infarction was based on a typical history of chest pain, characteristic electrocardiographic changes, and a rise in serum creatine kinase (CK). Thallium-201 myocardial perfusion scintigraphy was performed in the coronary care unit within 15 hours of the onset of infarction (range 3–15 hours; mean $\pm$ SD, 8 $\pm$ 4 hours) in the anterior and 40° and 60° left anterior oblique views.

Killip Class I was defined as the absence of any signs of left ventricular failure. Class IIA included patients with basilar rales or ventricular gallop on auscultation or an increase in upper lobe vascularity or interstitial edema on chest X-ray film. Class IIB consisted of patients with alveolar infiltrates due to pulmonary edema, but without the clinical syndrome of acute pulmonary edema.

Analysis of Thallium-201 Scintigrams

Thallium scintigrams were scored objectively by a technologist using a computer-assisted technique called "circumferential profiles" (FIG. 1).[16] Each view was independently analyzed after a single, nine-point, weighted smoothing without background subtraction. An ellipse was used to isolate the left ventricle from the rest of the image, and a computer-generated circumference was constructed around the outer edge of the left ventricle using an isocount criterion (usually about 50% of average activity in the ellipse) to provide a visual "best fit" to the outer edge of the left ventricle. Radii were then constructed by the computer from the automatically determined image center to each point on

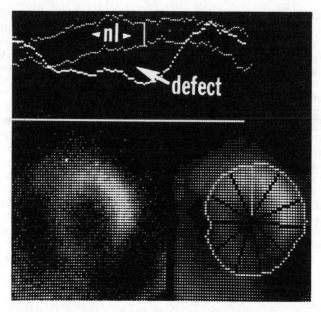

FIGURE 1. Computer-assisted scoring of defects. *Lower left:* unprocessed 40° left anterior oblique view showing markedly reduced septal, apical and distal lateral wall thallium uptake. *Lower right:* the image has been smoothed and an isocount outline generated around the left ventricle, and radii have been constructed from the center (computer-determined) to each circumference point; every tenth radius is shown in black, with the starting radius in white. *Upper panel:* whiter line is patient's normalized radial activity curve plotted against radial location, starting with the white radius and proceeding counterclockwise. The highest point shows highest activity in the upper posterolateral wall. The normal (nl) band is superimposed and aligned at the cardiac apex, marked with short white vertical bar. A defect is indicated where the patient's curve falls below normal limits. (From Silverman *et al.*[12] Reproduced by permission.)

the circumference (usually 75–125 radii). The average activity per pixel was calculated along each radius and normalized to the highest value. A curve was displayed of normalized thallium activity versus angular location, starting from the radius oriented upward and proceeding counterclockwise. A computer "defect score" was then determined by comparing the patient's profile curve with normal limits obtained by averaging the curves of 13 normal volunteers. The patient curve and normal curves were aligned about the radius corresponding to the apex. The lower limit of normal was defined as 2 standard deviations below the normal mean curve. An objective defect score was found for each view by integrating the area of the patient's curve below normal (percentage of radii with reduced activity multiplied by the average reduction in activity for these radii). This method of computer scoring has high intra- and inter-observer reproducibility.[16] Defect scores were summed for the three views to obtain a total defect score for each patient.

Follow-up and Analysis of Data

Thirty-five of 42 patients survived the initial hospitalization and were followed for 6 to 20 months (mean, 9 months). Kaplan-Meier survival curves were used to describe survival.[17] Differences in survival curves between patients with high and low thallium defect scores were evaluated by the Peto method [18] at three intervals: at the end of the hospitalization, 6 months after infarction, and at last follow-up. This method was also used to confirm that survival-curve differences were not due to other prognostic variables by the adjustment for each in turn.

Results

Fourteen of the 42 patients died, seven during hospitalization and seven after discharge 1.5 to 18 months after initial presentation. All of the deaths appeared to be cardiac in origin. Ten of the 14 deaths were sudden, although most appeared to involve a preceding ischemic episode. Three were attributed to acute left ventricular pump failure in the coronary care unit, and three other patients experienced chest pain before dying suddenly. The other four patients had unwitnessed sudden death, making it impossible to determine whether there was a preceding ischemic episode. Of the four non-sudden deaths, two were due to cardiogenic shock, one to reinfarction, and one occurred 1 day after bypass surgery.

Nonsurvivors had significantly larger thallium defects and a mean defect score of 14.3 versus a mean defect score of 2.3 in survivors ($p < 0.001$) (FIG. 2). Only one of 28 patients alive at last follow-up had a defect score of more than 7.0, while 12 of 14 patients who died had a score of 7.0 or more. A score of 7 generally corresponded to at least a moderate reduction

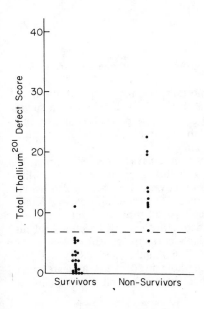

FIGURE 2. Retrospective study: thallium-201 defect scores for survivors and nonsurvivors. The dashed line is drawn at a score of 7.0. All but one of the survivors had a score less than 7.0 while all but two of the nonsurvivors had a score greater than 7.0 (From Silverman *et al.*[12] Reproduced by permission.)

of thallium uptake involving 40% or more of the left ventricle in two or more views. A severe reduction of uptake involving 60% of the left ventricle in a single view at times resulted in a score of this magnitude.

On the basis of the data in FIGURE 2, we defined thallium studies with a computer score of 7.0 or more as indicating high risk and those with a score of less than 7.0 as low risk. Actuarial survival curves for patients with high- and low-risk scintigrams are shown in FIGURE 3. The differences between the two curves was highly significant (p < 0.001) at 2 weeks, 6 months, and last follow-up. Mortality for the overall patient population and for high-risk and low-risk subgroups is compared during hospitalization, at 6 months, and at last follow-up in TABLE 1.

Mortality in high- and low-risk thallium scintigram groups was adjusted for age, sex, peak CK, history of previous myocardial infarction, anterior location of the acute infarct, and Killip Class IIB on admission. Analysis showed that after adjustment for each variable, mortality in the high-risk scintigraphic group was significantly higher than that in the low-risk group during hospitalization, at 6 months, and at last follow-up. Therefore, the

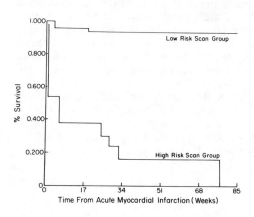

FIGURE 3. Retrospective study: actuarial survival curves for patients with high- and low-risk scintigrams. (From Silverman *et al.*[12] Reproduced by permission.)

greater mortality in the high-risk thallium group was not due to partial confounding by any of the variables examined.

Statistically significant predictors of mortality during hospitalization, at 6 months and at last follow-up are shown in TABLE 2. The ability of a single clinical variable to predict mortality was indexed by the percentage of patients whose mortality was correctly classified by the analysis. A high-risk thallium scintigram was the best predictor at each time interval.

Step-wise multivariate discriminant function analysis was performed to determine whether thallium scintigraphy was a better predictor of mortality than the best combination of clinical variables that were available on admission. Age, sex, history of previous infarct, location of the acute infarct and Killip class at admission were used for this analysis. At all three time intervals, the best combination of clinical variables included a history of infarction and an anterior location of the present infarct, which correctly classified 73.8% of cases for the initial hospitalization, 78.6% at 6 months, and 88.1% at last follow-up. Comparison of these values with those in TABLE 2 indicates that thallium scintigraphy was more predictive than the best combination of clinical

TABLE 1

RETROSPECTIVE STUDY: MORTALITY IN OVERALL POPULATION AND
HIGH-AND LOW-RISK SUBGROUPS

	Mortality		
	In-Hospital	At 6 Months	At Last Follow-up
Overall (n = 42)	17%	24%	33%
High-risk patients (n = 13) (score ≥ 7)	46%	62%	92%
Low-risk patients (n = 29) (score < 7)	3%	7%	7%

variables. Further, when the thallium defect score was added to this best combination of the multivariate analysis, predictiveness increased significantly at each interval.

PROSPECTIVE STUDY

Patients

The study group consisted of 92 consecutive patients with evident or strongly suspected acute myocardial infarction admitted to the hospital within 12 hours of the onset of symptoms in Killip Class I or II. A subsequent diagnosis of acute myocardial infarction was made in 77 patients. Fifteen patients lacked

TABLE 2

RETROSPECTIVE STUDY: SIGNIFICANT PROGNOSTIC VARIABLES FOR MORTALITY

In-Hospital	At 6 Months	At Last Follow-up
Thallium score (83.3%)*	Thallium score (83.3%)*	Thallium score (92.9%)*
Anterior location (78.6%)†	Anterior location (78.6%)‡	Anterior location (78.6%)*
	History of previous myocardial infarction (78.6%)†	History of previous myocardial infarction (78.6%)*
	Class IIB (78.6%)	Class IIB (73.8%)†
	Peak creatine kinase > 1000 (66.7%)†	Peak creatine kinase > 1000 (66.7%)†
	Age > 65 (78.6%)†	

NOTE: Numbers in parenthesis refer to "predictiveness" of each variable for mortality (percentage of patents classified correctly). Statistical significance of the predictiveness of each variable for mortality is:

$* p < 0.001$.
$† p < 0.05$.
$‡ p < 0.01$.

either diagnostic electrocardiographic or enzyme changes and were diagnosed as having unstable angina. As soon as possible after admission to the coronary care unit, thallium-201 myocardial perfusion scintigraphy was performed, followed immediately by technetium-99m gated blood pool scintigraphy using *in vivo* labelled erythrocytes. Scintigraphic studies were begun within 15 hours of the onset of chest pain (range, 3–15 hours; mean ± SD, 7 ± 4 hours). In one patient a gated blood pool scintigram was performed without a thallium study because thallium-201 was unavailable. In nine patients gated blood pool studies were either not done because of arrhythmias or were technically inadequate for analysis.

Analysis of the Scintigrams

Thallium scintigrams were scored objectively using the computer-assisted technique described earlier.[16] Gated blood pool scintigrams were analyzed by a commercial computer program ("MUGE")™. Semiautomatic regions of interest were generated over the left ventricle for each frame in the cardiac cycle using a combined second derivative and count threshold algorithm. A background region was automatically generated lateral and inferior to the left ventricle in the end-systolic frame. From these regions of interest, a background-corrected left ventricular time–activity curve was obtained and left ventricular ejection fraction calculated.

Results

Seventy-eight of 92 patients survived the first month after the acute event and were followed for 6 months. Two additional patients died between 1 month and 6 months. Thirteen of the 16 deaths appeared to be primarily cardiac in origin on the basis of clinical findings and postmortem examinations when available. The other three were tangentially related to the ischemic event, one patient dying of a cerebrovascular accident and the other two of probable pulmonary emboli. All deaths were included in the statistical analyses.

The results of thallium imaging in this prospectively identified group confirmed our previous findings. Nonsurvivors had significantly larger defects, with a mean score of 9.0 compared with a mean score of 2.4 in survivors ($p < 0.001$). A defect score of 7.0 was again found to be the best discriminator between high- and low-risk groups. Nine of the 16 nonsurvivors (56%) had a defect score of 7.0 or more, while 69 of the 75 6-month survivors (92%) had scores less than 7.

Global left ventricular ejection fraction was also useful for identifying a high-risk subset in this patient population. Nonsurvivors had a significantly lower mean ejection fraction compared with that of survivors (44.4% versus 60.2%, $p < 0.01$), and an ejection fraction of 35% appeared to provide the best discrimination for predicting mortality. Seven of the 15 nonsurvivors who had gated blood pool studies had ejection fractions less than or equal to 35%, while 65 of the 68 survivors at 6 months (96%) had ejection fractions greater than 35%. Mortality for high-risk and low-risk groups, as defined by thallium and gated blood pool scintigraphy, are shown in TABLE 3. It should be noted that these values are quite similar to those for the retrospective study given in TABLE 1.

TABLE 3

PROSPECTIVE STUDY: MORTALITY IN OVERALL POPULATION AND HIGH-RISK AND
LOW-RISK SUBGROUPS

	At 1 Month	At 6 Months
Overall (n = 92)	15%	17%
Thallium score ⩾ 7 (n = 15)	53%	60%
Thallium score < 7 (n = 76)	8%	9%
Left ventricular ejection fraction ⩽ 35% (n = 10)	50%	70%
Left ventricular ejection fraction > 35% (n = 73)	11%	11%

Taken singly, only three variables were significantly associated with mortality at 1 and 6 months. Thallium defect score and left ventricular ejection fraction each could be used to correctly classify 84–87% of cases, while transmural extent of infarction could be used to correctly classify 66%. Other variables including age, sex, Killip class on admission, location of infarction, history of previous infarction, and peak serum creatine kinase were not significantly associated with mortality, either at 1 month or at 6 months.

The sensitivity and specificity of the scintigraphic variables, transmural extent of infarction, and serum creatine kinase levels for predicting mortality at 1 month are shown in TABLE 4. Thallium defect score ≥ 7 had the best balance between sensitivity and specificity. Left ventricular ejection fraction $\leq 35\%$ had significantly lower sensitivity at a similar level of specificity. Sensitivity could be increased by raising the discriminating ejection fraction value, but specificity fell concomitantly. The combination of thallium score ≥ 7 and ejection fraction $\leq 35\%$ was highly specific, but sensitivity was low. Transmural extent of infarction and peak creatine kinase >1000 IU/liter both lacked adequate specificity. The values for sensitivity and specificity for prediction of mortality at 6 months were virtually identical, since only two further patients died.

Step-wise multivariate discriminant function analysis was performed to determine whether the variables studied were additively predictive. For this

TABLE 4

PROSPECTIVE STUDY: PREDICTION OF 1-MONTH MORTALITY BY SINGLE
SCINTIGRAPHIC AND CLINICAL VARIABLES

	Sensitivity	Specificity
Thallium defect score ≥ 7	57%	91%
Left ventricular ejection fraction ≤ 35%	38%	93%
Both thallium score ⩾ 7 and ejection fraction ≤ 35%	31%	99%
Transmural infarction	86%	63%
Peak creatine kinase > 1000 IU/liter	50%	76%

analysis thallium defect score and left ventricular ejection fraction were treated as continuous variables and mortality was examined at 6 months. The best prediction was obtained using a combination of thallium defect score, transmural extent of infarction, and history of previous infarction. Sensitivity was 73% and specificity 84%, and 82% of cases were classified correctly. Thallium score was selected as the most significant variable, after which left ventricular ejection fraction was no longer predictive, apparently because the two techniques tended to identify the same individuals as being at high risk. If thallium score was kept out of the analysis, the best combination of variables included left ventricular ejection fraction, transmural extent of infarction, and history of previous infarction. Sensitivity was 73%, specificity 75%, and 75% of cases were classified correctly. These values were not as good as when the thallium score was included.

Among the 14 patients with thallium defect score ≥ 7 having gated blood pool studies, left ventricular ejection fraction ranged widely from 28% to 62%. Five patients had ejection fractions $\leq 35\%$, six patients had values from 36 to 50%, and three patients had fractions $>50\%$. Mortality prediction was aided by combining the results from both scintigraphic studies. All five patients with thallium score ≥ 7 and ejection fraction $\leq 35\%$ died. Mortality was three of nine (33%) in those patients with thallium score ≥ 7 and ejection fraction $>35\%$. Among patients with thallium score <7, two of five (40%) with ejection fraction $\leq 35\%$ died compared with only five of 63 (8%) of those with ejection fraction $>35\%$. Thus, concordant results with thallium and gated blood pool scintigraphy identified subgroups with markedly different mortalities: 100% when both were high-risk and 8% when both were low-risk. When the results were discordant, mortality rate was intermediate at 33% and 40%.

AUTOPSY STUDY [15]

Patients and Methods

Twenty-four consecutive, autopsied patients were identified who had thallium scintigraphy during life and who at autopsy had coronary disease and recent or remote myocardial infarction. For each patient, we reviewed the clinical records, gross heart specimens, histologic sections, and postmortem coronary arteriograms. The age of the infarcts was determined by histologic evaluation. The infarctions were quantitated by examination of 1-cm thick transverse slices of ventricle, tracing each of the left ventricular slices on transparent plastic sheets, outlining the area of infarction on the tracings, and weighing each left ventricular slice minus the right ventricular free wall. The tracings were planimetered electronically and the percent of left ventricle involved by recent and old infarction and the total weight of the infarct in grams was determined.

The thallium scintigraphic defect scores, obtained by computer as noted earlier, were compared with percent total left ventricular necrosis by linear regression using the least-squares method. Large and small infarcts were examined in relation to high- and low-risk scintigrams and vice versa using the Fisher exact test.

Results

In 23 patients, coronary obstructive disease was present and in 22 there was >75% atherosclerotic narrowing of at least one major coronary artery. In one patient, an anterior wall myocardial infarction was related to an anomalous left coronary artery arising from the pulmonary trunk. In another patient, myocardial infarction occurred in the setting of a floppy mitral valve and recurrent ventricular tachycardia. Of the entire group, 13 had thallium imaging during an acute infarct; seven patients had imaging within 24 hours of the acute event, four patients within 1 week, and two within 3 weeks; of these, six had remote infarcts as well. All 13 of these patients died in the periinfarction period; the interval between the onset of infarction and death was 1–27 days (mean, 15 days). Eleven other patients with remote myocardial infarcts had imaging from 3 months to several years after the acute myocardial injury. Of these patients, two died of ventricular arrhythmias, two of heart failure, and seven in the setting of coronary bypass surgery. The intervals between thallium scintigraphy and death ranged from 36 hours to 65 days (mean, 19 days) in 23 of the 24 patients; one patient with a remote infarct died 6 months after imaging. There was no clinical or pathologic evidence of an infarct more recent than the date of the thallium scan.

Thallium defect scores in the 24 patients ranged from 0.1–41. There were 13 patients with high-risk (≥ 7) and 11 with low-risk scintigrams (<7) (FIG. 4). At autopsy, ten patients had infarcts involving >25% of the left ventricle, and 15 had infarcts involving $\leq 25\%$ of the left ventricle. The correlation between absolute thallium defect score and the percentage of necrosis was poor ($r = 0.27$). However, when we divided the patients into groups by high- and low-risk scintigrams and by "large" (>25% of the left ventricle) or "small" (<25% of the left ventricle) infarcts, a significant relationship between infarct size and thallium defect risk group was present. Among the 13 patients with high-risk scintigrams, eight (62%) had large infarcts and five (38%) small infarcts. Of the 11 patients with low-risk scores, ten patients (91%) had small infarcts and one (9%) had a large infarct. The mean percent necrosis was 36% for high-risk scores and 13% for low-risk scores ($p < 0.01$). Also, the association between scintigraphic score and infarct size was statistically significant by the Fisher exact test ($p < 0.01$).

There were six patients in whom defect score did not reflect infarct size. These discrepancies, however, clustered in one direction. Only one of the six errors occurred when a large infarct was assigned a low-risk defect score. The patient in whom this occurred had imaging 6 days after his acute infarct, while he was in severe heart failure and required vasopressors to maintain systemic blood pressure. He died 2 weeks after infarction and 7 days after thallium-201 scintigraphy. At autopsy there was no evidence of necrosis more recent than that seen on his thallium scan to account for the discrepancy. Therefore, the inability to detect a significant focal thallium defect appears to have been related to a diffuse decrease in thallium uptake by all myocardial segments, and increased uptake of tracer by the lungs, causing a low heart-to-background ratio. This is a technical limitation of thallium perfusion imaging as currently performed. If all myocardial segments are equally ischemic, the image may appear normally homogenous; this also represents a limitation of a computer method based on relative rather than absolute counts.

Most of the discrepancies occurred when the defect scores overestimated the infarct size. This was observed in five of six patients and the most marked example is shown in FIGURE 5. In this patient, a defect score of 10 was obtained shortly after he was admitted with an acute anteroseptal subendocardial myocardial infarct. Although recurrent chest pain and recurrent S-T segment depression in V_2–V_4 occurred over the next several days, the serum creatine kinase rose to a peak of only 230 IU/liter. Progressive left ventricular dysfunction, ventricular arrhythmias, and elevation of the pulmonary wedge pressure to 30 mm Hg developed, and he finally died in ventricular fibrillation. At autopsy, a remote high posterior infarct that involved about 3% of the left ventricle was identified, and there were also small foci of subendocardial necrosis in the anterior and anteroseptal myocardium that involved a little more than 1% of the left ventricle and were in the distribution of a critically narrowed proximal left anterior descending coronary artery. Thus, although the infarct was small, the clinical evidence suggested a large ischemic zone in the left anterior descending distribution that accounted for persistent electrocardiographic abnormalities, a large anteroseptal thallium defect, and severe left ventricular dysfunction and arrhythmias. The other four instances of discrepancy between scintigraphic defect and infarct size included one patient who had imaging while in cardiogenic shock 5 days after an acute infarct (this patient died 2 days later) and three patients who died with remote infarcts. One of the latter three patients had imaging after a cardiac arrest and was hemodynamically unstable, one had a ventricular septal defect and a low output state requiring placement of an intraaortic balloon, and one had Class IV angina pectoris, pending a coronary bypass procedure. In all five patients, therefore, there was at least some clinical history to suggest ischemia plus infarction as an explanation for large thallium defects and small infarct size.

The discrepancies between scintigraphic defect size and anatomic infarct size were present with the same frequency, regardless of the interval between the beginning of the infarct and the thallium scintigram. Seven patients were scanned within 24 hours of infarction, and the infarct size was overestimated in one (14%); six patients were scanned 1 to 21 days after infarction, and the infarct size was overestimated in one (17%) and underestimated in one (17%); 11 patients were scanned more than 30 days after infarction, and the infarct size was overestimated in two (18%).

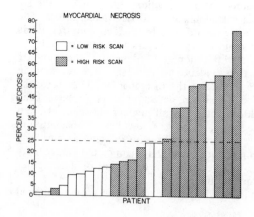

FIGURE 4. Each bar represents percentage of necrosis for a given patient. The dotted horizontal line is drawn at 25% necrosis. Patients with scores above the line are considered to have "large" infarcts and those with scores below to have "small" infarcts. (From Bulkley et al.[15] Reproduced by permission.)

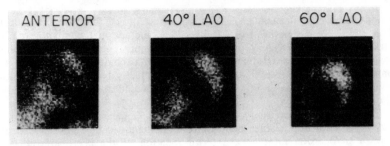

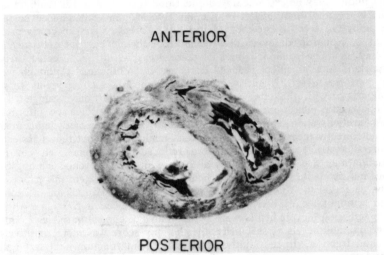

FIGURE 5. An example of a "high-risk" thallium scan (defect score 10) in a patient with a small infarct. The thallium scintigrams show defects in the apical and anteroseptal walls. At autopsy, focal subendocardial necrosis was evident anteroseptally and a small healed subendocardial posterior wall infarct was present, with a total injury to the left ventricle of about 4%. LAO = left anterior oblique. (From Bulkley *et al.*[15] Reproduced by permission.)

DISCUSSION

Our results indicate that in hemodynamically stable patients with acute myocardial infarction, thallium-201 scintigraphy performed within 15 hours of the onset of symptoms can be used to predict subsequent in-hospital and postdischarge mortality. In the retrospective study, overall mortality rate in our Killip Class I–II patients was 17% in-hospital, 24% at 6 months, and 33% at last follow-up (average, 9 months). In the prospective series, mortality was similar: 15% at 1 month and 17% at 6 months. These values are comparable with those of other series in which hospital mortality for Class I–II patients ranged from 13% to 18%.[4, 6, 19]

Other investigators have described prognostic indices in patients with acute myocardial infarction using a combination of clinical variables[2, 4–6] and invasive hemodynamic measurements.[3, 6] Although these indices improved stratification of risk, all were derived from studies that include patients admitted with marked hemodynamic compromise, including acute pulmonary edema or cardiogenic shock (Class III–IV). We specifically excluded these patients from our study because we felt that they were more likely to have already suffered irreversible myocardial injury and therefore would be poor candidates for infarct-limiting therapy.

The thallium defect score, as a single index, appeared to be better than a number of clinical variables believed to be prognostically important: history of prior myocardial infarction, anterior location of the acute infarct, higher peak levels of serum creatine kinase, and moderate left ventricular failure. This finding may be explained by the fact that the extent of the thallium defect reflects the total mass of left ventricular myocardium with reduced perfusion, including (1) areas of previous infarction, (2) areas of fresh necrosis, and (3) areas of jeopardized myocardium that are ischemic but not yet irreversibly injured.[7, 15] The combined mass of these areas would be expected to be an important determinant of reduced left ventricular function. Although we did not perform invasive hemodynamic measurements in our patients to allow comparison with thallium scintigraphy, earlier studies have suggested that hemodynamic measurements, while providing certain prognostic information, lack sensitivity and specificity.[3] This is probably because hemodynamic methods do not directly measure the size of the ischemic region, but reflect instead the depression of left ventricular function produced by ischemia. Left ventricular function may also be depressed by alterations in left ventricular loading conditions independent of myocardial ischemia. To a certain extent this may explain why we found the thallium defect score to be a better predictor of mortality than scintigraphically determined left ventricular ejection fraction. Although both scintigraphic predictors were better than the clinical variables examined, at comparable levels of specificity, the thallium score was more sensitive than ejection fraction. In the multivariate discriminant function analysis, thallium score was selected before ejection fraction. When thallium score was not used, ejection fraction was selected as the most predictive variable.

The two scintigraphic measurements appeared to provide additional predictive information when used together. When both tests indicated a high-risk situation, the mortality was 100%, compared with only 8% when both tests were low-risk. When the two tests gave discordant results, the mortality was intermediate.

The thallium defect score is prognostically useful because it reflects both the extent of necrosis that has already occurred and the amount of myocardium still jeopardized.[15] Most of the in-hospital deaths in both the retrospective and prospective series occurred suddenly with an acute deterioration in left ventricular pump function.[20] This may have been related to extensive areas of old and new necrosis or possibly to extension of the infarct process. Myocardial rupture was not found in any of the patients autopsied. The majority of post-discharge deaths also occurred suddenly, but the history in most cases suggested a new ischemic event. In these patients, the large perfusion defect found initially may have identified extensive areas of myocardium at risk for future ischemia. These same considerations almost certainly apply to the left ventricular ejection fraction as a prognostic indicator.

The patients in the prospective study with large thallium defects (score ≥ 7) and fair to normal left ventricular function (ejection fraction $>35\%$) form an interesting subgroup in this regard. Mortality was lower in this group than in the group with ejection fraction $\leq 35\%$, but was still considerably greater than what would be anticipated for Class I–II patients. We believe that these patients may have had relatively limited areas of myocardial necrosis combined with large surrounding areas of jeopardized ischemic tissue, as opposed to extensive areas of irreversibly damaged myocardium. Unfortunately, no autopsy studies were available on any of these patients. If the hypothesis is correct, patients in this subgroup should be ideal candidates for aggressive antiischemic therapy.

The value of a reliable prognostic index for patients suffering acute myocardial infarction is clear. Early, accurate identification of high-risk patients may permit improved and more selective medical care. High-risk patients can be closely monitored in the coronary care unit for a longer period of time, they can be allowed ambulation more slowly, and followed more closely after hospital discharge, whereas low-risk patients can be allowed ambulation more quickly and discharged from the hospital early. As new, more aggressive interventions are planned, it will be essential to identify high-risk patients quickly and reliably. These patients are the best candidates for aggressive treatment, provided they can be identified early, before hemodynamic deterioration and presumably before a sizable amount of ischemic myocardium progresses to infarction. By selecting high-risk patients, fewer patients would be required to prove a beneficial effect of therapy, and low-risk patients would not be unnecessarily exposed to the possible increased risk of these interventions.

REFERENCES

1. SCHULZE, R. A., JR., H. W. STRAUSS & B. PITT. 1977. Sudden death in the year following myocardial infarction. Relation to ventricular premature contractions in the late hospital phase and left ventricular ejection fraction. Am. J. Med. **62:** 192, 1977.
2. KILLIP, T. & J. T. KIMBAL. 1967. Treatment of myocardial infarction in a coronary care unit: A two year experience with 250 patients. Am. J. Cardiol. **20:** 457.
3. WEBER, K. T., J. S. JANICKI, R. O. RUSSELL & C. E. RACKLEY. 1978. Identification of high risk subsets of acute myocardial infarction. Am. J. Cardiol. **41:** 197.
4. NORRIS, R. M., P. W. T. BRANDT, D. E. CAUGHEY, A. J. LEE & P. J. SCOTT. 1969. A new coronary prognostic index. Lancet **1:** 274.
5. PEEL, A. A., T. SEMPLE, I. WANG, W. M. LANCASTER & J. L. G. DALL. 1962. A coronary prognostic index for grading the severity of infarction. Br. Heart J. **24:** 745.
6. HENNING, H., E. A. GILPIN, J. W. COVELL, E. A. SWAN, R. A. O'ROURKE & J. ROSS. 1979. Prognosis after acute myocardial infarction: A multivariate analysis of mortality and survival. Circulation **59:** 1124.
7. WACKERS, F. J. TH., E. B. SOKOLE, G. SAMSON, J. B. VAN DER SCHOOT, K. L. LIE, K. L. LIEM & H. J. J. WELLENS. 1976. Value and limitations of thallium-201 scintigraphy in the acute phase of myocardial infarction. N. Engl. J. Med. **295:** 1.
8. WACKERS, F. J. TH., A. E. BECKER, G. SAMSON, E. B. SOKOLE, J. B. VAN DER SCHOOT, A. J. T. M. VET, K. I. LIE, D. DURRER & H. WELLENS. 1977. Location and size of acute transmural myocardial infarction estimated from thallium-201 scintiscans. A clinicopathological study. Circulation **56:** 72.
9. HENNING, H., H. R. SCHELBERT, A. RIGHETTI, W. L. ASHBURN & R. A. O'ROURKE. 1977. Dual myocardial imaging with technetium 99m pyrophosphate and

thallium 201 for detecting, localizing, and sizing acute myocardial infarction. Am. J. Cardiol. **40:** 147.

10. BERGER, J. H., A. GOTTSCHALK & B. L. ZARET. 1978. Dual radionuclide study of acute myocardial infarction. Comparison of thallium-201 and technetium 99m pyrophosphate imaging in man. Ann. Intern. Med. **88:** 145.

11. SHAH, P. K., M. PICHLER, D. S. BERMAN, B. N. SINGH & H. J. C. SWAN. 1980. Left ventricular ejection fraction determined by radionuclide ventriculography in early stages of first transmural myocardial infarction. Relation to short-term prognosis. Am. J. Cardiol. **45:** 542.

12. SILVERMAN, K. J., L. C. BECKER, B. H. BULKLEY, R. D. BUROW, E. D. MELLITS, C. H. KALLMAN & M. L. WEISFELDT. 1980. Value of early thallium-201 scintigraphy for predicting mortality in patients with acute myocardial infarction. Circulation **61:** 996.

13. SILVERMAN, K. J., L. C. BECKER, B. H. BULKLEY, R. D. BUROW, D. MELLITS, C. KALLMAN & M. L. WEISFELDT. 1979. Scintigraphic predictors of mortality in stable patients with acute myocardial infarction: Thallium-201 versus gated blood pool scintigraphy. Circulation **60:** Suppl II: 11–149.

14. SILVERMAN, K. J., M. L. WEISFELDT, B. H. BULKLEY, R. D. BUROW & L. C. BECKER. 1979. Identification of high risk infarct patients with good left ventricular function. Circulation **60:** Suppl II: 11–69.

15. BULKLEY, B. H., K. SILVERMAN, M. L. WEISFELDT, R. BUROW, M. POND & L. C. BECKER. 1979. Pathologic basis of thallium-201 scintigraphic defects in patients with fatal myocardial injury. Circulation **60:** 785.

16. BUROW, R. D., M. POND, A. W. SHAFER & L. C. BECKER. 1979. Circumferential profiles: A new method for computer analysis of thallium-201 myocardial perfusion images. J. Nucl. Med. **20:** 771.

17. KAPAN, E. L. & P. MEIER. 1979. Nonparametric estimation from incomplete observations. Am. Stat. Assoc. J. **53:** 457.

18. PETO, R., M. C. PIKE, P. ARMITAGE, N. E. BRESLOW, D. R. COX, S. V. HOWARD, N. MANTEL, K. MCPHERSON, J. PETRO & P. G. SMITH. 1977. Design and analysis of randomized clinical trials requiring prolonged observation of each patient. II. Analysis and examples. Br. J. Cancer **35:** 1.

19. GOLDBERG, R., M. SZKLO, J. A. TONASCIA & H. L. KENNEDY. 1979. Time trends in prognosis of patients with myocardial infarction: A population based study. Johns Hopkins Med. J. **144:** 73.

20. RAIZES, G., G. S. WAGNER & D. B. HACKEL. 1977. Instantaneous nonarrhythmic cardiac death in acute myocardial infarction. Am. J. Cardiol. **39:** 1.

DISCUSSION

DR. MARCUS: Can the thallium score or ejection fraction be used to move a patient out of the coronary care unit, shortening the stay that the patient would ordinarily have? Do the tests you describe also predict complications such as ventricular tachycardia, ventricular fibrillation, or extension?

DR. BECKER: That's a good question. The prediction of complications would be a valid use of these tests, but we haven't used it for that as yet.

We have shown mortality data in this paper and that has been the main analysis. I can't say with certainty whether the other complications are present. As I remember these patients, I believe that there were few complications in the low-risk group.

THE CHRONOLOGY AND SUDDENNESS OF CARDIAC DEATH AFTER MYOCARDIAL INFARCTION *

Arthur J. Moss,† John DeCamilla, Jonathan Chilton, and
Henry T. Davis

*Heart Research Follow-up Program of the
Department of Preventive Medicine and Community Health
Department of Medicine
Division of Biostatistics
University of Rochester School of Medicine and Dentistry
Rochester, New York 14642*

Patients who survive the acute phase of myocardial infarction have a 1-year posthospital mortality of approximately 10%,[1-3] with a continued mortality rate of about 3 to 5% per year thereafter. Posthospital cardiac deaths may be sudden or nonsudden, with a heterogeneous combination of arrhythmic, mechanical, and ischemic factors playing a role in the terminal event. Recently, increasing emphasis has been placed on the identification and, it is hoped, the reduction of sudden cardiac death in postcoronary patients.[4-6] In fact, a national study of the efficiency of beta blocking agents has been mounted to determine whether the regular chronic administration of propranolol will reduce postinfarction mortality from any cause, and sudden death in particular, during a 4-year follow-up period.[7]

The present report is the outgrowth of a prospective postcoronary study initiated in Rochester, New York, in 1972 to better evaluate the posthospital clinical course of patients who survived one or more myocardial infarctions. During a 4-year enrollment of 978 patients with a variable follow-up period ranging from 1 to 5 years (average, 3 years), 117 patients died of cardiac cause. The purpose of this investigation is to identify the factors associated with the chronology and suddenness of cardiac death after myocardial infarction to better understand why postcoronary patients die. Such information should provide a useful data base for the planning of secondary intervention programs to reduce posthospital cardiac mortality.

METHODS

Population

The study population consisted of 978 Monroe County residents, 798 men and 180 women less than 66 years of age, who entered coronary care units in two Rochester community hospitals between January 1, 1973 and December 31, 1976 with either a definite or probable acute myocardial infarction and survived

* This work was supported in part by a grant from the Gebbie Foundation, Jamestown, New York, and by Research Grant HL–15790 from the National Heart, Lung, and Blood Institute, National Institutes of Health, Bethesda, Maryland.

† Address for correspondence: Arthur J. Moss, M.D., Box 653, University of Rochester Medical Center, 601 Elmwood Avenue, Rochester, New York 14642.

465

0077–8923/82/0382–0465 $01.75/0 © 1982, NYAS

hospitalization. Definite myocardial infarctions were substantiated by the presence of any two of the following: typical coronary-type chest pain, serial acute myocardial enzyme changes, or electrocardiographic documentation (an evolving Q wave abnormality with acute ST and T wave changes). Patients with probable myocardial infarctions had typical coronary-type chest pain with minor enzyme changes and/or electrocardiographically documented acute ST and T wave changes. Both the patient and the private physician had to give informed consent before the patient was entered into the study.

Data Acquisition

Nurse investigators interviewed the patients and reviewed their hospital charts during the last week of hospitalization. The patients' medical history prior to entry and their clinical course during the period in the coronary care unit (CCU) and subsequent hospitalization were recorded on prospectively designed forms as previously described.[8] In brief, clinical variables utilized in this study included: (1) demographic data; (2) history of concurrent morbidity, such as prior myocardial infarction, hypertension, angina pectoris, and diabetes mellitus; (3) severity of the acute coronary event in terms of the lowest systolic blood pressure, left ventricular dysfunction (roentgenographic evidence of interstitial or alveolar edema, significant pulmonary rales, or pitting edema), and arrhythmic complications; (4) myocardial infarct location, as determined by the Minnesota classification[9] of a 12-lead electrocardiogram categorized into anterior ($Q/QS = 1.11–1.12$), posterior ($Q/QS = 1.14$), and other (non Q/QS abnormality) locations; (5) usage of digitalis (digoxin or digitoxin), antiarrhythmic agents (procainamide or quinidine), diuretic agents, and beta blocking agent (propranolol) in the week prior to demise; and (6) ventricular arrhythmias on a predischarge 6-hour Holter-type electrocardiographic tape recording. All ventricular premature beats (VPB) were identified on each patient's record, and the VPB were categorized by frequency (number VPB/hr), prematurity (RR'/QT), and the presence of multiform, bigeminal, paired, and ventricular tachycardia (three or more VPB in a row) patterns. Complex VPB were defined by the occurrence of patterns of multiform, bigeminal, paired, or ventricular tachycardia beats.

Mortality

All patients who died before January 1, 1978 were identified. The 978 patients were exposed to the risk of dying from a minimum of twelve months (those who entered in December 1976) to a maximum of 60 months (those who entered in January 1973). When a nonsurvivor was identified, information was gathered from immediate family members, the personal physician, and witnesses to the terminal event. This information was evaluated by a mortality review committee, and a cause of death was assigned to each nonsurvivor, as previously described.[10] Patients dying from cardiac and noncardiac causes were identified. The suddenness of cardiac death was determined by the time elapsed between the onset of acute cardiac symptoms and demise. Unwitnessed deaths were separately categorized. During the period from January 1, 1973 through December 31, 1977, 136 of the patients died, and 117 of these deaths were from cardiac cause.

Missing Values

Of the 978 patients in the study population, 38 patients had the following missing values: 28 had technically unsatisfactory predischarge Holter recordings, 9 had missing data regarding roentgenographic evidence of interstitial or alveolar edema, and one had missing data for prior myocardial infarction. Among the 117 cardiac deaths, five had missing data regarding pertinent clinical data. Patients with missing values were excluded from specific analyses that included that variable.

Statistical Methods

Univariate analyses were performed using a Yates corrected Chi-square test for categorized variables and a two-tailed t test for continuous variables.

RESULTS

Description of the Cardiac Death Population

The clinical characteristics of the total cardiac death group (n = 112), the witnessed (n = 98) and the unwitnessed (n = 14) deaths, are presented in TABLE 1. More than half of the cardiac deaths occurred out-of-hospital or in the emergency department, and 56% of the witnessed deaths happened within 1 hour of onset of symptoms. The clinical characteristics of the witnessed and unwitnessed deaths were similar, except for a significantly younger age and a higher proportion of out-of-hospital mortality in the unwitnessed group.

Chronology and Suddenness of Cardiac Death

Because of the staggered enrollment and the censored follow-up, all members of the study population were exposed to a uniform mortality risk only during the first posthospital year. The frequency distribution of the chronologic occurrence of death (interval from hospital discharge to demise) and of the suddenness of cardiac death (elapsed time from the onset of terminal symptoms to demise) was evaluated in this 1-year cohort. The chronologic distribution of the number of sudden and nonsudden cardiac deaths occurring in the first posthospital year for three arbitrary definitions of sudden (≤ 5 minutes, ≤ 1 hour, ≤ 24 hours) is presented in FIGURE 1. For each temporal cutoff, sudden deaths were randomly distributed throughout the 12-month period, whereas nonsudden deaths were more frequent in the first month after hospital discharge. However, at progressively longer cutoffs for sudden (5 minutes, 1 hour, 24 hours), smaller percentages of nonsudden cardiac death occurred in the first few posthospital months, and the reverse was true for sudden cardiac death. The change in the chronologic distribution of sudden and nonsudden cardiac death was more marked between the 1-hour and 24-hour cutoffs than between the 5-minute and 1-hour times. For this reason, a 1-hour cutoff for sudden cardiac death was utilized in the remainder of the analyses. A graphic presentation of the 1-year cumulative mortality of the sudden (≤ 1 hour) and nonsudden

(>1 hour) cardiac deaths is presented in FIGURE 2. Fifty percent of the non-sudden deaths occurred within 1 month after hospital discharge, while only 16% of the sudden deaths occurred in this same period. A significant association exists between the chronology, dichotomized into early (≤1 month) and

TABLE 1

CLINICAL CHARACTERISTICS OF THE MORTALITY GROUPS

	All Cardiac Deaths (n=112)	Witnessed Deaths (n=98)	Unwitnessed Deaths (n=14)
Demographic Factors			
Age in years (mean ± SE)	54.6 ± 0.8	55.0 ± 0.8 †	51.7 ± 2.2 †
Sex, male (%)	82	84	71
Social class IV and V * (%)	68	70	50
Co-morbidity (%)			
History of cigarette-smoking	62	61	63
Hypertension	35	35	36
Angina pectoris	50	52	38
Prior myocardial infarction	39	39	43
NYHA functional class II, III, IV	55	57	43
Entry Coronary Event ‡			
Lowest systolic blood pressure in mm Hg (mean ± SD)	90 ± 2	90 ± 2	85 ± 8
Pulmonary congestion on X-ray film (%)	39	41	36
Left ventricular dysfunction (%)	63	66	43
Anterior infarct (%)	62	64	43
Holter VPB, any (%)	69	69	64
Holter VPB, complex (%)	28	31	14
Medications in Week Before Demise (%)			
Digitalis	65	67	50
Diuretics	57	59	43
Antiarrhythmics	27	27	29
Beta blocking agents	22	22	21
Mortality Event (%)			
Chronology ≤ 2 month posthospitalization	21	23	7
Suddenness ≤ 1 hour	—	56	—
Death out-of-hospital	53	47 †	93 †
Autopsy	19	19	23

* Derived from the Hollingshead [11] five-level occupational and educational class rank, where levels IV and V are the lowest two levels of social class.
† p < 0.01 witnessed versus unwitnessed deaths.
‡ See the METHODS section for criteria of pulmonary congestion, left ventricular dysfunction, anterior infarct, and complex VPB on Holter monitoring.

late (2–12 months) periods, and the suddenness of witnessed death (TABLE 2). A similar analysis was carried out for the full 60-month follow-up period, and comparable results were obtained for the relationship between the chronology (≤1 month, >2–60 months) and suddenness of cardiac death (Chi square =

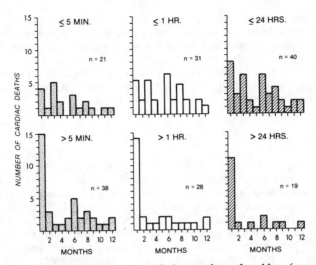

FIGURE 1. Chronologic occurrence of the number of sudden (upper panel) and nonsudden (lower panel) cardiac deaths in the first year after myocardial infarction for three arbitrary cutoff times: 5 minutes (*stippled*); 1 hour (*white*); and 24 hours (*hatched*).

6.75, $p < 0.01$) despite a variable risk exposure for those followed more than 12 months.

Clinical Associations with the Chronology and Suddenness of Cardiac Death

The clinical characteristics of the witnessed cardiac deaths ($n = 98$) were scrutinized to determine whether any significant associations exist between the variables listed in TABLE 1, including medication usage prior to demise and: (1) early (≤ 1 month) and late (>1 month) mortality; and (2) sudden

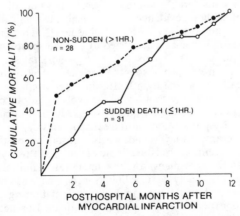

FIGURE 2. Cumulative occurrence of sudden (≤ 1 hour) and nonsudden (>1 hour) cardiac deaths during the first 12 months after myocardial infarction.

(≤ 1 hour) and nonsudden (>1 hour) death. No significant ($p < 0.05$) univariate associations were observed. That is, there were no individual clinical variables that distinguished between sudden and nonsudden death or between early or late death. In addition to the univariate analyses, various two- and three-factor combinations of physiologically meaningful variables (left ventricular dysfunction, complex VPB, and anterior wall infarction) were also evaluated, and no significant associations were found.

DISCUSSION

Prior reports from this laboratory [8, 10, 12] and the investigations of others [1, 4, 13-15] have emphasized the augmented mortality risk in the early posthospital period with a relatively diminished risk thereafter. The present report extends these observations by highlighting the chronologic predominance of nonsudden cardiac deaths in the first month after hospital discharge and the more uniform distribution of sudden cardiac deaths throughout the first posthospital year. No clinical variables identified those patients destined to die either early or late after hospital discharge or suddenly or nonsuddenly.

TABLE 2

ASSOCIATION BETWEEN CHRONOLOGY AND SUDDENNESS OF WITNESSED CARDIAC DEATHS IN THE FIRST YEAR AFTER MYOCARDIAL INFARCTION

| | Chronology | | |
	≤ 1 month	2–12 months	
Suddenness			
≤ 1 hour	5	26	31
> 1 hour	14	14	28
Total	19	40	59

NOTE: Chi square $= 6.25$; $p < 0.02$.

Presently, there is considerable interest in early hospital discharge in the uncomplicated patient without evidence of electrical, mechanical, or ischemic problems during the acute coronary care unit phase.[16, 17] This enthusiasm for early discharge frequently becomes generalized to a broad spectrum of coronary patients, and during the past few years the average hospital stay for patients with myocardial infarction has progressively shortened. The high incidence of nonsudden cardiac death in the first month after hospital discharge raises serious question about the early discharge trend which is evolving in our cost-conscious health-care delivery system. Certainly, infarct size reduction during the hyperacute phase,[18] longer hospitalization with reduced activity, and the use of afterload reduction therapy [19] may reduce early nonsudden posthospital mortality. Appropriate intervention trials are indicated to test this hypothesis.

There is no uniform agreement for the temporal definition for sudden death. The International Society of Cardiology proposed a 24-hour period [20] and a special committee of the American Heart Association agreed upon the following: "Sudden unexpected (natural) death is defined as death occurring instantaneously or within an estimated 24 hours of the onset of acute symptoms or signs." [21] Friedman *et al.*[22] dichotomized sudden death into instantaneous (prior to or within 30 seconds after the onset of any symptoms) and non-instantaneous (cardiac arrest occurring within minutes to 24 hours after the onset of symptoms or signs). Many investigators have used the practical definition of 1 hour for sudden death. In the current study three different time intervals (5 minutes, 1 hour, and 24 hours) were scrutinized for the cutoff between sudden and nonsudden death. With each time interval the frequency distribution of the chronology of death was strikingly different between the sudden and nonsudden groups (FIG. 1). However, when the chronologic occurrence of sudden and nonsudden cardiac death are compared and contrasted at the three time intervals, the change in the pattern distribution of these deaths (FIG. 1) was more marked between the 1-hour and 24-hour cutoffs than between the 5-minute and 1-hour times. These findings indicate that the 1-hour definition of "sudden" represents a reasonable clinical compromise between the electrophysiologic (5-minute) and epidemiologic (24-hour) definitions for sudden cardiac death.

It is of interest that the occurrence of predischarge VPBs and the use of various cardiac medications before demise were similar in the sudden and nonsudden death groups. The VPB finding was unexpected when viewed in the light of the recent report by Ruberman *et al.*[6] in which complex VPBs were associated with a three-fold increased risk of sudden death after myocardial infarction. However, close scrutiny of their report reveals that 50% of their patients were enrolled into the study 3 months or more after the infarction, that is, during the late posthospital period, when sudden death predominates.

This study indicates that routine clinical variables, including Holter-recorded VPBs prior to hospital discharge, do not differentiate postinfarction patients who subsequently die suddenly from those dying nonsuddenly. This conclusion is based on a limited number of witnessed cardiac deaths ($n = 98$) and is subject to a type II error (an erroneous conclusion that no difference exists when in fact a real difference was missed due to inadequate sample size). Other sources of error may be the failure to include pertinent clinical factors, such as a radionuclide ejection fraction, in the data base.[4] On the other hand, the findings may be valid, but difficult to accept. The current observations suggest a common pathophysiologic process underlying both sudden and nonsudden cardiac death. The time course of the terminal event is probably determined by a complex interplay of acute coronary, myocardial, ischemic, electrical, and neurogenic factors. The rapidity of the terminal event may bear little relationship to cardiac variables recorded in the remote past. If these observations and interpretations are correct, then more effective therapeutic results may be achieved by intervening to reduce total cardiac death rather than by preventing sudden cardiac death, as is currently emphasized.

SUMMARY

A prospective postinfarction study of 978 patients less than 66 years of age followed from 1 to 5 years was utilized to evaluate the chronology (interval from hospital discharge to demise) and suddenness (elapsed time from the onset of terminal symptoms to demise) of cardiac death. Clinical information including the patient's history and CCU, 6-hour Holter electrocardiographic, medication, and mortality event data was available on 112 cardiac deaths, with

56% of those with witnessed deaths dying suddenly (≤ 1 hour). During the first postinfarction year 50% of the nonsudden deaths occurred within the first month after hospital discharge, whereas 84% of the sudden deaths occurred in the 2 to 12 month period after infarction (Chi Square $= 6.25$, $p < 0.02$). There were no clinical variables including Holter-recorded ventricular premature beats that distinguished between early and late or sudden and nonsudden cardiac death. These findings indicate that the chronology and suddenness of the terminal cardiac event are more difficult to predict than had previously been appreciated. The therapeutic implications of these observations are discussed.

ACKNOWLEDGMENTS

We thank Lorrie Bayer for her programming assistance and Mrs. Nancy Kellogg and Mrs. Martha Jodoin for their secretarial assistance.

REFERENCES

1. VEDIN, A., C. WILHELMSSON, D. ELMFELDT, J. SAVE-SOLDERBERGH, G. TIBBLIN & L. WILHELMSEN. 1975. Deaths and non-fatal reinfarctions during two-years' follow-up after myocardial infarction. Acta Med. Scand. 198: 353–364.
2. LURIA, M. H., J. D. KNOKE, R. M. MARGOLIS, F. H. HENDRICKS & J. B. KUPLIC. 1976. Acute myocardial infarction: Prognosis after recovery. Ann. Intern. Med. 85: 561–565.
3. PELL, S. & C. A. D'ALONZO. 1964. Immediate mortality and five year survival of employed men with a first myocardial infarction. N. Engl. J. Med. 270: 915–922.
4. SCHULZE, R. A., H. W. STRAUSS & B. PITT. 1977. Sudden death in the year following myocardial infarction: Relation to ventricular premature contractions in the late hospital phase and left ventricular ejection fraction. Am. J. Med. 62: 192–199.
5. KOTLER, M. N., B. TABATZNIK, M. M. MOWER & S. TOMINAGA. 1973. Prognostic significance of ventricular ectopic beats with respect to sudden death in the late postinfarction period. Circulation. 47: 959–966.
6. RUBERMAN, W., E. WEINBLATT, J. GOLDBERG, C. FRANK & S. SHAPIRO. 1977. Ventricular premature beats and mortality after myocardial infarction. N. Engl. J. Med. 297: 750–758.
7. BETA-BLOCKER HEART ATTACK TRIAL STUDY PROTOCOL. 1978. Heart, Lung & Blood Institute, National Institutes of Health, Bethesda, Maryland. (June).
8. MOSS, A. J., J. DECAMILLA, H. DAVIS & L. BAYER. 1976. The early post-hospital phase of myocardial infarction: Prognostic stratification. Circulation 54: 58–64.
9. BLACKBURN, H. 1969. The electrocardiographic classification for population comparison: The Minnesota code. J. Electrocardiol. 2: 5–9.
10. MOSS, A. J., J. DECAMILLA & H. DAVIS. 1977. Cardiac death in the first six months after myocardial infarction: Potential for mortality reduction in the early posthospital period. Am. J. Cardiol. 39: 816–820.
11. HOLLINGSHEAD, A. B. & F. C. REDLICH. 1958. Social Class and Mental Illness. John Wiley. New York, NY.
12. MOSS, A. J., J. DECAMILLA, F. ENGSTROM, W. HOFFMAN, C. ODOROFF & H. DAVIS. 1974. The posthospital phase of myocardial infarction. Circulation. 49: 460–466.
13. FRANK, C. W. 1968. The course of coronary heart disease: Factors relating to prognosis. Bull. NY Acad. Med. 44: 900–915.

14. GAZES, P. C., J. R. KITCHELL, L. E. MELTZER, W. H. ROSENBLATT & O. ROTH. 1966. Death rate among 795 patients in first year after myocardial infarction. J. Amer. Med. Assoc. **197:** 906–908.
15. BIGGER, J. T., JR., C. A. HELLER, T. L. WENGER & F. M. WELD. 1978. Risk stratification after acute myocardial infarction. Am. J. Cardiol. **42:** 202–210.
16. HUTTER, A. M., JR., V. W. SIDEL, K. I. SHINE, *et al.* 1973. Early hospital discharge after myocardial infarction. N. Engl. J. Med. **288:** 1141–1144.
17. MCNEER, J. F., G. S. WAGNER, P. B. GINSBURG, *et al.* 1978. Hospital discharge one week after acute myocardial infarction. N. Engl. J. Med. **298:** 229–232.
18. MAROKO, P. R. & E. BRAUNWALD. 1973. Modification of myocardial infarction size after coronary occlusion. Ann. Intern. Med. **79:** 720–733.
19. FRANCIOSA, J. A., G. PIERPONT & J. N. COHN. 1977. Hemodynamic improvement after oral hydralazine in left ventricular failure. **86:** 388–393.
20. WORLD HEALTH ORGANIZATION EXPERT COMMITTEE. 1975. Services for cardiovascular emergencies. World Health Org. Tech. Rep. Ser. 562.
21. PAUL, O. 1971. On sudden death. Circulation **43:** 7–10.
22. FRIEDMAN, M., J. H. MANWARING, R. H. ROSENMAN, G. DONLON, P. ORTEGA & S. GRUBE. 1973. Instantaneous and sudden deaths: Clinical and pathological differentiation in coronary artery disease. J. Amer. Med. Assoc. **225:** 1319–1328.

SUDDEN CORONARY DEATH:
A LOOK TO THE FUTURE *

J. Thomas Bigger, Jr.

Department of Medicine
College of Physicians & Surgeons of
Columbia University, and the
Arrhythmia Control Unit
Columbia-Presbyterian Medical Center
New York, New York 10032

During this conference many areas related to sudden coronary death were reviewed. Most of the conference participants have indicated areas that need further elucidation in the future. I will summarize here some of the areas that, in my view, are most important to explore in the future from the perspective of the present. As research proceeds, the next step or experiment is generated by surveying the field of interest and then by planning experiments to answer the most important or most interesting questions. However, as this process unfolds, new and unexpected findings will emerge that may deflect the entire field or give rise to a new approach. As in the past, many disciplines will make significant contributions to our understanding of sudden coronary death in the future. Each discipline has its own responsibilities as well as the responsibility to interact with other groups who are working to solve the sudden death problem.

EPIDEMIOLOGY

Epidemiology already has contributed mightily to the field of sudden coronary death, but much work is still left. The primary and immediate risk factors must be better defined and confounding factors must be dealt with effectively. Analysis of existing trial results must be completed and the findings used to generate hypotheses that can be tested in additional prospective trials whether feasibility trials or full-scale observational or intervention trials. Also, epidemiologists must help to plan and conduct these studies. Populations that should be subjected to cardiologic screening at various levels of intensity need better definition.

As socioeconomic forces and lifestyles change, the epidemiologist must help us to adjust and interpret our data in the light of this knowledge. As many disciplines converge on this dreaded enemy with therapeutic programs, the epidemiologist will need to estimate the impact of multifactorial interventions designed to reduce the problem of sudden coronary death.

* Address for correspondence: J. Thomas Bigger, Jr., M.D., Arrhythmia Control Unit, Columbia-Presbyterian Medical Center, 630 West 168th Street, New York, New York 10032.

0077-8923/82/0382-0474 $01.75/0 © 1982, NYAS

ATHEROSCLEROSIS

Investigators in the field of atherosclerosis have many heavy responsibilities in the future. They must gather the information needed to give us a thorough understanding of the pathogenesis of the various types of coronary atherosclerosis. This effort is well under way, but is extremely complex. It is already obvious that smooth muscle cells, endothelial cells, platelets, physical trauma, and lipids, as well as many other factors, play a significant role in producing coronary atherosclerosis. However, the precise sequencing of events, the interreactions among factors, and the control of atherosclerosis need much clarification. Also, we need to know the potential for arresting or reversing the atherosclerotic process at various times in various types of lesions. In addition, experts in atherosclerosis will be indispensable in the effort to unravel the complex interactions between coronary arteries with significant atheromatous lesions and platelets or neurohumoral factors. New knowledge in this area should prompt many new and effective strategies for prophylaxis and therapy.

Similarly, new knowledge of what factors cause rupture or hemorrhage into atheromatous plaques may permit us to avoid these potentially lethal events in the future. And a better knowledge of the potential for regression of plaques, at various stages, will stimulate us to intensify our effort to identify persons with an atherogenetic diathesis before an irreversible stage is reached.

THROMBOSIS

Workers in the field of thrombosis in the future will have the opportunity to clarify which types of atheromatous lesions cause platelet aggregation and thrombosis. This effort will undoubtedly clarify the potential interreactions between platelets and various antigens and surfaces on atheroma or endothelial cells altered by underlying or adjacaent atheroma. The contribution of many other factors to coronary thrombosis needs to be clarified, such as the complement system, Hagemann factor, kinins, and thrombin generation. We should remember that some persons with very severe coronary atherosclerosis never have clinical symptoms or myocardial infarction. This fact encourages the hypothesis that prevention of thrombosis may have much to offer even in those persons with far-advanced and irreversible coronary atherosclerosis.

Obviously, workers in thrombosis will have to contribute to a better understanding of the role of platelets and thrombi in the early pathogenesis of coronary atherosclerosis. Sensitive tests of platelet activation, aggregation and release will facilitate the search for the role of the platelet both in clinical and in experimental studies. Sensitive immunoassays for peptides and proteins that are generated when clotting or kinin production are active are rapidly being developed and validated. Also, ultrasensitive HPLC-MS methods for prostaglandins and other substances are available. During the next decade, these tools will be put to good use in the study of thrombosis in the coronary circulation.

BIOCHEMISTRY

The field of biochemistry is very broad and many definitions would encompass some of the processes of atherosclerosis and thrombosis discussed earlier.

In addition to learning about the biochemical processes taking place in healthy or diseased arterial smooth muscle or platelets, we have much to learn about the biochemical processes in ischemic cells. Additional information on changes in the profile of substrate utilization in ischemia could be put to good use in designing approaches to management. In the same way, knowledge about myocardial energetics could have important implications for attempts to preserve myocardial function or attempts to forestall myocardial necrosis during ischemia.

Lesser degrees of ischemia may not lead to necrosis, but may have lethal consequences by severely impairing the electrical or mechanical function of the heart. Already we are beginning to learn about alterations of lipid metabolism in myocardial ischemia which may have profound effects on cardiac electrical properties and possibly lead to lethal arrhythmias. Sobel and his colleagues have shown that accumulation of acyl carnitine or lysophosphoglycerides can produce devastating electrophysiologic effects in the sarcolemma. The magnitude and time course of release of ampiphilic metabolites are congruent with the hypothesis that these substances may contribute to arrhythmogenesis in the ischemic heart.

Another interesting area for exploration is the effect of ischemia on turnover and regulation of receptors on myocardial cells. Recent work suggests that myocardial ischemia can importantly modulate the numbers of functioning beta-adrenergic receptors in the heart. The mechanisms and kinetics of this change need elucidation. All sorts of receptors—histaminergic, alpha-adrenergic, serotonergic and cholinergic—could be subject to a similar effect. Also, the affinity of receptors to their agonists and the linkage between agonist binding to subsequent biochemical events may be altered in ischemia. Binding of norepinephrine (NE) to beta-adrenergic receptors in an ischemic region might produce an unusually large or small increase in adenylate cyclase activity and phosphorylation of protein kinase. Analogous alterations may occur with alpha-adrenergic, cholinergic, and histaminergic receptors as well. Better understanding of these processes is of utmost importance to physiologists and pharmacologists.

PHYSIOLOGY

There are many problems in sudden coronary death which fall into the province of the physiologist. Much yet remains to be learned about rheology and vasomotion of coronary arteries that are afflicted with atheroma. Abnormalities of vasoconstriction and vasodilation are only partially understood at present. The full range of neurohumoral control mechanisms remains to be elucidated even in the normal coronary circulation. For example, the genesis, effects, and control of prostaglandin synthesis in the coronary vascular bed is a relatively new field and under active investigation. The role of nucleotides in the control of coronary circulation is still not completely defined. It seems likely that additional neurohumoral factors remain to be discovered. Much effort will be required to clarify the physiology and pharmacology of each newly discovered factor, and still more difficult will be the attempt to define the interrelations among control mechanisms, under normal circumstances and in coronary disease.

The interreactions between neural activity, ischemia, myocardial blood flow and function are complex and are currently the subject of intense investigation. Already a reasonable schema that accounts for these variables is emerging from animal and clinical investigation; this new knowledge is being used as the basis for guiding treatment of patients with myocardial ischemia or infarction. This area of investigation should continue to generate clinically useful information in the near future. The precise role of neural factors in producing coronary arterial spasm and myocardial ischemia needs further elucidation. Also, better measures of neural events occurring as a result of ischemia and infarction in man should clarify the clinical importance of these events and permit selective integration of experimental data with clinical problems.

There is new evidence that myocardial ischemia and infarction alter dramatically the turnover of receptors in the heart. We discussed earlier the responsibilities of biochemists in extending these preliminary findings. The physiologist will have a responsibility to quantitate the relationships between myocardial blood flow, neurohumoral regulators, and receptor changes. When these relationships are worked out, the pharmacologist will be greatly aided in his attempt to cope with the dynamic changes in receptors occurring during ischemia.

ELECTROPHYSIOLOGY

Electrophysiologists have worked actively for a long time on the problems of acute ischemic arrhythmias. Recently, a considerable body of knowledge has begun to emerge from studies in animal models of subacute or chronic ischemia. Electrical properties of the heart can be altered in a similar way by many different biochemical events. Better correlations of the biochemical and electrophysiologic events will aid plans to beneficially interrupt the pathophysiology of arrhythmias at different stages of coronary heart disease. These models also serve to screen potential therapies and to provide a rationale for clinical trials.

The electrophysiologist needs to dig deeper into the causes and pathogenesis of abnormal electrical processes during ischemia. To make rapid progress, he or she must cooperate with his or her associates, such as the biochemist, the pathologist, and the electrical engineer. Also, the electrophysiologist must borrow tools from physiologists interested in myocardial blood flow and the endocrine functions of the heart. Many of the electrical abnormalities in acute and chronic ischemia can undoubtedly be controlled when their pathogenesis is clearly understood.

Much new information about chronic ischemia arrhythmias has come from clinical electrophysiologic studies in the past 5 years. Workers at the University of Pennsylvania and elsewhere have studied the sustained ventricular tachycardia that occurs in patients with scarring and ventricular aneurysm due to advanced coronary artery disease. They have suggested mechanisms and approaches for pharmacologic or surgical control of ventricular tachycardia in this special group of patients. Also, new noninvasive means of evaluating patients with sustained ventricular activity are being explored. Sustained ventricular tachycardia in coronary heart disease seems to be a reentrant rhythm using pathways bordering on scarred tissue. In the future, this hypothesis will undoubtedly be better proven and the mechanism elucidated in more detail. The dependence of reentrant ventricular tachyarrhythmias on a large mass of scar tissue probably accounts for the striking success of surgery, even in patients with terrible left ventricular function. In the next 10 years these pioneering studies must be extended to a wider range of patients with arrhythmias. The mechanism of ventricular tachycardia in instances where no large scar exists must be worked out in the future. In coronary heart disease many lethal arrhythmias must depend upon an ischemic mechanism rather than scar-dependent reentry. The most efficient way to test the role of ischemia in a quantitative and reproducible way has yet to be discovered, but should be found during the foreseeable future.

CARDIOLOGY/PATHOLOGY

The cardiologist and cardiac pathologist working in sudden coronary death have especially weighty responsibilities in the future. Workers in experimental laboratories are finding many new potential mechanisms and treatments which must be judged for their utility in patients with ischemic heart disease. Only a few examples can be given here.

Recently, coronary vasospasm has been elevated from the status of a rare event to that of a common occurrence. Dynamic changes in coronary vascular resistance caused by neural and hormonal factors have been shown to occur in man, as in the cold pressor test where coronary blood flow can fall sharply despite a significant increase in mean arterial pressure. Thus, a new era in the study of the behavior and control of the human coronary circulation in health and disease has been ushered in. We have much to learn about what the system is capable of doing, and, more importantly, what it does under clinically relevant conditions. As new information is acquired about the control of coronary vasomotion, research in the field of sudden coronary death will almost certainly benefit.

It seems ludicrous that after all this time we still do not know the causes of coronary occlusion or how to diagnose a particular cause in a particular patient. But this is the sad state of affairs. Often, in medicine, we have a way of not bothering to learn those things that we do not need in our everyday practice. Now that we are attempting to reopen vessels that have been occluded for a few hours, we must know how they came to be occluded, what is occluding them, and how best to cope with a variety of occluding agencies. Already, coronary thrombolytic therapy has produced findings that are drastically re-shaping our thoughts about coronary occlusion, and much more will be learned as this effort and its derivatives are extended.

The current approach to coronary disease is to wait for crises to occur which then trigger vigorous action in a desperate attempt to rectify the situation. This approach is too expensive in terms of manpower and resources. We need the means to detect and quantitate silent coronary atherosclerosis. The method must be noninvasive and accurate, so that it can be used to measure progression or regression of coronary lesions. Such methods will provide better information on pathogenesis and the natural history of coronary atherosclerosis and will permit greater accuracy in evaluating medical or surgical treatment of coronary disease. Also, the status of atherosclerosis can be used as an end-point for pharmacologic studies. This will improve the efficiency and reduce the cost of secondary prevention studies. Also, it will permit better control of confounding variables. Armed with better knowledge of the status of the coronary vasculature, we can often practice *preventive* rather than *crisis* medicine.

In the past two decades three new means of restoring myocardial blood flow have been developed: coronary bypass surgery, transluminal coronary balloon angioplasty, and local infusion thrombolytic therapy. These and other new methods must be refined, simplified, and made less expensive so that adequate coronary blood flow can be restored without using half the gross national product to do so.

In cases where myocardial infarction does occur, effective means of minimizing its size must be found and made practical. It is becoming more and more clear that left ventricular dysfunction and potentially lethal ventricular arrhythmias play a major role in large myocardial infarctions. Therefore, a straightforward hypothesis is that much of the sudden cardiac death that occurs in the year after acute myocardial infarction could be avoided by limiting the infarct to a small area of myocardium. There is intense interest in testing of this hypothesis and generous support is available for this effort. We can expect significant progress in this area, and, probably, several totally new approaches will be forthcoming in the next decade. As a corollary of approaches to minimizing infarct size is the need to cope with ischemic jeopardy and to prevent recurrences or extension of acute myocardial infarction.

PHARMACOLOGY

Pharmacology has become a gigantic field. Both its academic and industrial arms continue to bring forward exciting new compounds at a gratifying rate. Think of the pharmacologic advances of the past 20 years: antiarrhythmic, antilipid, and antihypertensive drugs, thrombolytics, vasodilators, alpha- and beta-adrenergic blockers, calcium channel blocking agents, platelet antagonists, selective prostaglandin inhibitors, and nonglycoside cardiotonic drugs. The drug industry is a vital force in the fight against sudden coronary death and is always quick to respond as new pathogenetic sequences are clarified. We can count on new drugs to attack key steps in the pathogenetic sequences once these are established. A striking example is the recent introduction of converting enzyme inhibitors as a consequence of two decades of work which elucidated the renin–angiotensin system and its role in congestive heart failure. Also, new diagnostic reagents and new drug delivery systems continue to flow from this vital industry.

The drug industry has its work cut out for it in the area of sudden coronary death. We need convenient, safe and effective drugs to prevent or reverse atherosclerosis, coronary spasm, coronary thrombosis, effort-related ischemia, left ventricular dysfunction, and arrhythmias. We need agents to use during acute infarction that will reduce infarct size substantially, thus preventing ventricular aneurysm, left ventricular dysfunction, and arrhythmia. For patients who already have severe coronary disease with extensive myocardial scarring we need drugs for secondary prevention that are effective and safe to use.

I believe that developments in the next decade in cardiovascular pharmacology will be even more impressive than in the last two decades.

ELECTRONICS AND PHYSICS

The future contributions from the disciplines of electronics and physics promise to be even more exciting than those of the last 20 years, which gave us clinical electrophysiology, echocardiography, nuclear cardiology, nuclear magnetic resonance spectrography, computerized axial tomography, drug measurement with liquid chromatography or mass spectrography/fragmentography. We can expect greatly improved imaging technology using improved equipment to obtain higher resolution and quality of images as well as improved radiopharmaceuticals and/or other imaging reagents. Many of these imaging reagents are likely to be antibodies to proteins or smaller molecules that yield rather specific information about disease processes. Already antibodies for cardiac myosin can be used to quantitate myocardial infarct size. When the appropriate reagent is found, we will be able, by noninvasive methods, to localize and quantitate coronary atheroma. New immunopharmaceuticals will improve in quality, availability, and cost due to the industrialization of hybridoma technology.

More accurate, more available, and cheaper noninvasive methods for monitoring myocardial perfusion, arrhythmias, and ventricular function will become available in the next decade. This will help in the effort to detect factors that increase the risk of sudden coronary death. Early detection will be coupled to early prevention measures and better noninvasive measures of treatment effects.

Not the least of the contribution of the electronics and computer industry will be improved communications and improved data, word and information processing. Better communication systems could put all citizens within a few minutes of emergency medical services. Electronic data processing will not only speed the acquisition of biomedical data and its analysis but also will disseminate the new information faster and in a format more easily assimilated by the general physician and public. Thus, new validated research findings can become more quickly established as health policy and practice.

SURGERY

As workers in the field gain a better understanding of fundamental processes of coronary artery disease, the role of surgery as we now know it should diminish. However, a large residual group of patients who need surgical therapy will remain for a long time. During this period, changes ranging from refinement to major breakthroughs are needed. We need better ways of surgically improving myocardial perfusion and we need methods that are permanent, i.e., we need to avoid gradual closure of coronary artery vein grafts. Also, an artificial material for bypass grafts is needed for patients who have no veins available. For patients who have severe scarring and dysfunction of the myocardium, we need a practical, effective, totally implanted artificial heart, and the immunological problems that still plague cardiac transplantation dictate substantial improvement in cardiac immunology. Recent advances have launched arrhythmia surgery. Surgical treatment of arrhythmias is in its infancy. However, this approach clearly has much to offer patients with severe arrhythmias in many forms of heart disease. Also, catheter techniques, perhaps linked to communications technology, such as fiberoptic bundles and laser or cryotechnology, will likely be used to lessen arrhythmic foci in the future. Such techniques may find widespread use in the transluminal treatment of clinically important atheromatous lesions in coronary arteries.

Even though the use of present conventional coronary bypass surgery will probably decline over the next 30 years, there will still be an important role for surgery in the future. Surgery will be needed as an essential adjunct to many other forms of prevention and treatment of coronary heart disease and sudden death.

CONCLUSION

As amazing as the progress of the past 20 years has been, progress is likely to be even more spectacular in the future. Achievements of the past 20 years have led to a steady decline in the mortality rate from coronary heart disease. We should be able to extend this decline in mortality substantially in the future until sudden cardiac death can be declared controlled. To achieve this goal investigators in many disciplines must work vigorously and cooperatively. Both government and the private sector must allocate significant resources to this important target area.

Index of Contributors

(Italicized page numbers refer to comments made in discussion.)

Bahr, R., *21, 329, 422*
Baigrie, R., *222, 256*
Bär, F. W. H. M., 136–142
Bassett, A. L., 90–115
Becker, L. C., 450–464
Bigger, J. T., Jr., *134, 203, 227,* 229–237, *246, 255, 256, 286, 287, 322, 342,* 474–482
Brugada, P., 136–142
Bulkley, B. H., 450–464

Cabrol, C., 396–410
Cameron, J. S., 90–115
Case, R., *216*
Castellanos, A., 90–115
Chilton, J., 465–473
Cobb, L. A., *217, 222,* 330–342, *370, 380*
Colman, R. W., 190–203
Coutte, R., 396–410
Crampton, R., *38, 88, 89, 114–115, 134–135, 255,* 324–329

Davis, H. T., 465–473
DeBusk, R. F., 343–354, *421–422, 449*
DeCamilla, J., 465–473
DeSilva, R. A., 143–161, *255, 256*
Doyle, J., *437*
Dwyer, E. M., Jr., 1–2, *89, 288, 322, 342, 437*

El-Moraghi, N., *49*
Engelberg, H., *21*
Epstein, K., 90–115
Erikssen, J., 438–449

Frank, R., 396–410
Fontaine, G., 396–410

Gaide, M. S., 90–115
Gallerstein, P., *222, 257*
Gelband, H., 90–115
Gibson, J. K., 223–228
Gilmour, R. F., Jr., 258–288
Goldmann, M., *395*
Greenberg, H. M., 1–2, *181–182, 322*
Greenspan, A. M., 116–135

Grosgogeat, Y., 396–410
Guiraudon, G., 396–410

Hallstrom, A. P., 330–342
Hammill, S. C., 238–246
Harken, A. H., 381–395
Herling, I., *21, 75, 135, 222, 246, 256, 354, 421*
Herman, G. G., *160*
Hinkle, L. E., Jr., 22–38
Hirsh, J., *217,* 289–304
Hjalmarson, A., *21, 246,* 305–323
Horowitz, L. N., 116–135, 381–395
Hung, J., 343–354

Jacobson, S. K., 449
Johnson, W. D., 39–49
Josephson, M. E., 116–135, *142,* 381–395

Kallman, C., 450–464
Kannel, W. B., 3–21
Kastor, J. A., 76–77, *88, 113, 132, 133, 135, 141, 142, 160, 342, 410*
Kirk, E., *74*
Kupersmith, J., *132, 133*

Levy, R. I., 411–422
Lockhart, E. A., *38, 189*
Lown, B., 355–370
Lozner, E., *133, 227*
Lucchesi, B. R., *88, 114,* 223–228

Marcus, F., *75, 133, 464*
Marzullo, P., 204–217
Maseri, A., 204–217, *227*
Mellits, E. D., 450–464
Michelson, E. L., 78–89
Mirowski, M., 371–380
Moore, E. N., 78–89
Moss, A. J., *217, 287, 436, 437,* 465–473
Mower, M. M., 371–380
Mundal, R., 438–449
Myerburg, R. J., 90–115

Newman, W. P. III, 39–49

Oalmann, M. C., 39–49

Pitt, B., *217*, 218–222
Pritchett, E. L. C., 238–246

Reid, P. R., 371–380
Ribeiro, L. G. T., *20, 74, 287*
Rossi, L., 50–68, *395*

Salonen, J. T., 423–437
Schaper, W., 69–75
Scherlis, S., *68, 217*
Schwartz, A., 183–189
Schwartz, P. J., *75, 114,* 162–180, *227, 287, 288, 341, 342*
Severi, S., 204–217
Shand, D. G., 238–246, *304*
Silverman, K. J., 450–464
Sondik, E. J., 411–422
Spear, J. F., 78–89
Spielman, S. R., 116–135
Starget, W. W., 238–246

Stewart, J. R., 223–228, *322*
Stone, H. L., 162–180
Strong, J. P., 39–49

Thomas, H. E., Jr., 3–21
Tracy, R. E., 39–49
Tuckman, J., *437*

Vernon, S., *353*
Verrier, R. L., 355–370

Wagner, G. S., 238–246
Watkins, L., Jr., 371–380
Weisfeldt, M. L., 450–464
Weld, F. M., 229–237
Wellens, H. J. J., 136–142
Winkle, R. A., 247–257, *410*
Wong, S. S., 90–115

Zipes, D. P., *38, 75, 89, 142,* 258–288